Handbook of Urology

Handbook of Urology

Editor: Timothy Lawson

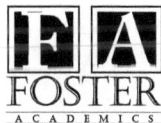

FA **FOSTER** ACADEMICS

www.fosteracademics.com

www.fosteracademics.com

FA FOSTER
ACADEMICS

Cataloging-in-Publication Data

Handbook of urology / edited by Timothy Lawson.
    p. cm.
Includes bibliographical references and index.
ISBN 978-1-63242-821-9
1. Urology. 2. Genitourinary organs--Diseases. I. Lawson, Timothy.
RC872.9 .H36 2019
616.6--dc23

Foster Academics,
118-35 Queens Blvd., Suite 400,
Forest Hills, NY 11375, USA

ISBN 978-1-63242-821-9 (Hardback)

Contents

Preface

I am honored to present to you this unique book which encompasses the most up-to-date data in the field. I was extremely pleased to get this opportunity of editing the work of experts from across the globe. I have also written papers in this field and researched the various aspects revolving around the progress of the discipline. I have tried to unify my knowledge along with that of stalwarts from every corner of the world, to produce a text which not only benefits the readers but also facilitates the growth of the field.

Urology is a branch of medicine, concerned with surgical as well as medical diseases related to the male and female urinary-tract system, and the male reproductive organs. Genitourinary disorders also fall under the domain of urology. Some of the common genitourinary disorders include hypospadias, labial fusion, epispadias and varicocele. Two of the most common and effective methods to treat urological diseases include robotic surgery and laparoscopic surgery. A robotic surgery is either performed through a direct telemanipulator or through computer control. In a laparoscopic surgery, small surgical incisions are made in the abdomen or pelvis. This book brings forth some of the most innovative concepts and elucidates the unexplored aspects of urology. The various advancements in urology are glanced at and their applications as well as ramifications are looked at in detail. Students, urologists, experts and all associated with urology will benefit alike from this book.

Finally, I would like to thank all the contributing authors for their valuable time and contributions. This book would not have been possible without their efforts. I would also like to thank my friends and family for their constant support.

Editor

Testicular histopathology, semen analysis and FSH, predictive value of sperm retrieval: supportive counseling in case of reoperation after testicular sperm extraction (TESE)

Lucio Gnessi[1*†], Filomena Scarselli[2†], Maria Giulia Minasi[2], Stefania Mariani[1], Carla Lubrano[1], Sabrina Basciani[1], Pier Francesco Greco[2], Mikiko Watanabe[1], Giorgio Franco[3], Alessio Farcomeni[4] and Ermanno Greco[2]

Abstract

Background: To provide indicators for the likelihood of sperm retrieval in patients undergoing testicular sperm extraction is a major issue in the management of male infertility by TESE. The aim of our study was to determine the impact of different parameters, including testicular histopathology, on sperm retrieval in case of reoperation in patients undergoing testicular sperm extraction.

Methods: We retrospectively analyzed 486 patients who underwent sperm extraction for intracytoplasmic sperm injection and testicular biopsy. Histology was classified into: normal spermatogenesis; hypospermatogenesis (reduction in the number of normal spermatogenetic cells); maturation arrest (absence of the later stages of spermatogenesis); and Sertoli cell only (absence of germ cells). Semen analysis and serum FSH, LH and testosterone were measured.

Results: Four hundred thirty patients had non obstructive azoospermia, 53 severe oligozoospermia and 3 necrozoospermia. There were 307 (63%) successful sperm retrieval. Higher testicular volume, lower levels of FSH, and better histological features were predictive for sperm retrieval. The same parameters and younger age were predictive factors for shorter time for sperm recovery. After multivariable analysis, younger age, better semen parameters, better histological features and lower values of FSH remained predictive for shorter time for sperm retrieval while better semen and histology remained predictive factors for successful sperm retrieval. The predictive capacity of a score obtained by summing the points assigned for selected predictors (1 point for Sertoli cell only, 0.33 points for azoospermia, 0.004 points for each FSH mIU/ml) gave an area under the ROC curve of 0.843.

Conclusions: This model can help the practitioner with counseling infertile men by reliably predicting the chance of obtaining spermatozoa with testicular sperm extraction when a repeat attempt is planned.

Keywords: Testicular sperm extraction (TESE), Testicular biopsy, FSH, Semen, Sperm retrieval

* Correspondence: lucio.gnessi@uniroma1.it
†Lucio Gnessi and Filomena Scarselli contributed equally to this work.
[1]Department of Experimental Medicine, Section of Medical Pathophysiology, Food Science and Endocrinology, Sapienza University of Rome, Policlinico Umberto I, 00161 Rome, Italy
Full list of author information is available at the end of the article

Background

The testicular biopsy has been for years one of the crucial investigations in the diagnosis and management of male infertility [1]. The advent of intracytoplasmic sperm injection (ICSI) made possible successful assisted reproduction with sperm derived from the testis in patients with non-obstructive azoospermia (NOA) through techniques of testicular sperm extraction (TESE). One of the major challenge with conventional TESE (cTESE) was to find indicators of the likelihood to recover spermatozoa. From time to time, circulating hormonal markers, testicular ultrasound and testicular biopsy have been used [2]. None of these procedures has proved particularly effective because often, due to the profound heterogeneity of the testicular tissue, spermatozoa were recovered even in the presence of indicators suggestive for adverse outcomes. Nevertheless, biopsy still seemed to be the best predictor of sperm recovery (SR). A further reduction in the use of forecasting techniques occurred with the advent of micro TESE (mTESE). Many groups have argued that the mTESE provides such a high SR compared to other techniques, even in case of severe histological diagnosis like agenesis of the germinal line, that cTESE and as a logical consequence all the procedures to predict the chances of SR, were put aside as techniques of historical interest not relevant to current reproductive technologies [3–7].

However, besides recent studies have questioned the superiority of mTESE compared to cTESE in the resilience of the sperm retrieved [8, 9], the question of being able to provide the patient and the doctor with a system to assess the likelihood of recovering sperm in cases of NOA retains all its meaning, particularly when a reintervention following an unsuccessful sperm retrival attempt is requested. Here we investigated retrospectively the correlations between clinical, laboratory, demographic characteristics, histolgical features and cTESE sperm retrieval outcomes. Predictive values of each one of these characteristics in the SR were scrutinized with the aim of providing elements to make a choice as conscious as possible in case of reintervention.

Methods

Four hundred eighty-six patients referring to the Centre for Reproductive Medicine, of the European Hospital (Rome, Italy) between january 2005 and june 2016, retrospectively identified to have undergone cTESE and ICSI, were studied. Concurrently with TESE all patients were subjected to testicular biopsy for histological analysis. All patients had a semen sample evaluated in at least two different occasions according to the WHO criteria [10]. Azoospermia was diagnosed when the absence of sperm was observed after 600 g centrifugation and screening at 400× magnification. Cryptozoospermia was

one of the conditions considered under the spectrum of NOA [11], defined as the absence of spermatozoa in fresh semen preparations but rare sperm in a centrifuged pellet [10]. Cryptozoospermia occurrence is attributed to fluctuations in spermatogenesis in cases of NOA [11]. Oligozoospermia and necrozoospermia were defined as less than 15 million sperm/ml and less than 5% viable spermatozoa in the ejaculate, respectively. Oligozoospermic patients were submitted to TESE after multiple ICSI failure with poor embryo quality and repeated implantation failure using motile ejaculatory spermatozoa on the basis of the reported better outcome in selected severe oligozoospermic patients when testicular spermatozoa were used [12].

A clinical history was recorded, including history of undescended testis, mumps orchitis, previous genito-urinary infection, radiotherapy, chemotherapy, surgical procedures or exposure to gonadotoxins. A clinical examination included secondary sexual characteristics, testicular size (measured with a Prader's orchidometer) and consistency, epididymal distension and varicocele. All patients had their serum follicle stimulating hormone (FSH), luteinizing hormone (LH) and testosterone (T) concentrations measured without any hormonal medical therapy within 2 months before cTESE. Karyotype and Y-chromosomal microdeletion analysis were performed on all patients. Patients with AZFa, AZFb, AZFab, AZFbc, AZFabc microdeletions were excluded.

Surgical technique

The surgical procedure was performed under general anesthesia. After scrotal disinfection, the spermatic cord and the scrotal skin were infiltrated with 8 ml of 7.5 mg/ml ropivacaine hydrochloride (Norepine, ASTA, Milan, Italy). The testicle on which the procedure was started was the one with larger volume. For cTESE, a small (5 mm) equatorial horizontal incision of the albuginea with extrusion of the testicular parenchima and scissors biopsy of approximately 5x2x3mm were performed. If no sperm was found, multiple conventional superficial biopsies (4–8 sampling) on the contralateral testicle was performed following the same procedure. A fragment of the testis removed from the testis used for the cTESE was processed for histology (see below). The surgical procedure was always performed by the same surgeon (GF) and the specimen processed by the same biological team. The time required to find sperm in the tissue was recorded.

Histology

A fragment of testicular parenchyma (2x2x2 mm) removed from the testis used for cTESE procedure was washed in buffered medium (Quinn's Advantages Medium with HEPES, SAGE, Cooper Surgical, Pasadena, USA) with 2.5% human serum albumin (HSA, Albutein, Alpha

Therapeutic Milan, Italy), fixed in Bouin's solution (1 ml) and sent to the pathology laboratory. All histological examinations were performed by the same pathologist. Based on the histopathological pattern, testicular histology was classified into: normal spermatogenesis (NormoS); hypospermatogenesis (HypoS, i.e. a reduction in the number of normal spermatogenetic cells); maturation arrest (MA, i.e. an absence of the later stages of spermatogenesis); and Sertoli cell only (SCO, i.e. the absence of germ cells).

Statistical analysis

Data are presented as mean ± standard deviation or median ± inter quartile range for non-symmetric continuous variables, and as counts and percentages for categorical ones.

The binary outcome (successful SR) was associated with potential predictors through logistic regression, with a Firth bias-reducing correction. The time-to-event outcome (time to successful SR) was associated with potential predictors through (univariate and multivariable) Cox regression modeling. In case of unsuccessfull SR, time-to-event was censored as the time spent on unsuccessful searching. Both for binary and time-to-event outcomes, the final multivariable model was selected by via forward-stagewise selection, based on Akaike Information Criterion (AIC) [13]. All potential predictors were initially considered for inclusion in the multivariable model, but only those leading to significant decrease in AIC (as sequentially considered) were finally included.

The final multivariable linear logistic regression model was used to build a score for successful SR. The points assigned to each indicator or unit for continuous predictors were obtained by rounding regression coefficients. The score obtained was evaluated by means of a receiver operating curve (ROC) analysis for a final model. The area under a curve (AUC) is a measure of predictive power. The value of 0.5 means that predictions are no better than random guessing and the value of 1.0 indicates a (theoretically) perfect test (i.e., 100% sensitive and 100% specific). A $p < 0.05$ was considered as statistically significant and all tests were two-sided. All statistical analyses were performed with the software R version 3.2.0.

Results

The present study includes 486 patients with a mean age of 37.2 ± 6.5 years (range 20–71 years): 430 with NOA (40 with cryptozoospermia), 53 severe oligozoospermic men who had previously failed to achieve paternity with assisted reproductive technology procedures and 3 with necrozoospermia.

In the NOA group, the mean patient age was 37.2 ± 6.6 years (range 20–71 years); in the severe oligozoospermia group, the mean patient age was 37.3 ± 6.0 (range

27–63); in the necrozoospermia group, the mean patient age was 42.0 ± 2.6 (range 39–44).

Table 1 shows the clinical parameters of the patients stratified according to SR. With the only exception of body mass index [BMI, weight (kg)/height (m^2)] and circulating T, all the other parameters differed significantly between the patients that experienced successfull SR compared to those that had unsuccessfull SR, including age that was older in the successfull SR group, FSH and LH whose values were higher in the unsuccessfull SR group, and testis volume that was lower in the unsuccessfull SR group.

Table 2 shows the clinical characteristics of the patients stratified according to histology. The sample size for the four groups of histological diagnosis was 205 for SCO, 75 MA, 149 HypoS, and 57 NormoS. Spermatozoa were recovered in 307 out of the 486 patients (63.17%). 60/205 (29.3%) from SCO, 58/75 (77.3%) from MA, 132/149 (88.6%) from HypoS, 57/57 (100%) from NormoS. The 57 NormoS were either oligozoospermic, necrozoospermic or cryptozoospermic. With the exception of BMI and T, all the clinical parameters were significantly different between the groups. Statistical difference in sperm retrieval rate was observed between all the groups with a pattern of increasing likelihood of SR from SCO to MA, HypoS and NormoS. The leves of FSH and LH were progressively lower and testicular volume was higher as much as the histological appearance was improving.

The univariate logistic regression analysis showed that four factors were associated with SR including semen analysis, histology, FSH values and testicular volume (Table 3A). As expected, the odds to recover spermatozoa from testicular specimens was significantly higher in both

Table 1 Clinical parameters and histopathological features of the patients stratified according to the SR

	Succesfull SR	No SR	P
Patients n.	307	179	
Age (years)	38.2±7.05	35.4±4.97	< 0.01
BMI (kg/m^2)	26.85±6.00	26.51±2.78	NS
FSH (mIU/ml)	15.70±12.22	22.51±12.11	< 0.01
LH (mIU/ml)	6.85±4.86	8.87±5.19	< 0.01
T (ng/ml)	4.57±1.94	4.39±3.11	NS
Testis vol. (right, ml)	9.77±6.46	7.11±4.66	0.010
Testis vol. (left, ml)	9.47±7.41	6.96±3.68	0.021
SCO n. (%)	60 (19.5%)	145 (81%)	< 0.01
MA n. (%)	58 (18.9%)	17 (9.5%)	< 0.01
HypoS n. (%)	132 (43.0%)	17 (9.5%)	< 0.01
NormoS n. (%)	57 (18.6%)	0 (0%)	< 0.01

SR sperm retrieval, BMI body mass index, FSH follicle stimulating hormone, LH luteinizing hormone, T testosterone, SCO Sertoli cell only, MA maturation arrest, HypoS hypospermatogenesis, NormoS normospermatogenesis, NS not significant

Table 2 Clinical characteristics of the patients and SR rate stratified according to testicular histology

	SCO	MA	HypoS	NormoS	P
Patients n.	205	75	149	57	
Age (years)	35.64±5.42	37.21±6.67	39.05±7.83	37.57±4.50	< 0.01
Azoospermia n. (%)	196 (95.6%)	60 (80.0%)	121 (81.2%)	13 (22.8%)	< 0.01
Criptozoospermia n. (%)	7 (3.4%)	10 (13.3%)	6 (4.0%)	17 (29.8%)	< 0.01
Oligozoospermia n. (%)	2 (1.0%)	5 (6.7%)	22 (14.8%)	24 (42.1%)	< 0.01
Necrozoospermia n. (%)	0 (0%)	0 (0%)	0 (0%)	3 (5.3%)	< 0.01
BMI (kg/m²)	25.86±2.90	27.71±3.54	27.66±7.80	25.5±2.42	NS
FSH (mIU/ml)	24.34±11.65	18.15±11.63	12.66±11.60	11.02±8.81	< 0.01
LH (mIU/ml)	9.80±6.00	7.25±4.08	5.63±3.25	5.18±2.90	< 0.01
T (ng/ml)	4.30±2.85	4.40±2.06	4.75±1.87	4.93±2.26	NS
SR	60 (29.3%)	58 (77.3%)	132 (88.6%)	57 (100%)	< 0.01
Testis vol. (right, ml)	7.24±4.58	7.75±3.39	11.05±8.52	12.38±5.15	< 0.01
Testis vol. (left, ml)	7.17±4.06	8.23±3.69	10.43±10.44	10.56±3.17	NS

SCO Sertoli cell only, *MA* maturation arrest, *HypoS* hypospermatogenesis, *NormoS* normospermatogenesis, *BMI* body mass index, *FSH* follicle stimulating hormone, *LH* luteinizing hormone, *T* testosterone, *SR* sperm retrieval, *NS* not significant

Table 3 Predictive factors of sperm recovery (A) and of time for recovery (B) by cTESE, univariate analysis

A. Sperm recovery

Predictor variable	OR	95% CI	P
Seminal fluid			
Criptozoospermic vs azoospermic	12.67	4.19–62.31	< 0.01
Oligo-astenozoospermic vs azoospermic	28.80	7.69–256.10	< 0.01
Histology			
MA vs SCO	8.04	4.44–15.19	< 0.01
HypoS vs SCO	18.21	10.41–33.49	< 0.01
FSH	0.96/mIU	0.94–0.97	< 0.01
Testis volume	1.05/ml	1.01–1.11	0.013

B. Time for sperm recovery

Predictor variable	HR	95% CI	P
Age	1.06/year	1.04–1.08	< 0.01
Seminal fluid			
Criptozoospermic vs azoospermic	3.34	2.05–5.45	< 0.01
Oligozoospermic vs azoospermic	6.64	0.88–46.15	NS
Histology			
MA vs SCO	4.61	2.84–7.49	< 0.01
HypoS vs SCO	9.10	6.03–13.74	< 0.01
FSH	0.95/mIU	0.93–0.96	< 0.01
Testis volume	1.02/ml	1.01–1.04	< 0.01

OR odds ratio, *HR* hazard ratio, *FSH* follicle stimulating hormone, *SCO* Sertoli cell only, *MA* maturation arrest, *HypoS* hypospermatogenesis, *NS* not significant

criptozoospermic and oligozoospermic patients compared to azoospermic patients. Analogously, the odds to recover spermatozoa was higher in MA and hypospermatogenic testes compared with testicular tissue specimens affected by SCO. Also significant was the odds of SR for each mIU increase of circulating FSH and for each ml increase of testicular volume. The same variables were significantly associated with the hazard ratio (HR) for time for SR with the exception of oligo-astenozoospermic versus azoospermic (Table 3B).

Multiple logistic regression analysis of variables, including semen and histology for SR and age, semen, serum FSH and testicular histology for sperm recovery time revealed that semen and testicular histology were both found to be significant variables to predict successful SR (Table 4A) while age, semen, histology and FSH were significant variables to predict time for sperm recovery (Table 4B).

We developed a model for the prediction of SR based on a score composed of three variables derived from logistic regression analyses, obtained by summing the points assigned for each predictor (1 point for SCO, 0.33 points for azoospermia and 0.004 points for each FSH mIU). The predictive ability of the score was evaluated by using the area under the ROC curve (Fig. 1) that gave a value of 0.843 with good discriminative performance. Therefore, we identified a cut-off value of the score ≤ 1.24 with a calculated specificity of 83.39% and sensitivity of 81.11% as suggestive of a good chance of SR upon further TESE.

Discussion

One of the major issues to be addressed in the management of male infertility by TESE is to have an indicator of

Table 4 Predictive factors of sperm recovery (A) and of time for recovery (B) by cTESE, multivariate analysis

A. Sperm recovery

Predictor variable	OR	95% CI	P
Seminal fluid			
Criptozoospermic vs azoospermic	8.00	2.24–42.64	< 0.01
Oligozoospermic vs azoospermic	6.55	1.56–63.11	< 0.01
Histology			
MA vs SCO	6.94	3.77–13.30	< 0.01
HypoS vs SCO	16.44	9.31–30.54	< 0.01

B. Time for sperm recovery

Predictor variable	HR	95% CI	P
Age	1.05/year	1.02–1.07	< 0.01
Seminal fluid			
Criptozoospermic vs azoospermic	1.51	0.87–2.62	NS
Oligozoospermic vs azoospermic	2.05	1.25–3.37	< 0.01
Histology			
MA vs SCO	4.07	2.36–7.02	< 0.01
HypoS vs SCO	6.60	3.96–10.99	< 0.01
FSH	0.98/mIU	0.96–0.99	0.030

OR odds ratio, *HR* hazard ratio, *FSH* follicle stimulating hormone, *SCO* Sertoli cell only, *MA* maturation arrest, *HypoS* hypospermatogenesis, *NS* not significant

the likelihood of recovery of sperm from the testis. This information is important for the couple to make a thoughtful choice about whether or not to undertake an in vitro fertilization procedure that can cause physical, psychological and financial consequences. It has recently been called into question the validity of predictive indicators of recovery of sperm from the testes of patients suffering from NOA, in particular the usefulness of diagnostic testicular biopsy [3–7]. The criticisms to the procedure are mainly based on two considerations. The first is that the histological appearance of a bioptic specimen does not mirror the condition of the testicular parenchyma as a whole and therefore it is not worth referring the patient to biopsy because even severe histological features such as SCO, do not rule out the presence of portions of tissue with intact spermatogenesis, generating false negatives. The second is that the mTESE, according to the proponents of the technique, substantially lowers the risk of not detecting preserved spermatogenesis areas, if present, ensuring almost total certainty of potential sperm recovery, reducing significantly the usefulness of diagnostic biopsy. These arguments have, in turn, limitations. It is clear that whatever the procedure, either diagnostic or therapeutic, it will never provide the absolute certainty of the absence of germ cells for fertilization, because in no case the entire tissue can be analized and

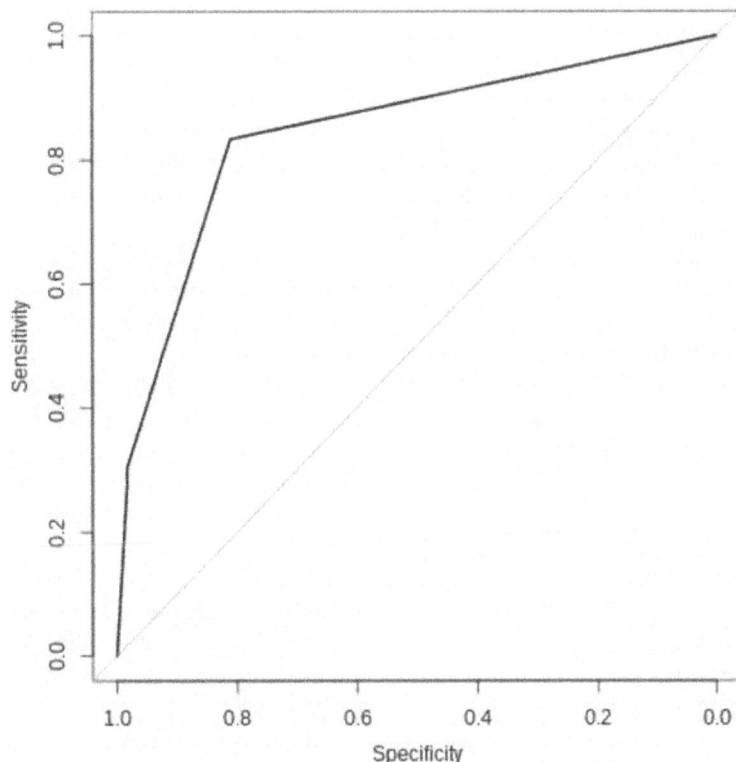

Fig. 1 ROC curve of pertinent parameters to discriminate successful and failed cTESE (AUC = 0.843). ROC = Receiver operating characteristic; cTESE = conventional testicular sperm extraction; AUC = area under a curve

the risk not to identify areas of tissue with intact spermatogenesis can not be eliminated. It is not clear, moreover, what is the real advantage of the mTESE in terms of recovery compared with cTESE because recent studies have not confirmed its superiority in all circumstances [8, 9, 14, 15]. Although, pseudo-randomized prospective data show more favourable sperm retrieval in NOA for mTESE compared to cTESE, especially in histological patterns of patchy spermatogenesis such as SCO, in patients with uniform histological patterns such as MA, the outcome of mTESE seems less favourable [14]. No secure clinical predictors of sperm retrieval are demonstrated for both procedures and clinical complication rate seems not to differ according to a systematic review [14]. A further systematic review with meta-analysis took into consideration fifteen studies with a total of 1890 patients [15]. In a direct comparison, performance of mTESE was 1.5 times more likely (95% confidence interval 1.4–1.6) to result in successful SR as compared with cTESE. The essential weakness of the studies and meta-analysis on mTESE is the lack of proper control groups. Also the studies comparing the success rate of mTESE against cTESE should be viewed with caution because due to the extreme variability of the spermatogenic process, clearly visible also in patients with normal spermatogenesis (seminal parameters in normozoospermic patient may vary profoundly a few days away), the success or failure of SR can change significantly from day to day.

There are only few exceptions to this methodological limit, namely studies in which both mTESE and cTESE were performed during the same recovery procedure in the same patient in comparison studies. Franco et al. showed that the outcome of mTESE did not improve SR as compared to single cTESE biopsy on the same testicle or to multiple contralateral cTESE [8]. Analogously, Marconi and colleagues found no difference between mTESE and cTESE in terms of sperm retrieval rates [9].

Whatever the best technique to recover spermatozoa, the opportunity to offer to both doctors and patients a likely indicator of success of SR rate is important. A situation that can occur in case of reoperation following a failure of TESE, provided that the information coming from the microscopic analysis of a testicular fragment is available.

The evidence for success rates of repeat sperm retrieval surgery in men with NOA is based on a very small number of retrospective case series with varying patient selection criteria and methodologies. The success rate of repeat TESE varied from 30% [16] to 41.6% in the first repeat attempt and the success rate increased to 100% for two patients with six attempts [17], there are limitations of this evidence as only 2 out of 628 patients in the study reached six attempts, hence it is difficult to generalise.

One retrospective case series of repeat mTESE showed a success rate of 82% [18]. The study identified lower FSH level and larger testicular volume to have a predictive value in determining the success of a second attempt. The findings of the study are limited by its retrospective, nonrandomized, non-controlled nature. In summary, there is low level evidence from retrospective case series that the cumulative success rate of repeat sperm retrieval increases with increasing numbers of attempts and is higher in males who have had a previous successful attempt. The results are not substantiated by other studies, hence the replicability of these results in other patients or settings is limited. These considerations substantiate the utility of the testicular biopsy, togheter with other potential predictors of SR, in dealing with assisted reproductive techniques that require TESE when further attempts of TESE are planned. Accordingly, our data suggest not to miss the opportunity to collect a testicular fragment in the course of TESE to perform histologic analysis. Clearly, histology should not be included as a predictive factor of SR at first TESE attempt since the TESE specimen, either conventional or micro, not a prior pure diagnostic biopsy is what is read for histology and a patient will know of succesful sperm retrieval before histology results are even available. Nevertheless, the diagnostic biopsy during cTESE or even mTESE, along with other indicators may help to make an informed choice in the hypothesis of a subsequent new attempt of SR. Therefore, the allegation that it is time to put testis biopsy aside as a technique of historical interest not relevant to current reproductive technologies should be called into question and the opportunity to collect a testicular specimen for histology during the course of TESE, for a better stratification of the SR chance in case of a subsequent attempt following a failure, should be taken. Accordingly, recent published evidences support the reliabilty of diagnostic biopsy as a predictor of positive sperm retrieval in men with NOA [19–23].

By performing TESE, the laboratory personnel should allow themselves enough time to dissect the testicular tissue and retrieve the sperm, particularly in the case of NOA patients, for whom spermatogenesis may be severely impacted and in whom it may take a long time to find sperm in the tissue [24]. Interestingly, the data presented here provide an estimate of what factors are expected to make sperm retrieval faster or slower. As expected, age, worst semen and histology and higher FSH values were all negative predictive factors in the multivariate analysis.

Our study does have limitations. Most importantly, a control population of men who were submitted to mTESE was not available. Other limitation includes the retrospective nature of the study.

Conclusions

Our data enable to construct a score which helps to provide a good approximation of the probability of SR with cTESE in case of reoperation because of failure in recovery of sperm, provided that a biopsy for microscopic analysis is harvested during the first TESE attempt. The biopsy, along with other parameters, enables a customization of the prognosis that would otherwise rely solely on literature data that often extend over a very wide range and still have the limitation of being strongly influenced by skill or experience of the team that created them and does not apply to all the peculiar situations that can bump into real life. Providing patients with a personalized, more clinically meaningful estimate of their likelihood of SR can aid in counseling and decrease anxiety for the patient and treating physician. Furthermore, consideration should be given to the variables found to be involved into the time required for sperm recovery. This individualized estimate is likely to improve the complex organisation of assisted reproductive technology procedures that may require multiple attempts, including repeated TESE.

Abbreviations

AIC: Akaike Information Criterion; AUC: Area under a curve; BMI: Body mass index; cTESE: Conventional TESE; FSH: Follicle stimulating hormone; HR: Hazard ratio; HypoS: Hypospermatogenesis; LH: Luteinizing hormone; MA: Maturation arrest; mTESE: Micro TESE; NOA: Non-obstructive azoospermia; NormoS: Normal spermatogenesis; ROC: Receiver operating curve; SCO: Sertoli cell only; SR: Sperm recovery; T: Testosterone; TESE: Testicular sperm extraction

Authors' contributions

LG had full access to all the data in the study and takes responsibility for the integrity of the data and the accuracy of the data analysis. *Study concept and design*: LG, FS, MGM, EG. *Acquisition of data*: FS, SM, MGM, MW, SB, GF, PFG. *Analysis and interpretation of data*: LG, FS, EG, SM, MW, AF, CL. *Drafting of the manuscript*: LG, FS, EG, SM, AF, CL. *Critical revision of the manuscript for important intellectual content*: LG, FS, EG. *Statistical analysis*: AF. All authors read and approved the final manuscript.

Competing interests

The authors declare that they have no competing interests.

Author details

¹Department of Experimental Medicine, Section of Medical Pathophysiology, Food Science and Endocrinology, Sapienza University of Rome, Policlinico Umberto I, 00161 Rome, Italy. ²Centre for Reproductive Medicine, European Hospital, Rome, Italy. ³Department Gynaecological-Obstetrical and Urological Sciences, Sapienza University of Rome, Policlinico Umberto I, 00161 Rome, Italy. ⁴Department of Public Health and Infectious Diseases, "Sapienza" University of Rome, Rome, Italy.

References

1. Dohle GR, Elzanaty S, van Casteren NJ. Testicular biopsy: clinical practice and interpretation. Asian J Androl. 2012;14:88–93.
2. Guler I, Erdem M, Erdem A, et al. Impact of testicular histopathology as a predictor of sperm retrieval and pregnancy outcome in patients with nonobstructive azoospermia: correlation with clinical and hormonal factors. Andrologia. 2016;48:765–73.
3. Schoor RA, Elhanbly S, Niederberger CS, Ross LS. The role of testicular biopsy in the modern management of male infertility. J Urol. 2002;167:197–200.
4. Ramasamy R, Schlegel PN. Microdissection testicular sperm extraction: effect of prior biopsy on success of sperm retrieval. J Urol. 2007;177:1447–9.
5. Berookhim BM, Palermo GD, Zaninovic N, Rosenwaks Z, Schlegel PN. Microdissection testicular sperm extraction in men with Sertoli cell-only testicular histology. Fertil Steril. 2014;102:1282–6.
6. Yildirim ME, Koc A, Kaygusuz IC, et al. The association between serum follicle-stimulating hormone levels and the success of microdissection testicular sperm extraction in patients with azoospermia. Urol J. 2014;11:1825–8.
7. Niederberger C. Re: microdissection testicular sperm extraction in men with sertoli cell-only testicular histology. J Urol. 2015;193:1605–6.
8. Franco G, Scarselli F, Casciani V, et al. A novel stepwise micro-TESE approach in non obstructive azoospermia. BMC Urol. 2016;16:20–7.
9. Marconi M, Keudel A, Diemer T, et al. Combined trifocal and microsurgical testicular sperm extraction is the best technique for testicular sperm retrieval in "low-chance" nonobstructive azoospermia. Eur Urol. 2012;62:713–9.
10. Cooper TG, Noonan E, von Eckardstein S, et al. World Health Organization reference values for human semen characteristics. Hum Reprod Update. 2010;16:231–45.
11. Bendikson KA, Neri QV, Takeuchi T, et al. The outcome of intracytoplasmic sperm injection using occasional spermatozoa in the ejaculate of men with spermatogenic failure. J Urol. 2008;180:1060–4.
12. Kim ED, Leibman BB, Grinblat DM, et al. Varicocele repair improves semen parameters in azoospermic men with spermatogenic failure. J Urol. 1999; 162(3 Pt 1):737–40.
13. Akaike H. A new look at the statistical model identification. IEEE Trans Autom Contr. 1974;19:716–23.
14. Deruyver Y, Vanderschueren D, Van der Aa F. Outcome of microdissection TESE compared with conventional TESE in non-obstructive azoospermia: a systematic review. Andrology. 2014;2:20–4.
15. Bernie AM, Mata DA, Ramasamy R, Schlegel PN. Comparison of microdissection testicular sperm extraction, conventional testicular sperm extraction, and testicular sperm aspiration for nonobstructive azoospermia: a systematic review and meta-analysis. Fertil Steril. 2015;104:1099–103.
16. Haimov-Kochman R, Lossos F, Nefesh I, et al. The value of repeat testicular sperm retrieval in azoospermic men. Fertil Steril. 2009;91(4 Suppl):1401–3.
17. Vernaeve V, Verheyen G, Goossens A, et al. How successful is repeat testicular sperm extraction in patients with azoospermia? Hum Reprod. 2006;21:1551–4.
18. Ramasamy R, Ricci JA, Leung RA, et al. Successful repeat microdissection testicular sperm extraction in men with nonobstructive azoospermia. J Urol. 2011;185:1027–31.
19. Abdel Raheem A, Garaffa G, Rushwan N, et al. Testicular histopathology as a predictor of a positive sperm retrieval in men with non-obstructive azoospermia. BJU Int. 2013;111:492–9.
20. Aydin T, Sofikerim M, Yucel B, Karadag M, Tokat F. Effects of testicular histopathology on sperm retrieval rates and ICSI results in non-obstructive azoospermia. J Obstet Gynaecol. 2015;35:829–31.
21. Xu T, Peng L, Lin X, Li J, Xu W. Predictors for successful sperm retrieval of salvage microdissection testicular sperm extraction (TESE) following failed TESE in nonobstructive azoospermia patients. Andrologia. 2016; https://doi org/10.1111/and.12642.
22. Caroppo E, Colpi EM, Gazzano G, et al. Testicular histology may predict the successful sperm retrieval in patients with non-obstructive azoospermia undergoing conventional TESE: a diagnostic accuracy study. J Assist Reprod Genet. 2016;34:149–54.
23. Güneri Ç, Alkibay T, Tunç L. Effects of clinical, laboratuary and pathological features on successful sperm retrieval in non-obstructive azoospermia. Turk J Urol. 2016;42:168–77.
24. Rajfer J. Timing of sperm harvesting: is there room for improvement? Rev Urol. 2008;10:170–1.

2

Risks and complications of transurethral resection of bladder tumors in patients receiving antiplatelet and/or anticoagulant therapy: a retrospective cohort study

Tsuzumi Konishi[1]* , Satoshi Washino[1], Yuhki Nakamura[1], Masashi Ohshima[1], Kimitoshi Saito[1], Yoshiaki Arai[2] and Tomoaki Miyagawa[1]

Abstract

Background: Information on the safety of transurethral resection of bladder tumors (TURBT) in patients receiving anti-thromboembolic drugs is currently lacking. This study aimed to evaluate the clinical safety of TURBT in patients receiving anti-thromboembolic agents compared with patients not taking these agents and patients who interrupted their use perioperatively.

Methods: We retrospectively analyzed data for patients who underwent TURBT at Jichi Medical University Saitama Medical Center from September 2013 to August 2016.Patients who underwent surgery while receiving antiplatelet and/or anticoagulant drugs were allocated to the continuation group, those who interrupted these drugs comprised the interruption group, and those who did not use these agents were designated as the control group. We compared the patient characteristics, hemoglobin levels, and complications among the three groups.

Results: A total of 174 patients were analyzed including 19, 18, and 137 in the continuation, interruption, and control groups, respectively. There were no significant differences in patient and tumor characteristics, apart from age, among the three groups. Decreases in hemoglobin levels were similar in the continuation, interruption, and control groups (−0.50 g/dl, −0.40 g/dl, and −0.50 g/dl, respectively).Significantly more patients in the continuation group experienced clot retention compared with the control group (21% vs 5%, $p = 0.03$). Large tumor size tended to be a risk factor for clot retention in the continuation group ($p = 0.07$). No patient in the continuation or interruption group required blood transfusion, compared with two patients (1%) in the control group. No patients in any of the groups experienced cardiovascular events during their hospital stay or required rehospitalization for hematuria after discharge.

Conclusions: TURBT can be performed safely in patients who continue to take antiplatelet and/or anticoagulant agents, without increasing the risks of severe hemorrhage and blood transfusion. However, the risk of postoperative clot retention may be increased in these patients.

Keywords: Anticoagulant, Antiplatelet, Turbt

* Correspondence: tsuzumi0203@gmail.com
[1]Department of Urology, Jichi Medical University Saitama Medical Center, 1-847 Amanuma-cho, Omiya-ku, Saitama 330-8503, Japan
Full list of author information is available at the end of the article

Background

Urologists are encountering increasing numbers of patients with multiple comorbidities associated with the progressive aging of the population. These include coronary artery disease requiring percutaneous coronary arterial intervention with angioplasty, together with the placement of bare metal (BMS) or drug-eluting stents (DES), and cardiac dysrhythmias such as valvular heart disease, deep vein thrombosis, or atrial fibrillation [1]. International guidelines recommend dual antiplatelet (AP) therapy (DAPT) for ≥4 weeks after implantation of BMS, and for 6–12 months after implantation of DES [2, 3], while anticoagulant (AC) agents are recommended in patients with cardiac dysrhythmias. Withdrawal of AP and/or AC agents is associated with a significantly increased risk of cardiac ischemic and/or thromboembolic events [4]. Surgeons, physicians, and patients thus face the dilemma of stopping these agents perioperatively to reduce the bleeding risk, and continuing them to avoid the risk of cardiovascular and cerebrovascular events [5]. There is currently no consensus among urologists regarding the perioperative management of patients taking AP/AC agents, and information on this issue is lacking [6]. A few recent reports have assessed the safety of continuing to use AP agents during transurethral resection of bladder tumors (TURBT) [5, 7], but there is little information on the safety of TURBT in patients receiving AC or combined AP/AC therapy. This study aimed to evaluate the clinical safety of TURBT in patients receiving AP/AC agents, compared with patients not taking these agents or patients who interrupted their use perioperatively.

Methods

Patients

This retrospective observational study was approved by our local institutional review board. Patients who underwent TURBT at Jichi Medical University Saitama Medical Center from September 2013 to August 2016 and who were followed-up for at least 3 months were eligible. Patients who underwent additional procedures at the same time as TURBT or who underwent second TURBT were excluded. Eligible patients were categorized into two groups: patients taking AP and/or AC drugs before surgery (AP/AC group) and those not taking these drugs (control group). Patients in AP/AC group were further categorized into two groups: patients who took AP/AC drugs during surgery (continuation group) and those who interrupted the drugs for the appropriate periods before, during, and after surgery (interruption group). The decision on whether to continue or interrupt AP/AC drugs was made after detailed discussions between patients and doctors (urologists, anesthesiologists, neurologist, and/or, cardiologists), mainly in light of the risk of cardiovascular events.

Device

TURBT was performed using a UES-40S (Olympus R, Tokyo, Japan) or ESG-400 (Olympus) endoscope.

Management

In principle, patients were not allowed to walk on the day of surgery, and started to walk the next morning. Blood tests, including hemoglobin levels, were performed on the first postoperative day. Patients were discharged from the hospital after removal of the urethral catheter and spontaneous voiding had been experienced.

Study endpoints

Patients' characteristics, decreases in hemoglobin levels, median catheter-indwelling duration after TURBT, and complications were compared among the three groups. The endpoints of our study were decrease in hemoglobin level and hemorrhagic complications after TURBT. Decreases in hemoglobin levels were determined as [preoperative hemoglobin level – hemoglobin level on first postoperative day]. Preoperative examinations were performed within 2 months before surgery.

Statistical analysis

Statistical analysis was performed using GraphPad Prism software version 6.0. Data were compared using Student's t-tests, Mann–Whitney U-tests, or χ^2 tests. All data are shown as medians and ranges. Statistical significance was set at $p < 0.05$.

Results

Patients and tumor characteristics

A total of 229 patients were eligible, of whom 31 patients who underwent additional procedures at the same time as TURBT and 24 who underwent second TURBT were excluded. A total of 174 patients were therefore analyzed, including 37 patients in the AP/AC group and 137 in the control group. Among the 37 AP/AC patients, 19 were in the AP/AC continuation group and 18 were in the interruption group.

Patient and tumor characteristics are shown in Table 1. The age in the interruption group was significantly higher than in the control group ($p = 0.003$), but gender, tumor size, tumor number, T classification at TURBT, and de novo/recurrence did not differ significantly among the three groups.

Details of medications and reasons for taking AP/AC agents

Among the 19 patients in the continuation group, seven, three, four, and five were taking a single AP, single AC, DAPT, and AP plus AC, respectively, prior to surgery (Table 2). Of the four patients taking DAPT, three interrupted clopidogrel during the perioperative period, and

Table 1 Patient and tumor characteristics

	AP/AC				Control (C) n = 137, n (%)		p value		
	Continuation (A) n = 19, n (%)		Interruption (B) n = 18, n (%)				A vs B	A vs C	B vs C
Median age (range)	77	(57–89)	81	(58–90)	72	(38–90)	0.14	0.12	0.00322
Sex									
Male	17	(88%)	14	(78%)	97	(71%)	0.40	0.10	0.78
Female	2	(12%)	4	(22%)	40	(29%)			
Tumor size									
< 1 cm	10	(53%)	8	(44%)	71	(52%)	0.75	1.0	0.62
≥ 1 cm	9	(47%)	10	(56%)	66	(48%)			
Tumor number									
Single	11	(58%)	12	(67%)	71	(52%)	0.74	0.81	0.32
Multiple	8	(42%)	6	(33%)	66	(48%)			
T classification at TURBT									
pT0–a	8	(42%)	7	(39%)	53	(39%)	0.43	0.71	0.35
pT1	9	(47%)	10	(56%)	59	(43%)			
Min. pT2	2	(11%)	1	(5%)	25	(18%)			
De novo	10	(53%)	10	(56%)	83	(61%)	>0.95	0.62	0.80
Recurrence	9	(47%)	8	(44%)	54	(39%)			

AP antiplatelet agents, *AC* anticoagulant agents, *Min* minimum

of the five patients taking AP plus AC, one interrupted the AC agent during the perioperative period. None of the other patients interrupted any AP/AC agents. At the time of surgery, 11, three, one, and four patients were taking a single AP, single AC, DAPT, and AP plus AC, respectively.

A heparin bridge was performed in nine patients in the interruption group, including four, two, and three patients taking a single AP, single AC, and AP plus AC, respectively, prior to surgery. In the heparin-bridged patients, heparin was started at a dose of 15,000 U/day, adjusted to achieve an activated partial thromboplastin time 1.5–2 times the control value, and then discontinued 4 h before surgery. Oral AP and/or AC drugs were re-started after no or little hematuria was achieved postoperatively.

The reasons for taking APs and/or ACs are shown in Table 3. Ischemic heart disease (51%), atrial fibrillation

(30%), and cerebral infarction (16%) were the three main reasons.

Anesthesia

Among the 19 patients in the continuation group, 17 underwent TURBT under general anesthesia and two under spinal anesthesia. In the interruption group, 11 and seven patients underwent TURBT under spinal and general anesthesia, respectively, while 104 and 33 patients in the control group underwent TURBT under spinal and general anesthesia, respectively.

Complications

Complications during and after TURBT in the three groups are shown in Table 4. Decreases in hemoglobin levels were similar in all three groups (–0.50 g/dl, –0.40 g/dl, and –0.50 g/dl in the continuation, interruption, and control

Table 2 Details of medication before surgery

		Continuation, n = 19 n (%)				Interruption, n = 18 n (%)		
		Before surgery		During surgery		Before surgery		During surgery
Single agent	Aspirin	7	(37)	11	(58)	11	(61)	–
	Clopidogrel	–		–		1	(5)	–
	AC	3	(16)	3	(16)	3	(17)	–
Combination	DAPT	4	(21)	1	(5)	0	(0)	–
	AP + AC	5	(26)	4	(21)	3	(17)	–

AP antiplatelet agents, *AC* anticoagulant agents, *DAPT* dual antiplatelet therapy

Table 3 Reasons for medication

	Continuation n = 19, n (%)		Interruption n = 18, n (%)		Total n = 37, n (%)	
IHD	12	(63%)	7	(39%)	19	(51)
AF	5	(26%)	6	(33%)	11	(30)
CI	0	(0%)	6	(33%)	6	(16)
Primary prevention	2	(11%)	1	(6%)	3	(8)
Others	3	(16%)	0	(0%)	3	(8)

IHD ischemic heart disease, *AF* atrial fibrillation, *CI* cerebral infarction

groups, respectively). Significantly more patients (21%, 4/19) in the continuation group experienced clot retention compared with the control group (5.0%, 7/140) (*p* = 0.03). All four patients with clot retention in the continuation group were only taking aspirin (Table 5). Two of them experienced clot retention during catheterization (postoperative day [POD] 1 and POD3) and required surgical reintervention, while the other two experienced clot retention after catheter removal (POD3 and POD21), which was improved by bladder drainage and catheter replacement. Two (11%) and three patients (2%) in the continuation and control groups required surgical reintervention to stop bleeding, respectively. The median duration of catheter-indwelling was significantly longer in the continuation group (2 days) compared with the control group (1 day) (*p* = 0.03). However, there was no significant difference in hospitalization days after surgery among the three groups. No patient in the continuation or interruption group required blood transfusion, compared with two patients (1%) in the control group. No patients in any of the groups experienced cardiovascular events during their hospital stay, or required rehospitalization for hematuria during the 3 months after discharge.

Risk factors for clot retention in patients continuing AP/AC

We evaluated the risk factors for clot retention in patients continuing AP/AC drugs by comparing patients in the continuation group with (*n* = 4) and without clot retention (*n* = 15) (Table 6). Large tumors tended to be a risk factor for clot retention (*p* = 0.07), though the difference was not significant. However, age, tumor number, T classification at TURBT, and type and number of AP/AC agents were unrelated to clot retention (*p* > 0.1).

Discussion

The American Urologic Association and the International Consultation on Urological Disease produced a collaborative review of Anticoagulation and Antiplatelet Therapy in Urologic Practice [1], which stated that urologists need to understand the factors affecting the safe and effective use of AP and AC prophylaxis, as well as the risks posed by their withdrawal. These risks include venous and arterial thromboembolism, as well as major adverse cerebrovascular and cardiac events, which may be more life-altering than hemorrhage. Although the review also considered the management of AP/AC drugs during various urologic procedures, including shock wave lithotripsy, ureteroscopy with laser lithotripsy, percutaneous nephrolithotomy, laser prostatectomy, transurethral resection of the prostate, ultrasound-guided prostate biopsy, radical prostatectomy, and surgical renal procedures, it did not discuss the appropriate management of patients undergoing TURBT. A review of AP therapy in patients with coronary stents who underwent urologic surgery [8] included TURBT as a high risk procedure for bleeding. This review recommended that APs should be discontinued in patients at low thromboembolic risk undergoing TURBT, while elective surgery should be postponed if possible in patients at intermediate or high risk. In non-

Table 4 Surgical outcomes and complications

	AP/AC							p value		
	Continuation (A) n = 19, n (%)		Interruption (B) n = 18, n (%)		Control (C) n = 137, n (%)			A vs B	A vs C	B vs C
Median Hb decrease g/dL (range)	−0.5	(−−2.8–0.6)	−0.4	(−1.6–1.2)	−0.5	(−3.1–2.6)		0.27	0.20	0.48
Median catheter indwelling days (range)	2	(1–8)	1	(1–5)	1	(0–20)		0.06	0.03	0.50
Clot retention	4	(21)	0	(0)	7	(5)		0.11	0.03	>0.95
Surgical reintervention	2	(11)	0	(0)	3	(2)		0.49	0.11	>0.95
Transfusion	0	(0)	0	(0)	2	(1)		>0.95	>0.95	>0.95
Cardiovascular events	0	(0)	0	(0)	0	(0)		>0.95	>0.95	>0.95
Median days of hospital stay after surgery (range)	5	(3–12)	5	(3–7)	5	(2–14)		0.57	0.18	0.50
Re-admission	0	(0)	0	(0)	0	(0)		>0.95	>0.95	>0.95

AP antiplatelet agents, *AC* anticoagulant agents, *Hb* hemoglobin

Table 5 Cases with clot retention in AP/AC continuation group

	Sex	Medication	Tumor no.	Tumor size (cm)	pT stage	POD at catheter removal	Onset of clot retention (POD)	Treatment
Case 1	M	Aspirin	2	1.5	a	(−)	1	Surgical reinterventiom
Case 2	M	Aspirin	2	3	1	(−)	3	Surgical reinterventiom
Case 3	M	Aspirin	1	2	1	1	21	Bladder drainage
Case 4	M	Aspirin	6	2	1	2	3	Bladder drainage and irrigation

AP antiplatelet agents, *AC* anticoagulant agents, *no* number, *POD* postoperative day, *M* male

deferrable cases, aspirin should be continued if possible, P2Y12 inhibitors should be discontinued 5 days before surgery and resumed within 24–72 h with a loading dose, and bridge therapy with glycoprotein IIb/IIIa inhibitors is recommended if aspirin is discontinued, though these agents may be clinically unavailable, as in Japan. However, no replacement therapy has yet been validated prospectively [9].

International guidelines for percutaneous cardiovascular intervention advocate DAPT for ≥4 weeks after BMS implantation and for 6–12 months after DES implantation [2], and premature withdrawal of AP agents was shown to be related to a higher risk of cardiac ischemic or thromboembolic events associated with stent thrombosis [3]. This rare but life-threatening complication usually manifests as acute myocardial infarction, with a mortality of 10%–40%, though the incidence of stent thrombosis can be increased up to 90-fold following premature discontinuation of DAPT [10]. APs provide effective long-term secondary prevention of vascular events and ischemic stroke after acute or transient ischemic stroke. A systematic review of 287 randomized trials in patients at high risk of vascular occlusive events found that AP agents significantly decreased the risk of stroke by 31% [11]. Interruption of aspirin therapy was a significant risk factor for a stroke event within 4 weeks after aspirin discontinuation (odds ratio 3.4), with the main reasons for interrupting aspirin therapy being surgery, the treating physician's decision that the therapy had no clear clinical benefit, and bleeding complications [12]. Five of 493 (1%) patients who stopped continuous ACs to allow the performance of dental procedures developed severe embolic complications, resulting in four deaths [4]. Overall, discontinuation of AP/AC agents is associated with severe thrombotic events and these drugs should be continued if at all possible.

Piccozi et al. recently demonstrated that continued use of aspirin monotherapy did not increase overall bleeding or reintervention risks in patients undergoing TURBT (2.8% in the aspirin group vs 1.9% in the control group) [5]. Camignani et al. assessed 12 patients receiving DAPT who underwent TURBT and demonstrated that no patients required reintervention for hemostatic purposes, but three (25%) of the 12 patients experienced clot retention after removal of the bladder catheter, all of which cases were resolved by replacing the catheter [7]. In the current study, we demonstrated that continuing AP/AC agents did not lead to increased blood loss or an increased incidence of blood transfusion compared with patients not taking or interrupting AP/AC agents. However, the incidence of clot retention was significantly increased in the AP/AC continuation group (21%) compared with the control group (5%). Interestingly, all four patients with clot retention received aspirin monotherapy, whereas patients

Table 6 Risk factors for clot retention in AP/AC continuation group

		Clot retention (+) $n = 4$, n (%)		Clot retention (−) $n = 15$, n (%)		p value
Median age (range)		77	(63–89)	77	(57–85)	0.76
Median tumor size, cm (range)		2	(1.5–3)	0.8	(0.5–3)	0.07
Tumor number	Single	1	(25)	10	(67)	0.26
	Multiple	3	(75)	5	(33)	
T classification at TURBT	pTa	1	(25)	7	(47)	0.43
	pT1	3	(75)	6	(40)	
	Min. pT2	0	(0)	2	(13)	
AP/AC drugs	Single AP	4	(100)	7	(47)	0.16
	Single AC	0	(0)	3	(20)	
	Combination	0	(0)	5	(33)	

AP antiplatelet agents, *AC* anticoagulant agents, *Min* minimum taking AC agents or combined AP/AC agents did not experience clot retention. Large tumor size appeared to be a risk factor for clot retention, though the result was not statistically significant. Overall, these results suggest that TURBT can be performed in patients continuing to take AP/AC agents, including a combination of AP/AC agents, without increasing the risk of severe hemorrhage, though the risk of clot formation after surgery might be increased, especially in patients with large tumors. However, the incidence of complications in patients who interrupted AP/AC agents was similar to that in patients not taking these drugs, suggesting that it might be preferable to interrupt AP/AC agents in patients with a low thromboembolic risk, with a heparin bridge in patients taking ACs. However, the use of heparin-bridging therapy is controversial, and a recent study found that it did not reduce the risk of arterial thromboembolism compared with no bridging therapy in patients with stable nonvalvular atrial fibrillation [13]. In patients taking novel oral ACs, short-term interruption of these agents during the perioperative period might be possible because of their rapid offset and onset of anticoagulant activity [14].

There were several limitations to the present study. Notably, the retrospective nature of the study increased the risk of patient selection bias, and the sample size was small because of the small portion of patients taking AP and/or AC agents undergoing TURBT, which might underestimate the risk of taking these agents while undergoing TURBT. However, to the best of our knowledge, this is the first study to compare complications among patients who continued AP/AC, those who interrupted the treatment, and those not taking these agents, and to demonstrate that major bleeding complications were relatively rare, even in patients taking DAPT or a combination of AP and AC agents. However, further large prospective studies are therefore needed to verify these results.

Conclusion

TURBT can be performed safely in patients who continue to use AP and/or AC agents without increasing the risks of severe hemorrhage and blood transfusion. However, the risk of clot retention after surgery may be increased in these patients.

Abbreviations

AC: anticoagulant; AP: antiplatelet; BMS: bare metal stents; DAPT: dual antiplatelet therapy; DES: drug-eluting stents; M: male; Min: minimum; POD: postoperative day; TURBT: transurethral resection of bladder tumors

Acknowledgments
We would like to thank the cardiologists and anesthesiologists at Jichi Medical University Saitama Medical Center for their cooperation and insightful comments. We thank Susan Furness, PhD, from Edanz Group (www.edanzediting.com/ac) for editing a draft of this manuscript.

Funding
None

Authors' contributions
TK was a major contributor to the conception and design of the study and in drafting the manuscript. SW and MT analyzed and interpreted the patient data. YN, MO, KS, and YA provided administrative and technical support, including data acquisition. All of the authors read and approved the final manuscript.

Competing interests
The authors declare that they have no competing interests.

Author details
[1]Department of Urology, Jichi Medical University Saitama Medical Center, 1-847 Amanuma-cho, Omiya-ku, Saitama 330-8503, Japan. [2]Department of Urology, Nishi-Omiya Hospital, 1-1173 Mihashi, Omiya-ku, Saitama 330-0856, Japan.

References
1. Culkin D, Exaire E, Green D, Soloway M, Gross A, Desai M, White J, Lightner D. Anticoagulation and Antiplatelet therapy in urological practice: ICUD/AUA review paper. J Urol. 2014;192(4):1026–34.
2. Kolh P, Wijns W, Danchin N, Di Mario C, Falk V, Folliguet T, Garg S, Huber K, James S, Knuuti J, Lopez-Sendon J, Marco J, Menicanti L, Ostojic M, Piepoli M, Pirlet C, Pomar J, Reifart N, Ribichini F, Schalij M, Sergeant P, Serruys P, Silber S, Uva M, Taggart D, Torracca L, Valgimigli M, Wijns W, Witkowski A. 2014 ESC/EACTS guidelines on myocardial revascularization: the task force on myocardial revascularization of the European Society of Cardiology (ESC) and the European Association for Cardio-Thoracic Surgery (EACTS). Developed with the special contribution of the European Association of Percutaneous Cardiovascular Interventions (EAPCI). Eur J Cardiothorac Surg. 2014;46(4):517–92.
3. Biondi-Zoccai G, Lotrionte M, Agostoni P, Abbate A, Fusaro M, Burzotta F, Testa L, Sheiban I, Sangiorgi G. A systematic review and meta-analysis on the hazards of discontinuing or not adhering to aspirin among 50 279 patients at risk for coronary artery disease. Eur Heart J. 2006;27(22):2667–74.
4. Wahl M. Dental surgery in anticoagulated patients. Arch of Intern Med. 1998;158(15):1610–6.
5. Picozzi S, Marenghi C, Ricci C, Bozzini G, Casellato S, Carmignani L. Risks and complications of transurethral resection of bladder tumor among patients taking antiplatelet agents for cardiovascular disease. Surg Endosc. 2014; 28(1):116–21.
6. Eberli D, Chassot P, Sulser T, Samama C, Mantz J, Delabays A, Spahn D. Urological surgery and Antiplatelet drugs after cardiac and Cerebrovascular accidents. J Urol. 2010;183(6):2128–36.
7. Carmignani L, Picozzi S, Stubinski R, Casellato S, Bozzini G, Lunelli L, Arena D. Endoscopic resection of bladder cancer in patients receiving double platelet antiaggregant therapy. Surg Endosc. 2011;25(7):2281–7.
8. Naspro R, Rossini R, Musumeci G, Gadda F, Da Pozzo L. Antiplatelet therapy in patients with coronary stent undergoing urologic surgery: is it still no Man's land? Eur Urol. 2013;64(1):101–5.
9. Samama C, Bastien O, Forestier F, Denninger M, Isetta C, Juliard J, Lasne D, Leys D, Mismetti P, Grp E. Antiplatelet agents in the perioperative period: expert recommendations of the French Society of Anesthesiology and Intensive Care (SFAR) 2001 - summary statement. Can J Anaesth. 2002;49(6):S26–35.
10. Iakovou I, Schmidt T, Bonizzoni E, Ge I, Sangiorgi G, Stankovic G, Airoldi F, Chieffo A, Montorfano M, Carlino M, Michev I, Corvaja N, Briguori C, Gerckens U, Grube E, Colombo A. Incidence, predictors, and outcome of thrombosis after successful implantation of drug-eluting stents. JAMA. 2005; 293(17):2126–30.
11. Straus S, Majumdar S, McAlister F. New evidence for stroke prevention - scientific review. JAMA. 2002;288(11):1388–95.
12. Llinas R. Could discontinuation of aspirin therapy be a trigger for stroke? Nat Clin Pract Neurol. 2006;2(6):300–1.
13. Bouillon K, Bertrand M, Boudali L, Ducimetiere P, Dray-Spira R, Zureik M. Short-Term Risk of Bleeding During Heparin Bridging at Initiation of Vitamin K Antagonist Therapy in More Than 90 000 Patients with Nonvalvular Atrial Fibrillation Managed in Outpatient Care. J Am Heart Assoc. 2016;5(11).

3

Impact of a protein-based assay that predicts prostate cancer aggressiveness on urologists' recommendations for active treatment or active surveillance: a randomized clinical utility trial

John W. Peabody[1,2]*, Lisa M. DeMaria[1], Diana Tamondong-Lachica[1], Jhiedon Florentino[1], M. Czarina Acelajado[1], Othman Ouenes[1], Jerome P. Richie[3] and Trever Burgon[1]

Abstract

Background: Of the more than 1.1 million men diagnosed worldwide annually with prostate cancer, the majority have indolent tumors. Distinguishing between aggressive and indolent cancer is an important clinical challenge. The current approaches for assessing tumor aggressiveness are recognized as insufficient. A validated protein-based assay has been shown to predict tumor aggressiveness from prostate biopsy. The main objective of this study was to measure the clinical utility of this new assay in the management of early-stage prostate cancer.

Methods: One hundred twenty nine board-certified urologists were asked to participate in a randomized, two-arm experiment. We collected data over 2 rounds using simulated clinical cases administered via an online platform. The cases were all newly diagnosed Gleason 3 + 3 or 3 + 4 prostate camcer patients. Urologists in the intervention arm received a 15-min webinar on this protein-based assay and given assay test results for their simulated patients in round 2. Each case had a preferred recommendation of either active surveillance or active treatment. The measured outcome was rate of preferred recommendation, defined as urologists who recommended the proper treatment course. Analyses were done using difference-in-difference estimations.

Results: Using multinomial logistical regression, urologists who were given the assay results were significantly more likely to choose the preferred recommendation (active surveillance or active treatment) compared to controls ($p = 0.004$). These urologists were also significantly more likely to involve their patients in the treatment decision compared to controls ($p = 0.001$).

Conclusions: By providing additional information to inform the physician's treatment plan, a protein-based assay shows demonstrable clinical utility confirmed through a rigorous randomized controlled study design and regression analyses to test for effects.

Keywords: Proteomic biomarker, Protein-based assay, Gleason score, Active surveillance, Active treatment, Simulated patients, Evidence-based treatment

* Correspondence: jpeabody@qurehealthcare.com
[1]QURE Healthcare, 450 Pacific Ave, Suite 200, San Francisco, CA, USA
[2]University of California, San Francisco, 500 Beale Street, San Francisco, CA, USA
Full list of author information is available at the end of the article

Impact of a protein-based assay that predicts prostate cancer aggressiveness on urologists'...

15

Background

Worldwide, prostate cancer is the most commonly diagnosed solid organ tumor and the second deadliest, with more than 1.1 million new cases in 2012 [1]. Depending on emphasis of early detection and/or treatment, wide variation exists in mortality rates in various countries [2]. Over recent decades, however, widespread use of prostate-specific antigen (PSA) testing has led to a pronounced shift toward identification of early-stage tumors, many of which are likely indolent and ultimately present little or no risk to the patient [3]. Simultaneously, treatment advances in robotic surgery and advanced radiation therapy have opened up additional opportunities to aggressively treat localized tumors, which may subject some patients to unnecessary treatment and the risks. These advances are key drivers in the rising cost of prostate cancer treatment [4]. Because of this, active surveillance is increasingly being recommended as a treatment option [5].

Distinguishing between aggressive and indolent cancer, and delivering the appropriate level of care to each group, is thus an important clinical and economic challenge. Active surveillance (AS) protocols, which emphasize identification of low-risk patients and monitoring of the tumor in lieu of aggressive treatment, have been incorporated into U.S. and European guidelines [6, 7], are linked with the highest quality-adjusted life expectancy [8], but appear to be underutilized [9], with significant variation in adoption that cannot be explained by clinical characteristics [10]. The decision to pursue AS is a complex process where clinical risk stratification, physician recommendation, and patient preference all play roles [11–14]. In a recent review [14], the researchers noted that while a uniform approach to AS would be appealing, "current diagnostic and prognostic tools lack the precision needed to reliably monitor men... [who have] varying risks and preferences."

Evaluation of appropriate use of AS and active treatment (AT) is plagued by subtle differences in patient presentation *and* differences in clinical treatment decisions. If, however, patient level variability could be controlled, the (expected high level of) variability in clinical decision making between AS and AT, defined as providing a clinical intervention [11, 15], could be understood.

Given the wide variation in prostate cancer treatment decisions, a key question is whether better diagnostic tests for assessing tumor aggressiveness leads to better treatment decisions and better clinical utility. Given the preponderance of low risk patients, diagnostics that increase confidence in risk assessment will also likely result in reduced health care spending. A new quantitative immunofluorescent protein-based assay (ProMark) that predicts tumor aggressiveness at biopsy has been described for patients with Gleason grades 3 + 3 or 3 + 4 prostate cancer, wherein aggressiveness is difficult to distinguish using existing clinical and pathological parameters [16].

The objective of this study is to measure the variability of treatment decisions of AT or AS and determine the impact of adding a protein-based risk assessment assay to current standard of care risk classification approaches in the management of early-stage prostate cancer. To overcome patient-level (case-mix) variability, this study uses validated case simulations of early stage prostate cancer, among a large cohort of urologists.

Methods
Design

A "before-and-after" design was utilized in a longitudinal randomized controlled study of board-certified urologists practicing in the U.S. Urologists were asked to care for online simulated patients with underlying but undiagnosed prostate cancer, using Clinical Performance and Value (CPV®) vignettes via web-based interactive 'patient visits.' All patients had a Gleason Score of 3 + 3 = 6 or 3 + 4 = 7. CPVs are simulated cases wherein clinicians are asked to interview and examine patients and order investigational studies including biopsies and blood tests. Clinicians taking care of the simulated patient are provided with responses to all history and physical items and results for any tests or procedures they choose to order. They are asked to diagnose the patient and make a treatment plan based on their investigations.

Physicians were randomized into control or intervention study arms and completed three vignettes at baseline (Round 1) and another three 6 to 8 weeks later (Round 2). In Round 1, no urologist received any information about the protein-based assay test, and none of the vignettes included these results. Between Rounds 1 and 2, intervention group urologists were introduced to the protein-based assay via a 15-min informational video. Intervention participants were then provided with these results for each Round 2 vignette. Protein-based assay information and results were not made available to the control group. The study design was approved by Chesapeake IRB (Columbia, MD). All participants provided written consent to participate.

The protein-based assay

The protein-based assay is a novel 8-biomarker proteomic test, using quantitative multiplex immunofluorescence to measure protein levels on prostate biopsy tissue. The assay produces a prognostic risk score scaled from 0 to 100 and stratifies patients into low (0–33), intermediate (34–60) or high risk (61–100). These scores independently predict final disease pathology and assess disease aggressiveness [16]. This test supplements current prostate cancer risk assessment methods, especially in cases where existing tools do not clearly delineate the appropriateness of AS or AT.

Eligibility and selection of physicians

Physicians had to (1) be currently practicing board-certified urologists, (2) have practiced (as a board-certified urologist) for greater than 2 or less than 30 years, (3) be English-speaking, (4) practice in a community/non-academic setting, (5) have ≥50 prostate cancer patients under care annually, (6) have Internet access, (7) have no prior experience with the protein-based assay test and (8) provide consent to participate in the study. Potential participants were contacted from a list of approximately 5100 practicing urologists who were randomly selected and invited to participate. Eligibility requirements, screening tools and study information presented during recruitment were identical for both groups. Eligible urologists were invited to participate in the study and 261 initially consented (Fig. 1). These were randomized into one of two arms: 138 in intervention and 123 in control. Of those initially randomized, 82 intervention and 69 control physicians participated at baseline, and 67 intervention and 62 control physicians completed the second round of CPVs. Statistical analysis yielded no significant differences between the physicians recruited in either of the two strategies nor among those who dropped out of the study or were lost to follow up.

Clinical Performance and value® vignettes

Treatment choice and treatment utility were measured at baseline (Round 1) and after 6–8 weeks (Round 2) using Clinical Performance and Value (CPV®) vignettes. CPVs are a validated means for assessing differences in clinical practice and inherent variation in care, independent of case-mix [17, 18]. All providers care for the same patients and patient types, eliminating patient variability or observed and unobserved patient heterogeneity from the analysis and allowing for whether a test changes clinical practice; both of which are difficult to completely overcome through chart review analysis.

The CPVs were designed around the evidence-base with clear appropriate recommendations for treatment courses. The vignettes simulated clinical encounters involving men presenting with suspected early stage prostate cancer, verifiable by ordering a biopsy. In each vignette, the urologists were asked to 'care for the patient' by answering open-ended questions regarding the clinical care they would provide. Responses were requested and scored in: taking a medical history, performing a physical examination, ordering appropriate diagnostic tests (including laboratory tests, imaging studies and procedures), determining a diagnosis, and outlining a treatment plan (i.e., AS or AT). Explicit scoring criteria were established prior to study administration and were derived from a literature review, National Comprehensive Cancer Network guidelines, and expert opinion. Completed vignettes were scored as a percentage of physician answers matching these evidence-based criteria.

Three groups of three (9 total) CPV vignettes, representing typical cases for practicing urologists, were written to evaluate the variability of AS versus AT and the impact of protein-based assay test results on patient management (Table 1). All nine cases were undiagnosed Gleason 3 + 3 and 3 + 4 prostate cancer patients, Stage T1c or T2a, specified by their activity level, an elevanted PSA and risk categories such that each case had a preferable treatment course that was either AS or AT (Table 2). The primary outcome measure was the appropriate recommendation according to the individual case.

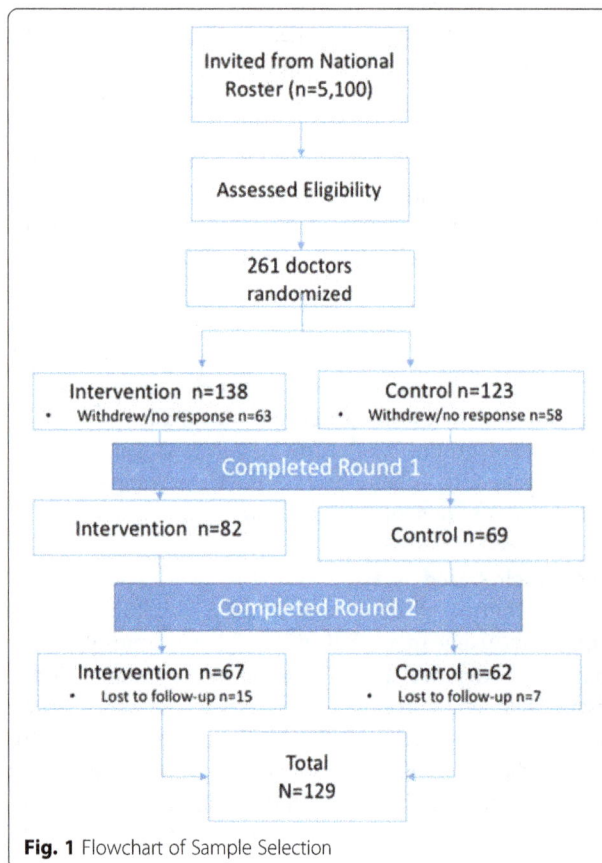

Fig. 1 Flowchart of Sample Selection

Table 1 List of Case Types, 3 CPV Cases within Each Type

Case Type	Standard	Standard + Protein-based Assay
A	Evidence-based treatment[a]	Assay confirms treatment
B	Evidence-based treatment[a]	Assay recommends switch (e.g., AS to AT)
C	Ambiguous treatment course	Assay resolve ambiguity

[a]Either AS or AT (depending on individual case) and based on age, PSA, Gleason score, etc

Table 2 CPV Case Details

CPV Case	Presenting History	Stage	Gleason	Cores	PSA	NCCN Risk Category	PBA score	PBA Risk Category	Preferred Option
1	Active 60 year old M with increasing urinary frequency	T1c	3 + 3	2_12 (<50%)	<10	Very Low	15	Low	AS
2	Sedentary 78 year old M with hematuria	T1c	3 + 3	4_12 (<50%)	7.1	Very Low	15	Low	AS
3	Moderately active 73 year old M with urinary frequency and hesitancy	T2a	3 + 4	3_12 (20% tumor in 4 s)	14	Intermediate	17	Low	AS
4	Quite active 57 year old M with erectile dysfunction and recent prostatitis	T2a	3 + 4	7_12	21	High	17	Low	AS
5	Moderately active 55 year old M with rising serum PSA levels	T1c	3 + 3	4_12	9.8	Very Low	35	Intermediate	AS
6	63 year old M, no longer active due to knee osteoarthritis, with suspicious digital rectal examination	T1c	3 + 3	6_12	8.9	Low	60	Intermediate	AT
7	Active 62 year old M with gross hematuria	T1c	3 + 4	3_12 (10% showing)	10.4	Intermediate	20	Low	AS
8	Lightly active 75 year old M seen for follow-up of suspicious nodularity on prostate	T2a	3 + 4	6_12	8.7	Intermediate	77	High	AT
9	Moderately active77 year old M seen in referral for nodule on prostate and high serum PSA	T2a	3 + 4	6_12	22.1	High	77	High	AT

PBA protein-based assay

The intervention

Prior to Round 2, the intervention group was given information about the protein-based assay via a 15-min informational video that provided an overview of the test and interpretation of the scores. 87.5% of the intervention group watched the video webinar. The intervention group then received hypothetical protein-based assay scores and disease aggressiveness risk estimates for each patient case in the Round 2 vignettes.

Analysis

The analysis determined how frequently did, urologists caring for Gleason 3 + 3 and 3 + 4 prostate cancer patients, recommend the preferred treatment pathway, and did this increase with the introduction of the protein-based assay? The preferred treatment pathway, defined on a case-by-case basis, was either AS or AT. Physician treatment was classified into four mutually exclusive categories: preferred treatment for the case; suboptimal treatment, defined as recommending AS when the case presentation and clinical guidelines indicated AT or recommending AT when AS was indicated; involving the patient in the treatment decision without making a recommendation for either AS or AT; and no cancer treatment recorded. If, for example, a urologist both recommended AS and involved the patient, then their response would be marked (depending on the case) as either preferred or suboptimal treatment.

Analyses used difference-in-difference estimations for intervention versus control in choosing the preferred treatment pathway. Multinomial multivariate regressions modeled choosing the preferred treatment pathways versus each of the other three possibilities for this variable (suboptimal, indeterminate, or no treatment). We included variables for round and the intervention arm. The interaction terms of round and arm measure the differential change in the odds ratio of a physician ordering the preferred treatment (compared to suboptimal treatment) after the intervention compared to Round 1. Physician and practice characteristics were included as control variables, consisting of: CPV case, physician age, prostate cancer patient load, overall urology patient load, in-practice access to robotic surgery capability, and proportion of patients covered by Medicare and Medicaid.

We also examined the impact of protein-based assay on the overall rates of AT, both in cases where surveillance was the preferred management pathway or where treatment was preferred. This analysis provided an additional perspective of the protein-based assay's clinical utility and role in modifying treatment patterns in clinical use.

Analyses were performed in Stata 13.0 (College Station, TX). The sample size of physicians was sufficient to detect a difference of 10% with an alpha of 0.05 and a beta of 0.80.

Results

Physician and practice characteristics

Participating urologists were typically in single specialty (86.3%), physician-owned (89.3%) group practices (85.9%). More than three-quarters (75.6%) have 11 or more years in practice post-fellowship and more than half (55.5%) have onsite robotic surgical capability. When looking at payor mix, these providers care for the same percentage of public versus private insurance. There were no significant differences between the two groups except a greater proportion of the intervention group reported seeing over 20 prostate cancer patients in a week (68.6%) versus the control group (46.8%) (Table 3).

We evaluated the physicians' AS or AT treatment choice for each case. The choices recorded in the CPVs were categorized as 1) either having appropriately recommended either AS or AT based upon guidelines for

Table 3 Baseline Physician and Practice Characteristics

	Overall	Intervention	Control	Int vs, Control p-value
	n = 129	n = 67	n = 62	
Age (Average / SD)	50.1 (8.9)	49.0 (8.9)	51.2 (8.9)	0.133
Number of years post-fellowship				
0–5	7.2%	10.2%	3.8%	0.410
6–10	17.3%	18.1%	16.3%	
11–20	45.1%	47.5%	42.3%	
21+ years	30.5%	24.1%	37.7%	
Number of MD's associated with practice				
1–3	33.9%	34.8%	32.8%	0.816
4–10	35.5%	33.9%	37.4%	
10+	30.6%	31.3%	29.8%	
Single Specialty Practice (%)	86.3%	85.7%	87.0%	
Practice type (% breakdown)				
Group/Staff	85.9%	82.1%	90.2%	0.410
IPA	4.6%	4.8%	4.3%	
Mixed	7.9%	10.2%	5.4%	
Network	1.5%	2.9%	0.0%	
Practice Ownership (% breakdown)				
Physician-Physician group	89.3%	93.1%	85.1%	0.246
Hospital	6.3%	4.1%	8.9%	
Community Health Center	3.4%	1.4%	5.7%	
Other	0.9%	1.4%	0.3%	
Employed by practice (% Yes)	65.3%	66.7%	63.8%	0.713
Average days worked per week (%)				
4	11.0%	14.3%	7.2%	0.568
5+	89.0%	85.7%	92.8%	
On-site robotic surgery capability (%)	55.5%	51.9%	59.4%	0.364
Number of urology patients seen in 1 week				
< 50	1.6%	1.4%	1.9%	0.861
51–100	49.6%	48.9%	50.4%	
> 100	48.7%	49.6%	47.7%	
Number of prostate cancer patients seen in 1 week				
0–20	58.3%	47.3%	70.8%	0.005
> 20	41.7%	52.7%	29.2%	
Proportion of all patients covered by (sd)				
Medicare	47.6 (11.6)	48.4 (11.8)	46.7 (11.5)	0.379
Commercial	41.3(13.3)	40.3 (13.0)	42.5 (13.6)	0.316
Medicaid	6.1(6.4)	6.1 (5.9)	6.2 (6.9)	0.966
Self-pay	3.7 (4.0)	3.7 (3.8)	3.7 (4.3)	0.989

Table 4 Treatment Mode by Study Arm and Round (%)

Overall	Correct Treatment		Incorrect Treatment		MDs asks patient preference (PP) (%)		No prostate cancer treatment (NT) (%)	
	Cont.	Interv.	Cont.	Interv.	Cont.	Interv.	Cont.	Interv.
Round 1	17.9%	21.6%	22.4%	29.1%	25.5%	22.0%	34.2%	27.3%
Round 2	18.5%	29.1%	25.3%	21.1%	40.4%	32.7%	15.7%	17.1%
D in D estimation	6.9%		−10.8%		−4.3%		8.2%	
p-value	0.001		0.028		0.210		0.021	

that case, 2) incorrectly choosing, 3) presenting both options equally (AS and AT) to the patients (shared decision-making), or 4) no treatment specified (no AS, AT, or shared decision-making recommended). At baseline, we found that 19.7% of the participants chose the preferred treatment, 26.0% the suboptimal treatment, 23.6% left the choice to the patient, and 30.5% did not recommend one treatment or the other, with a nonsignificant difference between control and intervention physicians ($p = 0.645$). We observed that those urologists who did not specify either AS or AT treatment were more likely to misdiagnose the patient ($p < 0.001$) or not order a biopsy ($p < 0.001$) (data not shown).

Treatment recommendations

In bivariate analyses across all nine cases, after the protein-based array was introduced in the intervention group, the optimal treatment was selected 29.1% by the intervention arm versus 21.6% for controls (Table 4). Intervention urologists saw a 6.9% greater increase in correct treatment than the controls ($p = 0.001$) over the two rounds of data collection. Similarly, suboptimal treatment choice declined by 10.8% in the intervention group, compared to the controls ($p = 0.028$). The percentage of urologists recommending that the patient choose, decreased in the intervention group by 4.3%.

In multinomial logistic regression, compared to controls, urologists in the intervention group were significantly more likely to recommend the preferred treatment (AS or AT) in Round 2, with an odds ratio of 2.84 (95% CI 1.39, 5.82) ($p = 0.004$). The multinomial logit accounts for the four different recommendations (preferred versus suboptimal versus patient choice versus no treatment recommendation), controlling for the individual case types and other variables of interest (Table 5).

The same model found that the introduction of a protein-based assay prompted urologists to involve their patients in treatment discussions more often than controls (OR 2.72; 95%CI 1.47, 5.05) ($p = 0.001$). Urologists treating more than 20 prostate cancer patients in a week were less likely to involve their patients in deciding the treatment for their cancer ($p = 0.001$).

Changes in use of active surveillance and treatment

We specifically evaluated urologists who made either an AS or AT recommendation in Round 1 (excluding those who would counsel their patients or those who did not provide a treatment plan), grouping the cases by whether a preferred AS (6 of the 9 cases developed) or AT (3 cases) strategy was preferable. Overall, for those six cases where AS is the preferable treatment, the percentage of providers recommending AT decreased by 28.9% more in the intervention group compared to controls (Fig. 2). This decrease is observed across all three case types.

Table 5 Multinomial logistic regression analysis by treatment category

	Correct Treatment			Physician counsels patient on all treatment options			No Prostate Cancer Treatment		
	Odds ratio	95% Confidence Interval	P-value	Odds ratio	95% Confidence Interval	P-value	Odds ratio	95% Confidence Interval	P-value
Intervention	0.94	(0.47,1.82)	0.860	0.57	(0.338,1.00)	0.050	0.99	(0.56,1.72)	0.960
Interaction Round with Study Arm	2.84	(1.39,5.82)	0.004	2.72	(1.47, 5.05)	0.001	0.98	(0.50,1.89)	0.946
Onsite robotics capacity	0.87	(0.51,1.49)	0.608	0.92	(0.59,1.44)	0.716	0.78	(0.49,1.26)	0.318
More than 20 prostate cancer patients per week	0.64	(0.35,1.15)	0.138	0.43	(0.26,0.70)	0.001	0.56	(0.33,0.95)	0.031
More than 100 urology patients per week	1.14	(0.64,2.03)	0.652	1.10	(0.69,1.78)	0.682	1.36	(0.81,2.26)	0.243
Greater than 50% public payors	0.99	(0.97,1.01)	0.400	1.00	(0.98,1.02)	0.889	1.00	(0.98,1.02)	0.768
Age over 40	1.02	(0.99,1.05)	0.217	1.01	(0.98,1.04)	0.435	1.05	(1.02,1.08)	0.000
Physician-owned practice	1.21	(0.49,2.95)	0.678	0.82	(0.41,1.64)	0.572	1.20	(0.55,2.64)	0.648
Constant	0.56	(0.05,6.03)	0.636	4.27	(0.63,28.78)	0.136	0.38	(0.05,2.92)	0.354

Incorrect treatment is the baseline treatment mode. Model also controls for CPV case type

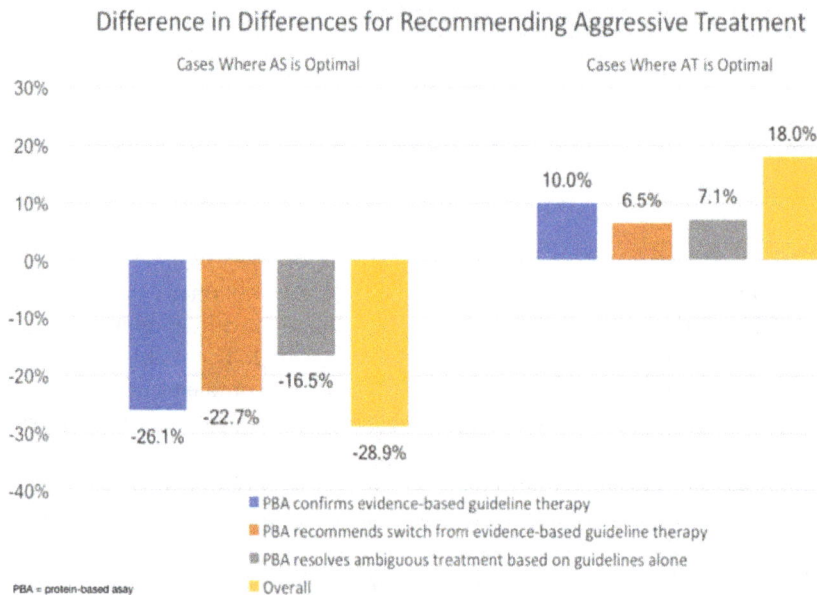

Fig. 2 Change in AT Recommendations across Rounds, by AS and AT Cases

For the 3 cases where AT was preferred, urologists in the intervention group increased the recommendation for AT by 18% in Round 2 compared to controls.

Discussion

As understanding of prostate cancer disease progression increases, the evidence indicates over-treatment with many men undergoing unnecessary prostatectomies [4]. The addition of a diagnostic tool to assess disease aggressiveness empowers clinicians to make more informed decisions on the recommended course of treatment.

This study confirms that care of prostate cancer patients, similar to many other disease states, is highly variable [18, 19]. Despite the variability in care, the results show that a protein-based assay had a positive impact on physician practice, improving treatment domain scores, and more specifically, moving patients from suboptimal to preferred recommendations, thereby providing the right treatment recommendation for the right patient.

Physicians provided with protein-based assay results changed their practice from "no recommendation" and "suboptimal recommendation" categories to either the preferable treatment pathways or engaging the patient in a conversation about their options. Importantly, this movement from the suboptimal to preferred recommendation categories by the intervention physicians maintained significance in the difference-in-differences model.

Limitations exist in this study. Since physicians responded to open-ended questions, we could not explore the counseling process for those who would present both AS and AT options to their patients. Thus,

we could not determine their ultimate course of action. Likewise, a proportion of urologists did not identify the case as one of prostate cancer, and as a result, they recommended neither active treatment nor surveillance. We cannot know from these cases their treatment plan if they were presented with a prostate cancer patient.

Conclusions

A protein-based assay provided physicians with additional prognostic information that resulted in a change to more appropriate recommendations for management, particularly in those cases where biopsy findings did not indicate a clear and precise treatment pathway. The additional information encouraged physicians to change their treatment plans. Thus, this protein-based assay shows demonstrable clinical utility, confirmed through a rigorous randomized controlled study design and regression analyses testing for effects.

Abbreviations
AS: Active Surveillance; AT: Active Treatment; CPV: Clinical Performance and Value

Acknowledgements
None.

Funding
QURE Healthcare received an unrestricted research grant from Metamark Genetics to support the costs of this study.

Authors' contributions
JWP contributed to project design and development, data collection/management, data analysis, and manuscript writing/editing. LMD contributed

to project development, data management, data analysis, and manuscript writing. DTL contributed to project design and development, data collection, and manuscript editing. JF contributed to data analysis and manuscript writing. MCA contributed to project development, data collection/management, and manuscript writing. OO contributed to project design, data management, and manuscript writing. JPR contributed to project design and development, data collection, and manuscript writing/editing. TB contributed to project development, data management, data analysis, and manuscript editing. All authors have read, edited, and given approval of the final version of the manuscript.

Competing interests
Dr. Richie is Chief Medical Officer at Metamark Genetics, the company which developed the protein-based assay used in this study. Dr. Peabody developed the CPVs and is president of CPV Technologies, LLC, which owns the quality measurement tool used in this study. For the remaining authors, no competing interests were declared.

Author details
[1]QURE Healthcare, 450 Pacific Ave, Suite 200, San Francisco, CA, USA.
[2]University of California, San Francisco, 500 Beale Street, San Francisco, CA, USA. [3]Metamark Genetics, 245 First Street, 10th Floor, Cambridge, MA, USA.

References
1. Ferlay J, Soerjomataram I, Ervik M, et al. GLOBOCAN 2012 v 1.1. Cancer Incidence and Mortality Worldwide: IARC CancerBase No.11 Lyon, France. International Agency for Research on Cancer; 2014.
2. Center MM, Jemal A, Lortet-Tieulen J, et al. International variation in prostate cancer incidence and mortality rates. Eur Urol. 2012;61:1079–92.
3. Lu-Yao GL, Albertsen PC, Moore DF, et al. Outcomes of localized prostate cancer following conservative management. JAMA. 2009;302:1202–9.
4. Nguyen PL, Gu X, Lipsitz SR, et al. Cost implications of the rapid adoption of newer technologies for treating prostate cancer. J Clin Onc. 2011;29:1517–24.
5. Cooperberg MR, Carroll PR. Trends in management for patients with localized prostate cancer, 1990-2013. JAMA. 2015;314:80–2.
6. Mohler JL, Kantoff PW, Armstrong AJ, et al. Prostate cancer, version 2.2014. J Natl Compr Cancer Netw. 2014;12:686–718.
7. Heidenreich A, Bastian PJ, Bellmunt J, et al. EAU guidelines on prostate cancer. Part 1:screening, diagnosis, and local treatment with curative intent - update 2013. Eur Urol. 2014;65:124–37.
8. Hayes JH, Ollendorf DA, Pearson SD, et al. Active surveillance compared with initial treatment for men with low-risk prostate cancer: a decision analysis. JAMA. 2010;304:2373–80.
9. Overholser S, Nielsen M, Torkko K, et al. Active surveillance is an appropriate management strategy for a proportion of men diagnosed with prostate cancer by prostate specific antigen testing. J Urol. 2015;194:680–4.
10. Chamie K, Williams SB, Hu JC. Population-based assessment of determining treatments for prostate cancer. JAMA Onc. 2015;1:60–7.
11. Aizer AA, Paly JJ, Zietman AL, et al. Multidisciplinary care and pursuit of active surveillance in low-risk prostate cancer. J Clin Onc. 2012;30:3071–6.
12. Loeb S, Carter HB, Berndt SI, et al. Is repeat prostate biopsy associated with a greater risk of hospitalization? Data from SEER-Medicare. J Urol. 2013;189:867.
13. Xu J, Dailey RK, Eggly S, et al. Men's perspectives on selecting their prostate cancer treatment. J Nat Med Assoc. 2011;103:468–78.
14. Tosoian JJ, Carter HB, Lepor A, Loeb S. Active surveillance for prostate cancer: current evidence and contemporary state of practice. Nat Rev Urol. 2016;13:205–15.
15. Filson CP, Schroeck FR, Ye Z, et al. Variation in use of active surveillance among men undergoing expectant treatment for early stage prostate cancer. J Urol. 2004;192:75–81.
16. Blume-Jensen P, Berman DM, Rimm DL, et al. Development and clinical validation of an in situ biopsy-based multimarker assay for risk stratification in prostate cancer. Clin Canc Res. 2015;21:2591–600.
17. Peabody JW, Luck J, Glassman P, et al. Comparison of vignettes, standardized patients, and chart abstraction: a prospective validation study of 3 methods for measuring quality. JAMA. 2000;283:1715–22.
18. Peabody JW, Luck J, Glassman P, et al. Measuring the quality of physician practice by using clinical vignettes: a prospective validation study. Ann Int Med. 2004;141:771–80.
19 Peabody JW, Strand V, Shimkhada R, et al. Impact of rheumatoid arthritis disease activity test on clinical practice. PLoS One. 2013;8:e63215.

4

Simultaneous antegrade and retrograde endoscopic treatment of non-malignant ureterointestinal anastomotic strictures following urinary diversion

Weiguo Hu, Boxing Su, Bo Xiao, Xin Zhang, Song Chen, Yuzhe Tang, Yubao Liu, Meng Fu and Jianxing Li[*]

Abstract

Background: The ureterointestinal anastomosis stricture (UAS) is a common complication of urinary diversion after radical cystectomy. For decades, open anastomotic revision remained the gold standard for the treatment of UAS. However, with the advancement in endoscopic technology, mini-invasive therapeutic approaches have been used in its management. Here, we report our experience with and long-term results of combined simultaneous antegrade and retrograde endoscopy (SARE) in the treatment of non-malignant UASs after urinary diversion in a consecutive series of patients.

Methods: From March 2012 to January 2015, there were 32 consecutive patients with 32 non-malignant UASs following radical cystectomy and urinary diversion. Twenty-nine patients were treated with SARE technique and comprised the study group. Using simultaneous antegrade flexible ureteroscope combined with retrograde semi-rigid ureteroscope or nephroscope, partial or complete strictures were managed with laser incision and balloon dilation under direct visualization. A 7/12 Fr graded endopyelotomy stent was left for 3–6 months after the procedure. Success was defined as symptomatic improvement and radiographic resolution of obstruction.

Results: With a median followup of 22 months (6–36), the overall success rate for SARE was 69.0%. Twenty patients with partial stricture had a success rate of 85%, and 9 patients with complete stricture had a success rate of 33.3%. Renal function, hydronephrosis grade, stricture type, and stricture length were significant influences on the outcome ($P < 0.05$). No complication was observed.

Conclusions: The SARE is a safe and effective treatment for UAS, and may be the only endoscopic treatment approach for complete UAS. While success rate for complete strictures is low compared to open revision, it should be considered as an initial approach given its low overall morbidity. For partial strictures, prudent patient selection results in higher success rates that are nearly comparable to open revision.

Keywords: Ureterointestinal anastomotic stricture, Antegrade, Retrograde, Endourology, Urinary diversion

* Correspondence: ljx1@sina.com
Department of Urology, Beijing Tsinghua Changgung Hospital, Tsinghua University, No. 168 Litang Road, Changping District, Beijing 102218, China

Background

Despite the advances and modifications in urinary diversion after radical cystectomy, the ureterointestinal anastomosis stricture (UAS) is still a common complication of this procedure. The reported incidence of UAS following urinary diversion ranges from 3 to 10% [1, 2], depending on clinical factors such as patient series, intestinal segment and anastomosis type [3]. Standard management of UAS involves open surgical revision of the anastomosis with reimplantation of the viable ureter into the urinary diversion. Despite a high success rate of greater than 80%, open anastomotic revision is often a technically challenging procedure, leading to considerable morbidity and prolonged hospitalization [4].

In the recent decades, treatment for UAS has changed drastically as a result of advances in endoscopic techniques and instrumentation [5]. Various endoscopic methods have been employed to treat UAS, such as balloon dilation [2], or endoureterotomy using cold-knife [6], electrocautery [7] or laser [8]. However, in most previously published studies, endourologic treatment of ureterointestinal strictures have employed either an antegrade or retrograde access exclusively. It is always challenging to identify the ureterointestinal anastomosis in the retrograde approach. The antegrade approach has been limited to treating only partial UAS.

In the current series, we describe a surgical endoscopic technique performed by adopting a simultaneous percutaneous antegrade flexible ureteroscope combined with retrograde semi-rigid ureteroscope or nephroscope. We retrospectively reviewed 29 partial and complete nonmalignant UASs treated with this technique to evaluate its efficacy and safety during the long-term followup.

Methods

From March 2012 to January 2015, there were 32 consecutive patients (19 males and 13 females) with 32 non-malignant UASs following radical cystectomy and urinary diversion. Of these patients 3 with complete stricture longer than 2 cm were excluded from analysis. Open surgery had to be performed on these patients. The remaining 29 people were treated with combined simultaneous antegrade and retrograde endoscopy (SARE) technique and comprised the study group. The mean age was 55.7 years (range 39–73 years). The indications for these urinary diversions were transitional cell carcinoma of the bladder. Patients with extrinsic ureteral compression, or tumor at the anastomotic site were not included.

The main symptoms were flank pain (n = 8) and urinary infection (n = 4). Fourteen patients were asymptomatic at presentation. Three patients presented with biochemical and/or clinical evidence of renal failure. Of all the patients, 20 had partial strictures and the remaining 9 had complete strictures. Twenty-six had a Bricker urinary diversion and 3 had a Studer orthotopic neobladder. Four patients received initial drainage with a nephrostomy tube, and antibiotics were used in 9 patients prior to definitive treatment, other patients were treated initially with this combined approach after the UAS were diagnosised. The mean interval between the urinary diversion and the initial diagnosis of UAS formation was 22 months (ranged 3–51). In all patients, UAS was diagnosed by computerized tomography urography (CTU) and/or antegrade pyelography. Complete stricture was diagnosised if the contrast can't pass the strictured anastomosis. Abdominal CT was performed preoperatively in all patients to exclude tumor metastasis or local recurrence. Neobladder cystoscopy was performed to rule out urethral or neobladder neck stricture or tumor recurrence. When poor renal function was suspected on radiographic imaging, renal scan was performed. Stricture site, length and degree of patency were obtained from the preoperative adjunct imaging studies or the operative notes. Biopsy of the strictured anastomosis area was obtained when necessary. Preoperative hydronephrosis was found in all patients by sonographical and radiological studies. Hydronephrosis was graded asI- mild pelvic dilatation only, grade II- moderate caliceal dilatation, grade III- severe caliceal dilatation and grade IV- caliceal dilatation with renal parenchymal atrophy.

Under general anesthesia, the patients with Bricker bladders were placed in a modified oblique supine position with raised (approximately 20–30°) nephrostomy side. Patients with orthotopic neobladders were placed in the modified lithotomy position with access to the flank region for nephrostomy. Optimal percutaneous access was performed under ultrasonographic guidance using the two-step method as we mentioned previously [9].

After percutaneous access was achieved, concurrent renal or ureteral calculi were removed firstly. Then, an 8.5–9 Fr flexible ureteroscope was passed antegrade over a guidewire to the strictured area. Under direct vision, the guidewire was passed through the stricture down to the pouch. If the anastomosis was obstructed completely, the modified cut-to-the-light technique was employed. Briefly, we turned off the light of the flexible ureteroscope, and performed the incision towards another illuminated endoscope placed retrograde to the distal end of the stricture using a 200 μm holmium: YAG laser fiber. The incision was usually made in the depression of the mucosa located in proximal end of the stricture. When the stiff end of the 0.032-in. hydrophilic guidewire (Bard Medical Division) passed through the stenotic segments, it was extracted ureteroscopically or nephroscopically from the intestinal urinary pouch with a grasp to get through-and-through access. The X Force®

U30 balloon dilator (Bard Medical Division) was then placed in UAS segment in retrograde way and inflated under direct visual guidance. We typically dilated the balloon to 21 Fr (25 atm) and left it inflated for 5 min. Endoureterotomy was performed following balloon dilation using the 200 μm, end firing, pulsed, 80 W holmium: YAG laser (energy 0.6–2.0 J and rate 10–15 Hz) under direct vision.

Pulsations at the stricture area were evaluated prior to the endoureterotomy. The incision was made anteriorly over the iliac vessels, anteromedially over the internal iliac vessels to avoid vascular injury. A full-thickness incision was made into the periureteral adipose tissue, extending about 5 mm above and below the strictured segment. In severe strictures, the stenotic segments can be pre-dilated with fascial dilators before retrograde balloon dilation.

A 7/12 Fr graded endopyelotomy stent (Urovision, Germany) was left in situ for 3–6 months postoperatively. Routine followup consisted of history, physical examination and renal ultrasound every 3 months in year 1 and biannually thereafter. CT and/or diuretic renography were performed if necessary. Success was defined as radiographic resolution of obstruction and symptomatic improvement without the need for ureteral stents or nephrostomy tubes.

Time to the last followup in successfully treated patients was considered a censor point and time to failure was considered as end points for assessment using Kaplan-Meier analysis. Associations between different clinicopathological factors and success were analyzed to predict the outcome, using Student t or Wilcoxon rank sum test t for continuous data and the standard chi-square or Fisher's exact test for categorical data with $p < 0.05$ considered statistically significant.

Results

The median followup time was 22 months (range 6–36), and the overall success rate was 69.0% (20 of 29 UASs). No serious perioperative complications or urinary tract infections were noted. With a median followup of 27 months (range 10–36) for patients with partial strictures, the success rate was 85% (17 out of 20). For the patients with complete strictures, after a median followup of 12 months (range 6–28), the success rate was 33.3% (3 out of 9). Figure 1 shows a Kaplan-Meier curve of success rate of SARE treatment for the complete and partial UAS respectively. The average operation time was 26 min (ranged 15–60), with minimal blood loss. The average hospital stay was 3.7 days (ranged 3–5). In the 9 failed patients, restenosis occurred 5.6 (range 1–9) months after the removal of the ureteral stent. Failure was managed by open anastomotic revision in 4, permanent indwelling stent drainage in 2 and nephrostomy

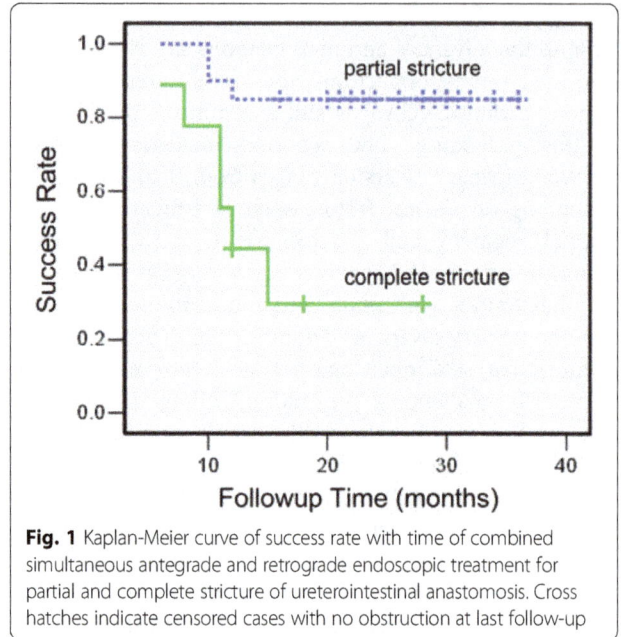

Fig. 1 Kaplan-Meier curve of success rate with time of combined simultaneous antegrade and retrograde endoscopic treatment for partial and complete stricture of ureterointestinal anastomosis. Cross hatches indicate censored cases with no obstruction at last follow-up

in 3. Table 1 lists the categorical data for patient and stricture characteristics, and the success rates are presented accordingly. The UAS located in 16 ureterorenal units (URU) on the left side and 13 on the right. Nine of the patients had stricture associated with ureteral calculi. While kidney function, hydronephrosis grade, and stricture type significantly influence the results of the treatment ($p < 0.05=$, side of the stricture, history of endoscopic therapy, co-existence of ureteral calculi or urinary diversion type seem to be independent of the outcome of endourological treatment ($p > 0.05$). We didn't find a statistically significant association between prior radiation and outcome, this maybe due to limited number of patients (only 2 with radiation history) included in our analysis. Table 2 shows the continuous data for patient and stricture characteristics. Our analysis suggested that the age of the patients, postoperative stent duration (3–6 months) or the period to the diagnosis of UAS after original conduit creation had no influence on the outcome. However, our data demonstrated that the stricture length was significantly associated with the prognosis of outcome.

Discussion

The non-malignant UAS can be caused by anastomotic technique associated ischemia, avascular necrosis or perianastomotic fibrosis due to chronic inflammation, edema or urine leakage [10]. For many decades, open surgical revision of the anastomosis remained the gold standard for the management of ureterointesitinal stricture with an 80–91% reported success rate [4, 11]. However, the open surgical procedures can be difficult to perform, and associated with considerable morbidity,

Table 1 Statistical analysis of categorical data for patient and stricture characteristics (n=29)

Characteristics	No. Successes /No. Patients (%)	P^a value
Gender:		0.454
Male	10/16 (62.5)	
Female	10/13 (61.5)	
Side:		1.000
Left	11/16 (68.8)	
Right	9/13 (69.2)	
Irradiation:		0.089
Yes	0/2 (0)	
No	20/27 (74.1)	
% Preop ipsilateral renal function:		0.002
≥25	17/19 (89.5)	
<25	3/10 (9.1)	
Hydronephrosis grade:		0.003
I—II	15/16 (93.8)	
III—IV	5/13 (38.5)	
Diversion type:		1.000
Studer orthotopic neobladder	2/3 (66.7)	
Bricker	18/26 (69.2)	
Stricture type:		0.010
Complete	3/9 (33.3)	
Partial	17/20 (85.0)	
Past therapy:		0.287
Endoscopic	2/5 (40)	
None	18/24(75.0)	
Co-existence of ureteric calculi:		0.088
Yes	4/9 (44.4)	
No	16/20 (80.0)	

[a]Fisher's exact test

due to dense adhesions or fibrosis caused by previous surgery or radiotherapy. The advancement in urologic endoscopic technology has facilitated minimally invasive therapeutic approaches for the treatment of ureterointe-sitinal stricture, leading to less complications and shorter convalescence time. Although there were plenty of reports describing different endourological techniques

for treatment of UAS, most of them employed either an antegrade or retrograde approach alone and currently there is no report suggests that any modality is superior to another (Table 3).

The concept of combined simultaneous antegrade and retrograde endoscopic approach offers several advantages over either modality used alone. Firstly, in the SARE approach, antegrade placement of the flexible ureteroscope permits cooperative treatment of the stenotic lesion with retrograde modality over through-and-through guidewire, which provided the control required to ensure full-thickness and full-length stricture incision under direct visualization. The 85% success rate nearly comparable to open revision in patients with partial strictures in our analysis further proved that the SARE is an effective treatment approach. Secondly, the SARE permits the using of "cut-to-the-light" technique to get the through-and-through access, which may be the only way to endoscopically treat the complete obstruction. In our patient series, the success rate for complete obstruction is 33%. Long-term and large-scale studies are needed to further explore this method. However, given its low morbidity compared with open revision, the SARE treatment should be considered initially in patients with complete strictures.

Cut-to-the-light technique had been described to establish through and through access in complete obliteration of ureteral strictures [12]. However, few studies have been done to evaluate the long term results of this procedure. Goda et al. [13] described a case of complete ureteral stricture managed by endoscopic recanalization using the cut-to-the-light technique through potassium titanyl phosphate (KTP) laser ureterotomy. No signs of restenosis were observed 24 months after endoscopic treatment. In our series, this technique was successfully performed in 9 patients with complete strictures shorter than 2 cm, and 3 complete UASs remain patent after a median followup of 12 months. To our knowledge this is the first series of patients with complete UAS treated by this modified technique with long term followup.

Our analysis shows that factors associated with success rate are renal function, hydronephrosis grade, stricture type, and stricture length. Decreased ipsilateral renal function has been reported in several studies as a risk

Table 2 Statistical analysis of continuous data for patient and stricture characteristics (n=29)

Variable	Total	Success	Failure	P Value
Age (yr)	55.72 (8.61)	56.45 (8.48)	54.11 (9.19)	0.508[a]
Interval to stricture formation (mo)	21.52 (11.06)	21.10 (9.84)	22.44 (14.04)	0.768[a]
Stricture length (cm)	1.29(0.34)	1.12 (0.25)	1.67 (0.14)	0.0001[a]
Stent duration (mo)	4.66 (1.47)	4.50 (1.54)	5.00 (2.32)	0.501[b]

Data presented as the mean, with the standard deviation in parentheses
[a]Student's t test
[b]Wilcoxon rank sum test

Table 3 Endoscopic management of non-malignant ureterointestinal anastomotic strictures

Technique	Study	Procedures	Approach[a]	Mean follow-up (mo)	Success rate (%)
Balloon dilation	Nassar et al. [3]	16	A	43	50
	Yagi et al. [19]	13	A	47.1	77
	Ravery et al. [17]	14	A	16	61
	DiMarco et al. [2]	52	A/R	24	15
	Kwak et al. [20]	18	A	6	28
Laser incision	Mihoua et al. [18]	15	A	11.5	33
	Laven et al. [4]	16	A	35	50
	Watterson et al. [8]	24	A	22.5	70.8
Cold-knife incision	Nassar et al. [3]	21	A	43	52.3
	Poulakis et al. [6]	43	Combined	38.8	60.5
	Poulakis et al. [7]	22	A	23.5	74
Electrocautery incision	Lovaco et al. [5]	25	Combined	51	80
	Meretyk et al. [21]	14	R	28.6	57
Acucise cutting balloon device	Cornud et al. [22]	37	A	25	67.5
	Lin et al. [23]	10	A	13	32
	Babayan et al. [24]	9	A	3	33
Multiple modalities	Wolf et al. [16]	30	A	13	32

[a]A antegrade, R retrograde, A/R antegrade or retrograde

factor for failure of endoscopic treatments of the ureteral stricture disease [14, 15]. Wolf et al. found that no patient with renal function less than 25% had successful endoureterotomy in a series of 47 ureteral strictures [16]. Poulakis et al. reported that all the patients who failed in treatment with cold knife incision had less than 25% ipsilateral renal function in a series of 22 UASs [7]. In our series, 11 patients had less than 25% renal function and treatment failed in 10. Few groups have examined the impact of hydronephrosis on the success rate of endoscopic treatment of non-malignant UAS. Our study shows that significant hydronephrosis predicts a higher failure rate. 94.4% of UAS were successfully treated in patients with renal hydronephrosis leveled gradeI—II verse 21.4% in patients leveled grade III—IV.Similar results were also reported by Poulakis and his colleagues in a series of 40 patients with 43 UASs underwent cold-knife endoureterotomy [6].

Several studies found ureteral stricture length to have statistically significant influence on the result of endourological intervention with decreasing ureteroscopic success rate as the stricture length increases [15]. One series of 18 patients with 22 non-malignant UASs who underwent antegrade cold-knife endoureterotomy found that 72.7% of the patients with strictures>1.5 cm failed the endoscopic management, while all patients with stricture lengths ≤1.5 cm succeed [7]. In our analysis, the length of the stenotic portion of the ureterointestinal anastomosis ranged from 0.5 to 1.8 cm, and our results showed shorter stricture length strongly correlated with higher success rates (Table 2).

Regarding postoperative stenting, a stent duration of 6–8 weeks is widely accepted in many published studies [7], however, there is no large scale randomized clinical trial published to date demonstrating the optimum stent duration after endoureterotomy. Ravery et al. postulated that the prolonged ureteral stenting might have promoted ureteric healing and attributed the high success rate of 61% to the increased duration of stenting (4–30 months) [17]. Wolf et al. proved statistically that the stent duration (≤4 Vs.>4 weeks) did not influence the short- and long-term success rate of endoureterotomy in cases of both benign ureteral strictures and ureteroenteric ones [16]. In our analysis, we found that prolonged stent duration (range 3–6 months) had no beneficial effects on the clinical outcome.

Our study has several limitations. First, it is limited by its retrospective and single-institution study design. Future prospective, large-scale and long-term studies are needed in multiply centers. Secondly, the stent duration in our series is 3–6 months postoperatively based on our experiences, however, our data showed that prolonged stent duration was not significantly associated with high success rate, further study should be proposed to find the optimum stent duration and its correlation with clinical outcome. Thirdly, our study can't explain the influence of failed balloon dilation and laser incision, especially for complete UAS obstruction, on the success rate of subsequent open surgical revision. However, the previously published data have showed that there was no statistically significant difference in open surgical revision outcomes for patients with and without prior endoureterotomy [4, 18]. Fourthly, due to the small cohort size and limited number of events, we were unable to perform multivariate analyses to identify independent predictors of success. Further study is needed to explore this.

Conclusions

Conventional endourologic interventions for UAS, such as antegrade balloon dilation, have lower success rates and have been limited to treating only partial strictures. Our study is the first series of patients with partial and complete UASs treated with endoscopic method. Although the success rates of SARE for complete strictures are low compared to open revision, it should be considered initially as it may be the only endoscopic treatment approach for complete strictures. For incomplete strictures, selection of patients with the most favorable prognostic factors, such as better renal fuction, lower hydronephrosis grade and shorter stricture length, will lead to excellent success rates nearly comparable to open revision. Further perspective studies with more patients and longer followups are needed in order to validate our conclusion regarding the practice of SARE in patients with non-malignant UASs after urinary diversion.

Abbreviations
CTU: Computerized tomography urography; SARE: Simultaneous antegrade and retrograde endoscopy; UAS: Ureterointestinal anastomotic stricture; URU: Ureterorenal units

Acknowledgements
None.

Funding
The capital health research and development of special Award Number: 2016-2-2242.

Authors' contributions
LJX and HWG conceived and designed this study. LJX, HWG, XB, ZX and CS carried out surgeries on patients. SBX, LYB, TYZ and FM contributed to the follow-up questionnaire. LJX, SBX, HWG and LYB participated in data acquisition and interpretation. SBX and HWG performed the statistics analyses and drafted the manuscript. LJX, LYB, TYZ and FM critically reviewed the manuscript. All the authors read and approved the final manuscript.

Competing interests
The authors declare that they have no competing interests.

References
1. Gburek BM, Lieber MM, Blute ML. Comparison of studer ileal neobladder and ileal conduit urinary diversion with respect to perioperative outcome and late complications. J Urol. 1998;160:721–3.
2. DiMarco DS, LeRoy AJ, Thieling S, Bergstralh EJ, Segura JW. Long-term results of treatment for ureteroenteric strictures. Urology. 2001;58:909–13.
3. Nassar OA, Alsafa ME. Experience with ureteroenteric strictures after radical cystectomy and diversion: open surgical revision. Urology. 2011; 78:459–65.
4. Laven BA, O'Connor RC, Gerber GS, Steinberg GD. Long-term results of endoureterotomy and open surgical revision for the management of ureteroenteric strictures after urinary diversion. J Urol. 2003;170: 1226–30.
5. Lovaco F, Serrano A, Fernandez I, Perez P, Gonzalez-Peramato P. Endoureterotomy by intraluminal invagination for nonmalignant ureterointestinal anastomotic strictures: description of a new surgical technique and long-term followup. J Urol. 2005;174:1851–6.
6. Poulakis V, Witzsch U, De Vries R, Becht E. Cold-knife endoureterotomy for nonmalignant ureterointestinal anastomotic strictures. Urology. 2003;61:512–7.
7. Poulakis V, Witzsch U, de Vries R, Becht E. Antegrade percutaneous endoluminal treatment of non-malignant ureterointestinal anastomotic strictures following urinary diversion. Eur Urol. 2001;39:308–15.
8. Watterson JD, Sofer M, Wollin TA, Nott L, Denstedt JD. Holmium: YAG laser endoureterotomy for ureterointestinal strictures. J Urol. 2002;167: 1692–5.
9. Li J, Xiao B, Hu W, et al. Complication and safety of ultrasound guided percutaneous nephrolithotomy in 8, 025 cases in China. Chin Med J. 2014; 127:4184–9.
10. Banner MP, Pollack HM, Ring EJ, Wein AJ. Catheter dilatation of benign ureteral strictures. Radiology. 1983;147:427–33.
11. Vandenbroucke F, Van Poppel H, Vandeursen H, Oyen R, Baert L. Surgical versus endoscopic treatment of non-malignant uretero-ileal anastomotic strictures. Br J Urol. 1993;71:408–12.
12. Thomas MA, Ong AM, Pinto PA, Rha KH, Jarrett TW. Management of obliterated urinary segments using a laser fiber for access. J Urol. 2003;169: 2284–6.
13. Goda K, Kawabata G, Yasufuku T, et al. Cut-to-the-light technique and potassium titanyl phosphate laser ureterotomy for complete ureteral obstruction. Int J Urol. 2004;11:427–8.
14. Gnessin E, Yossepowitch O, Holland R, Livne PM, Lifshitz DA. Holmium laser endoureterotomy for benign ureteral stricture: a single center experience. J Urol. 2009;182:2775–9.
15. Lane BR, Desai MM, Hegarty NJ, Streem SB. Long-term efficacy of holmium laser endoureterotomy for benign ureteral strictures. Urology. 2006;67:894–7.
16. Wolf JJ, Elashry OM, Clayman RV. Long-term results of endoureterotomy for benign ureteral and ureteroenteric strictures. J Urol. 1997;158:759–64.
17. Ravery V, de la Taille A, Hoffmann P, et al. Balloon catheter dilatation in the treatment of ureteral and ureteroenteric stricture. J Endourol. 1998;12:335–40.
18. Milhoua PM, Miller NL, Cookson MS, Chang SS, Smith JA, Herrell SD. Primary endoscopic management versus open revision of ureteroenteric anastomotic strictures after urinary diversion–single institution contemporary series. J Endourol. 2009;23:551–5.
19. Yagi S, Goto T, Kawamoto K, Hayami H, Matsushita S, Nakagawa M. Long-term results of percutaneous balloon dilation for ureterointestinal anastomotic strictures. Int J Urol. 2002;9:241–6.
20. Kwak S, Leef JA, Rosenblum JD. Percutaneous balloon catheter dilatation of benign ureteral strictures: effect of multiple dilatation procedures on long-term patency. AJR Am J Roentgenol. 1995;165:97–100.
21. Meretyk S, Clayman RV, Kavoussi LR, Kramolowsky EV, Picus DD. Endourological treatment of ureteroenteric anastomotic strictures: long-term followup. J Urol. 1991;145:723–7.
22. Cornud F, Chretien Y, Helenon O, et al. Percutaneous incision of stenotic uroenteric anastomaoses with a cutting balloon catheter: long-term results. Radiology. 2000;214:358–62.
23. Lin DW, Bush WH, Mayo ME. Endourological treatment of ureteroenteric strictures: efficacy of acucise endoureterotomy. J Urol. 1999;162:696–8.
24. Babayan RK. Use of the Acucise balloon catheter. In: Smith AD, editor. Controversies in Endourology. Philadelphia: WB Saunders; 1995. p. 309.

5

Clinical utility of computed tomography Hounsfield characterization for percutaneous nephrolithotomy: a cross-sectional study

Andrea Gallioli[1]*[iD], Elisa De Lorenzis[1], Luca Boeri[1], Maurizio Delor[2], Stefano Paolo Zanetti[1], Fabrizio Longo[1], Alberto Trinchieri[3] and Emanuele Montanari[1]

Abstract

Background: Computed Tomography (CT) is considered the gold-standard for the pre-operative evaluation of urolithiasis. However, no Hounsfield (HU) variable capable of differentiating stone types has been clearly identified. The aim of this study is to assess the predictive value of HU parameters on CT for determining stone composition and outcomes in percutaneous nephrolithotomy (PCNL).

Methods: Seventy seven consecutive cases of PCNL between 2011 and 2016 were divided into 4 groups: 40 (52%) calcium, 26 (34%) uric acid, 5 (6%) struvite and 6 (8%) cystine stones. All images were reviewed by a single urologist using abdomen/bone windows to evaluate: stone volume, core (HUC), periphery HU and their absolute difference. HU density (HUD) was defined as the ratio between mean HU and the stone's largest diameter. ROC curves assessed the predictive power of HU for determining stone composition/stone-free rate (SFR).

Results: No differences were found based on the viewing window (abdomen vs bone). Struvite stones had values halfway between hyperdense (calcium) and low-density (cystine/uric acid) calculi for all parameters except HUD, which was the lowest. All HU variables for medium-high density stones were greater than low-density stones ($p < 0.001$). HUC differentiated the two groups (cut-off 825 HU; specificity 90.6%, sensitivity 88.9%). HUD distinguished calcium from struvite (mean $\pm$ SD 51 ± 16 and 28 ± 12 respectively; $p = 0.02$) with high sensitivity (82.5%) and specificity (80%) at a cut-off of 35 HU/mm. Multivariate analysis revealed HUD $\geq$ 38.5 HU/mm to be an independent predictor of SFR (OR = 3.1, $p = 0.03$). No relationship was found between HU values and complication rate.

Conclusions: HU parameters help predict stone composition to select patients for oral chemolysis. HUD is an independent predictor of residual fragments after PCNL and may be fundamental to categorize it, driving the imaging choice at follow-up.

Keywords: Hounsfield, Kidney stone, Percutaneous nephrolithotomy, Computed tomography

* Correspondence: andrea.gallioli@gmail.com
[1]Fondazione IRCCS Ca' Granda Ospedale Maggiore Policlinico, Department of Urology, University of Milan, Via della Commenda 15, 20122 Milan, Italy
Full list of author information is available at the end of the article

Background

Computed Tomography (CT) is the gold standard for the pre-operative study of stones and influences the choice of surgical strategy [1]. Hounsfield Units (HU) indicate the hardness of renal calculi and identify high density stones to be excluded from shockwave lithotripsy (SWL) [2]. Several in vitro studies have demonstrated the utility of CT in predicting stone composition [3–6]. The use of different HU parameters, such as Hounsfield Density (HUD), has been proposed to distinguish stone groups in vivo [7–12]. In order to further improve the differentiation of stones, scans conducted with the bone window setting have been attempted [13] and, recently, the mean HU value has been suggested as a predictor for the stone-free rate (SFR) after percutaneous nephrolithotomy (PCNL) [14]. To the best of our knowledge, no study has evaluated the role of a wide range of HU parameters in vivo. The aim of this study is to evaluate the clinical significance and utility of the HU parameters determined during pre-operative CT study, using bone and soft tissue window (=abdomen), to be predictive factors of stone composition, SFR and complication rate in a cohort of patients submitted to PCNL.

Patients and methods

We retrospectively reviewed the institutional stone registry between January 2011 and April 2016. 284 patients submitted to PCNL were found. Inclusion criteria were: I) the availability of a pre-operative CT-scan, II) a maximum stone diameter > 4 mm, III) the availability at our Institution of the biochemical analysis of the stones, IV) a prominent stone component >50% in mixed stones. Patients with pre-operative urinary stents were excluded.

CT scans were performed with a 64-detector row Lightspeed VCT scanner (General Electric Healthcare, Milwaukee, WI) with tube voltage 120 kV, energy >100 mA, pitch 1:1, slice thickness comprised between 0.6 and 5 mm. CT scans were evaluated by the same Urologist (M.D.), blinded to the stone composition, using PACS Synapse Fujifilm version 4.0 software at 4× zoom. Both bone (X_B) and soft tissue (X_{ST}) windows were analyzed. The slice with the stone's largest diameter (D_1) on the axial plane was selected and the following variables were recorded: perpendicular diameter (D_2), HU value at the center of the stone (HUC) and the mean HU value (HUM) which was calculated by generating an extensive circular Region Of Interest (ROI). The HU value at the stone's periphery (HUP) was obtained from the mean of HU values at extremities of D_1 and D_2 (Fig. 1). HUD was defined as the ratio between HUM and D_1. The absolute HU difference between the stone center and periphery was calculated as HUC minus HUP (ΔHU). The stone's Area (A) and Volume (V) were estimated using Tiselius formulas [15]. D_3 was determined as the maximum diameter at coronal plane CT scans.

PCNL was performed by the same surgeon (E.M.) for all cases. The procedure was conducted in the supine position. An open-ended ureteral catheter was positioned before an ultrasound-guided renal puncture. A one-shot dilatation of the percutaneous access tract was conducted using an Amplatz 24 Charrier dilator [16]. Lithotripsy was performed with ballistic, ultrasound or holmium laser energy while fragments were removed with an endoscopic nipper or basket. An 8 Ch nephrostomy was positioned at the conclusion of each procedure.

The evaluated peri-operative parameters were surgical time (from the access puncture to nephrostomy), reduction of hemoglobin, fever, need for transfusion and hospital stay. Complications were classified using the Clavien-Dindo score modified by the Clinical Research Office of Endourological Society (CROES) and divided in three groups: no complications, slight complications (Clavien-Dindo 1/2), severe complications (Clavien-Dindo ≥3) [17].

SFR, defined as the absence of residual fragments, was assessed by US or CT after 3 months. Stone composition was determined by infrared spectrophotometry (Thermo Scientific Nicolet™ iS™ 10) and stones were categorized into 4 groups: 40 (52%) calcium, 26 (34%) uric acid, 6 (8%) cystine and 5 (6%) struvite. The patient group was composed of 52 (67%) men and 25 (33%) women with a mean age of 57 (range 14–92) years. No differences in terms of sex and age were found between stone composition groups, with the exception of patients with cystine stones who had a younger average age (32 years) (Additional file 1: Table S1).

Statistical analysis was performed utilizing GraphPad Prism v 5 (GraphPad Software Inc., California, USA) and SPSS v 13.0 (IBM Cor., Armonk, NY, USA). T-tests and one-way analysis of variance (ANOVA) tests were used for group comparisons. Chi-Square and logistic regressions were calculated for categorical parameters. Receiver Operating Characteristic (ROC) curves were generated to find HU value cut-offs (defined as Youden J Index) to predict stone composition and SFR. Statistically significant differences were assumed for p values less than 0.05.

Results

Analysis of the groups showed that stone dimensions appeared generally larger using the CT soft tissue window, but no significant differences in D_1, A and V were observed. On the contrary, HU values were higher using the CT bone window (Table 1).

Comparisons were made between the stone groups on the results obtained for 4 variables (HUM, ΔHU, HUC, HUD) using both the bone and soft tissue windows. Calcium stones were consistently hyperdense while uric acid and cystine stones had lower HU values. Struvite had intermediate values on all variables with the exception of HUD, which was the lowest among all stone groups (Fig. 2).

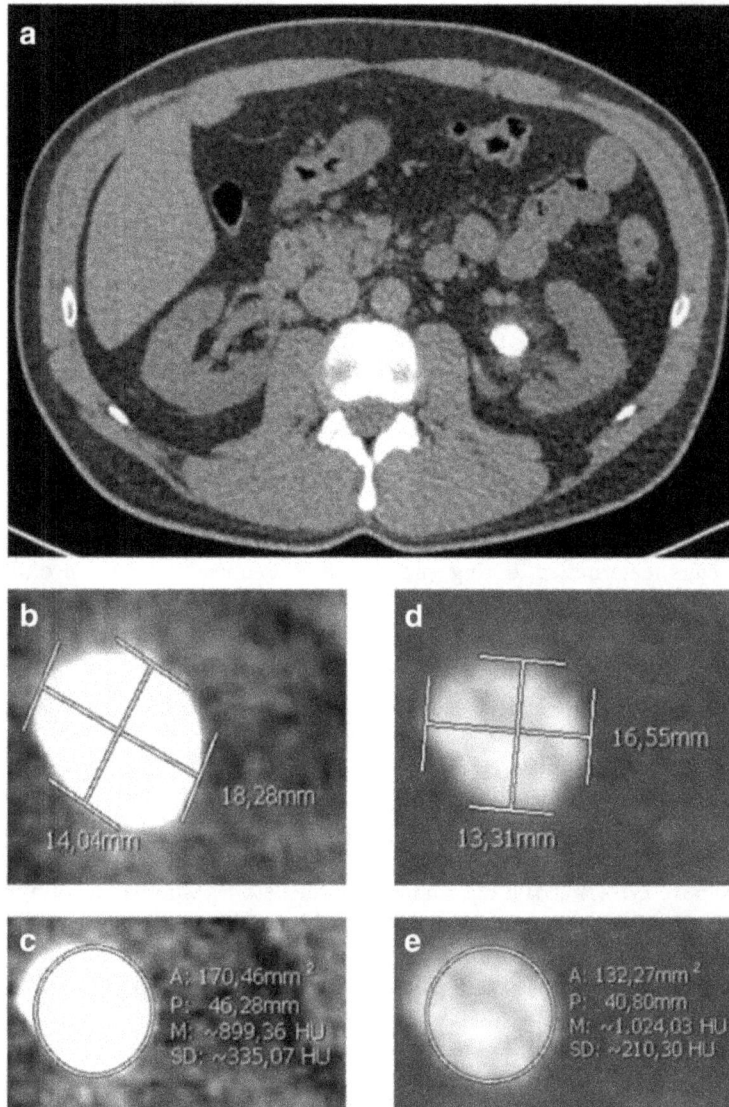

Fig. 1 Calculus of left renal pelvis (**a**). Maximum/perpendicular diameters and ROI of the stone on soft tissue (**b**, **c**) and bone (**d**, **e**) window scans. Legend: A = area; P = perimeter; M = mean Hounsfield; SD = standard deviation

Table 1 Stone characteristics on soft tissue/bone window CT (mean ± SD)

	Soft tissue (Bone) windows	p	Calcium	Uric acid	Cystine	Struvite
D_1 (mm)	19 ± 7 (17 ± 7)	0.34	18 ± 6 (16 ± 6)	19 ± 8 (18 ± 8)	18 ± 8 (17 ± 8)	24 ± 6 (23 ± 6)
Area (mm²)	188 ± 137 (164 ± 126)	0.26	174 ± 122 (148 ± 111)	190 ± 150 (168 ± 137)	204 ± 168 (185 ± 160)	275 ± 152 (250 ± 143)
Volume (mm³)	2914 ± 3481 (2438 ± 3084)	0.37	2495 ± 3072 (2024 ± 2669)	3097 ± 4034 (2612 ± 3563)	4178 ± 4228 (3714 ± 3964)	3792 ± 2964 (3318 ± 2637)
HUC	942 ± 378 (986 ± 389)	0.48	1190 ± 251 (1240 ± 259)	606 ± 276 (638 ± 271)	683 ± 75 (708 ± 66)	1010 ± 394 (1090 ± 439)
HUP	314 ± 55 (395 ± 93)	<0.001	*330 ± 59 (426 ± 85)*[a]	*287 ± 41 (358 ± 98)*[a]	300 ± 45 (358 ± 49)	340 ± 42 (390 ± 96)
HUM	687 ± 265 (761 ± 306)	0.11	835 ± 233 (941 ± 270)	500 ± 203 (531 ± 216)	542 ± 86 (608 ± 86)	650 ± 235 (700 ± 255)
ΔHU	628 ± 356 (590 ± 347)	0.5	860 ± 234 (814 ± 245)	319 ± 266 (280 ± 216)	383 ± 75 (350 ± 45)	670 ± 411 (700 ± 434)
HUD	41 ± 19 (50 ± 26)	*0.01*	*51 ± 16 (63 ± 22)*[a]	31 ± 18 (36 ± 22)	35 ± 14 (43 ± 21)	28 ± 12 (33 ± 16)

[a] Significant difference ($p \leq 0.01$) between HU values at soft tissue versus bone windows

Legend: D_1 = stone's largest diameter at axial plane; HUC = HU at the center; HUP = HU value at periphery; HUM = HU mean value; ΔHU = HUC-HUP; HUD = ratio between HUM and D_1

The mean values for calcium stones differed from those of the uric acid calculi on every parameter considered while cystine stones did not differentiate from struvite/uric acid calculi.

The values for HUC, HUM and ΔHU, but not HUD, differed between calcium and cystine stones. Struvite calculi had significantly higher values than uric acid stones for HUC and ΔHU, with ΔHU_B being the parameter that best differentiated them (mean ± SD 700 ± 434 vs 280 ± 216; $p = 0.004$).

Calcium and struvite stones differed significantly for HUD_{ST} (mean ± SD 51 ± 16 and 28 ± 12 respectively; $p = 0.02$). For a HUD_{ST} cut-off of 35 HU/mm, sensitivity was 82.5%, specificity 80%, negative predictive value (NPV) 36% and positive predictive value (PPV) 97%.

In order to apply these results in a clinical setting we grouped hypodense stones (uric acid, cystine) and compared them with hyperdense stones (calcium, struvite), finding that the hypodense had statistically lower HU values ($p < 0.001$). HUC_{ST} more accurately differentiated the two groups with a specificity of 90.6%, sensitivity 88.9%, PPV 93% and NPV 85.3% at a cut-off of 825 HU (Additional file 2: Figure S1).

Mean surgical time was 123 (40–240) minutes, medium hospital stay was 6 (1–15) days. Linear regression revealed that hospital stay was inversely correlated with HUD_{ST} ($p = 0.04$) and HUD_B ($p = 0.02$).

In 42 (55%) patients no complications were recorded, in 24 (32%) and 11 (13%) Clavien-Dindo grade 1–2 and grade ≥ 3 complications were observed, respectively. A hemoglobin drop necessitating blood transfusion was observed in 6 (7.8%) cases. HUD values in patients requiring transfusion, irrespective of the window used, were generally higher (mean HUD_{ST} 54.89 ± 10.58 vs. 40.13 ± 2.14, $p = 0.06$; mean HUD_B 69.78 ± 14.63 vs 48.6 ± 2.86, $p = 0.05$). The other evaluated peri-operative data were not related to HU values. SFR was 61% with no differences according to stone composition ($p = 0.37$). However, SFR was significantly higher in patients with stones <2 cm compared to those with stones deemed to be ≥2 cm using soft tissue (71% vs 40%; $p < 0.009$) and bone scans (70% vs 42%; $p < 0.01$). To evaluate whether an HU parameter was predictive of SFR we analyzed each variable, generating ROC curves. HUD_{ST} (cut-off 38.5 HU/mm) was the best SFR predictive factor (AUC 0.66, sensitivity 70%, specificity 63.8%, OR 4.12, $p = 0.005$; Table 2). Multivariate analysis revealed HUD_{ST} to be a significant predictor of SFR regardless of stone diameter (OR = 3.1, $p = 0.03$).

Discussion

The current study evaluates the clinical applications of HU characterization using bone and soft tissue window CT scans in a cohort of patients treated with PCNL.

At present, there is no proven method to differentiate stone types prior to endosurgery or SWL. However, the treatment choice for intrarenal stones is based on stone dimension, location and HUM [18].

Mostafavi et al. has shown the predictive value of HU obtained from CT scans to differentiate uric acid, struvite and calcium oxalate kidney stones, while Dual-Energy CT has been proposed, albeit with controversial results, to

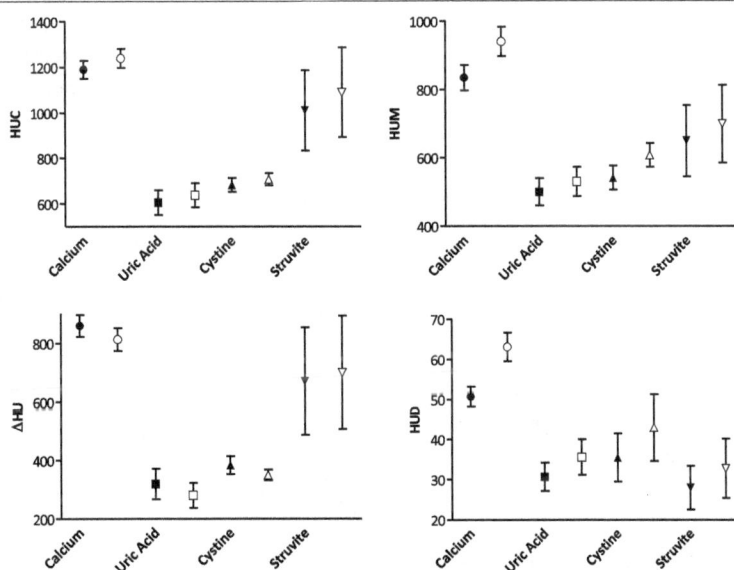

Fig. 2 Visual distribution of HUC (1a), HUM (1b), ΔHU (1c), HUD (1d) evaluated in soft tissue (●) and bone (○) scans for all stone types. Legend: HUC = HU at the center of the stone; HUM = HU mean value; ΔHU = difference between HUC and HU at stone's periphery; HUD = ratio between HUM and stone's largest diameter at axial plane

Table 2 Specificity and sensitivity of HUD in predicting stone-free rate at 3 months and relative univariate analysis

	Cut-off	ROC curve				Stone free		Univariate analysis		
		AUC	Sens	Spec	p	no (%)	yes (%)	OR	(95%- CI)	p
HUD$_{ST}$	<38.5					21 (55)	17 (45)	1.00 Ref		
	≥38.5	0.66	70%	63.8%	0.016	9 (23)	30 (77)	4.12	(1.54–10.99)	0.005
HUD$_B$	<49					21 (54)	18 (46)	1.00 Ref		
	≥49	0.67	70%	61%	0.015	9 (24)	29 (76)	3.76	(1.42–9.99)	0.008

Legend: *HUD* ratio between HU mean value and stone's largest diameter at axial plane on soft tissue (ST) or bone (B) CT window, *OR* Odds ratio, *CI* Confidence interval

improve HU power to predict stone composition [5, 9, 19]. However, this procedure is impractical as it is not available in the majority of the hospitals.

Eisner et al. explored the precision of bone and abdomen window scans in measuring ureteral stones that were then spontaneously passed and physically measured. They concluded that the bone window offers a substantially more accurate estimate than the abdomen window [13]. Our study shows that stone diameter is smaller and HU values are higher when observed with the bone window, probably due to the better contrast provided by this window. However, such differences are clinically irrelevant.

Torricelli et al. analyzed the predictive power of HUC to differentiate uric acid ($n = 47$), calcium oxalate ($n = 36$) and cystine ($n = 30$) stones and concluded that HUC of calcium oxalate stones is significantly higher than that of uric acid stones [11]. Two studies have explored the possibility of dividing the HU value by the stone's maximum diameter to reduce the bias derived from the observation that the bigger the stone, the higher the HU, regardless of the type of calculi. Nakada et al. reported the utility of the maximum HU/size ratio in discriminating uric acid versus calcium stones (28.8 ± 27.2 vs 49.1 ± 85.2; $p = 0.0001$) in a cohort of 99 patients [7].

Motley et al. confirmed the utility of the HU/size ratio (HUD), showing that it discriminated calcium ($n = 87$; mean $\pm$ SD = 105 ± 43), uric acid ($n = 7$; 50 ± 24), cystine ($n = 2$; 45 ± 4) and struvite ($n = 4$; 53 ± 28) stones [8].

Our study further confirms the capability of HU parameters to differentiate uric acid and cystine stones from calcium stones, regardless of the type of HU variable analyzed. Uric acid calculi have lower ΔHU and HUC values than struvite stones, while cystine calculi have HU values similar to stones composed of uric acid and struvite. However, the diagnosis of cystine stones is also guided by laboratory and epidemiological data (Brand's test, urinary pH, crystals, uricosuria, uricemia, patient age).

HU measurements are useful if they first provide differentiation of medium-high (calcium, struvite) from low dense (uric acid, cystine) stones and then distinguish calcium from struvite stones. HUC$_{ST}$ is the best predictor of stone density at a cut-off of 825 HU with a PPV of 93% and a NPV of 85.3%. Our study also demonstrates that struvite has low HUD, which differentiates it from calcium with a high sensitivity (82.5%) and specificity (80%).

These results suggest the utility of creating a flow-chart based on HUC and HUD values with integrated laboratory and demographic data to pre-operatively recognize stone composition (Fig. 3). The possibility to characterize uric

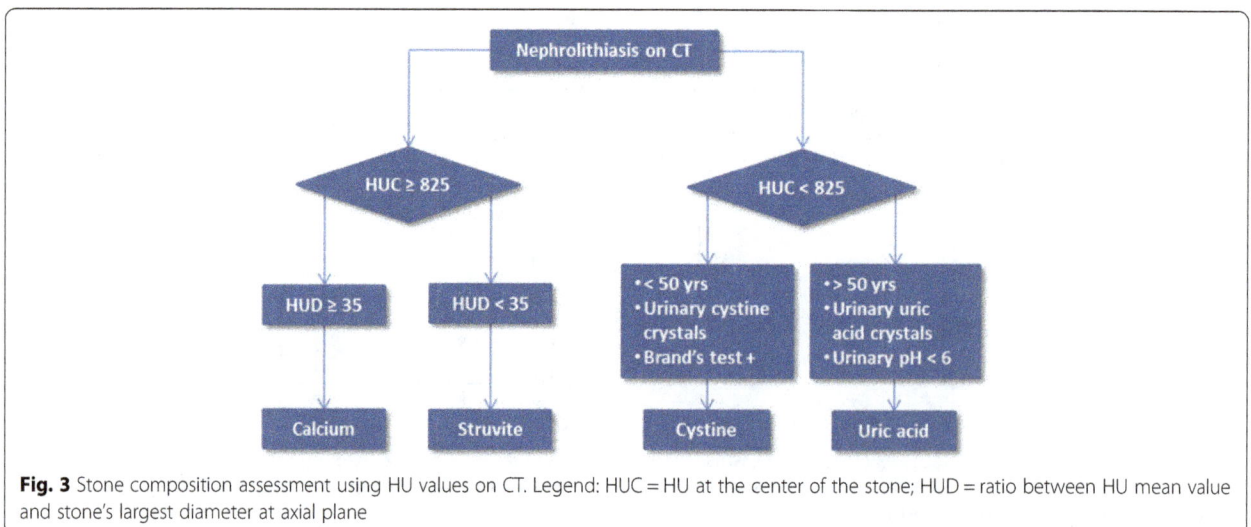

Fig. 3 Stone composition assessment using HU values on CT. Legend: HUC = HU at the center of the stone; HUD = ratio between HU mean value and stone's largest diameter at axial plane

acid stones with such accuracy may help to individuate candidates for oral chemolysis.

HU measurements are also known to be predictive factors of SFR after PCNL as described by CROES in a cohort of 5803 patients. Gücük et al. demonstrated that a HUM lower than 677.5 HU is a predictor of PCNL failure, even if the AUC was only 0.299 [14, 20]. In our study HUD_{ST} is an independent predictor of PCNL failure when lower than 38.5 HU/mm, indicating a 3.1 folds higher risk of residual stones. This may be due to the low sensitivity of intra-operative fluoroscopy in detecting stones less dense than 500 HU as reported by Chua et al. [21]. Furthermore, low HUD also indicates a large stone, which is one of the best-known predictive factors of PCNL failure. HUD, evaluated with other data such as the number of stones, their dimensions and the intraoperative stone clearance impression, can help categorize the risk of residual fragments. For high risk cases, a non-contrast CT should be requested at follow-up; otherwise an abdominal ultrasound might be preferred.

HU values were also correlated with peri-operative data. Our study shows that the higher the HUD, the shorter the hospitalization time. This result is in line with generally lower complication rates for hyperdense calculi, as described by CROES [20]. In contrast, the need for transfusion was directly related to HUD values, consistent with the data of Gücük et al. who reported a larger decrease in hemoglobin in cases of high HUM [14]. This can be explained by the energy needed to break hard stones into fragments, which can increase the risk of mucosal damage.

Our study has some limitations. First, it is a retrospective study with relatively few patients. We did not differentiate between calcium oxalate monohydrate and dihydrate stones because of the limited number of patients. Furthermore, the CT collimation varied between 0.6 and 5 mm; however, we tried to reduce this limit by only evaluating stones larger than 4 mm to increase the precision of each procedure.

For these reasons perspective studies should be conducted to confirm the results we describe.

Conclusions

HU measurements at CT scan may help predict stone composition, regardless of the window setting (i.e. bone or abdomen) used. HUC accurately differentiates medium to high (struvite, calcium) from low (uric acid, cystine) density stones, a factor that can aid in selecting patients for oral chemolysis, while HUD distinguishes struvite from calcium calculi. Of note, HUD is an independent predictor of stone-free status after PCNL at three-month follow-up. Thus, it may be a useful tool for categorizing the risk of residual fragments and planning imaging follow-up.

Abbreviations
ΔHU: difference between HUC and HUP; A: area; D_1: stone's largest diameter at axial plane; D_2: D_1 perpendicular diameter; D_3: maximum diameter at coronal plane; HU: Hounsfield units; HUC: HU value at the center of the stone; HUD: ratio between HUM and D_1; HUM: HU mean value; HUP: HU value at stone's periphery; PCNL: percutaneous nephrolithotomy; SFR: stone-free rate; SWL: shockwave lithotripsy; V: volume; X_B: bone window scans; X_{ST}: soft tissue window scans

Acknowledgements
The Authors would thank Dana Kuefner for language revision.

Funding
None.

Authors' contributions
A.G.: project development, data management, data analysis, manuscript writing E.D.L.: manuscript writing/editing L.B.: data analysis M.D.: data collection S.P.Z.: project development F.L.: project development A.T.: manuscript editing E.M.: project development, manuscript editing. All authors read and approved the final manuscript.

Competing interests
The authors declare that they have no competing interests.

Author details
[1]Fondazione IRCCS Ca' Granda Ospedale Maggiore Policlinico, Department of Urology, University of Milan, Via della Commenda 15, 20122 Milan, Italy. [2]Istituto Europeo di Oncologia, Department of Urology, University of Milan, Via Giuseppe Ripamonti 435, 20141 Milan, Italy. [3]Department of Urology, Ospedale Alessandro Manzoni Lecco, Via dell'Eremo 9/11, 23900 Lecco, Italy.

References
1. Turk C, Petrik A, Sarica K, et al. EAU guidelines on diagnosis and conservative Management of Urolithiasis. Eur Urol. 2016;69:468–74. https://doi.org/10.1016/j.eururo.2015.07.040.
2. Hounsfield GN. Computerized transverse axial scanning (tomography). 1. Description of system. Br J Radiol. 1973;46:1016–22.
3. Mitcheson HD, Zamenhof RG, Bankoff MS, Prien EL. Determination of the chemical composition of urinary calculi by computerized tomography. J Urol. 1983;130:814–9.
4. Newhouse JH, Prien EL, Amis ES Jr, et al. Computed tomographic analysis of urinary calculi. Am J Roentgenol. 1984;142:545–8.
5. Mostafavi MR, Ernst RD, Saltzman B. Accurate determination of chemical composition of urinary calculi by spiral computerized tomography. J Urol. 1998;159:673–5.
6. Saw KC, McAteer JA, Monga AG, et al. Helical CT of urinary calculi: effect of stone composition, stone size, and scan collimation. Am J Roentgenol. 2000; 175:329–32.
7. Nakada SY, Hoff DG, Attai S, et al. Determination of stone composition by noncontrast spiral computed tomography in the clinical setting. Urology. 2000;55:816–9.
8. Motley G, Dalrymple N, Keesling C, et al. Hounsfield unit density in the determination of urinary stone composition. Urology. 2001;58:170–3.
9. Deveci S, Coskun M, Tekin MI, et al. Spiral computed tomography: role in determination of chemical compositions of pure and mixed urinary stones -an in vitro study. Urology. 2004;64:237–40.
10. Marchini GS, Remer EM, Gebreselassie S, et al. Stone characteristics on noncontrast computed tomography: establishing definitive patterns to discriminate calcium and uric acid compositions. Urology. 2013;82:539–46. https://doi.org/10.1089/end.2012.0470.
11. Torricelli FC, Marchini GS, De S, et al. Predicting urinary stone composition based on single-energy noncontrast computed tomography: the challenge of cystine. Urology. 2014;83:1258–63. https://doi.org/10.1016/j.urology.2013.12.066.
12. Marchini GS, Gebreselassie S, Liu X, et al. Absolute Hounsfield unit measurement on noncontrast computed tomography cannot accurately predict struvite stone composition. J Endourol. 2013;27:162–7. https://doi.org/10.1089/end.2012.0470.

13. Eisner BH, Kambadakone A, Monga M, et al. Computerized tomography magnified bone windows are superior to standard soft tissue windows for accurate measurement of stone size: an in vitro and clinical study. J Urol. 2009;181:1710–5. https://doi.org/10.1016/j.juro.2008.11.116.

14. Gucuk A, Uyeturk U, Ozturk U, et al. Does the Hounsfield unit value determined by computed tomography predict the outcome of percutaneous nephrolithotomy? J Endourol. 2012;26:792–6. https://doi.org/10.1089/end.2011.0518.

15. Tiselius HG, Andersson A. Stone burden in an average Swedish population of stone formers requiring active stone removal: how can the stone size be estimated in the clinical routine? Eur Urol. 2003;43:275–81.

16. Frattini A, Barbieri A, Salsi P, et al. One shot: a novel method to dilate the nephrostomy access for percutaneous lithotripsy. J Endourol. 2001;15:919–23.

17. De la Rosette JJ, Opondo D, Daels FP, et al. Categorisation of complications and validation of the Clavien score for percutaneous nephrolithotomy. Eur Urol. 2012;62:246–55. https://doi.org/10.1016/j.eururo.2012.03.055.

18. Turk C, Petrik A, Sarica K, et al. EAU guidelines on interventional treatment for Urolithiasis. Eur Urol. 2016;69:475–82. https://doi.org/10.1016/j.eururo.2015.07.041.

19. Manglaviti G, Tresoldi S, Guerrer CS, et al. In vivo evaluation of the chemical composition of urinary stones using dual-energy CT. Am J Roentgenol. 2011;197:76–83.

20. De la Rosette J, Assimos D, Desai M, et al. The clinical research Office of the Endourological Society Percutaneous Nephrolithotomy Global Study: indications, complications, and outcomes in 5803 patients. J Endourol. 2011;25:11–7.

21. Chua ME, Gatchalian GT, Corsino MV, Reyes BB. Diagnostic utility of attenuation measurement (Hounsfield units) in computed tomography stonogram in predicting the radio-opacity of urinary calculi in plain abdominal radiographs. Int Urol Nephrol. 2012;44:1349–55.

6

Life after prostate cancer treatment: a mixed methods study of the experiences of men with sexual dysfunction and their partners

Jeffrey A. Albaugh[1][*] , Nat Sufrin[2], Brittany R. Lapin[3], Jacqueline Petkewicz[1] and Sandi Tenfelde[4]

Abstract

Background: Prostate cancer is the most common non-skin cancer in men and sexual dysfunction is the most frequently reported long-term side effect of prostate cancer surgery or radiation. The aim of this study was to examine the experiences of men with sexual dysfunction and their partners following prostate cancer treatment.

Methods: Men with sexual dysfunction from either surgical removal or radiation therapy 1-5 years after treatment were interviewed, as well as their partners. A mixed method design was used to determine the lived experience of men with sexual dysfunction. Open-ended questions guided the interviews.

Results: Twenty seven men completed the study with a mean age of 61 years (SD = 8.0; range = 44-77 years). Nine partners also participated. The majority of men (92.6%) had surgery. The average time from treatment to the interview was 23.5 months (SD = 11.7). Themes were frustration with sexual dysfunction, importance of support and understanding from others, depression and anxiety related to sexual dysfunction, importance of intimacy with partner, factors that impact treatment satisfaction, and education and comprehensive information about sex.

Conclusions: Prostate cancer survivors and partners need accurate information about sexual side effects before during and after treatment. Men and partners required individualized help and guidance to manage sexual dysfunction. Support and understanding from partners, family, and others was also identified as an important aspect of healing and adjustment after prostate cancer treatment. Prostate cancer education/support groups played a key role in helping men and partners gain advocacy, education, and support. Psychological problems such as depression and anxiety need to be identified and addressed in men after prostate cancer treatment. Men and partners need assistance in understanding and navigating their way through intimacy to move forward with connectedness in their relationship. Satisfaction with treatment and with providers is dependent on patient education and understanding of all aspects of prostate cancer treatment including sexual side effects and incontinence.

Keywords: Prostate cancer, Male cancers, Sexual dysfunction, Qualitative research, Phenomenology, Survivorship

* Correspondence: jalbaugh@northshore.org
[1]John and Carol Walter Center for Urological Health, NorthShore University HealthSystem, 2180 Pfingsten Road, Suite 3000, Glenview, Illinois 60026, USA
Full list of author information is available at the end of the article

Background

One out of eight men will be diagnosed with prostate cancer during their lifetime, making the disease the most common non-skin cancer in the male population [1]. Although the majority of men will not die from prostate cancer, with survivorship as high as 93% for 15 years after diagnosis [1], treatment can have long-term side effects that greatly impact quality of life. Notably, sexual dysfunction is the most common side effect of both surgical removal of the prostate and radiation therapy [2]. While erectile dysfunction (ED) is not an immediate result of radiation therapy, a multicenter study has shown that sexual function in men who have undergone external beam radiation continues to decline to levels similar to men who had radical prostatectomy [3]. The incidence of ED has been reported as high as 79-88% after radical prostatectomy [4], despite advances in nerve sparing surgical techniques, and 67-72% after external beam radiation [5]. Helping men and their partners adjust to potential side effects such as sexual dysfunction following prostate cancer treatment is an important part of holistic care.

Erectile dysfunction impacts quality of life, with the majority of men reporting quality of life as either severely or moderately affected by ED [3, 6]. Several broad qualitative studies have been done to examine the lived experience of men with prostate cancer and have identified the challenges of sexual dysfunction after treatment in these men [7, 8], but little research was found looking at the lived experience of men specifically examining sexual dysfunction after prostate cancer treatment. Researchers examined the struggle towards the new normal with psychosexual adjustment after prostate cancer treatment in Australian men [7]. They found three main themes: Men were impacted by distressing sexual and urinary difficulties which negatively impacted self-perception and intimate relationships; receiving adequate information and support and good communication with providers and partners facilitated better adjustment; coming to terms with the side effects of prostate cancer treatment involved making lifestyle changes, coping and emotional struggles, while striving to accept/integrate the new normal self/life. Since an extensive Medline search did not reveal previous research to specifically examine the lived experience of men with sexual dysfunction after prostate cancer treatment and/or partners, the powerful descriptions from this study will provide new information on this phenomenon.

Methods

Sample/Study population

Participants were men who had undergone prostate cancer treatment within the last 1-5 years, with resulting sexual dysfunction. These men, and their partners, were asked to describe their experience with sexual dysfunction and prostate cancer treatment. Men and/or partners of men with prostate cancer were recruited through prostate cancer awareness/support/information groups or from the urology clinic of the principal investigator's academic medical center. Recruitment was done through word of mouth and a recruitment flyer.

Inclusion criteria

(1) Men and/or partners of men with sexual dysfunction who underwent treatment for prostate cancer at least 1 year ago and no more than 5 years ago through either radical prostatectomy or radiation therapy.
(2) Sexually active prior to and at the time of prostate cancer treatment.
(3) Command of verbal and written English.

Procedures

The IRB-approved study used a mixed methods design to determine the lived experience of men with sexual dysfunction and their partners. Participants individually, verbally answered open-ended questions about their treatment and experience. Interview sessions lasted as long as the participant needed (most lasting approximately 25 min) and were audio-recorded and transcribed. As is the norm with qualitative research, accrual stopped when the saturation level was achieved (when no new themes were emerging from the descriptions). In addition to open-ended interviews, participants, excluding partners, also completed quantitative questionnaires about erection hardness, erectile function and orgasm/climax quality.

Analysis

Interview transcriptions were randomly spot checked for accuracy. Qualitative thematic text coding with a concentrated examination of the transcripts was performed using Dedoose [9, 10]. A code book was developed after two staff independently reviewed several transcripts to determine appropriate codes. The two coders met with a third coder to discuss and reconcile the codes in the code book. At this point, inter-rater reliability was assessed for all three coders, with a pooled Kappa value of 0.66. New codes were added by each of the three coders as they emerged, which were communicated to other coders. After initial coding was completed by the three independent coders, the coders met again to revisit and discuss all codes. The transcripts were re-assigned to different coders and further coding was done to increase inter-relater reliability, accuracy and comprehension. Following this phase, the group met to review codes and organize into emerging higher-order themes.

All three reviewers submitted quotes from the interviews associated with the various themes. For the manuscript, the group reached consensus on 1-3 quotes for each theme that exemplified that particular theme. Quantitative data were analyzed using SAS version 9.3 (SAS Institute Inc., Cary, NC), which included calculation of descriptive statistics and measures of central tendency.

Measures

Phenomenological Open Ended Questions: This qualitative study used open-ended questions to explore the experience of men with sexual dysfunction after prostate cancer treatment. Each man and/or partner was interviewed separately and asked an open-ended question: Please describe your journey with sexual dysfunction after prostate cancer treatment and/or how has sexual dysfunction impacted your life after prostate cancer treatment? Other guiding statements were used to help participants describe their lived experience such as: Is there anything else you want to tell us about your experience or that you think other people going through this or treating people going through this should know?

Erection Hardness Grading Score: Men were asked to grade the strength of their erections with the Erection Hardness Score, which is a validated measure. Erection strength was rated on a scale ranging from 0 to 4 with 0 (representing a 0% erection) being no erection at all and 4 (representing a fully hard 100% erection) being a completely hard erection [11].

The International Index of Erectile Function (IIEF) including the IIEF 5 and Overall Sexual Satisfaction: Sexual function was determined using the International Index of Erectile Function, which consists of a 15-item questionnaire measuring five domains including erectile function, orgasmic function, sexual desire, intercourse satisfaction, and overall sexual satisfaction, which were determined by principal components analysis [12]. Higher scores indicate higher functioning and satisfaction.

The Self-Esteem and Relationship Questionnaire (SEAR): Self-Esteem, sexual self confidence and participants' relationship satisfaction were measured using the Self-Esteem and Relationship Questionnaire, which is a 14-item instrument developed as a patient-reported tool to assess sexual confidence and intimacy in a sexual relationship [13]. Higher scores indicate better satisfaction.

Orgasm/climax: In addition to questions used from the IIEF in the orgasm domain, orgasm/climax quality was evaluated by asking participants a single question to compare the quality of their orgasm to orgasms experienced prior to treatment. Men could respond to the question by circling a response of absent, diminished, normal or better as compared to prior to prostate cancer treatment.

Other Questions: The participants were asked demographic questions, if they had erectile dysfunction prior to prostate cancer treatment, if they had pain or leakage with orgasm, and about the type and length of time since prostate cancer treatment.

Results

Twenty seven men completed the study, mean age 61 (±8) years (range 44-77 years). Nine partners of the men also participated in the interview process. Partners did not complete any forms. The large majority of men (93%) had surgical treatment. The average time from treatment to completion of study was 24 (±12) months (range 12-52 months). The majority of men did not report erectile dysfunction prior to prostate cancer (74%), however men reported post treatment erectile dysfunction with an average erection hardness of 1.48 (±1.2) (0-4 scale). The erectile dysfunction domain of the IIEF revealed a mean score of 16.1 (±5.8) out of a possible score of 30. All men except for two reported the ability to climax, but most men reported diminished orgasm quality (55.6%). Although the overall relationship satisfaction scores mean was high on the SEAR (76.9 ± 24.4), mean sexual relationship satisfaction was low (49.1 ± 26.3). For complete quantitative results including the results for IIEF and SEAR, see Table 1. Emergent themes from the qualitative interviews were the importance of education/comprehensive information about sex and/or sexual dysfunction, frustration with sexual dysfunction, the importance of support and understanding from others, the importance of intimacy in a relationship, the psychological ramifications of sexual dysfunction, and prostate cancer treatment provider satisfaction and/or dissatisfaction.

Theme 1: Importance of education/comprehensive information

The men in our study spoke about the importance of education and comprehensive information before and throughout the process of prostate cancer treatment. Many men who were dissatisfied with their care were upset when they were given misinformation or they felt the information about sexual dysfunction after prostate cancer treatment was not accurate. Although the men who were most unhappy about sexual dysfunction after prostate cancer did not feel well-prepared in terms of their understanding of the impact of prostate cancer treatment on sexual function, the men who had come to terms with their sexual dysfunction felt they had been well-prepared for the sexual side effects of treatment. Men recommended that information be repeated before, during, and after treatment due to challenges in terms of readiness to learn immediately after the cancer diagnosis. They also talked about the challenges of dealing with a stigmatized topic such as sexual dysfunction. The participants said the following:

Table 1 Sample characteristics

Characteristics	N (%)
Total # of participants	27
Age (years), mean ± SD (range)	60.9 ± 8.0 (44-77)
Race	
Caucasian	22 (81.5)
Asian	1 (3.7)
African-American	4 (14.8)
Non-Hispanic	27 (100.0)
Education	
Master's and above	12 (44.4)
Bachelor's and above	21 (77.8)
Some college	27 (100.0)
Doctorate	5 (18.5)
Prior ED	7 (25.9)
Effective medications taken before prostate cancer (n = 9)	6 (66.7)
Time since	
Surgery (months) (n = 25), mean ± SD	23.5 ± 11.7
Radiation (months) (n = 5), mean ± SD	18.2 ± 13.1
Surgery	25 (92.6)
Robotic	20 (80.0)
Open	5 (20.0)
Nerve-sparing (vs. partial) (n = 24)	21 (87.5)
Hormone treatment	4 (14.8)
Surgery followed by radiation	5 (18.5)
Erection hardness score (n = 26), mean ± SD	1.48 ± 1.18
Orgasm quality	
Absent	2 (7.4)
Diminished	15 (55.6)
Normal	6 (22.2)
Better	3 (11.1)
Unknown	1 (3.7)
Pain with orgasm (n = 25)	0 (0.0)
Urine leakage during sex	
Never	7 (25.9)
Occasionally	14 (51.9)
Always	6 (22.2)
IIEF (n = 16), mean ± SD	
Erectile function	16.1 ± 5.8
Orgasmic function	6.6 ± 3.0
Sexual desire	7.3 ± 2.2
Intercourse satisfaction	8.3 ± 3.3
Overall satisfaction	5.5 ± 2.4

Table 1 Sample characteristics (Continued)

SEAR, mean ± SD	
Sexual relationship satisfaction	49.1 ± 26.3
Confidence about self-esteem	66.2 ± 24.8
Overall relationship satisfaction	76.9 ± 24.4

Man 21: "I was not prepared for what was to follow… I think everybody – all the medical staff starting with nursing and support staff and the doctors themselves, they really need to inform the patient with what's going to happen after the surgery with complications and side effects and on the surgical end and the physical end, but also then that the effects from the surgery should be talked about from the get go so that patients are not surprised, that they know what's going to be heading their way and if it's – give them the full information…And I'm very, very emotionally upset about because if I would have known I think I would have been in a better place through the first year and following that first year if I knew."

Man 16: "I was fully informed by everybody. All the doctors that were involved fully informed me that these were things that I was up against if they removed my prostate… So definitely – you definitely must keep everybody informed about what's going on…It's really-that's extremely important "

Theme 2: Frustration with sexual dysfunction
The men in our study spoke about their frustration with sexual dysfunction. The men described being upset with the change in their sexual functioning and the impact it had on their intimate relationships. Some men described feelings of loss and grief with changes in orgasm/climax. Three men in the study were pleased to have more intense climax after surgery. The participants said the following:

Man 12: "If you have a lack of sensation you don't have any nocturnal erections. You don't wake up with an erection and I miss that. I miss it a lot. I miss the sensations of how I used to feel down there, how my body used to feel…I don't feel whole and I think about it every single day…It's the first thing I think about in the morning when I wake up and it's the last thing I think about at night…"

Man 16: "I have not – I do not have any recall of having orgasm like I have now. And honest to God there has to be – I mean sometimes I go into mini convulsions because the orgasm lasts and it's so strong and lasts for probably two minutes."

Theme 3: Importance of support and understanding

Not surprisingly, the men and partners we interviewed impressed upon us the need and importance of support and understanding, from their partner and from others in their lives, including their families and support groups like the Us TOO International Prostate Cancer Education and Support Network. An essential element of this support was communication, especially with the partner, which could be very difficult for both parties. To enable this communication, it was crucial for men and their partners to be open about their intimate feelings and concerns. The participants said the following:

Man 13: "I'm in a great relationship really for the first time in my life with a woman who really I don't think doesn't care what we do as long as we're together. We enjoy sex a lot not just to be active, just to have intercourse. Without her I don't think I would be as far along in getting my sex life back to where I want it to be. It's got to do with her and she's put up with so much."

Partner 1: "And I think in the beginning he felt we weren't there for him, the family, because the family – again, the family does think that the man or father or the husband is strong, is – he doesn't get sick. He's there, he has the answer, this is how he is. Go, go, go, I'm here, whatever. And then he gets sick and it's like, okay, you're done, you're fine, you had the surgery, it's okay. But it wasn't okay to him, but we felt, no, you're strong, you're okay. You're okay. And that kind of wasn't good because he felt we didn't care. And we really didn't understand him."

Man 9: "I come here (prostate cancer support group) shaking like a leaf, man. I get in here with a bunch of guys that had been where I was about to go and man they gassed me up with that strength. And like I said, when I came in I was shaking like a leaf. When I left out I was empowered. "

Theme 4: Importance of intimacy

Intimacy, both physical and emotional, was a priority for men and their partners. Participants discussed the importance of non-penetrative sex. Most men and their partners felt that non-penetrative sex was a helpful way to maintain intimacy. Some participants felt the relationship was stronger after prostate cancer treatment. The participants said the following:

Man 21: "I was fortunate to find this woman and it just enhances every single aspect, whatever, if you're going to a social event, you're going on a vacation, you are just being intimate around the house, you're

sharing thoughts and dreams. It just encompasses what life is all about. Some people don't care about it, but for the men that do it's devastating."

Partner 5: "Anything I could tell anybody going through this is like, "If you guys are not intimate, and able to talk with each other now you'd better get that straight before the surgery. Better get it straight because you're gonna need each other, and you're gonna need the intimacy more than you've ever had it..."

Man 15: "I miss the holding of hands. I miss hugging and things like that. I don't – that's not sex in the definition of this survey. But that's what is available to me in my current physical condition...and so yes, it's important."

Theme 5: Psychological ramifications of sexual dysfunction

Some of the men we interviewed reported psychological issues due to the sexual dysfunction that resulted from prostate cancer treatment. This included many reports of depression and anxiety, in addition to some suicidal ideation. One man reported that he'd rather have his legs cut off than exist in his current state of sexual dysfunction. Men who might not have used clinical terms like "depression" or "anxiety" nevertheless reported the psychologically devastating effects of feeling abnormal, unnatural, and less of a man due to their sexual dysfunction. There was a sense from men and their partners that sexual dysfunction has a great impact on every aspect of life. Like depression, it can change the very lens with which men and their partners view and experience their whole existence. The participants said the following:

Man 14: "And that made me very depressed. I was really surprised about that because nowhere in our research prior to my surgery did I run across that a whole lot about how one of the side effects mentally would be depression. And even now I still have some issues with depression, but it's been over a year and a half and I think I've adjusted somewhat because I found that to combat depression I need to stay active, find things that I used to enjoy that I still enjoy and not focus so much on the depression aspect because I had a lot to be pleased about."

Man 12: "The other thing that happened, and again I was not told to expect this, was depression. I had a very serious bout of depression, post op, when I found out the things that were going on with me physically and the time it was taking to get to what I hoped would be healing. I didn't understand depression. I didn't know I had it but I suffered with it for several months until I got to the point where I became suicidal."

Theme 6: Treatment/provider satisfaction/dissatisfaction

Some men reported dissatisfaction with the treatment they received, while others were happy with the treatment and the care they received around the treatment. The majority of men talked about being happy they were cancer free. Several men talked about their frustration with their provider's sole focus on the surgery and the lack of resources or help with side effects from treatment. Men who were dissatisfied talked about the lack of support and help from their providers; while men who were satisfied with their care commented on the support and help they got from the provider throughout treatment. Some men felt the provider did not really understand them in terms of their priorities and their feelings about sexual function. Some patients regretted the particular treatment they received or that they received treatment at all. The participants said the following:

> **Man 17:** "Uh, we're alive, ok? I was Gleason 7. My statistical life expectancy would be about 12 years, you know, that's average. Could be less, could be more. If I did not get treatment. And, uh, my mentality– and still is—I got it out, out of my body."

> **Man 16:** "I mean, this guy gave us an appointment and sat down with us for two full hours in his office... He sent me home and said do this kind of research and to call him if I had additional questions. Well, after I did a little bit of research, I did have additional questions so I called and he called me back. I mean, I couldn't believe it. I got a call at home from a doctor. And then he spent another 45 minutes after having spent this two, two and a half hours with me – a half hour after ___ (partner) left and then spent another 40 minutes with me on the telephone. I just thought that was awesome."

> **Man 1:** "I think back. Maybe I shouldn't have done it (the surgery). And go with the shorter quality of life rather than a long life – a longer life with the situation."

> **Partner 1:** "Because he would always say, maybe I shouldn't have done that. And I'm like; you did it, so let's live on and not live in the past...It got better, yeah. He felt like he was just – didn't want to live because it was – he didn't feel like a man. He felt like, oh, God, this is a mess.

Discussion

This study was carried out using an open-ended inquiry into men and their partners' journeys with sexual dysfunction after prostate cancer treatment. Unlike many qualitative studies that interview with a semi-structured model [7, 14–17] or focus-group model [18], an open-ended question was used to learn the experiences of men and their partners. The majority of the men underwent surgical removal of the prostate (93%). The themes were salient and common across men and partners.

Men emphasized the importance of education and comprehensive information about sexual dysfunction throughout the course of prostate cancer treatment. Men described the need to be better informed about the negative sexual side effects, in order to proactively manage the sexual dysfunction consequences more easily. Yet, this reality was sometimes complicated by the fact that some men were not ready to learn about sexual side effects upon first hearing their cancer diagnosis, as M Ball, et al. [15] found in a study of men post rectal cancer treatment. Nonetheless, similar to findings by M Ball, et al. [15] and N Hanly, S Mireskandari and I Juraskova [7], we found that men insisted that more education at the outset and throughout the process would alleviate anxiety surrounding side effects. The men in our study articulated a clear need for comprehensive information before, during, and after prostate cancer treatment. Men who felt well-prepared and informed reported satisfaction with their care, while the men and partners who did not feel well prepared and informed were unhappy with the care they received.

Some men reported the importance of seeking out information on one's own, through books, the internet, and support groups such as Us TOO International. They urged their fellow men and partners to do the same. This finding is echoed in KA Krumwiede and N Krumwiede [17] who reported no complaints about a lack of information. Rather, there was a proactive sense of men seeking out information on their own, particularly from men who had already gone through the treatment. This helped men with treatment choices, as it did in our study.

Not surprisingly, another major theme was the distress and frustration caused by sexual dysfunction, which included erectile dysfunction, changes in orgasm and ejaculate, and penile rehabilitation and its accompanying challenges. These frustrations affected both men and their partners and led to a whole range of negative feelings, most notably feeling like less of a man. However, men often assumed their partners were more upset over their sexual dysfunction than they actually were. Few partners reported being upset about their male partners' sexual dysfunction, although they were aware of the men's own dissatisfaction. Our study benefited by separately interviewing both men and their partners, as we were able to directly compare what men said to what their partners said. A small minority of men (n = 3) reported a more intense climax after surgery, which they found to be a positive experience.

The theme of negative emotions caused by sexual dysfunction is common in the literature [7, 8, 16–19]. In a quantitative study, T Zaider and colleagues [19] showed that regardless of level of sexual function, men who perceive a loss of masculinity following treatment are more likely to be distressed by ED. As most men tied their ED to "feeling like less of a man," our study confirms this finding. Helping men deal with negative emotions, including grief and loss, is an important part of care.

The psychological ramifications of sexual dysfunction following prostate cancer treatment were articulated by many participants. The majority of men we spoke to reported psychological distress resulting from post-treatment sexual dysfunction, including depression, anxiety, and suicidal ideation. Some sought outside professional counseling or prostate cancer support groups to remedy their situation, and reported positive results in this endeavor. Other studies in the field report similar psychological ramifications as a result of sexual dysfunction [7, 8, 17, 18, 20]. Some men reported the same need to seek outside psychological help, since the primary care provider was not available for such services [7, 20]. N Hanly, S Mireskandari and I Juraskova [7] found not only that the men in their study struggled with depression, but this depression acted as a catalyst for psychological distress due to un-related issues, such as retirement. Offering comprehensive mental health services may be beyond the scope of practice for many urology clinics, yet having a strong referral network of mental health professionals and sexual therapists available will strengthen the care and provide a team-based approach.

The frustration and psychological suffering from sexual dysfunction led men to talk about the importance of support and understanding from others. Others included their partners, their families, and support groups like Us TOO International. Communication was at the heart of this support. Fueling the communication was a sense of openness. Neither communication nor openness was easily achieved. KA Krumwiede and N Krumwiede [17] uncovered the same theme, with a particular emphasis on the gratitude men felt for this support, especially from partners. N Hanly, S Mireskandari and I Juraskova [7], MW Kazer, J Harden, M Burke, MG Sanda, J Hardy and DE Bailey [14], CJ Nelson, S Lacey, J Kenowitz, H Pessin, E Shuk, AJ Roth and JP Mulhall [18] also found this theme. At the heart of this support and understanding from their partners, the men in our study spoke of the importance of intimacy. Romantic relationships are often driven by intimacy, but perhaps our more

surprising finding is that many men said that after diagnosis, and especially after treatment, they grew closer to their partners. They were not romanticizing cancer, or wishing it upon others, but some men did say that their relationship to their partner is now better than it was prior to being diagnosed. The process and possibility for physical intimacy was an integral element of this post-treatment emotional intimacy, as men and their partners struggled to resume their sexual lives in the face of men's post-treatment sexual dysfunction. However, the men reported greater concern with physical intimacy and sex than their partners. To maintain physical intimacy, many couples turned to non-penetrative sex or "outercourse," such as oral sex, manual stimulation, handholding, and cuddling. N Hanly, S Mireskandari and I Juraskova [7], L Jakobsson, L Persson and P Lundqvist [21] found a similar deepened relationship with spouse. However, many partners in N Hanly, S Mireskandari and I Juraskova [7] were unwilling to engage in outercourse and less supportive with side effects from treatment. Partners that interviewed in our study were positive about outercourse and supportive with side effects from treatment.

Finally, we found a range of experiences with treatment and treatment provider satisfaction. Many men were angry at their providers for being overly optimistic about their post-treatment sexual and urinary functions. Others felt wronged by a lack of care or attention by their surgeons. Some of these men regretted their particular treatment or that they received treatment at all. These findings were echoed in CJ Nelson, S Lacey, J Kenowitz, H Pessin, E Shuk, AJ Roth and JP Mulhall [18]. On the other hand, some men in our study expressed no illusions about the role of the surgeon. The removal of the cancer was the primary job. Other care needs were met with a team based approach, including doctors, nurses, and support staff. Some men expressed deep gratitude towards their doctors and nurses for meeting with them for extended periods of time and answering all their questions and concerns with depth and patience. These patients felt well-informed about all side effects, including sexual side effects. N Hanly, S Mireskandari and I Juraskova [7] also found that men placed trust in doctors who provided ample info and answered lots of questions. MW Kazer, J Harden, M Burke, MG Sanda, J Hardy and DE Bailey [14] reported that men cited their confidence in the healthcare team as one of their reasons for a good recovery. Many men in our study were satisfied with the reality of being cancer-free, with or without sexual dysfunction. Even those men and partners who were frustrated with sexual dysfunction felt grateful to be free of prostate cancer. L Jakobsson, L Persson and P Lundqvist [21] found men expressed a similar gratitude for life, as well as anxiety about death.

The health care team plays a crucial role in establishing expectations for care and recovery, and guiding patients and their partners through the journey.

Although this study involved a relatively large group of men and partners from across the country, there were limitations to this study. Men who had been treated for prostate cancer were invited to speak about their experience with sexual dysfunction from the clinic of the principal investigator and from prostate cancer support groups. Thus, men self-selected to participate in the study and their views may not represent the views of other men who did not self-select to participate. Although the sample size is fairly large for a qualitative study, this sample of men was rather homogeneous in race, socio-economic status, and education. The majority of the men in this study underwent surgical removal of the prostate and this is consistent with the most common treatment choice in America. Only 7% of the men in this study had radiation without surgery. Additionally, men were asked post-treatment to describe their pre-treatment sexual function which can lead to recall bias. Future research might include a more diverse sample of men including more men who underwent radiation therapy as a primary treatment. It might also be beneficial to collect information prior to and following treatment.

Conclusion

This study provides qualitative descriptions of men's and partners' journeys with sex and intimacy after prostate cancer treatment. Prostate cancer survivors and their partners report a need for accurate information about sexual side effects before, during, and after prostate cancer treatment. Men and their partners want providers to be sensitive to their sexuality and assist them in finding appropriate help to deal with sexual dysfunction. Men with sexual dysfunction after prostate cancer treatment report not only frustration with sexual problems, but depression and anxiety. Men identified support and understanding from partners, family, and prostate cancer support groups as an important aspect of the healing process. Involving and engaging partners when disseminating information about intimacy and sex after prostate cancer treatment is also important.

Understanding the impact of the anticipated side effects, like erectile dysfunction, and assisting patients with treating erectile dysfunction, is imperative to treatment satisfaction. Results of this study can be used by healthcare providers to improve care and promote intimacy for the man and his partner by providing comprehensive information about sexual issues throughout and after treatment and providing resources addressing sexual dysfunction and depression and anxiety.

Abbreviations

ED: Erectile dysfunction; IIEF: International Index of Erectile Function; SEAR: Self-Esteem and Relationship Questionnaire

Acknowledgements

Expertise in qualitative research methods was provided by David Victorson, PhD, Northwestern University and the authors wish to thank him for his help.

Funding

Funding was provided by the NorthShore University HealthSystem Foundation and the William D. and Pamela Hutul Ross Clinic for Sexual Health.

Authors' contributions

JA conceived the study, conducted interviews, analyzed the data, and drafted the manuscript. NS conducted interviews, analyzed the data, and drafted the manuscript. BL performed the statistical analysis. JP helped analyze the data and draft the manuscript. ST helped draft the manuscript. All authors have read and approved the final manuscript.

Authors' information

Jeffrey Albaugh is the principle investigator and Director of Sexual Health at NorthShore University Healthsystem. Inquiries can be made to Dr. Albaugh by email at jalbaugh@northshore.org. Nat Sufrin is a student at The Doctoral Program in Clinical Psychology, The City College of the City University of New York, New York, NY, USA. Brittany Lapin is affliated with Cleveland Clinic, Cleveland, OH, USA. Sandi Tenfelde is affliated with The Marcella Niehoff School of Nursing, Loyola University of Chicago, Maywood, IL, USA. Jacqueline Petkewicz is affiliated with NorthShore University HealthSystem.

Competing interests

The authors declare that they have no competing interests.

Author details

[1]John and Carol Walter Center for Urological Health, NorthShore University HealthSystem, 2180 Pfingsten Road, Suite 3000, Glenview, Illinois 60026, USA. [2]The Doctoral Program in Clinical Psychology, The City College of the City University of New York, New York, NY, USA. [3]Cleveland Clinic, Cleveland, OH, USA. [4]The Marcella Niehoff School of Nursing, Loyola University of Chicago, Maywood, IL, USA.

References

1. American Cancer Society: Cancer facts and figures. American Cancer Society. 2017. Atlanta, GA, USA. Retrieved from https://www.cancer.org/research/cancer-facts-statistics/all-cancer-facts-figures/cancer-facts-figures-2017.html.
2. Yarbro CH, Ferrans CE. Quality of life of patients with prostate cancer treated with surgery or radiation therapy. Oncol Nurs Forum. 1998;25(4):685–93.
3. Potosky AL, Davis WW, Hoffman RM, Stanford JL, Stephenson RA, Penson DF, et al. Five-year outcomes after prostatectomy or radiotherapy for prostate cancer: the prostate cancer outcomes study. J Natl Cancer Inst. 2004;96(18):1358–67.
4. Korfage IJ, Essink-Bot ML, Borsboom GJ, Madalinska JB, Kirkels WJ, Habbema JD, et al. Five-year follow-up of health-related quality of life after primary treatment of localized prostate cancer. Int J Cancer. 2005;116(2):291–6.
5. Mols F, Korfage IJ, Vingerhoets AJ, Kil PJ, Coebergh JW, Essink-Bot ML, et al. Bowel, urinary, and sexual problems among long-term prostate cancer survivors: a population-based study. Int J Radiat Oncol Biol Phys. 2009;73(1):30–8.
6. Meyer JP, Gillatt DA, Lockyer R, Macdonagh R. The effect of erectile dysfunction on the quality of life of men after radical prostatectomy. Br J Urol Int. 2003;92(9):929–31.
7. Hanly N, Mireskandari S, Juraskova I. The struggle towards 'the new Normal': a qualitative insight into psychosexual adjustment to prostate cancer. BMC Urol. 2014;14:56.
8. Hedestig O, Sandman PO, Tomic R, Widmark A. Living after radical prostatectomy for localized prostate cancer: a qualitative analysis of patient narratives. Acta Oncol. 2005;44(7):679–86.
9. Creswell JW. Qualitative inquiry and research design: choosing among five traditions. Thousand Oaks: Sage Publications; 1998.
10. Braun V, Clarke V. Using thematic analysis in psyhology. Qual Res Psychol. 2006;3(2):77–101.

11. Mulhall JP, Goldstein I, Bushmakin AG, Cappelleri JC, Hvidsten K. Validation of the erection hardness score. J Sex Med. 2007;4(6):1626–34.

12. Rosen RC, Riley A, Wagner G, Osterloh IH, Kirkpatrick J, Mishra A. The international index of erectile function (IIEF): a multidimensional scale for assessment of erectile dysfunction. Urology. 1997;49(6):822–30.

13. Cappelleri JC, Althof SE, Siegel RL, Shpilsky A, Bell SS, Duttagupta S. Development and validation of the Self-Esteem And Relationship (SEAR) questionnaire in erectile dysfunction.[Article]. Int J Impot Res. 2004;16(1): 30–8.

14. Kazer MW, Harden J, Burke M, Sanda MG, Hardy J, Bailey DE. The experiences of unpartnered men with prostate cancer: a qualitative analysis. J Cancer Surviv. 2011;5(2):132–41.

15. Ball M, Nelson CJ, Shuk E, Starr TD, Temple L, Jandorf L, et al. Men's experience with sexual dysfunction post-rectal cancer treatment: a qualitative study. J Cancer Educ. 2013;28(3):494–502.

16. Iyigun E, Ayhan H, Tastan S. Perceptions and experiences after radical prostatectomy in Turkish men: a descriptive qualitative study. Appl Nurs Res. 2011;24(2):101–9.

17. Krumwiede KA, Krumwiede N. The lived experience of men diagnosed with prostate cancer. Oncol Nurs Forum. 2012;39(5):E443–50.

18. Nelson CJ, Lacey S, Kenowitz J, Pessin H, Shuk E, Roth AJ, et al. Men's experience with penile rehabilitation following radical prostatectomy: a qualitative study with the goal of informing a therapeutic intervention. Psycho-Oncology. 2015;24:1646–54.

19. Zaider T, Manne S, Nelson C, Mulhall J, Kissane D. Loss of masculine identity, marital affection, and sexual bother in men with localized prostate cancer. J Sex Med. 2012;9(10):2724–32.

20. O'Brien R, Rose PW, Campbell C, Weller D, Neal RD, Wilkinson C, et al. Experiences of follow-up after treatment in patients with prostate cancer: a qualitative study. BJU Int. 2010;106(7):998–1003.

21. Jakobsson L, Persson L, Lundqvist P. Daily life and life quality 3 years following prostate cancer treatment. BMC Nurs. 2013;12:11.

7

A prospective study of magnetic resonance imaging and ultrasonography (MRI/US)-fusion targeted biopsy and concurrent systematic transperineal biopsy with the average of 18-cores to detect clinically significant prostate cancer

Yuji Hakozaki[1]* (iD), Hisashi Matsushima[1], Jimpei Kumagai[4], Taro Murata[1], Tomoko Masuda[1], Yoko Hirai[1], Mai Oda[2], Nobuo Kawauchi[2], Munehiro Yokoyama[3] and Yukio Homma[4]

Abstract

Background: This study compared the detection rates for clinically significant prostate cancer (CSPC) between magnetic resonance imaging and ultrasonography (MRI/US)-fusion-targeted biopsy (TB), systematic biopsy (SB) and combination of TB and SB.

Methods: This prospective study evaluated simultaneous TB and SB for consecutive patients with suspicious lesions that were detected using pre-biopsy multiparametric MRI. A commercially available real-time virtual sonography system was used to perform the MRI/US-fusion TB with the transperineal technique. The prostate imaging reporting and data system version 2 (PI-RADS v2) was assigned to categorize the suspicious lesions.

Results: A total of 177 patients were included in this study. The detection rate for CSPC was higher using SB, compared to TB (57.1% vs 48.0%, $p = 0.0886$). The detection rate for CSPC was higher using the combination of TB and SB, compared to only SB (63.3% vs 57.1%, $p = 0.2324$). Multivariate analysis revealed that PIRADS v2 category 4 and an age of <65 years were independent predictors for TB upgrading (vs. the SB result).

Conclusions: PI-RADS v2 category 4 and an age of <65 years were predictive factors of upgrading the Gleason score by MRI/US-fusion TB. Thus, MRI/US-fusion TB may be appropriate for patients with those characteristics.

Keywords: Clinically significant prostate cancer, Targeted biopsy, MRI/US fusion biopsy, PI-RADS version 2 score, Extended biopsy

* Correspondence: yhakozaki11012@gmail.com
[1]Department of Urology, Tokyo Metropolitan Police Hospital, #4-22-1 Nakano, Nakano-ku, Tokyo 164-0001, Japan
Full list of author information is available at the end of the article

Background

There is increasing evidence that multiparametric magnetic resonance imaging (mpMRI) of the prostate can improve the detection rates of clinically significant prostate cancer (CSPC) and prevent unnecessary biopsies. Extensive research has recently evaluated the efficacy of magnetic resonance imaging and ultrasonography (MRI/US)-fusion targeted biopsy (TB), although it remains unclear whether MRI/US-fusion TB could replace systematic biopsy (SB) [1–3].

We performed a prospective study to compare the diagnostic value of MRI/US-fusion TB and concurrent SB. Imaging-guided biopsy can be classified into three categories such as cognitive targeting without any technological guidance, targeting in the MRI gantry and real-time MRI/US-fusion guided biopsies. However, there is no visual feedback in the absence of technological guidance, and TB in the MRI gantry is time-consuming, so we adopted MRI/US-fusion guided biopsies using the transperineal technique in our hospital.

Methods

Study design

This was a prospective study approved by an institutional review board, and all participants provided written informed consent. All patients who presented to our hospital for prostate biopsy were recommended to undergo pre-biopsy multiparametric MRI (mpMRI) of the prostate. Patients with suspicious prostate lesions were subsequently recruited to undergo MRI/US-fusion TB and concurrent SB.

Multiparametric MRI and biopsy methods

The mpMRI (Achieva 3.0 T TX: Philips Medical Systems, Best, Netherlands) was used to obtain T2-weighted fast spin-echo images in the transverse, sagittal and coronal planes, as well as diffusion-weighted (DW) images and dynamic-contrast enhanced (DCE) images. The detailed MRI parameters are shown in Table 1. For MRI/US-fusion TB, T2-weighted 3-D/sagittal images (70 slices with a thickness of 1 mm) were reconstructed. A commercially available real-time virtual sonography (RVS) system (Hitachi Medical Corporation, Tokyo, Japan) was used for the

present study. The time resolution of the DCE images was 27.1 s. Suspicious lesions were marked using a circle on the axial images, and the corresponding sagittal images were automatically marked. Transperineal biopsies were performed with the patient under general or spinal anesthesia. For the TBs, a linear transrectal probe (HI VISION, Ascendus, Hitachi) and magnetic position sensors (3D Guidance Trakstar, Ascension) were used to obtain at least 2 cores from the targeted lesion [4]. After the TB, extended SB was performed in a prostate volume dependent manner along the parasagittal and far lateral lines with a 5 mm interval from 1 cm above the echo probe to the top of the prostate.

Clinically significant prostate cancer

We defined CSPC as cancers that did not fulfill all of the Epstein criteria for clinically insignificant cancer [5]: (i) prostate-specific antigen (PSA) density of <0.15, (ii) ≤50% involvement of any 1 core, (iii) a Gleason score of ≤3 + 3, and (iv) <3 positive biopsy cores. PSA value was not included.

Statistical analysis

The Student t test and Pearson's chi-square test were used for comparing detection rates. Univariate and multivariate analyses were performed using the logistic regression model. All statistical analyses were performed using JMP® 12.2.0 (SAS Institute Inc., Cary, NC, USA).

Image interpreting

One experienced radiologist (M.O.) scored the suspicious lesions according to the Prostate Imaging Reporting and Data System version 2 (PI-RADS v2) in a blinded fashion. The highest score of suspicious lesions was defined as the patient's score.

Upgrade

The highest Gleason score from the SB and TB specimens was considered the patient's score. Pathology results were obtained for MRI/US-fusion TB and SB specimens, and cases were considered upgraded if one method provided a higher Gleason score, or if one method detected prostate cancer (PC) when the other did not detect PC.

Table 1 The magnetic resonance imaging parameters

	Sequence type	Slice thickness, mm	No. of slices	TR, ms	TE, ms	b-values	Voxel size, mm
T2 sagittal	TSE	1	80	571	155	–	$0.75 \times 0.75 \times 1$
T2 coronal	TSE	3	20	4000	100	–	$0.57 \times 0.71 \times 3$
T2 axial	TSE	3	20	4000	100	–	$0.57 \times 0.72 \times 3$
DWI	SE-EPI	3	20	3773	84	2000 s/mm^2	$2.5 \times 3.1 \times 3$
T1 DCE	FFE	0.85	85×6	6.6	3.4	–	$0.85 \times 0.85 \times 0.85$

DWI diffusion-weighted imaging, DCE dynamic contrast enhanced, TR repetition time, TE echo time, TSE turbo spin echo, SE-EPI spin echo-echo planar imaging, FFE fast field echo

Results

Between January 2014 and March 2016, 177 consecutive patients were included in this study. Of these, 163 patients had one suspicious lesion on MRI and 14 patients had two. The patients' profiles are shown in Table 2. The mean number of biopsied cores per patient was 3.8 by TB and 18.4 by SB. The median age and PSA were 68 (48–89) years and 7.42 (1.65–218) ng/mL, respectively. One patient was under active surveillance and had a Gleason score of 3 + 3.

A total of 116 patients (65.5%) were found to have PC. The detection rates of total prostate cancer were 49.7% for TB, 58.7% for SB and 65.5% for the combination of TB and SB (Table 3). The detection rates of CSPCs were 48.0% for TB, 57.1% for SB and 63.3% for the combination of TB and SB. The combination of SB and TB showed a statistically higher CSPC detection rate than that of TB (Fig. 1). The detection rate for CSPC was non-significantly higher for SB over TB and the combination over SB, since the p-values were >0.05. The detection rates of both total cancer and CSPCs were highest for the combination of SB and TB.

Regarding CSPC, approximately 10% (11/112) were not detected using SB. In contrast, 22%(25/112) were not detected using TB (Table 4).

There was agreement between the Gleason scores for the TB and SB specimens in 62.7% (111/177) of all patients, and in 43.1% (50/116) of the patients with cancers

Table 2 The patients overall clinical and histological characteristics

Patients, n	177
Age, years	68.3 (48–89)
Prebiopsy prostate-specific antigen level, ng/mL	10.9 (1.65–218)
Prostate volume, mL	42.4 (11–134)
Positive digital rectal examination result, %	51 (28.8)
Systematic cores per prostate, n	18.4 ± 2.1
Targeted cores per prostate, n	3.84 ± 0.4
Patients without prior biopsy, n	145
Patients with prior biopsy negative for cancer, n	31
Patients under active surveillance, n	1
Previous prostate-related treatment, n	0
Gleason score, n	
6 (3 + 3)	19
7 (3 + 4)	16
7 (4 + 3)	14
8 (4 + 4)	48
≥ 9 (4 + 5, 5 + 4, or 5 + 5)	19
Clinically significant prostate cancer, %	112 (63.3)

Data were reported as mean (range) or mean ± standard deviation

Table 3 The detection rates of prostate cancer and clinically significant prostate cancer

	TB + SB	SB	TB
Prostate cancer	116/177 (65.5%)	104/177 (58.7%)	88/177 (49.7%)
95%CI	58.2 to 72.1	51.4 to 65.7	42.4 to 57.0
CSPC	112/177 (63.3%)	101/177 (57.1%)	85/177 (48.0%)
95%CI	56.0 to 70.0	49.7 to 64.1	40.8 to 55.3

TB Targeted biopsies, *SB* Systematic biopsies, *CSPC* Clinically significant prostate cancer, *CI* Confidence interval

(Table 5). 16 patients were diagnosed with prostate cancers using only TB or upgraded using TB (vs. the SB results). Univariate and multivariate regression analysis revealed that the PI-RADS v2 category 4 and an age of <65 years were independent predictors for TB-based upgrading (vs. the SB results) (Table 6). Receriver operating characteristics curve analysis indicated that PSA density > 0.17 was the strongest predictor of TB-based upgrading (area under curve = 0.582). However, univariate analysis showed PSA density was not a predictor for TB-based upgrading using this cut-off value.

Discussion

PSA has been used for PC screening for over 20 years and TRUS-guided 10–12-core biopsy is still a standard diagnostic method as the number of biopsy cores is associated with improved PC detection rates. However, this approach can also detect indolent cancers. The US Preventive Service Task Force (USPSTF) recommended against PSA screening for PC to avoid over-diagnosis and over-treatment, which led to a decrease in the American use of the prostate biopsy. Recent studies have

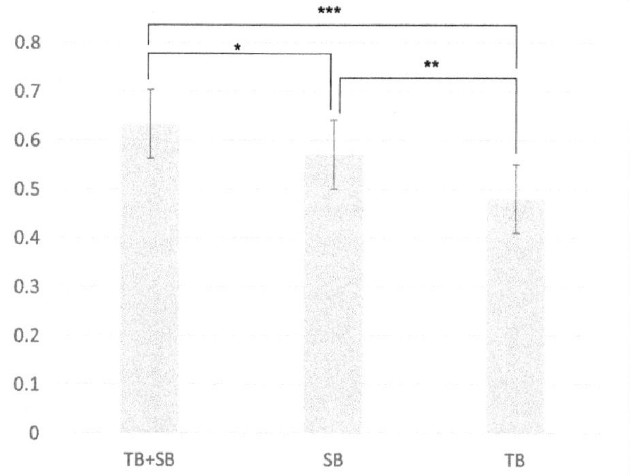

Fig. 1 The detection rates for clinically significant prostate cancer with targeted biopsy (TB), systematic biopsy (SB), and the combination of both (TB + SB). *statistically insignificant with a p value of 0.2324. **statistically insignificant with a p value of 0.0886. ***statistically significant with a p value of 0.0039

Table 4 The correspondence table of the diagnosis between targeted biopsies and systematic biopsies

Diagnosis of TB	Diagnosis of SB		
	CSPC, n	Clinically insignificant Pca, n.	No cancer, n.
CSPC, no.	74	0	11
Clinically insignificant Pca, no.	2	0	1
No cancer, no.	25	3	61

TB targeted biopsy, *SB* Systematic biopsy, *Pca* Prostate cancer, *CSPC* Clinically significant prostate cancer

revealed that MRI/US-fusion TB provides higher detection rates of CSPC and is less invasive than PSA-based SB. However, it is unclear whether MRI/US-fusion TB can replace SB. In this study, we compared the detection rates of PC between MRI/US-fusion TB and concurrent extended SB with the transperineal technique. To the best of our knowledge, this is the first prospective study to compare MRI/US-fusion TB and extended SB with an average of 18 cores.

The results indicate that SB provided a higher detection rate of CSPC, compared to TB (57.1% vs 48.0%), and that only SB was able to diagnose 25 patients with CSPC. In contrast, some previous studies have indicated that TB provides high rates of PC detection [6, 7].

There are two reasons why SB provided higher rates of PC and CSPC detection in the present study. The first reason is that we performed transperineal biopsy along the parasagittal and far lateral lines with an interval of 5 mm and a prostate volume- dependent number of biopsy cores. This technique is similar to the template biopsy technique, and the PROMIS study revealed that the template biopsy technique was able to detect PC (119/452, 26.3%) in some cases that were missed by standard TRUS [8]. Hossack et al. reported that transperineal biopsy detected more anterior tumors than transrectal biopsy [9]. Although we did not perform template biopsy, our transperineal SB technique may have provided better

Table 5 Agreement in the Gleason scores for the targeted and systematic biopsies

Histology of TB	Histology of SB					
	No cancer	3 + 3	3 + 4	4 + 3	4 + 4	≥9
No cancer	61	8	7	4	7	2
3 + 3	4	7	2	2	5	0
3 + 4	1	0	6	1	5	0
4 + 3	2	0	0	5	2	0
4 + 4	4	1	0	1	23	5
≥9	1	0	0	0	2	9

TB targeted biopsy, *SB* Systematic biopsy

PC detection, compared to standard 10–12-core random biopsy or transrectal biopsy. The second reason is that we used the Epstein criteria, which only define insignificant cancer to be present in cases with a Gleason score of 3 + 3, and only a few patients in the present study had insignificant cancers. Baco et al. used the same definition for significant/insignificant PC, and reported that 12-core random biopsy provided a higher detection rate, compared to MRI/TRUS-guided TB (49% vs 38%) [2].

We also detected CSPC using SB when TB provided negative results in 15.3% of the patients (27/177). It is possible that TB can fail to detect PC, as Ahmed et al. reported that CSPC was detected using template biopsy in 10.8% of patients (17/158) who had negative MRI findings [8]. Cash et al. reported that TB failure is the main cause of negative TB findings [10]. In this context, SB may detect PC in areas where MRI failed to do so or where TB did not effectively target the PC. This under-detection of PC could be caused by a lack of conspicuity on MRI because of image quality, which may result from image noise using very high b-values for DWI, or low temporal resolution for dynamic contrast-enhanced imaging. It could also result from misregistration and mistargeting when MRI correctly identifies suspicious areas [11, 12]. Histopathological results from radical prostatectomy are needed to address this issue, although only a few patients in the present study underwent radical prostatectomy.

Twelve patients were diagnosed with PC using TB but not using SB. To assess the utility of TB, we compared the Gleason scores from TB and SB respectively. There were 116 PC patients who were diagnosed using the combination of TB and SB. However, only 50 patients had the same Gleason scores for the TB and SB specimens. Furthermore, 16 patients were upgraded based on the TB results (vs. the SB results), and 34 patients were upgraded based on the SB results. A previous study revealed TB upgrading (vs. SB) in 22% of cases (43/198) [3], while the result was much lower in the present study (9.0%, 16/177). On the other hand, Muthigi et al. reported the upgrading rate for SB (vs. TB) as 23.9% of the cases (135/564) [13]. The upgrading rate for SB was a similar rate in the present study (28.2%, 50/177).

We assigned the PI-RADS v2 category to all lesions retrospectively and blindly. The PI-RADS v2 score provides a good prognostic value for PC and CSPCs [14, 15]. This scoring system was established in 2012 by the ESUR guidelines [16] and version 2 was updated in 2014. A consensus statement from the American Urological Association and the Society of Abdominal Radiology's Prostate Cancer Disease-Focused Panel about the reporting system of MRI recommends the use of the PI-RADS v2 score and states that categories 3 to 5 should be targeted by image-guided biopsies [17].

Table 6 Univariate and multivariate analyses of upgrading predictions for targeted versus systematic biopsies

		Univariate analysis			Multivariate analysis		
		OR	95% CI	p-value	OR	95% CI	p-value
PI-RADS v2 category	5	1.14	0.37–3.45	0.8215	–	–	–
	4	4.24	1.40–12.8	0.0064[a]	4.33	1.46–14.6	0.0077[a]
PSAD >0.17 (yes vs. no)		2.71	0.74–9.91	0.1179	–	–	–
DRE (yes vs. no)		0.79	0.24–2.57	0.6910	–	–	–
Number of biopsies per PV ≥0.5 (yes vs. no)		1.77	0.62–5.11	0.2836	–	–	–
Age < 65 years (yes vs. no)		3.64	1.28–10.4	0.0111[a]	3.73	1.28–11.4	0.0165[a]
Repeat biopsy (yes vs. no)		1.05	0.28–3.92	0.9417	–	–	–

OR odds ratio, *CI* confidence interval, *PSAD* prostate-specific antigen density, *DRE* digital rectal examination, *PV* prostate volume
[a]statistically significant

To identify cases that would benefit from TB, we evaluated the factors that might predict TB upgrading. Univariate and multivariate analyses revealed that the PI-RADS v2 category 4 and an age of <65 years were independent predictive factors for upgrading for TB. The PI-RADS v2 category 5 was not a significant predictive factor. It is probably because the suspected lesions were larger than PI-RADS v2 category 4 lesions and CSPCs from category 5 lesions were easily detected using SB. It is unclear why an age of <65 years predicted upgrading for TB, although it is possible that interpreting MRI and targeting may be more difficult in older patients who have prostatic hypertrophy or prostatitis. The number of cores by SB was not a predicting factor of upgrading by TB, so increasing the number of SB cores should not be recommended to decrease upgrading of TB.

There are some limitations in our study. First, only one experienced radiologist assigned the PI-RADS v2 scores with the lesions. However, the inter-radiologist reproducibility of the PI-RADS v2 is good for experienced radiologists [18] and the PI-RADS v2 score has moderate inter-reader agreement. As the radiologist had over 10 year-career of interpreting PC imaging, it is likely that the results of this study are reliable. Second, only a few patients underwent radical prostatectomy. It will be important to collect more histological data from the radical prostatectomies with upgrading for TB. Third, the PI-RADS v2 categories were retrospectively assigned. Prospective scoring is necessary to assess the accuracy of the PI-RADS v2 category, although there was no bias for the urologists to perform the biopsies based on the PI-RADS v2 category in this study.

Conclusion

In conclusion, the combination of TB and SB was a good tool to detect CSPCs. MRI/US-fusion TB might not be a suitable replacement for systematic transperineal biopsies. Nevertheless, 16 patients were upgraded based on TB findings. The PI-RADS v2 category 4 and an age

of <65 years were predictive factors of upgrading for MRI/US-fusion TB, so MRI/US-fusion TB should be recommended in such patients. To the best of our knowledge, this is the first prospective study to compare MRI/US-fusion TB and extended SB with an average of 18 cores.

Abbreviations
CSPC: Clinically significant prostate cancer; DCE: Dynamic-contrast enhanced; DW: Diffusion-weighted; mpMRI: Multiparametric MRI; MRI/US: Magnetic resonance imaging and ultrasonography; PC: Prostate cancer; PI-RADS v2: Prostate imaging reporting and data system version 2; RVS: Real-time virtual sonography; SB: Systematic biopsy; TB: Targeted biopsy

Acknowledgments
None.

Funding
None.

Authors' contributions
HM and JK conceived of the study. Taro M, Tomoko M, and Yoko H collected the data. MO assigned the PI-RADS v2 scores to the images. MY performed the pathological diagnose. YH analyzed the data. YH, HM, NK and Yukio H wrote the manuscript. All authors read and approved the final manuscript.

Competing interests
The authors declare that they have no competing interests.

Author details
[1]Department of Urology, Tokyo Metropolitan Police Hospital, #4-22-1 Nakano, Nakano-ku, Tokyo 164-0001, Japan. [2]Department of Radiology, Tokyo Metropolitan Police Hospital, Tokyo, Japan. [3]Department of Pathology, Tokyo Metropolitan Police Hospital, Tokyo, Japan. [4]Department of Urology, The University of Tokyo Graduate School of Medicine, Tokyo, Japan.

References

1. Rais-Bahrami S, Siddiqui MM, Turkbey B, Stamatakis L, Logan J, Hoang AN, et al. Utility of multiparametric magnetic resonance imaging suspicion levels for detecting prostate cancer. J Urol. 2013;190:1721–7.

2. Baco E, Rud E, Eri LM, Moen G, Vlatkovic L, Svindland A, et al. A randomized controlled trial to assess and compare the outcomes of two-core prostate biopsy guided by fused magnetic resonance and Transrectal ultrasound images and traditional 12-core systematic biopsy. Eur Urol. 2016;69:149–56.

3. Siddiqui MM, Rais-Bahrami S, Truong H, Stamatakis L, Vourganti S, Nix J, et al. Magnetic resonance imaging/ultrasound-fusion biopsy significantly upgrades prostate cancer versus systematic 12-core transrectal ultrasound biopsy. Eur Urol. 2013;64:713–9.

4. Miyagawa T, Ishikawa S, Kimura T, Suetomi T, Tsutsumi M, Irie T, et al. Real-time virtual sonography for navigation during targeted prostate biopsy using magnetic resonance imaging data. Int J Urol. 2010;17:855–60.

5. Epstein JI, Walsh PC, Carmichael M, Brendler CB. Pathologic and clinical findings to predict tumor extent of nonpalpable (stage T1c) prostate cancer. JAMA. 1994;271:368–74.

6. Panebianco V, Barchetti F, Sciarra A, Ciardi A, Indino EL, Papalia R, et al. Multiparametric magnetic resonance imaging vs. standard care in men being evaluated for prostate cancer: a randomized study. Urol Oncol. 2015;33(17):e1–7.

7. Pokorny MR, de Rooij M, Duncan E, Schröder FH, Parkinson R, Barentsz JO, et al. Prospective study of diagnostic accuracy comparing prostate cancer detection by transrectal ultrasound-guided biopsy versus magnetic resonance (MR) imaging with subsequent MR-guided biopsy in men without previous prostate biopsies. Eur Urol. 2014;66:22–9.

8. Ahmed HU, El-Shater Bosaily A, Brown LC, Gabe R, Kaplan R, Parmar MK, et al. Diagnostic accuracy of multi-parametric MRI and TRUS biopsy in prostate cancer (PROMIS): a paired validating confirmatory study. Lancet. 2017;389:815–22.

9. Hossack T, Patel MI, Huo A, Brenner P, Yuen C, Spernat D, et al. Location and pathological characteristics of cancers in radical prostatectomy specimens identified by transperineal biopsy compared to transrectal biopsy. J Urol. 2012;188:781–5.

10. Cash H, Günzel K, Maxeiner A, Stephan C, Fischer T, Durmus T, et al. Prostate cancer detection on transrectal ultrasonography-guided random biopsy despite negative real-time magnetic resonance imaging/ultrasonography fusion-guided targeted biopsy: reasons for targeted biopsy failure. BJU Int. 2016;118:35–43.

11. Wang X, Qian Y, Liu B, Cao L, Fan Y, Zhang JJ, et al. High-b-value diffusion-weighted MRI for the detection of prostate cancer at 3 T. Clin Radiol. 2014; 69:1165–70.

12. Othman AE, Falkner F, Weiss J, Kruck S, Grimm R, Martirosian P, et al. Effect of temporal resolution on diagnostic performance of dynamic contrast-enhanced magnetic resonance imaging of the prostate. Investig Radiol. 2016;51:290–6.

13. Muthigi A, George AK, Sidana A, Kongnyuy M, Simon R, Moreno V, et al. Missing the mark: prostate cancer upgrading by systematic biopsy over magnetic resonance imaging/Transrectal ultrasound fusion biopsy. J Urol. 2017;197:327–34.

14. Zhao C, Gao G, Fang D, Li F, Yang X, Wang H, et al. The efficiency of multiparametric magnetic resonance imaging (mpMRI) using PI-RADS version 2 in the diagnosis of clinically significant prostate cancer. Clin Imaging. 2016;40:885–8.

15. Vargas HA, Hötker AM, Goldman DA, Moskowitz CS, Gondo T, Matsumoto K, et al. Updated prostate imaging reporting and data system (PIRADS v2) recommendations for the detection of clinically significant prostate cancer using multiparametric MRI: critical evaluation using whole-mount pathology as standard of reference. Eur Radiol. 2016;26:1606–12.

16. Barentsz JO, Richenberg J, Clements R, Choyke P, Verma S, Villeirs G, et al. ESUR prostate MR guidelines 2012. Eur Radiol. 2012;22:746–57.

17. Rosenkrantz AB, Verma S, Choyke P, Eberhardt SC, Eggener SE, Gaitonde K, et al. Prostate magnetic resonance imaging and magnetic resonance imaging targeted biopsy in patients with a prior negative biopsy: a consensus statement by AUA and SAR. J Urol. 2016;196:1613–8.

18. Schimmöller L, Quentin M, Arsov C, Lanzman RS, Hiester A, Rabenalt R, et al. Inter-reader agreement of the ESUR score for prostate MRI using in-bore MRI-guided biopsies as the reference standard. Eur Radiol. 2013;23:3185–90.

8

Upper urinary tract stone disease in patients with poor performance status: active stone removal or conservative management?

Shimpei Yamashita[1*], Yasuo Kohjimoto[1], Yasuo Hirabayashi[2], Takashi Iguchi[1], Akinori Iba[1], Masatoshi Higuchi[3], Hiroyuki Koike[4], Takahito Wakamiya[1], Satoshi Nishizawa[1] and Isao Hara[1]

Abstract

Background: It remains controversial as to whether active stone removal should be performed in patients with poor performance status because of their short life expectancy and perioperative risks. Our objectives were to evaluate treatment outcomes of active stone removal in patients with poor performance status and to compare life prognosis with those managed conservatively.

Methods: We retrospectively reviewed 74 patients with Eastern Cooperative Oncology Group performance status 3 or 4 treated for upper urinary tract calculi at our four hospitals between January 2009 and March 2016. Patients were classified into either surgical treatment group or conservative management group based on the presence of active stone removal. Stone-free rate and perioperative complications in surgical treatment group were reviewed. In addition, we compared overall survival and stone-specific survival between the two groups. Cox proportional hazards analysis was performed to investigate predictors of overall survival and stone-specific survival.

Results: Fifty-two patients (70.3%) underwent active stone removal (surgical treatment group) by extracorporeal shock wave lithotripsy ($n = 6$), ureteroscopy ($n = 39$), percutaneous nephrolithotomy (n = 6) or nephrectomy ($n = 1$). The overall stone-free rate was 78.8% and perioperative complication was observed in nine patients (17.3%). Conservative treatment was undergone by 22 patients (29.7%) (conservative management group). Two-year overall survival rates in surgical treatment and conservative management groups were 88.0% and 38.4%, respectively ($p < 0.01$) and two-year stone-specific survival rates in the two groups were 100.0% and 61.3%, respectively (p < 0.01). On multivariate analysis, stone removal was not significant, but was considered a possible favorable predictor for overall survival ($p = 0.07$). Moreover, stone removal was the only independent predictor of stone-specific survival (p < 0.01).

Conclusions: Active stone removal for patients with poor performance status could be performed safely and effectively. Compared to conservative management, surgical stone treatment achieved longer overall survival and stone-specific survival.

Keywords: Poor performance status, Urolithiasis, Extracorporeal shock wave lithotripsy, Ureteroscopy, Percutaneous nephrolithotomy, Prognosis

* Correspondence: keito608@wakayama-med.ac.jp
[1]Department of Urology, Wakayama Medical University, 811-1 Kimiidera, Wakayama City, Wakayaka 641-0012, Japan
Full list of author information is available at the end of the article

Background

The rate of aging (65 years of age or older) worldwide is expected to rise from 7.6% in 2010 to 18.3% in 2060 as the population increases [1]. As the rate of aging rises, patients with poor performance status (PS) are also expected to increase worldwide. These patients have increased risk of urolithiasis because of various factors, including hypercalciuria associated with osteoporosis, urinary stasis, urinary tract infection and low fluid intake. Therefore, management of urolithiasis in patients with poor PS is emerging as a crucial issue in urology.

However, debate exists as to whether active stone removal should be performed in patients with poor PS. One of the reasons for such debate is that patients with poor PS have poor prognoses because of their comorbidities [2–4]. In addition, active stone removal for poor PS patients is introduced to deal with various problems, such as risks involved in their comorbidities, decreased immune competence, coexisting urinary tract infection and restriction on surgical positioning. Nonetheless, it is necessary to investigate whether active stone removal for patients with poor PS is beneficial.

To date, there have been few reports concerning the optimal management of urolithiasis in these patients. In this study, we evaluate treatment outcomes of active stone removal in patients with poor PS and compared life prognosis with those managed conservatively.

Methods

Patients

Between January 2009 and March 2016, 81 patients with Eastern Cooperative Oncology Group (ECOG) PS 3 or 4 were hospitalized for upper urinary tract calculi at the Wakayama Medical University Hospital, Hashimoto Municipal Hospital, Kinan Hospital and Rinku General Medical Center. Of these, seven patients who experienced spontaneous stone expulsion were excluded and 74 patients were enrolled in this study. This retrospective study was approved by the Institutional Review Board of Wakayama Medical University (approval number 1922).

Clinical information including age, gender, ECOG PS, medical history, Charlson Comorbidity Index (CCI), serum creatinine on admission, coexisting acute pyelonephritis, urinary drainage and stone characteristics were collected retrospectively from medical records. Urinary drainage was defined as placement of ureteral stent or nephrostomy tube on admission. Stone characteristics, including size, location and number, were assessed by non-contrast computed tomography (NCCT) and stone size was defined as the largest diameter of the major stone. In addition, data were collected on the management of any stones, such as active stone removal, including shock wave lithotripsy (SWL), ureteroscopy (URS) and percutaneous nephrolithotomy

(PCNL), and observation without operation. Patients were classified into two groups, surgical treatment group and conservative management group, based on occurrence of active stone removal. The treatment policy was left to the judgment of attending physicians, patients and their families.

Outcomes

We investigated the stone-free rate (SFR) and perioperative complications (Clavien-Dindo system grade II or more) in the operation group. Stone-free status was determined using NCCT within 3 months after operation and was defined as the absence of stones or residual fragments of less than 4 mm. We also investigated stone-related event-free survival (EFS), with events defined as stone-related symptoms and interventions, and recurrence-free survival (RFS), with recurrence defined as new stone formation and/or regrowth of residual fragments on imaging studies as well as any stone-related events. In addition, we defined stone-specific survival (SSS) as a net survival measure representing urolithiasis survival in the absence of other causes of death, and compared overall survival (OS) and SSS between the surgical treatment group and the conservative management group.

Statistical analyses

Chi-square test, Fisher's exact test and Mann-Whitney U test were used for univariate analyses to compare variables between surgical treatment group and conservative management group. EFS, RFS, OS and SSS rates were calculated by the Kaplan-Meier method with the hospitalization date as the starting point. Univariate and multivariate analyses of OS and SSS were performed to compare the prognostic factors in a Cox proportional hazards analysis. Any P values less than 0.05 were considered significant. All statistical analyses were performed using JMP Pro 12 (SAS Institute, USA).

Results

Patient demographics

Patient demographics and stone characteristics are summarized in Table 1. The median age was 82 years (range: 36–98 years) and 51 (68.9%) patients were females. ECOG PS was 3 in 19 (25.7%) patients and 4 in 55 (74.3%) patients. Sixty-one (82.4%) patients presented acute pyelonephritis. The median stone size was 11.5 mm (range: 2–53 mm). More information about patient demographics and stone characteristics can be found in Additional file 1: Table S1.

Of 74 patients included in this study, 22 patients (29.7%) did not undergo stone removal and were classified as conservative management group. In conservative management group, 15 patients (68.2%), three patients

Table 1 Patient demographics

	Total	Management		p value (surgical treatment vs. conservative management)
		Surgical treatment	Conservative management	
No. patients (%)	74	52 (70.3)	22 (29.7)	
Age, years	82 (36–98)	76 (36–92)	86 (68–98)	<0.01
Female, n (%)	51 (68.9)	33 (63.5)	18 (81.8)	0.17
ECOG PS, n (%)	19 (25.7)	16 (30.8)	3 (13.6)	0.15
3	55 (74.3)	36 (69.2)	19 (86.4)	
4				
Charlson comorbidity index	2 (0–8)	2 (0–6)	2 (0–8)	0.82
Serum creainine on admission, mg/dL	1.01 (0.33–5.49)	0.89 (0.44–5.49)	1.26 (0.33–3.83)	0.28
History of urinary calculi, n (%)	20 (27.0)	16 (30.8)	4 (18.2)	0.39
Coexisting acute pyelonephritis, n (%)	61 (82.4)	40 (76.9)	21 (95.5)	0.09
Urinary drainage	61 (82.4)	43 (82.7)	18 (81.8)	1.00
Bilateral stone, n (%)	7 (9.5)	7 (13.5)	0 (0.0)	0.09
Stone position, n (%)				
Kidney	17 (23.0)	14 (26.9)	3 (13.6)	
Ureter	44 (59.5)	28 (53.9)	16 (72.7)	
Kidney and ureter	13 (17.6)	10 (19.2)	3 (13.6)	
Stone size, mm	11.5 (2–53)	12 (2–53)	10.5 (4–35)	0.82
Multiple stones, n (%)	41 (55.4)	28 (53.9)	13 (59.1)	0.79

Abbreviations: ECOG, Eastern Cooperative Oncology Group, *PS* performance status
Continuous variables are shown in "median (range)" form

(13.6%) and four patients (18.2%) had a ureteral stent, a nephrostomy tube and neither of these, respectively. A further 52 (70.3%) patients underwent active stone removal and were classified as surgical treatment group patients. The median interval between first admission and definitive therapy in surgical treatment group was 41 days (range: 2–243 days). The patients with acute pyelonephritis at admission underwent surgical treatment after improvement of infections. Comparing patients in surgical treatment group and those in conservative management group, the median age of patients in conservative management group was 86 years and significantly older than in surgical treatment group ($p < 0.01$). Coexisting acute pyelonephritis and unilateral stones seemed to be more frequently observed in conservative management group compared with surgical treatment group ($p = 0.09$ and p = 0.09, respectively).

Treatment outcomes in surgical treatment group
Patients in operation group were treated by SWL ($n = 6$, 8.8%), URS ($n = 39$, 52.7%), PCNL ($n = 6$, 8.1%) or nephrectomy ($n = 1$, 1.4%). All PCNL cases were performed in a prone split-leg position and combined with retrograde flexible ureteroscopy. Overall SFR in operation group was 78.8% and by the operative treatment

method, 50.0% in SWL, 87.2% in URS and 50.0% in PCNL (Table 2). Nine patients (17.3%) experienced perioperative complications. Postoperative pyelonephritis (Clavien-Dindo system grade II) were observed in eight patients (one out of six SWL patients, six out of 39 URS patients and one out of six PCNL patients) and other complication, namely pseudoaneurysm (Clavien-Dindo system grade III), was observed in one out of six PCNL patients (Table 2).

Two-year and five-year RFS rates in surgical treatment group were 60.2% and 42.1%, respectively (Fig. 1a). On the other hand, two-year and five-year EFS rates were 86.0% and 75.4%, respectively (Fig. 1b).

Comparison of overall survival and stone-specific survival rates between surgical treatment group and conservative management group
In entire cohort, nine patients (12.2%) died of pyelonephritis or renal failure associated with urolithiasis and 17 patients (23.0%) died of other causes during the observation period (median 23 months, range: 1–78 months). A total of 15 patients in conservative management group died and, of these patients, 12 patients (80.0%), 1 patient (6.7%) and 2 patients (13.3%) had a ureteral stent, a nephrostomy tube and neither of these,

Table 2 Stone-free rates and perioperative complications in operation group

| | No. pts. | Stone-free pts., n = (%) | Perioperative complications, n = (%) | | |
			Postoperative pyelonephritis	Others	Total
SWL	6	3 (50.0)	1 (16.7)	0 (0.0)	1 (16.7)
URS	39	34 (87.2)	6 (15.4)	0 (0.0)	6 (15.4)
PCNL	6	3 (50.0)	1 (16.7)	1 (16.7)	2 (33.3)
Nephrectomy	1	1 (100.0)	0 (0.0)	0 (0.0)	0 (0.0)
Total	52	41 (78.8)	8 (15.4)	1 (1.9)	9 (17.3%)

respectively. Two-year OS rates in surgical treatment and conservative management groups were 88.0% and 38.4%, respectively ($p < 0.01$, Fig. 2a), while two-year SSS rates in surgical treatment and conservative management groups were 100.0 and 61.3% ($p < 0.01$, Fig. 2b).

Associations between various parameters and overall survival

Univariate and multivariate Cox proportional hazards regression models were used to investigate predictors of OS (Table 3). Among several predictors, age ($p < 0.01$), female ($p = 0.02$) and stone removal ($p < 0.01$) were identified as significant predictors for OS on univariate analysis. Furthermore, CCI trended toward significance ($p = 0.06$). Of these factors, age (HR 1.08, 95% CI 1.02–1.15) and CCI (HR 1.36, 95% CI 1.10–1.68) were independent unfavorable predictors of OS on multivariate analysis. Stone removal was not significant, but was considered a possible favorable predictor of OS (HR 0.43, 95% CI 0.16–1.09).

Associations between various parameters and stone-specific survival

Table 4 shows the results of univariate and multivariate Cox proportional hazards regression models of factors which predict SSS. Age ($p < 0.01$) and stone removal ($p < 0.01$) were significantly associated with SSS in univariate analysis. Female gender trended toward significance ($p = 0.08$). Of the factors, stone removal was the only independent predictor of SSS in multivariate analysis (HR 0.06, 95% CI 0.00–0.43).

Discussion

We analyzed the treatment outcomes of active stone removal in patients with poor PS and compared life prognosis with those managed conservatively. In this study, we made three important clinical observations.

First, if patients who are suitable for active stone removal are appropriately selected, active stone removal could be performed safely, in spite of their poor PS. One of the main reasons for avoiding surgical treatment for patients with poor PS is the risk of perioperative complications, especially infectious disease. A review of the current literature on the management of urolithiasis in patients with spinal cord injury showed that the overall complication rate in patients with spinal cord injury is higher than in the general population, and the majority of these are infectious in nature are due to the associated medical comorbidities and chronic bacteriuria [5]. In our study, postoperative pyelonephritis was observed in 16.7% (1/6 cases), 15.4% (6/39 cases) and 16.7% (1/6 cases) of the patients who underwent SWL, URS and PCNL, respectively. This was higher than previously reported [6–9]. However, major perioperative complications (Clavien-Dindo system grade III or more) were

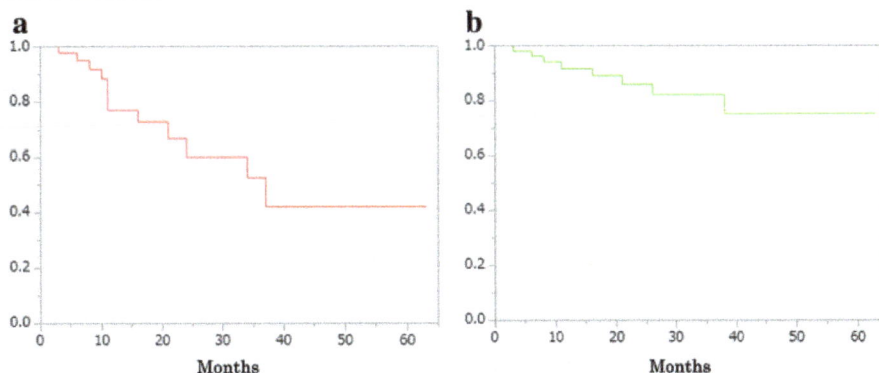

Fig. 1 a Stone recurrence-free survival rate and **b** Stone-related event-free survival rate in operation group

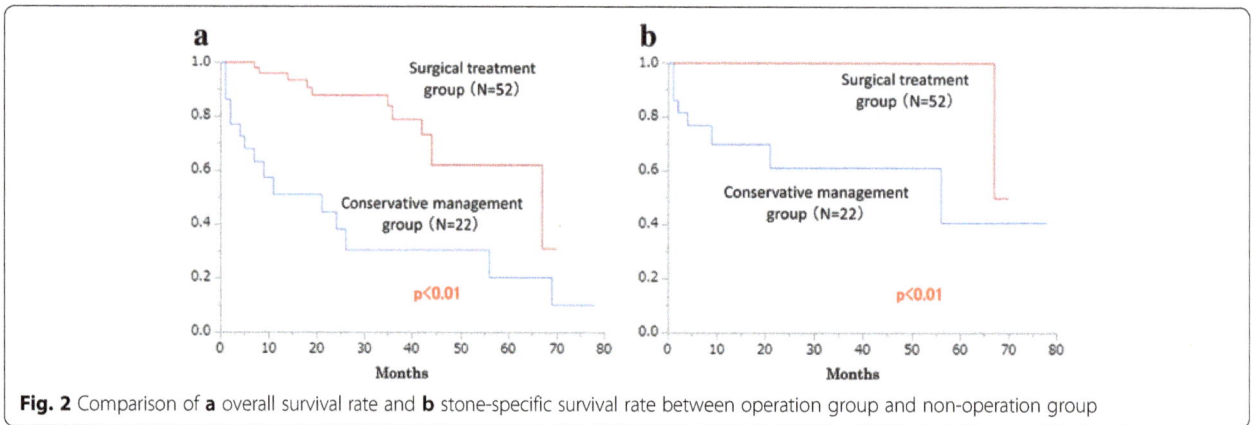

Fig. 2 Comparison of **a** overall survival rate and **b** stone-specific survival rate between operation group and non-operation group

observed in only one patient and no patients expired perioperatively. These results suggest that perioperative complications were acceptable, given the comorbidities in patients with poor PS. In spite of this, these results do not necessarily mean that active stone removal, even for patients in conservative management group, could be performed safely. Patient backgrounds are different between surgical treatment and conservative management groups. We suggest that active stone removal for patients with poor PS could be performed safely as long as perioperative risks are assessed and managed carefully.

Second, results of the survival analyses suggested that patients who had active interventions achieved longer survival in spite of their poor PS. Another reason why physicians choose conservative treatment for patients with poor PS is the assumption that they have poor prognoses because of the multiple comorbidities. Slot et al. reported that the median survival of patients with poor PS resulting from ischaemic stroke was 2.5 years after the stroke [3]. Xie et al. reported that the median survival of patients with dementia was 4.5 years after the onset [2]. Hossain et al. reported that approximately one in five people with spinal cord injury who are wheelchair-dependent die within 2 years of discharge from hospital [10]. Considering the results of these

studies, it is questionable whether active stone removal is recommended for patients with poor PS. However, to our knowledge, there are no published studies related to the influence of stone removal on patients with poor PS.

In the present study, the two-year OS rate in the surgical treatment group (88.0%) was better than that in the conservative management group (38.4%). Multivariate Cox proportional hazards regression model shows that stone removal is the only independent predictor of SSS. In addition, stone removal is not significant, but is considered a possible favorable predictor of OS. These survival analyses showed that the patients who had active interventions achieved their longer survival in spite of their poor PS. However, these results do not necessarily suggest that active stone removal in patients with poor PS could prevent stone-related death and may improve their prognosis, because patient characteristics are different between two groups. The median age of patients in the conservative management group was 86 years, significantly older than that in the surgical treatment group ($p < 0.01$). Moreover, preoperative pyelonephritis seemed to be more frequently observed in the conservative management group compared with the surgical treatment group ($p = 0.09$). Although we adjusted the patient backgrounds using various factors, such as age, sex,

Table 3 Univariate and multivariate analyses of associations between various parameters and overall survival

Variable	Univariate analysis			Multivariate analysis		
	HR	95% CI	p value	HR	95% CI	p value
Age, year	1.09	1.05–1.15	<0.01	1.08	1.02–1.15	<0.01
Female (vs Male)	3.10	1.17–10.70	0.02	1.92	0.63–7.41	0.26
Charlson Comorbidity Index	1.28	0.98–1.64	0.06	1.36	1.10–1.68	<0.01
Coexisting acute pyelonephritis	1.53	0.58–5.26	0.42			
Urinary drainage	0.94	0.38–2.83	0.90			
Stone size, mm	0.99	0.94–1.03	0.52			
Multiple stones	0.89	0.41–1.96	0.75			
Stone removal	0.22	0.10–0.49	<0.01	0.43	0.16–1.09	0.07

Table 4 Univariate and multivariate analyses of associations between various parameters and stone-specific survival

Variable	Univariate analysis			Multivariate analysis		
	HR	95% CI	p value	HR	95% CI	p value
Age, year	1.10	1.02–1.22	<0.01	1.01	0.91–1.14	0.90
Female (vs Male)	4.59	0.83–85.69	0.08	3.80	0.39–95.67	0.27
Charlson Comorbidity Index	1.21	0.79–1.78	0.36			
Coexisting acute pyelonephritis	1.99	0.36–37.98	0.47			
Urinary drainage	0.43	0.11–2.07	0.26			
Stone size, mm	0.97	0.86–1.04	0.45			
Multiple stones	1.55	0.40–7.39	0.53			
Stone removal	0.05	0.00–0.27	<0.01	0.06	0.00–0.43	<0.01

coexisting acute pyelonephritis and CCI, as possible in multivariate Cox proportional hazards regression model, other differences which are not reflected in these factors could have a strong influence on the patients' prognosis. Therefore, randomized controlled trials or a large-scale propensity score matching analysis using even more factors are necessary to make clear whether active stone removal in patients with poor PS could prevent stone-related death and could improve their prognosis.

Third, active stone removal for patients with poor PS could prevent stone-related events. In the present study, overall SFR in the surgical treatment group was 78.8%. This is acceptable considering the adverse conditions specific to patients with poor PS. However, when new stone formation and regrowth of residual fragments were included in the definition of recurrence, two-year and five-year RFS rates were low at 60.2% and 42.1%, respectively. This might be because of risks of stone formation specific to patients with poor PS such as hypercalciuria associated with osteoporosis, urinary stasis, urinary tract infection and low fluid intake. In addition, prevention of stone recurrence is also difficult in these patients because of decreased accessibility to medical services and compliance to fluid intake and medication. However, given the fact that their life expectancy is generally short, we believe that it is more important to prevent stone-related symptoms and avoid further interventions for stones, rather than preventing radiographic recurrence. From that point of view, two-year EFS rate of 86.0% and five-year EFS rate of 75.4% were considered to be satisfactory.

To reduce the recurrence rate, the achievement of stone-free status is important. In our study, by the operative treatment method, SFR was 50.0% in SWL, 87.2% in URS and 50.0% in PCNL, respectively. The main cause of the low SFR in PCNL cases was considered to be larger stone size (median 27.5 mm, range 9–53 mm) compared with other operations. On the other hand, the reasons for the low SFR in SWL might include the difficulty of spontaneous expulsion of fragments after

lithotripsy because of low fluid intake and physical activities in patients with poor PS. Therefore, our results suggest that URS is preferable to SWL in the treatment of patients with poor PS.

There are several limitations to the present study. First, this was a retrospective study undertaken at several centers with a relatively small number of patients. Second, treatment policy was left to the judgment of attending physicians, patients and their families. In addition, this study targeted only hospitalized patients and did not include most patients with asymptomatic calculi.

Despite these limitations in our study, we were able to demonstrate that active stone removal for patients with poor PS could be performed safely and the patients who had active interventions achieved their longer survival with infrequent stone-related events as long as perioperative risks are assessed and managed carefully. To establish the guideline for the optimal management of urolithiasis in these patients, further prospective analysis involving a multicenter approach is required. In addition, an effective method to prevent stone recurrence is essential as it has been a challenge particularly for the patients with poor PS.

Conclusions

Active stone removal for patients with poor PS could be performed safely and effectively. Compared to conservative management, surgical stone treatment achieved longer OS and SSS.

Abbreviations

CCI: Charlson Comorbidity Index; ECOG: Eastern Cooperative Oncology Group; EFS: Stone-related event-free survival; NCCT: Non-contrast computed tomography; OS: Overall survival; PCNL: Percutaneous nephrolithotomy; PS: Performance status; RFS: Recurrence-free survival; SFR: Stone-free rate; SSS: Stone-specific survival; SWL: Shock wave lithotripsy; URS: Ureteroscopy

Acknowledgements
We would like to thank Prof Shimokawa for assistance in statistical analysis.

Funding
This study was supported by third research grant from the Japanese Society on Urolithiasis Research. The study protocol has been peer-reviewed by the funding body.

Authors' contributions
SY and YK designed the study. YH, TI, AI, MH, HK, TW and SN acquired the data. SY performed statistical analyses and drafted the manuscript. SY, YK and IH interpreted study results and finalized the manuscript. All authors read and approved the final manuscript.

Competing interests
The authors declare that they have no competing interests.

Author details
[1]Department of Urology, Wakayama Medical University, 811-1 Kimiidera, Wakayama City, Wakayaka 641-0012, Japan. [2]Department of Urology, Hashimoto Municipal Hospital, 2-8-1 Ominedai, Hashimoto City, Wakayama 648-0005, Japan. [3]Department of Urology, Kinan Hospital, 46-70 Shinjyo, Tanabe City, Wakayama 646-8588, Japan. [4]Department of Urology, Rinku General Medical Center, 2-23 Rinkuouraikita, Izumisano City, Osaka 598-8577, Japan.

References
1. United Nations World Population Prospects:The 2012 Revision (http://esa.un.org/unpd/wpp/).
2. Xie J, Brayne C, Matthews FE. Survival times in people with dementia: analysis from population based cohort study with 14 year follow-up. BMJ (Clinical research ed). 2008;336(7638):258–62.
3. Slot KB, Berge E, Dorman P, Lewis S, Dennis M, Sandercock P. Impact of functional status at six months on long term survival in patients with ischaemic stroke: prospective cohort studies. BMJ (Clinical research ed). 2008;336(7640):376–9.
4. Mitchell SL, Teno JM, Kiely DK, Shaffer ML, Jones RN, Prigerson HG, Volicer L, Givens JL, Hamel MB. The clinical course of advanced dementia. N Engl J Med. 2009;361(16):1529–38.
5. Nabbout P, Slobodov G, Culkin DJ. Surgical management of urolithiasis in spinal cord injury patients. Current urology reports. 2014;15(6):408.
6. Guidelines on Urolithiasis.European Association of Urology. (http://uroweb.org/guideline/urolithiasis/).
7. Logarakis NF, Jewett MA, Luymes J, Honey RJ. Variation in clinical outcome following shock wave lithotripsy. J Urol. 2000;163(3):721–5.
8. Labate G, Modi P, Timoney A, Cormio L, Zhang X, Louie M, Grabe M, Rosette On Behalf Of The Croes Pcnl Study Group J. The percutaneous nephrolithotomy global study: classification of complications. Journal of endourology/Endourological Society. 2011;25(8):1275–80.
9. Seitz C, Desai M, Hacker A, Hakenberg OW, Liatsikos E, Nagele U, Tolley D. Incidence, prevention, and management of complications following percutaneous nephrolitholapaxy. Eur Urol. 2012;61(1):146–58.
10. Hossain MS, Rahman MA, Herbert RD, Quadir MM, Bowden JL, Harvey LA. Two-year survival following discharge from hospital after spinal cord injury in Bangladesh. Spinal Cord. 2016;54(2):132–6.

9

Expression of cannabinoid 1 and, 2 receptors and the effects of cannabinoid 1 and, 2 receptor agonists on detrusor overactivity associated with bladder outlet obstruction in rats

Sung Dae Kim[1], Kang Jun Cho[2] and Joon Chul Kim[2*]

Abstract

Background: This study investigated changes in the expression of cannabinoid (CB) receptors and the effects of CB1 and CB2 agonists on detrusor overactivity (DO) associated with bladder outlet obstruction (BOO) in rats.

Methods: Male Sprague Dawley rats were randomly assigned to four groups ($n = 10$) in each group. The control group comprised sham-operated rats. A animals in the BOO, CB1 agonist and CB2 agonist groups all underwent BOO surgery. Three weeks postoperatively, cystometrography (CMG) was performed on all rats. After confirming the presence of DO in the CB1 and CB2 agonist groups, a CB1 agonist (WIN 55,212–2) and a CB2 agonist (CB65) were instilled intravesically, and CMG was repeated. CMG parameters, including the contraction interval (CI) and contraction pressure (CP) were then analyzed. The bladders of rats in all four groups were excised following CMG. Immunofluorescence staining and Western blotting were performed to localize CB1 and CB2 and measure their expression levels in the urothelium and detrusor muscle.

Results: The CI was significantly longer and the CP was significantly lower in the CB1 agonist group than in the BOO group. CI and CP in the CB2 agonist group showed the same results. CB1 receptor immunofluorescence staining signals and immunoreactive bands in Western blotting were increased in the BOO group compared with results in the control group. Similarly, results for the CB2 receptor were also increased in the BOO group, although this difference was not significant. The CMG parameters in the BOO group were significantly improved by the inhibitory effects of CB1 and CB2 agonists on BOO-associated DO. The expression of CB1 was significantly increased in the urothelium and detrusor muscle in BOO-associated DO, but no significant change in CB2 expression was observed.

Conclusions: CB1 and CB2 receptors, especially CB1, play a role in the pathophysiology of BOO-associated DO, and could serve as therapeutic targets.

Keywords: Bladder outlet obstruction, Cannabinoid, Overactive, Receptor, Urinary bladder

* Correspondence: kjc@catholic.ac.kr
[2]Department of Urology, Bucheon St. Mary's hospital, College of Medicine,
The Catholic University of Korea, Sosa-Ro 327, Wonmi-gu, Bucheon-si,
Gyeonggi-do, Seoul 14647, South Korea
Full list of author information is available at the end of the article

Background

Detrusor overactivity (DO) seen in patients with overactive bladder (OAB) symptoms appears accompanied with bladder -outlet obstruction (BOO) in approximately 52% of cases [1]. The main causes of DO have been suggested to be associated with functional changes in the urothelium of the bladder. The importance of the urothelium as a physicochemical organoleptic cell layer has been shown to be significant because of the associations among urothelium, sensory neurons and smooth muscle cells, therefore, the development of a new drugs based on these interrelationships among in progress at an active area of research. Various receptors of the urothelium in the bladder, such as cannabinoid, acetylcholine, transient receptor potential vanilloid 4, and calcium-activated potassium channel receptors, mediate the pathophysiology of DO [2–6].

Cannabinoids, chemical components of marijuana, have been used to treat pain and vomiting for a long time. In recent years, cannabinoid receptors were found in the urothelium and detrusor muscle in the bladder, and it is believed that they are closely related to pain and sensory neurotransmission [7]. In addition, beneficial effects have been associated with the cannabinoid receptors cannabinoid-1 (CB1) and cannabinoid-2 (CB2) [8], which are known to be expressed in the urothelium and detrusor muscle in the bladder. Activation of these receptors could modulate bladder afferent activity and the micturition reflex [9]. It has been reported that many patients with multiple sclerosis and OAB showed improved after the administration of cannabinoid-based extracts [10]. Results from an animal model of spinal cord injury with the administration of a CB agonist and antagonist show that CB receptors play a key role in neurogenic bladder dysfunction [11]. Therefore, CB1 and CB2 receptors may function in the urinary bladder to help control bladder function. Recently, experimental studies have shown that CB receptors appear to be involved in afferent signaling pathways. Specially, Gratzke et al. noted that in rats with partial BOO treated with a CB agonist, the ability to empty the bladder was preserved, while non-voiding contraction frequency was decreased compared to that in controls [12]. In addition, Walczak et al. showed that the co-localization of CB1 receptors and P2X3 receptors in the bladders of mice declined in response to mechanically evoked bladder afferent activity in the pelvic nerve after the intravesical administration of a CB agonist [13]. Our study was designed based on the research findings discussed above.

We investigated changes in the expression of CB1 and CB2 receptors and the effects of CB1 and CB2 agonists on DO associated with BOO in male rats.

Methods

Experimental animals

This study was carried out using 16-week-old male Sprague Dawley rats weighing 250–300 g (Orient Bio Co., Seongnam, Korea). The rats were housed at room temperature (20–26 °C) under a 12-hlight/dark cycle with unlimited access to food. 40 rats were randomly assigned to four groups. The control group ($n = 10$) comprised sham-operated rats. The remaining three groups were the BOO group ($n = 10$), CB1 agonist group ($n = 10$) and CB2 agonist group ($n = 10$), all of which underwent BOO surgery. We used WIN55,212–2, and CB65 as representative CB1 and CB2 receptor agonists, respectively. For the CB1 and CB2 agonist groups, drugs were instilled into the bladder of each rat.

BOO procedure

Experimental rats were anesthetized using an intramuscular injection of 5 mg/kg xylazine and 15 mg/kg ketamine. A suprapubic midline incision was made in the lower abdomen of rats. The bladder neck and periurethral areas were dissected out. A 25-G needle sheath was inserted into the urethra, and the bladder neck was ligated using 3–0 silk, after which the sheath was removed. In the sham-operated control animals, the bladder neck was very loosely ligated so as to not cause any obstruction.

Cystometrography (CMG)

CMG was performed on all rats 3 weeks postoperatively, when we confirmed the presence of DO in the all three groups undergoing BOO surgery. A 25-G needle connected to polyethylene tubing was inserted into the bladder dome. The tubing was connected to a pressure transducer and an infusion pump using 3-way stopcock. The bladder was emptied and then continuously filled with warm saline using a Harvard syringe pump. CMG parameters including contraction interval (CI) and contraction pressure (CP) were recorded using a polygraph apparatus (Grass 7D, Grass Institute Co., Quincy, USA). In addition, the bladder was emptied in the CB1 and CB2 agonist groups, and a penile clamp was used to impede urination. Then 50 µM/kg of a CB1 receptor agonist (WIN55,212–2) and 10 µM/kg CB2 receptor agonist (CB65) in 0.2 mL of saline was injected through a needle into the bladder of each rat in these two groups. Then, we repeated CMG 1 h after the administration of each drug, with the bladder filled with saline.

Bladder collection and immunofluorescence staining

After CMG was completed, the bladders of all rats were excised, cut vertically and dissected under a microscope into the urothelium and detrusor muscle. Bladder sections were frozen in liquid nitrogen for further analysis. Using optimal cutting temperature solution and, polyethylene glycol, the frozen tissues were cut into 3-µm sections. The tissue sections were then rinsed with phosphate-buffered saline (PBS). To inhibit nonspecific immunofluorescence staining, slides were exposed to a blocking solution (1.5% normal goat serum, 1.5% normal horse serum, 1% bovine serum albumin, 0.1% Triton X-100 in PBS) at room temperature for 1 h. Immunolabelling was performed by incubating samples with antibodies against CB1 and CB2 (1:100 dilution, Abcam Ltd., Cambridge, UK) in PBS for 2 h at room temperature. The slides were rinsed three times with PBS and then incubated with the secondary antibody, Alexa Fluor 488-labelled goat anti-rabbit IgG (1:300 dilution, Molecular Probes, Eugene, USA) at room temperature for 1 h. After washing in PBS, the slides were stained with 4′,6-diamidino-2-phenylindole (Vector Laboratories, Burlingame, USA), and mounted for examination using light microscopy (BX50, Olympus, Tokyo, Japan). Staining was visualized using fluorescence microscopy, and digital images were captured. Because CB1 and CB2 receptor-expressing cells were stained green, their immunoreactivity was evaluated as the percentage of green-stained area in three random fields per image using an imaging analysis program (IMTi-Solution ver.10.1, IMTi-Solution Inc., Montreal, Canada).

Western blotting

Western blotting was performed to compare the expression levels of CB and CB2 receptors in the urothelium and detrusor muscle layer in rats from each group. Frozen tissue samples were pulverized and then homogenized at 4°C using a Qproteome Mammalian Protein preparation kit (Qiagen, Hilden, Germany). The homogenates were centrifuged at 900 g for 20 min at 4°C. The pellets were discarded, and the supernatant was either used immediately or stored at −70°C. Total protein was measured using a Bradford dye-binding protein assay kit (Bio-Rad Laboratories, Hercules, USA) according to the manufacturer's instructions, and the equivalent of 50 mg of total protein was loaded onto polyacrylamide gels with primary antibodies against CB1 and CB2 receptors. The samples were electrophoresed using a Mini-Protean 3 Cell system (Bio-Rad Laboratories) under constant voltage. After electrophoresis, the proteins were transferred to polyvinylidene fluoride membranes for 2 h at 4°C using a transblot semidry transfer cell (Mini-Protean 3Cell, Bio-Rad). Nonspecific binding sites were blocked

by incubating the membranes with Tris-Tween-buffered saline (TBS-T) containing 10% skim milk and 0.1% Tween 20 for 1 h at 4°C. The membranes were then incubated overnight at 4°C with a biotinylated antibody against either the CB1 or CB2 receptor (1:5000 dilution in TBS-T, Abcam PLC). After washing with TBS-T, the membranes were incubated for 30 min at room temperature with goat anti-rabbit IgG horseradish peroxidase (1:5000 dilution) and then washed. Immunoreactive proteins were detected and visualized using a chemiluminescence reagent (ECL, Amersham International, Bucks, UK).

Statistical analysis

All data were analyzed using Sigma Stat for windows (Version 3.0, SPSS Inc., Chicago, IL, USA). The data are expressed as the mean ± SEM. For comparisons among the groups, one-way analysis of variance (ANOVA) and Newman-Keuls multiple comparison tests were performed with $P < 0.05$ as an indication of statistical significance.

Results

CMG showed that BOO group had a significantly higher CP (28.03 ± 3.94 cmH$_2$O vs. 23.03 ± 3.07 cmH$_2$O, $p < 0.05$) and significantly shorter CI (4.42 ± 0.76 min, vs. 10.52 ± 1.07 min, $p < 0.05$) than the control group, as shown in Table 1. Three weeks postoperatively, the CB1 agonist group had a significantly longer CI (8.61 ± 0.61 min vs. 4.42 ± 0.76 min, $p < 0.05$) and lower CP (19.88 ± 3.14 cmH$_2$O vs. 28.03 ± 3.94 cmH$_2$O, $p < 0.05$) than the BOO group, as did CB2 agonist group (CI 9.51 ± 0.55 min vs. 4.42 ± 0.76 min, $p < 0.05$; CP 23.76 ± 4.78 cmH$_2$O vs. 28.03 ± 3.94 cmH$_2$O, $p < 0.05$). Moreover, the immunofluorescence signal for CB1 receptors was significantly increased in urothelium and detrusor muscles of the BOO group compared with that of control group. The immunofluorescence signal for CB2 receptors was also increased in the BOO group, but this increase was not statistically significant (Fig. 1).

Immunoreactive bands from Western blotting indicated that the expression of both CB1 and CB2 receptors were present in the urothelium and detrusor muscle of rats in all groups. CB1 receptor expression was

Table 1 Cystometrography results for the experimental groups

	Control group (n = 10)	BOO group (n = 10)	CB1 agonist group (n = 10)	CB2 agonist group (n = 10)	P value[a] control vs BOO	BOO vs CB1 agonist	BOO vs CB2 agonist
Contraction Pressure Mean(SD)cmH$_2$O	23.03 (3.07)	28.03 (3.94)	19.88 (3.14)	23.76 (4.78)	< 0.05	< 0.05	< 0.05
Contraction Interval Mean(SD) min	10.52 (1.07)	4.42 (0.76)	8.61 (0.61)	9.51 (0.55)	< 0.05	< 0.05	< 0.05

BOO bladder outlet obstruction, *CB* cannabinoid
[a]analysis of variance test showed significant difference in all 3 parameters among all 3 groups

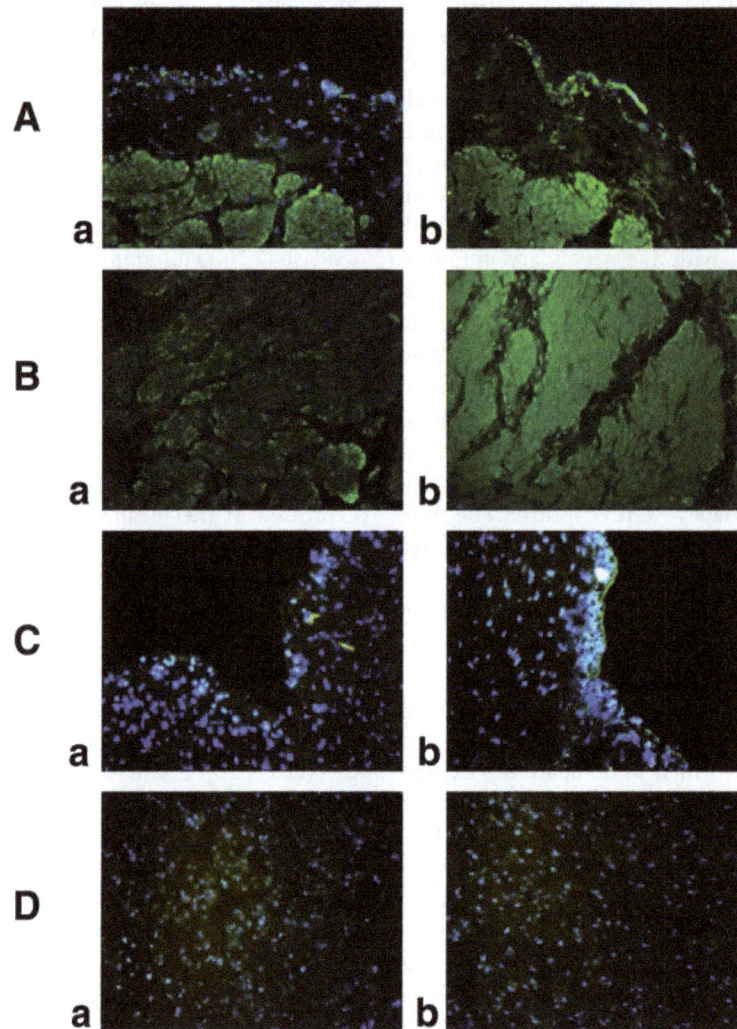

Fig. 1 Immunofluorescence staining of CB1 and CB2 receptors. **a** and **b** show that there were significant increases in CB1 receptor immunoreactivity in the urothelium (*a*) and detrusor muscle (*b*) of rats in the BOO group. **c** and **d** show that there were no differences in CB2 receptor immunoreactivity in the urothelium (*a*) and detrusor muscle (*b*) between the control group and the BOO group. Green shows CB1 or CB2 receptor expressing cells and blue dots show DAPI staining of nuclei. BOO:bladder outlet obstruction. CB:cannabinoid

significantly increased in the BOO group compared with expression in the control group ($p < 0.05$). However, although the immunoreactive bands for the CB2 receptor were also increased in the BOO group, this increase was not statistically significant ($p > 0.05$) (Fig. 2).

Discussion

The animal model used in this study, does not completely represent patients with OAB, but it has been demonstrated in several studies as the best animal model of OAB [14, 15]. The methods used here are based on previous finding, as discussed below. Hedlund et al. reported on CB1 and CB2 receptors, and showed that CB1 and CB2 agonists inhibit nerve-mediated contractions of the mouse bladder [16]. Representative CB1 agonists include, CP55244, WIN55,212–2, delta-9-tetrahydrocannabinol

(THC), arachidonyl-2'-chloroethylamide (ACEA), and nabilone. CB2 agonists, CP55940, CB65. In this study, we used WIN55,212–2 and, CB65 as CB1 and CB2 agonists, respectively. Systemically administered cannabinoids can act at multiple sites, including the bladder and many sites in the central nerve system. Intravesical activation of CB1 does block Nerve Growth Factor-induced increased bladder activity [17]. In addition, according to Tyagi et al., CB1 and CB2 receptors have higher expression rates in the bladder urothelium, and bladder strips incubated for 15 min CB agonists show a decreased detrusor muscle contraction amplitude [8]. Therefore, we thought that intravesically instilling these drugs into the urothelium of bladder could affect detrusor contraction.

We interpret the experimental results of this study as follows. First, the CMG findings of a higher CP and

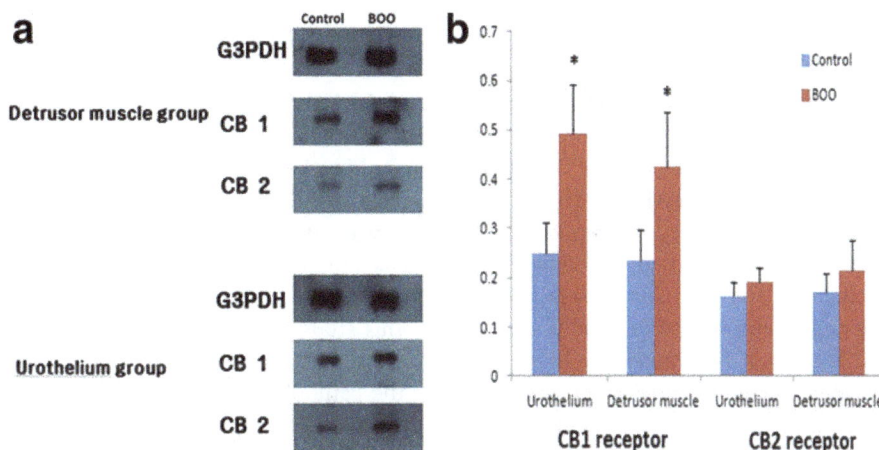

Fig. 2 Comparison of CB1 and CB2 receptors expression levels from Western blot analysis between the control group and the BOO group. CB1 receptor expression was significantly increased in the BOO group compared to the control group ($p < 0.05$). Immunoreactive bands for the CB2 receptor were also increased in the BOO group, but the difference was not significant ($p > 0.05$) **a**: Western blotting **b**: densitometry results relative to G3PDH. Data are expressed as the mean ± SD. * < 0.05 compared with the BOO group. BOO:bladder outlet obstruction, G3PDH:glyceraldehyde-3-phosphate dehydrogenase, CB:cannabinoid

shorter CI in the BOO group than in the control group provided clear evidence that DO was present in the BOO group. The results also showed that DO was significantly improved by the inhibitory effects of CB1 and CB2 receptor agonists. Second, the expression of the CB1 receptor was significantly increased in the urothelium and detrusor muscle in rats with BOO-associated DO, but no significant change in the expression of the CB2 receptor was observed. These findings suggest a key role for CB1 and CB2 receptors, particularly the CB1 receptor, in the regulation of bladder function in rats with BOO-associated DO. Many previous studies have shown that cannabinoids affect bladder DO in patients with OAB symptoms and CMG parameters reflecting sensory function, and they reduce the sensory activity of isolated tissues, and induce antihyperalgesia in animal studies of bladder inflammation [16]. Endocannabinoids relax the detrusor muscle during filling of the bladder by binding to CB1 and CB2 receptors, possibly modulating sensory afferent signals [18]. However, there are also contradictory results from previous studies of the expression and function of CB receptors, thus, the mechanism of this effect remains unclear.

In our study, both Western blotting and immunofluorescence showed that in BOO-associated DO, CB1 receptor expression in the urothelium and detrusor muscle was significantly increased, while CB2 receptor expression was not significantly changed. These results are consistent with those of Tyagi et al. [8], who suggested that both CB1 and CB2 receptors are expressed in the urothelium and detrusor muscle and that CB1 receptor expression was significantly higher than that of CB2 receptor. They also suggested that

CB2 receptor expression did not increase at the onset of DO or an inflammatory response because CB2 receptors are mainly expressed in peripheral immune cells; our results support their hypothesis. In a study using CB1 receptor-knockout mice, Füllhase et al. reported that the pathophysiologic role of CB1 receptors, but not that of CB2 receptors, is related to central and peripheral nervous control of micturition [19, 20].

In contrast to these studies, there are reports that it is not CB1 receptors, but rather CB2 receptors that play an important role. For example, Gratzke et al. [21] reported that increased CB2 receptor expression, but not increased CB1 receptor expression, was present in the urothelium and sensory nerves, and that a CB2 agonist improved the micturition interval and threshold, suggesting that the CB2 receptor mediate afferent signals in the bladder. Another study reported that the CB2 receptor was upregulated in a rat model of bladder inflammation [22]. Lastly, it was recently reported by Bakali et al. [23, 24] that in both rat and human bladders, CB1 receptors were localized in the urothelium, detrusor muscle, and nerve fiber structures of the subendothelium, and have both pre- and post-synaptic inhibitory effects, whereas CB2 receptors were localized in the same sites in the human bladder, but only in the detrusor muscle in rat bladders, suggesting that CB2 receptors only have postsynaptic inhibitory effects.

The differences between our study and previous studies could be due to the different methodologies. In our study, we used intravenous ketamine and xylazine to anesthetize rats, whereas Gratzke et al. [21] used intraperitoneal administration of isoflurane and urethane and performed CMG on conscious rats. It has been reported that ketamine inhibits the micturition reflex [25].

This study had several limitations. First, we used one dose and type of agonist for CB1 and CB2 receptors, however, these doses and types may not produce the maximal effect on the bladder of rats. Definitive characterization of CB receptor expression in tissues depends on the availability of selective agonists and antagonists. Further studies are warranted to examine these receptors in the urothelium and detrusor muscle and to develop drugs targeting these receptors. Such studies would be helpful for regulating DO caused by BOO and to control OAB symptoms. Second, we did not measure residual urine volume or functional bladder capacity in the rat model used here. CB1 and CB2 agonists may reduce the resistance provided by external sphincter, thereby indirectly reducing bladder CP. Therefore, we can not exclude the possibility that reduction in CP was because of a decrease in urethral resistance after the administration of CB1 and CB2 agonists. Third, although we attempted to measure non-voiding contractions, we were unable to do so; in this study, CP and CI were measured at voiding. It is also possible that our conclusions are not valid for technical reasons. We considered that the changes in CP and CI suggested the presence of DO, and may therefore provide information regarding changes in bladder status related to DO. Fourthly, both immunofluorescence staining and Western blotting showed that CB2 receptor density was not significantly higher in the BOO group than in the control group. The cause to explain this discrepancy is not precisely known, but it is presumed that CB2 receptors are involved in the mechanisms discussed in this study but to a lesser degree than CB1 receptors. The factors underlying these differences were not revealed by the methods used here. However, there was a statistically significant difference in the control, CB1 agonist, and CB2 agonist group for CMG parameters relative to the BOO group ($p < 0.05$).

In addition, although treatment with CB1 and CB2 agonists can have beneficial effects on DO, they can also cause complications or side effects during long-term administration. However, our study did not reveal any serious complications. Complications may have been avoided because agonists were administered intravesically, which is a local injection rather than a systemic injection. A potential problem is that it may be difficult to determine the most appropriate method of administration and dosage of CB agonist in future clinical studies of human patients.

Ultimately, CB1 receptor expression was upregulated in the bladder in BOO-associated DO. A possible explanation for this may be feedback activation via decreased levels of endocannabinoid ligands. The concentration of endocannabinoids in the bladder, which have

inhibitory effects, may decrease during BOO-associated DO.

Conclusions
CMG parameters in the BOO group were significantly improved by the inhibitory effect of CB1 and CB2 receptor agonists on DO associated with BOO. The expression of CB1 was significantly increased in the urothelium and detrusor muscle in DO associated with BOO, but no significant change in CB2 expression was observed. The results of this study suggest that CB1 and CB2 receptors in the bladder, particularly CB1 receptors, play a significant role in the pathophysiology of BOO-associated DO, and could serve as diagnostic biomarker and therapeutic targets in this disorder.

Abbreviations
BOO: Bladder outlet obstruction; CB: Cannabinoid; CI: Contraction interval; CMG: Cystometrography; CP: Contraction pressure; DO: Detrusor overactivity; G3PDH: Glyceraldehyde-3-phosphate dehydrogenase; PBS: Phosphate-buffered saline

Acknowledgements
Not applicable.

Funding
This work was supported by a research grant from Jeju National University Hospital in 2014. (No. 2014-03).

Authors' contributions
JCK was involved in protocol, project development, data collection and management and manuscript editing; SDK performed the experiment and involved in manuscript writing and editing; KJC was involved in data collection and analysis. All authors read and approved the final version of the manuscript.

Competing interests
The authors declare that they have no competing interests.

Author details
Department of Urology, Graduate School of Medicine, Jeju National University, Jeju, South Korea. ²Department of Urology, Bucheon St. Mary's hospital, College of Medicine, The Catholic University of Korea, Sosa-Ro 327, Wonmi-gu, Bucheon-si, Gyeonggi-do, Seoul 14647, South Korea.

References
1.   de Nunzio C, Franco G, Rocchegiani A, Iori F, Leonardo C, Laurenti C. The evolution of detrusor overactivity after watchful waiting, medical therapy

and surgery in patients with bladder outlet obstruction. J Urol. 2003;169: 535–9.

2. Andersson KE. Bladder activation: afferent mechanisms. Urology. 2002;59(5 Suppl 1):43–50.

3. Fowler CJ. Bladder afferents and their role in the overactive bladder. Urology. 2002;59(5 Suppl 1):37–42.

4. Kim HS, Park WJ, Park EY, Koh JS, Hwang TK, Kim JC. Role of nicotinic acetylcholine receptor α3 and α7 subunits in detrusor Overactivity induced by partial bladder outlet obstruction in rats. Int Neurourol J. 2015;19:12–8.

5. Cho KJ, Park EY, Kim HS, Koh JS, Kim JC. Expression of transient receptor potential vanilloid 4 and effects of ruthenium red on detrusor overactivity associated with bladder outlet obstruction in rats. World J Urol. 2014;32: 677–82.

6. Kim DY, Yang EK. 17 Beta-estradiol inhibits calcium-activated Potassium Channel expressions in rat whole bladder. Int Neurourol J. 2016;20:18–25.

7. Ben Amar M. Cannabinoids in medicine: a review of their therapeutic potential. J Ethnopharmacol. 2006;105:1–25.

8. Tyagi V, Philips BJ, Su R, Smaldone MC, Erickson VL, Chancellor MB, et al. Differential expression of functional cannabinoid receptors in human bladder detrusor and urothelium. J Urol. 2009;181:1932–8.

9. Boudes M, De Ridder D. Cannabinoid receptor 1 also plays a role in healthy bladder. BJU Int. 2014;113:142–3.

10. Brady CM, DasGupta R, Dalton C, Wiseman OJ, Berkley KJ, Fowler CJ. An open-label pilot study of cannabis-based extracts for bladder dysfunction in advanced multiple sclerosis. Mult Scler. 2004;10:425–33.

11. Goonawardena AV, Plano A, Robinson L, Platt B, Hampson RE, Riedel G. A Pilot Study into the Effects of the CB1 Cannabinoid Receptor Agonist WIN55,212-2 or the Antagonist/Inverse Agonist AM251 on Sleep in Rats. Sleep Disord. 2011. https://doi.org/10.1155/2011/178469.

12. Gratzke C, Streng T, Stief CG, Alroy I, Limberg BJ, Downs TR, et al. Cannabinor, a selective cannabinoid-2 receptor agonist, improves bladder emptying in rats with partial urethral obstruction. J Urol. 2011;185:731–6.

13. Walczak JS, Price TJ, Cervero F. Cannabinoid CB1 receptors are expressed in the mouse urinary bladder and their activation modulates afferent bladder activity. Neuroscience. 2009;159:1154–63.

14. Parsons BA, Drake MJ. Animal models in overactive bladder research. Handb Exp Pharmacol. 2011;202:15–43.

15. Fry CH, Daneshgari F, Thor K, Drake M, Eccles R, Kanai AJ, et al. Animal models and their use in understanding lower urinary tract dysfunction. Neurourol Urodyn. 2010;29:603–8.

16. Hedlund P. Cannabinoids and the endocannabinoid system in lower urinary tract function and dysfunction. Neurourol Urodyn. 2014;33:46–53.

17. Wang ZY, Wang P, Bjorling DE. Activation of cannabinoid receptor 1 inhibits increased bladder activity induced by nerve growth factor. Neurosci Lett. 2015;589:19–24.

18. Freeman RM, Adekanmi O, Waterfield MR, Waterfield AE, Wright D, Zajicek J. The effect of cannabis on urge incontinence in patients with multiple sclerosis: a multicentre, randomised placebo-controlled trial (CAMS-LUTS). Int Urogynecol J Pelvic Floor Dysfunct. 2006;17:636–41.

19. Füllhase C, Campeau L, Sibaev A, Storr M, Hennenberg M, Gratzke C, et al. Bladder function in a cannabinoid receptor type 1 knockout mouse. BJU Int. 2014;113:144–51.

20. Füllhase C, Russo A, Castiglione F, Benigni F, Campeau L, Montorsi F, et al. Spinal cord FAAH in normal micturition control and bladder overactivity in awake rats. J Urol. 2013;189:2364–70.

21. Gratzke C, Streng T, Park A, Christ G, Stief CG, Hedlund P, et al. Distribution and function of cannabinoid receptors 1 and 2 in the rat, monkey and human bladder. J Urol. 2009;181:1939–48.

22. Merriam FV, Wang ZY, Guerios SD, Bjorling DE. Cannabinoid receptor 2 is increased in acutely and chronically inflamed bladder of rats. Neurosci Lett. 2008;445:130–4.

23. Bakali E, Elliott RA, Taylor AH, Willets J, Konje JC, Tincello DG. Distribution and function of the endocannabinoid system in the rat and human bladder. Int Urogynecol J. 2013;24:855–63.

24. Bakali E, McDonald J, Elliott RA, Lambert DG, Tincello DG. Cannabinoid receptor expression in the bladder is altered in detrusor overactivity. Int Urogynecol J. 2016;27:129–39.

25. Ozkurkcugil C, Ozkan L. Effects of anesthetics on cystometric parameters in female rats. Int Urol Nephrol. 2010;42:909–13.

10

Transcutaneous electrical stimulation of somatic afferent nerves in the foot relieved symptoms related to postoperative bladder spasms

Chanjuan Zhang[1], Zhiying Xiao[1], Xiulin Zhang[1], Liqiang Guo[1], Wendong Sun[1], Changfeng Tai[2,3], Zhaoqun Jiang[1] and Yuqiang Liu[1*]

Abstract

Background: Bladder spasm is a common side effect of urological surgery. Main treatment modalities include opioids or anticholinergic medication; however, bladder spasms still occur even after these interventions. Recent studies indicate that transcutaneous stimulation of the foot can result in 50% increase in bladder capacity in healthy adults, and inhibit bladder detrusor overactivity in spinal cord injured patients. In this study, we examined the effects of transcutaneous electrical stimulation of the foot on bladder spasms related symptoms.

Methods: Sixty-six male patients who underwent prostate or bladder surgeries due to benign prostatic hyperplasia or bladder diseases were randomly divided into two groups: the control group ($n = 36$) and the treatment group ($n = 30$). The control group received the routine postoperative care. The treatment group received daily transcutaneous electrical stimulation of the foot during 3 days after surgery; each time lasted for 60 min. All patients were evaluated by the Visual Analogue Scale for pain sensation, frequency of bladder spasm episodes, and a total score of bladder spasms symptoms.

Results: In the control group, the patients with bladder surgery had a higher Visual Analogue Scale score than patients with prostate surgery ($P = 0.024$). In both treatment and control groups, the Visual Analogue Scale score, spasm frequency, and total score of bladder spasm symptoms decreased from day 1 to day 3 ($P < 0.001$). The Visual Analogue Scale score at day 2, total score of bladder spasm symptoms at day 2 and day 3 were significantly lower in the treatment group than in the control group ($P < 0.05$).

Conclusion: These results provided preliminary evidence suggesting beneficial effects of stimulating somatic afferent nerves in the foot on postoperative bladder spasms.

Keywords: Transcutaneous electrical stimulation, Afferent nerve, Bladder spasm

* Correspondence: zcj810515@163.com
[1]Department of Urology, The Second Hospital of Shandong University, 247 Beiyuan Street, Jinan 250033, China
Full list of author information is available at the end of the article

Background

Postoperative bladder spasms are involuntary movements of the detrusor muscle that can cause a sudden onset of pain in the region of bladder, a sensation of urgency to void, intermittent abdominal cramps, perineal pain, and/or urinary leakage around a urethral catheter after surgical procedures [1–3]. The intermittent bladder pain is usually short, lasting 30 s or more with an interval about several minutes or hours. Bladder spasm is a common side effect of urological surgery; it could result in not only postoperative pain but also hemorrhage and therefore may prolong bladder recovery. Current treatment modalities include opioids [4], anticholinergic medication [5], bladder smooth muscle relaxants [3] and sedation [6]. However, bladder spasms still occur even though the patients are treated by these interventions.

Transcutaneous electrical nerve stimulation is a non-pharmacological and non-invasive method that delivers electrical pulses to the nerve via skin surface electrodes and widely used for pain relief [7–9]. Recent studies indicate that transcutaneous stimulation of the foot can result in more than 50% increase in bladder capacity in healthy adults [10], and inhibit bladder detrusor over-activity in spinal cord-injured patients [11]. Therefore, we hypothesize that transcutaneous electrical stimulation of the foot might partially or completely relieve the symptoms caused by postoperative bladder spasms. To test this hypothesis, this study examined the effects of electrical stimulation of the foot in patients who underwent surgical procedures for benign prostate hyperplasia (BPH) or bladder diseases.

Methods

This prospective and randomly controlled study was reviewed and approved by the ethical committee of the second hospital of Shandong University in China(20150024), and was conducted in the urology department of the hospital. The written informed consent was obtained from each participant prior to enrollment and the study was registered with Chinese Clinical Trial Registry (http://www.chic-tr.org.cn/) (Identifier: ChiCTR-INR-16008635).

Patients and study design

Male patients who underwent operations for BPH ($n = 41$) or bladder diseases ($n = 25$) were enrolled between June 2016 and August 2016. Patients mean age was 64.5 years ranged from 54 to 79 years. The inclusion criteria include patients: (1) with BPH diagnosed preoperatively by urosonography, prostate specific antigen, digital rectal examination and urodynamic tests, or with bladder disease confirmed preoperatively by cystoscopy; (2) can complete the three times stimulation without missing anyday; (3) without neurogenic bladder, urinary tract infection, urinary incontinence, and/or cardiac pacemaker. In 41 patients

with BPH, transurethral holmium laser enucleation of the prostate were performed by one experienced surgeon and his assistants under epidural anesthesia, In 25 patients with bladder diseases, transurethral vaporization of bladder lesions with laser or transurethral electro-resection of bladder lesions was performed under epidural anesthesia by the same experienced surgeon. All patients had indwelling catheters (22 F) during the study period, and the anticholinergics or antibiotics were not applied.

The current study was reported according to CONSORT guidelines (Fig. 1). Initially, seventy patients were enrolled in this study, 4 patients declined to participate, 66 patients met the inclusion criterion, and were randomly divided into two groups: the control group ($n = 36$) and the treatment group ($n = 30$) following a computer generated randomization list. A simple random allocation sequence was generated and concealed by a trained nurse. There were 22 patients who underwent prostate surgery and 14 patients had bladder surgery in control group, while in the treatment group, the numbers were 19 and 11, respectively.

The control group patients received routine postoperative care including health education for diet plan, postoperative body positioning and catheterization, and management of adverse effects after surgery. For patients in treatment group all the interventions are the same as control group except they underwent daily electrical stimulation of the foot for 3 days after surgery; each time lasted for 60 min. The first stimulation was given at 12 h postoperatively and repeated at day 2 and 3, respectively. After each stimulation, patients were evaluated by the Visual Analogue Scale (VAS, from 0 to 10) for pain, spasm frequency and total score of bladder spasms symptoms. Data were collected at the same time points in control group and treatment group, i.e. 12, 36 and 60 h after surgery in the patient bedside.

Electrical stimulation protocol

We referred a report from Dr. Chen for the stimulation method [10]. Briefly, two skin surface electrodes (LGMedSupply, Cherry Hill, New Jersey, USA) were placed over the bottom of foot and connected to a TEC Elite transcutaneous electrical nerve stimulator (LGMedSupply, New Jersey, USA) which provided constant current, rectangular pulses of 5 Hz frequency and 0.2 millisecond pulse width (Fig. 2). The stimulation threshold was defined as the minimal intensity for inducing toe twitching. Stimulation intensity was then increased to the maximal level (ranging from 35 to 105 mA, or 2-6 times of the stimulation threshold) comfortable to the subject for the entire 60 min stimulation. The stimulation was conducted in the hospital, and was finished by one tester who was also responsible for data collection.

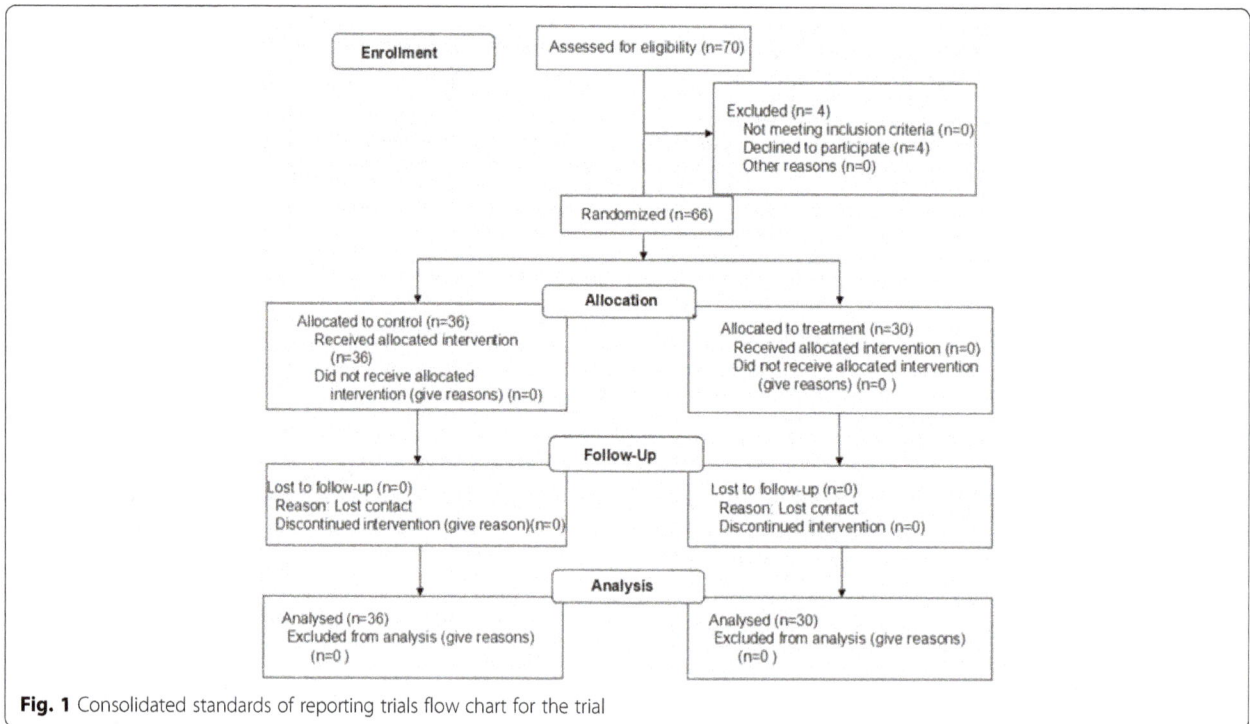

Fig. 1 Consolidated standards of reporting trials flow chart for the trial

Assessment of bladder spasm and pain

Visual Analogue Scale (VAS, from 0 to 10) for pain was used to measure bladder spasm-related pain. In addition to pain sensation, patients with bladder spasm usually have other presentations including urgency, urinary leakage. To comprehensively assess the symptom severity of bladder spasm, a questionnaire, which was based on the answers to five questions including urination feeling, urgency incontinence, spasm episodes, bladder pain, and

urinary leakage around catheter, was developed and used in this study. The total score of bladder spasm symptoms was calculated by adding the five sub-scores as shown in Table 1.

Primary and secondary outcomes

The primary outcomes were bladder spasm frequency and VAS score, the secondary outcome was the total score of spasm.

Statistical analysis

All data were expressed as mean $\pm$ SD. The Sigmaplot program was used for the data analysis. The sample size was calculated to be at least 30 patients in each group with $\alpha = 0.05$, $\beta = 0.10$, a desired statistical power level of 90% and 60% reduction of spasm episode at day 2 in treatment group relative to control group. In both control and treatment groups, the time course of spasm severity (time effect), the effects of electrical stimulation and interactions between stimulation and time were analyzed by two-tailed repeated measures ANOVA followed by Holm-Sidak post hoc tests to detect the statistical significance ($P < 0.05$).

Results

The final number of patients analyzed for control group was 36, and it was 30 for treatment group (Fig. 1). There was no significant difference in subject distribution of the two different surgeries (prostate/bladder) between control and treatment groups (22/14

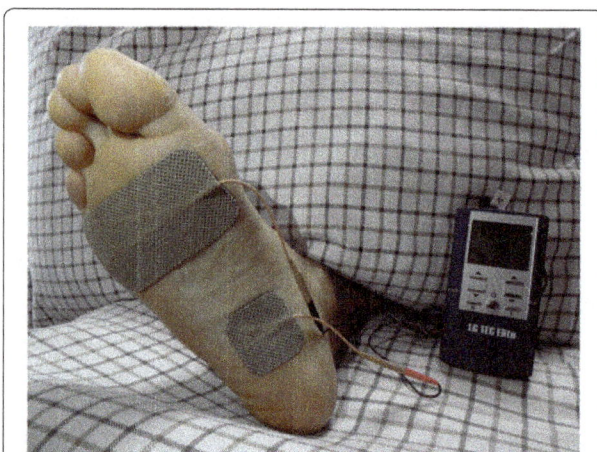

Fig. 2 The position of two skin surface electrodes and the connection with the stimulator. A large cathodal electrode (2 × 3.5 in.) was placed on the front of the foot and a small anodal electrode (2 × 2 in.) was placed between the inner foot arch and the heel. A written consent was obtained from the patient for publication of the image in the journal

Table 1 The total score of bladder spasms symptoms was calculated by adding scores from every sub-symptom

Score	0	2	4	6
Sub-symptoms				
Urgency	Never	Mild	Moderate	Severe
Bladder pain	Never	<30 min/day	30-60 min/day	>60 min/day
Urgent incontinence	Never	1/day	2-4/day	>4/day
Urinary leakage around catheter	Never	Rarely	Sometimes	Often
Spasm episode	<2/day	2-5/day	5-7/day	>7/day

for control and 19/11 for treatment, χ^2 test, $P > 0.05$). In the control group, patients with bladder surgery had higher VAS score than those with prostate surgery ($P = 0.024$), spasm frequency and total score of bladder spasms symptoms were also higher for bladder surgery but did not reach significance ($P > 0.05$) (Table 2).

In both treatment and control groups, the VAS score ($P < 0.001$), the spasms frequency ($P = 0.003$), and total score of bladder spasms ($P < 0.001$) symptoms are all significantly decreased from day 1 to 3 (Table 3). There was no interaction between foot stimulation and time in treatment group for VAS ($P = 0.194$), bladder spasms ($P = 0.418$), and total score of bladder spasms ($P = 0.864$).

Our data revealed a lower VAS score in treatment group than control group on day 2 ($P = 0.027$, Table 3). A lower total score of bladder spasm symptoms in treatment group was revealed at day 2 ($P = 0.020$) and day 3 ($P = 0.045$) when compared to control group (Table 3). Patients who received foot stimulation tended to have less bladder spasm episodes than those in control group on day 2 and day 3, but the

Table 2 Comparison of VAS score, spasm frequency and total symptom score between prostate and bladder surgery in control group

	Prostate surgery (n = 22)	Bladder surgery (n = 14)	P
VAS score			
Day 1	3.76 ± 0.42	5.23 ± 0.47	0.014
Day 2	3.53 ± 0.44	4.54 ± 0.54	0.031
Day 3	1.94 ± 0.36	3.00 ± 0.65	0.027
Spasm episode			
Day 1	1.18 ± 0.42	2.00 ± 0.55	>0.05
Day 2	1.18 ± 0.42	2.15 ± 0.53	>0.05
Day 3	0.47 ± 0.36	0.92 ± 0.49	>0.05
Total score			
Day 1	9.06 ± 1.59	11.54 ± 2.20	>0.05
Day 2	8.59 ± 1.66	12.00 ± 2.34	>0.05
Day 3	4.71 ± 1.31	6.62 ± 2.23	>0.05

Table 3 Comparison of VAS score, spasm frequency and total score between control and treatment groups

	Control group (n = 36)	Treatment group (n = 30)	P
VAS score			
Day 1	4.48 ± 0.37	4.12 ± 0.37	>0.05
Day 2	3.85 ± 0.38	2.85 ± 0.23	0.027
Day 3	2.26 ± 0.38	1.38 ± 0.21	>0.05
Spasm episode			
Day 1	1.63 ± 0.37	1.51 ± 0.34	>0.05
Day 2	1.48 ± 0.36	0.38 ± 0.16	0.065
Day 3	0.59 ± 0.32	0.08 ± 0.08	0.086
Total score			
Day 1	10.30 ± 1.44	11.38 ± 1.59	>0.05
Day 2	9.41 ± 1.47	5.54 ± 0.75	0.020
Day 3	5.26 ± 1.30	2.15 ± 0.52	0.045

difference did not reach significant level ($P = 0.065$ and $P = 0.086$, respectively) (Table 3).

Discussion

The management modalities for post operative bladder spasms include opioids [4], anticholinergic medication [5], bladder smooth muscle relaxants [3], sedation [6] and anaesthesia [1]. This study examined the effects of transcutaneous foot stimulation on patients with bladder spasms after prostate or bladder surgeries. It showed that foot stimulation could significantly reduce pain sensation and alleviate the symptoms of bladder spasms. These results provided preliminary evidence suggesting beneficial effects of stimulating somatic afferent nerves in the foot after bladder or prostate surgeries.

Previous studies showed that bladder and posterior urethral injuries associated with invasive procedures, postoperative catheterization, and bladder irrigation could induce involuntary contraction of detrusor muscle [1, 2, 12, 13]. In consistent with these reports bladder spasms were noticed in patients who underwent resection of the prostate or bladder lesions in our study. The mechanism underlying bladder spasm still remains unclear. It is well known that bladder mucosa, especially at the trigone is extremely sensitive to temperature, pressure and mechanical stimulation [14]. A higher VAS score was found in patients after bladder surgery than those after prostate surgery (Table 2), suggesting that bladder surgeries may result in more irritation of the bladder mucosa and trigone than prostate surgeries. There was a similar distribution of the bladder and prostate patients in the control and treatment groups. Therefore, the surgical effects on bladder spasm should be comparable between the two groups.

To our knowledge, there are no internationally recognized criteria for assessing bladder spasm. Currently, spasm frequency and VAS score are the most commonly used criteria to evaluate bladder spasm [1–3]. In this study, we combined these two parameters together with urination feeling, urgent incontinence and urinary leakage around catheter in order to measure the symptom severity of bladder spasm (Table 1). The total score of bladder spasm symptoms provided more comprehensive information than VAS score or spasm frequency alone, which could help clinicians better understand and manage postoperative bladder spasms.

The effects of foot stimulation was only observed on days 2 and 3 but not on day 1, indicating that repeated stimulation might be required in order to accumulate the therapeutic effects. Meanwhile, the stimulation was only applied 1 time/day but the effects seem sustained during the whole day, indicating that the stimulation must have induced post-stimulation effects. The post-stimulation inhibitory effects on bladder spasms are in agreement with previous studies showing that a post-stimulation inhibition of the micturition reflex can be induced by stimulation of the foot or tibial nerve in rats [15] and cat [16, 17]. In both treatment and control groups, the VAS score, spasm frequency, and total score of bladder spasm symptoms decreased from day 1 to day 3 (Table 3), which might be due to the natural healing process postoperatively.

Even though we did not know exactly which nerves were activated by foot stimulation, it is highly likely that it activates afferent axons in the lateral and medial plantar nerves of the foot, because the 2 skin surface electrodes were placed along the passage of these nerves (Fig. 2). A large body of animal studies indicated that tibial nerve neuromodulation inhibited bladder overactivity by activating spinal inhibitory neurotransmitters (opioid, gamma aminobutyric acid) and metabolic glutamate receptor 3 [16, 18, 19]. Inhibition of bladder spasm in the present study may also involve these inhibitory neurotransmitters. The activation of sensory nerves at foot might induce the release of inhibitory neurotransmitters that in turn produce an inhibitory interaction between somatic peripheral neuropathway and autonomic micturition reflex to suppress bladder hyperactivity and pain.

Neuromodulation is widely used as an alternative approach for treatment of bladder dysfunctions [18, 20]. Sacral neuromodulation is the most effective method, but it is invasive and requires high cost. Tibial neuromodulation is minimally invasive, that involves inserting a needle electrode near the ankle to stimulate the tibial nerve, there were no reports indicate the beneficial effects of tibial nerve stimulation on bladder spasm, however, it was proved as efficacious as antimuscarinic drugs for many bladder dysfunctions such as detrusor overactivity [21], a full-scale randomized trial (RCT) conducted in older adults in residential care homes suggested transcutaneous tibial nerve stimulation (PTNS) could reduce the number of episodes of urinary and fecal incontinence [22]; another RCT study conducted on overactive bladder patients demonstrated 12 month weekly PTNS had effectiveness on overactive bladder symptom improvement [23]. There are several advantages of foot stimulation used in this study over tibial neuromodulation: compeletely noinvasive, without adverse effects and can be conducted by patients themselves.

It should be noted that there are some limitations in the present study such as the absence of placebo controls. It is hard to design a placebo control for foot stimulation, since managements such as simply turning off the stimulation would be easily noticed by the patient.

Conclusion

In summary, electrical foot stimulation could relieve the symptoms of bladder spasms and pain after BPH or bladder surgeries. Since foot stimulation is non-invasive, convenient for patients to use, and has no side effect, it could be considered as an additional modality for the control of postoperative bladder spasms and/or pain.

Abbreviations
BPH: Benign prostate hyperplasia; VAS: Visual analogue scale

Acknowledgement
The authors thank all our participants for their gracious participation in this study.

Funding
This research was supported by Youth Fund of the Second Hospital of Shandong University(Y2015010054), Natural Science Foundation of Shandong Province (CN) (ZR2014HL025) and Science Innovation Plan for Clinical Medicine of Jinan (201602150).

Authors' contributions
YL and CT designed and conducted the study. CZ and ZX contributed to the data analysis and interpretation. LG and XZ contributed to data collection, data analysis, data interpretation and editing manuscript. WS and ZJ conceived the project, contributed to data collection and writing manuscript. All authors read and approved the final manuscript.

Competing interests
The authors declare that they have no competing interests.

Author details
[1]Department of Urology, The Second Hospital of Shandong University, 247 Beiyuan Street, Jinan 250033, China. [2]Department of Urology, University of Pittsburgh, Pittsburgh, PA, USA. [3]Department of Pharmacology and Chemical Biology, University of Pittsburgh, Pittsburgh, PA 15213, USA.

References

1. Chiang D, Ben-Meir D, Pout K, et al. Management of post-operative bladder spasm. J Paediatr Child Health. 2005;41:56–8.

2. Park JM, Houck CS, Sethna NF, et al. Ketorolac suppresses postoperative bladder spasms after pediatric ureteral reimplantation. Anesth Analg. 2000;91:11–5.

3. Chen TD, Wang YH, Yang LY, et al. Safe and effective for the prevention of bladder spasm after TURP. Zhonghua Nan Ke Xue. 2010;16(11):1004–6.

4. Olshwang D, Shapiro A, Perlberg S, et al. The effect of epidural morphine on ureteral colic and spasm of the bladder. Pain. 1984;18:97–101.

5. Paulson DF. Oxybtynin chloride in control of post-transurethral vesical pain and spasm. Urology. 1978;11(3):237–8.

6. Matthews RD, Nolan JF, Libby-Straw JA, et al. Transurethral surgery using intravesical bupivacaine and intravenous sedation. J Urol. 1992;148(5):1475–6.

7. Zimmerman MB, Geasland K, Embree J, et al. Transcutaneous electrical nerve stimulation for the control of pain during rehabilitation after total knee arthroplasty: A randomized, blinded, placebo-controlled trial. Pain. 2014;155(12):2599–611.

8. Ahmed HE, White PF, Craig WF, et al. Use of Percutaneous electrical Nerve stimulation (PENS) in the short-term management of headache. Headache. 2000;40:311–5.

9. Evron S, Schenker JG, Olshwang D, et al. Postoperative analgesia by percutaneous electrical stimulation in gynecology and obstetrics. Eur J Obstet Gynecol Reprod Biol. 1981;12:305–13.

10. Chen ML, Chermansky CJ, Shen B, et al. Electrical stimulation of somatic afferent nerves in the foot increases bladder capacity in healthy human subjects. J Urol. 2014;191(4):1009–13.

11. Chen G, Liao L, Li Y. The possible role of percutaneous tibial nerve stimulation usin-1013 g adhesive skin surface electrodes in patients with neurogenic detrusor overactivity secondary to spinal cord injury. Int Urol Nephrol. 2015;47(3):451–5.

12. Grass JA, Sakima NT, Valley M, et al. Assessment of ketorolac as an adjuvant to fentanyl patient-controlled epidural analgesia after radical retropubic prostatectomy. Anesthesiology. 1993;78:642–8.

13. Nazarko L. Bladder pain from indwelling urinary catheterization: case study. Br J Nurs. 2007;16(9):511–2.

14. Yoshimura N, de Groat WC. Neural control of the lower urinary tract. Int J Urol. 1997;4:111–25.

15. Matsuta Y, Roppolo JR, de Groat WC. Poststimulation inhibition of the micturition reflex induced by tibial nerve stimulation in rats. Physiol Rep. 2014;2(1):1–6.

16. Xiao Z, Reese J, Schwe Z, et al. Role of spinal GABAA receptors in pudendal inhibition of nociceptive and non-nociceptive bladder reflexes in cats. Am J Physiol Renal Physiol. 2014;306:F781–9.

17. Chen G, Larson JA, Ogagan PD, et al. Post-stimulation inhibitory effect on reflex bladder activity induced by activation of somatic afferent nerves in the foot. J Urol. 2012;187(1):338–43.

18. de Groat WC, Tai C. Impact of bioelectronic medicine on the neural regulation of pelvic visceral function. Bioelectron Med. 2015;22:25–36.

19. Zhang Z, Slater RC, Ferroni MC, et al. Role of μ, κ, and δ opioid receptors in tibial inhibition of bladder overactivity in cats. J Pharmacol Exp Ther. 2015; 355(2):228–34.

20. Liberman D, Ehlert MJ, Siegel SW. Sacral Neuromodulation in Urological Practice. Urology. 2016;S0090-4295(16):30277–1.

21. Peters KM, Macdiarmid SA, Wooldridge LS, et al. Randomized trial of percutaneous tibial nerve stimulation versus extended-release tolterodine: results from the overactive bladder innovative therapy trial. J Urol. 2009;182:1055.

22. Booth J, Hagen RS, McClurg D, et al. A Feasibility study of transcutaneous posterior tibial nerve stimulation for bladder and bowel dysfunction in elderly adults in residential care. JAMDA. 2013;14:270–4.

23. MacDiarmid SA, Peters KM, Shobeiri SA, et al. Long-term durability of percutaneous tibial nerve stimulation for the treatment of overactive bladder. J Urol. 2010;183:234–40.

11

Lymphoepithelioma-like, a variant of urothelial carcinoma of the urinary bladder: a case report and systematic review for optimal treatment modality for disease-free survival

Andy W. Yang[*], Aydin Pooli, Subodh M. Lele, Ina W. Kim, Judson D. Davies and Chad A. LaGrange

Abstract

Background: Lymphoepithelioma-like carcinoma (LELC) is a rare high-grade carcinoma that resembles nasopharyngeal lymphoepithelioma and can occur throughout the body. First reported in 1991, bladder LELC has an incidence of about 1% of all bladder carcinomas. Due to its rare occurrence, prognoses and ideal treatment guidelines have not been clearly defined.

Methods: A PubMed search was performed using two terms, "lymphoepithelioma-like carcinoma" and "bladder." Review articles, articles in foreign languages, expression studies, and studies not performed in the bladder were excluded. We report a case of LELC of the bladder including treatment and outcome and performed a systematic review of all 36 available English literatures from 1991 to 2016 including the present case to identify factors affecting disease-free survival.

Results: One hundred forty cases of bladder LELC were analyzed. The mean age of the patients was 70.1 years ranging from 43 to 90 years with 72% males and 28% females. Pure LELC occurs most often at 46% followed by mixed LELC 28% and predominant LELC 26%. EBV testing was negative in all cases tested. Mean follow-up length for all cases was 33.8 months with no evidence of disease in 62.2%, while 11.1% died of disease, 10.4% alive with metastasis, and 8.2% died without disease. 5.0% of cases had recurrence at an average of 31.3 months. Prognosis is significantly favorable for patients presenting with pure or predominant forms of LELC compared to mixed type ($p < 0.0001$). The treatment significantly associated with the highest disease mortality and lowest disease-free survival was TURBT alone when compared to any multi-modality treatment ($p < 0.01$).

Conclusion: We conclude that the best treatment modality associated with the highest disease-free survival is multi-modal treatment including radical cystectomy.

Keywords: Lymphoepithelioma-like carcinoma, Bladder tumor, Systematic review, Case report

* Correspondence: ayang@unmc.edu
Division of Urologic Surgery, University of Nebraska Medical Center, Omaha, NE, USA

Background

Lymphoepithelioma-like carcinoma (LELC) is a rare high-grade carcinoma that resembles nasopharyngeal lymphoepithelioma and has been reported to occur in other sites of the body such as gastrointestinal tract [1], liver [2], lung [3], skin [4], uterus [5], gallbladder [6], pancreas [7], kidney [8], and breast [9]. First reported in 1991 [10], LELC of the bladder appears to resemble LELC histologically in the nasopharynx but is actually a variant of urothelial carcinoma and has an incidence of about 1% of all bladder carcinomas [11]. Unlike other sites of the body, LELC in the bladder has not been associated with the presence of Epstein-Barr Virus to date [12]. Due to its rare occurrence, prognoses and ideal treatment guidelines have not been clearly defined. We report a case of LELC in the bladder and performed a systematic review of all available English literature including the present case to evaluate factors affecting disease-free survival.

Methods

A PubMed search was performed using two terms, "lymphoepithelioma-like carcinoma" and "bladder." Of the 63 results generated as of July 18th, 2016, 27 review articles, articles in foreign languages, expression studies, and studies not performed in the urinary bladder were excluded. Attempts were made to translate foreign articles to minimize bias but it was unsuccessful. Potential bias due to language barrier should be minimal. A total of 140 patients, including the present case, were collected from 36 published English articles from 1991 to 2016 [10, 11, 13–46]. Preferred reporting items for systematic review and meta-analysis protocols (PRISMA-P) 2015 guidelines were followed including creation of a protocol available upon request [47]. Patient data collected include gender, age, chief complaint, LELC type, TNM staging, EBV status, primary treatment, secondary treatment, neoadjuvant therapy used, follow-up time in months, recurrence time in months, and outcome. Studies with insufficient information for particular data were excluded from that particular statistical analysis to reduce bias. LELC classification criteria was described by Amin et al. with pure being 100% of the tumor showed LELC pattern, pre-dominant being ≥ 50% mixed with another type of tumor pattern, and mixed being < 50% mixed with another type of tumor pattern. *Student's t-test* was performed for statistical analysis.

Case report

A 69-year-old African American female presented in February 2015 in our department with the chief complaint of gross hematuria and dysuria that started in December 2014. Prior to urology evaluation, she had received two courses of antibiotics without resolution for her presenting symptoms. The patient denied history of urologic trauma, nephrolithiasis, chronic Foley catheter, family history of genitourinary (GU) malignancy, or previous GU surgeries. The patient had a history of stage IA adenocarcinoma of the right upper lung in 2011 and a 20-pack year history of smoking.

Cystoscopy revealed a large complex bladder mass on the right lateral wall and right trigone involving the right ureteral orifice. Abdominal and pelvic CT scan revealed right-sided bladder mass involving the right ureterovesical junction, right hydronephrosis and right-sided pelvic lymphadenopathy. Transurethral resection of the bladder tumor (TURBT) was performed and pathologic examination showed a prominent inflammatory background with admixed high-grade undifferentiated tumor cells arranged in sheets with ill-defined cytoplasmic borders imparting a syncytial appearance diagnostic of the LEL variant of urothelial carcinoma (Fig 1a and b). Foci of urothelial carcinoma in situ were also noted involving the surface urothelium. Muscularis propria invasion was present.

Patient was treated with four cycles of neoadjuvant chemotherapy of gemcitabine and cisplatin. Repeat CT two weeks after the last round of chemotherapy revealed smaller right-sided bladder mass (6.1 x 2.9 cm vs. 6.9 x 3.4 cm). Two months after the last round of chemotherapy, the patient underwent a radical cystectomy with ileal conduit diversion and pelvic lymph node dissection in July 2015. The operation was complicated by extensive adhesions from previous appendectomy, hysterectomy, and hernia repair with ventral mesh placement necessitating small bowel resection.

Final pathology report showed three high-grade tumor foci in the bladder with the largest being high-grade urothelial carcinoma located in the right lateral wall measuring 2.8 cm, another tumor located in the posterior wall measuring 0.9 cm with areas of squamous differentiation, and the smallest tumor located at the dome measuring 0.6 cm with pathology consistent with LEL urothelial carcinoma. The LEL variant of urothelial carcinoma is rare and diagnosed by the presence of high-grade/poorly differentiated tumor cells admixed with a prominent inflammatory cell infiltrate. The tumor cells have high nuclear:cytoplasmic ratios and indistinct cytoplasmic borders imparting a syncytium-like appearance. The overall appearance is similar to the lymphoepitheliomas typically seen in the nasopharyngeal region. They can be seen in the bladder either in the pure form or admixed with more usual forms of high-grade urothelial carcinoma, as seen in the present case. One obturator lymph node was positive for metastatic urothelial carcinoma (1/17 nodes positive). All surgical margins were negative. Final pathology staging was pT3bN1MX.

Patient had an uneventful recovery and was discharged on post-operative day 12 to a skilled nursing facility.

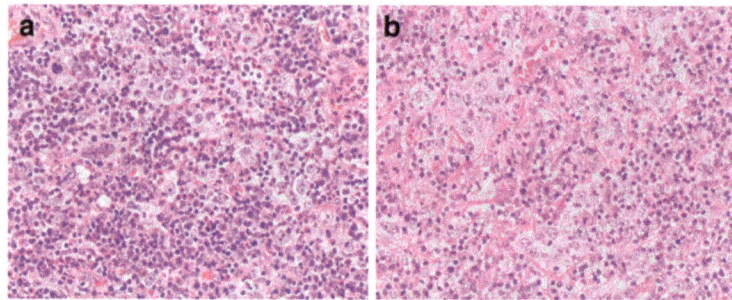

Fig. 1 Note the (**a**) high-grade carcinoma cells with large nuclei, irregular nuclear borders and prominent nucleoli present in small aggregates and also (**b**) singly with ill-defined cytoplasmic borders imparting a syncytium-like pattern and admixed with numerous inflammatory cells, typical of a lymphoepithelioma-like urothelial carcinoma. Original magnification X400; hematoxylin and eosin stain

Repeat abdominal and pelvis CT at 9 weeks post-op showed no mass, lymphadenopathy, or destructive osseous lesions. Patient reported improvement in appetite and normal bowel movement with persistent mild abdominal pain. However, lung cancer follow-up chest CT in September 2015 revealed a new 3 mm left upper lobe nodule not present in preoperative chest CT in June 2015. Repeat chest CT in February 2016 showed left upper lobe nodule enlarged to 12 mm. CT-guided needle biopsy showed CK7+, p40+, and GATA3+ tumor cells similar to morphology of previous bladder cancer, consistent with metastatic urothelial carcinoma. Multiple

new liver lesions were present on repeat CT in April 2016. Patient unfortunately died with metastases in October 2016.

Results

One hundred forty cases of LELC in the bladder including the present case were reported between 1991 and 2016. The mean age of the patients was 70.1 years ranging from 43 to 90 years with 57% males, 22% females, and 21% unknown; of those with known genders, 72% were male and 28% female (Table 1). Primary presentation was gross hematuria in 53% of patients. Mean

Table 1 LELC cases from 36 published English literature from 1991–2016 including the present case with demographic breakdown

Reference	Case(s)	Reference	Case(s)
Zukerberg et al., 1991 [10]	1	Guresci et al., 2009 [22]	1
Young et al., 1991 [44]	1	Singh et al., 2009 [35]	1
Dinney et al., 1993 [19]	3	Trabelsi et al., 2009 [39]	1
Amin et al., 1994 [13]	11	Yun et al., 2010 [45]	1
Bianchini et al., 1996 [14]	1	Kozyrakis et al., 2011 [26]	6
Holmang et al., 1998 [23]	9	Williamson et al., 2011 [41]	33
Constantinides et al., 2001 [18]	3	Pantelides et al., 2012 [32]	1
Lopez-B et al., 2001 [11]	13	Mori et al., 2013 [30]	1
Ward et al., 2002 [40]	1	Spinelli et al., 2013 [36]	1
Porcaro et al., 2003 [33]	1	Yoshino et al., 2014 [43]	1
Chen et al., 2003 [16]	2	Ziouziou et al., 2014 [46]	1
Izuquierdo et al., 2004 [24]	3	Kushida et al., 2015 [27]	1
Guresci et al., 2005 [21]	1	Kessler et al., 2015 [25]	1
Yaqoob et al., 2005 [42]	1	Mina et al., 2015 [29]	1
Mayer et al., 2007 [28]	1	Raphael et al., 2015 [34]	1
Tamas et al., 2007 [38]	29	Nagai et al., 2016 [31]	1
Cai et al., 2008 [15]	2	Stamatiou et al., 2016 [37]	1
Chikwava et al., 2008 [17]	1	Yang et al., 2017	1
Fadare et al., 2009 [20]	1	Total	140
Age Range	43–90	Male	72%
Average Age	70.1	Female	28%

follow-up length for all cases was 33.8 months with no evidence of disease in 62.2%, while 11.1% died of disease, 10.4% alive with metastasis, 8.2% died without disease, and 8.2% lost to follow-up. 5.0% of cases had recurrence at an average of 31.3 months. Pure LELC occurs most often at 46% (62 cases) followed by mixed LELC 28% (38 cases) and predominant LELC 26% (36 cases). Pathological staging of the tumor was pT1 in 10.1% (14 cases), pT2 in 56.1% (78 cases), pT3 in 30.9% (43 cases), and pT4 in 2.9% (4 cases). Lymph node metastasis was present in 13.6% of patients, with distant metastasis noted in 5.7%. EBV testing was performed in 51.4% of the cases and was negative in all cases.

Comparing treatment modality, 50% of the cases utilized one treatment modality only with radical cystectomy being the most common (58.6%) followed by TURBT (30.0%), partial cystectomy (7.1%), and intravesical chemotherapy (1.4%) with outcomes of no evidence of disease (55.7%), died of disease (12.9%), alive with metastasis (10.0%), and died without disease (7.1%). Of the multi-modality treatments, primary treatments were diverse and included TURBT (49.9%), radical cystectomy (41.0%), partial cystectomy (6.0%), intravesical chemotherapy (1.5%), chemotherapy (0.8%), and radiation therapy (0.8%). Secondary treatments included chemotherapy (51.8%), radiation therapy (28.2%), TURBT (7.1%), intravesical chemotherapy (7.1%), radical cystectomy (4.7%), and thermal ablation (1.2%). Outcomes for those receiving multi-modal treatments include no evidence of disease (67.2%), alive with metastasis (10.5%), died without disease (9.0%), and died of disease (7.5%) (Table 2).

Comparing surgical resection methods, TURBT alone has the lowest disease-free survival rate (33.3%) when compared to any combination therapy (67.9%) ($p < 0.01$); TURBT alone also carries the highest mortality rate (23.8%) when compared to any combination therapy (7.1%, $p < 0.05$). Radical cystectomy is associated with the highest disease-free survival rate at 67.8% and is significant when compared to TURBT alone at 33.3% ($p < 0.01$) but not significant when compared to partial cystectomy at 50%.

Systematic chemotherapy treatments utilized are varied with 24 cases documenting detailed regiments. Of those, eight cases specified MVAC treatments while 16 cases specified GC treatments. Neoadjuvant chemotherapy was

administered in 4.3% of cases with an average disease-free survival of 41 months and did not significantly impact outcome. Comparing subtypes of LELC, the treatment regiments reported did not significantly differ; of those with pure and predominant LELC, 71.0% and 75.0% had no evidence of disease, respectively, while only 31.6% of mixed LELC patients had the same outcome ($p < 0.0001$, Table 3). In addition, patients who underwent radical cystectomy had the highest disease-free survival (67.8%, $p < 0.01$) when compared to partial cystectomies (50%) or TURBT only (33.3%). However, patients receiving TURBT combined with any type of secondary treatment have a 71.1% disease-free survival rate.

Discussion
LELC of the bladder is a rare cancer that most often presents with painless hematuria occurring in older males. By the time of presentation, most LELCs have invaded the muscularis propia but have not metastasized outside of the bladder. Even though LELC in other organ systems has been shown to be associated with EBV, no case of LELC in the bladder has been associated with the presence of EBV. The subtypes of LELC appear to significantly impact outcome, as disease-free survival is higher in predominant and pure LELC than mixed LELC. Highest mortality is mixed LELC followed by predominant and pure LELC and this could suggest that LELC itself is not as aggressive as high-grade urothelial carcinoma.

As for treatment impacting outcome, TURBT alone should not be recommended, as it is associated with both lowest disease-free survival and highest mortality rate. Radical cystectomy is associated with the highest disease-free survival rate, whereas partial cystectomy was only utilized as the main surgical resection method in eight cases its impact is unknown. As for neoadjuvant chemotherapy, it was administered in six cases and while it had a longer

Table 3 Outcomes for LELC types and treatment modalities

LELC Type	Cases	NED	p-value	DOD	p-value
Pure	62	71.0%	0.00002	1.6%	0.0001
Predominant	36	75.0%	0.00002	5.6%	0.002
Mixed	38	31.6%	-	28.9%	-
Treatment	Cases	NED	p-value	DOD	p-value
MM	112	67.9%	0.002	7.1%	0.04
RC+	59	67.8%	0.002	10.2%	0.08
PC+	8	50.0%	0.21	12.5%	0.22
TURBT+	45	71.1%	0.002	2.2%	0.012
TURBT-	21	33.3%	-	23.8%	-

p-values calculated against mixed type and against TURBT-only
NED no evidence of disease, DOD died of disease, MM multi-modality overall treatments including RC+, PC+, and TURBT+; RC+ radical cystectomy + adjuvant therapy, PC+ partial cystectomy + adjuvant therapy, TURBT+ transurethral resection of the bladder + adjuvant therapy, TURBT- transurethral resection of the bladder only

Table 2 Outcomes of all cases comparing single vs. multi-modal treatment modality

Treatments	NED	AWM	DOD	DWD
Single	55.7%	10.0%	12.9%	7.1%
Multi	67.2%	10.5%	7.5%	9.0%
Overall	62.2%	10.4%	11.1%	8.2%

NED no evidence of disease, AWM alive with metastasis, DOD died of disease, DWD died without disease

disease survival, it was not significant, perhaps also due to the small sample size. As for chemotherapy regiment, it appears to have evolved over time and without significant difference as all eight cases of MVAC were before 2003 and all 16 cases of GC were after.

To define best treatment strategy for rare diseases is difficult as rare diseases are best evaluated in a prospective registry. Even though LELC in the bladder is rare and there is currently no clear treatment guideline, our study suggests that a combination therapy including radical cystectomy would possibly yield the best outcome.

Conclusion

LELC of the bladder is a rare cancer that most often occurs in older males. Of the three subtypes, mixed LELC carries the highest mortality rate and TURBT alone or any single treatment is not recommended for therapy as it is associated with both the highest mortality rate and the lowest disease-free survival rate. Prognosis is favorable for patients presenting with pure or predominant forms of LELC and those undergoing combination therapies that include radical cystectomy while the impact of neoadjuvant chemotherapy is yet undetermined.

Abbreviations
GU: Genitourinary; LELC: Lymphoepithelioma-like carcinoma; TURBT: Transurethral resection of bladder tumor.

Acknowledgement
Not applicable.

Authors' contributions
AWY collected and compiled the data, performed the analysis, drafted, prepared, edited, and submitted the manuscript. AP contributed to the manuscript. SML performed the pathology study and prepared the images and pathological sections of the manuscript. IWK contributed to the manuscript and treated the patient. JDD treated the patient and performed the surgery. CAL contributed to the manuscript and directed the project. All authors read and approved the final manuscript.

Competing interests
The authors declare that they have no competing interests.

References
1. Kang BW, Seo AN, Yoon S, Bae HI, Jeon SW, Kwon OK, Chung HY, Yu W, Kim JG. Prognostic value of tumor-infiltrating lymphocytes in Epstein-Barr Virus-associated gastric cancer. Ann Oncol. 2016;27(3):494–501.
2. Wei J, Liu Q, Wang C, Yu S. Lymphoepithelioma-like hepatocellular carcinoma without Epstein-Barr Virus infection: A case report and a review of the literature. Indian J Pathol Microbiol. 2015;58(4):550–3.
3. Wang L, Lin Y, Cai Q, Long H, Zhang Y, Rong T, Ma G, Liang Y. Detection of rearrangement of anaplastic lymphoma kinase (ALK) and mutation of epidermal growth factor receptor (EGFR) in primary pulmonary lymphoepithelioma-like carcinoma. J Thorac Dis. 2015;7(9):1556–62.
4. Lee J, Park J, Chang H. Lymphoepithelioma-like carcinoma of the skin in the cheek with a malignant metastatic cervical lymph node. Arch Plast Surg. 2015;42(5):668–71.
5. Makannavar JH, KishanPrasad HL, Shetty JK. Lymphoepithelioma-like carcinoma of endometrium: A rare case report. Indian J Surg Oncol. 2015;6(2):130–4.
6. Sinha PK, Mangla V, Behari C, Rastogi A, Chattopdhyay TK. Lymphoepithelioma-like carcinoma: An unusual gall bladder tumor. Trop Gastroenterol. 2014;35(3):182–3.
7. Samdani RT, Hetchman JF, O'Reilly E, DeMatteo R, Sigel CS. EBC-associated Lymphoepithelioma-like carcinoma of the pancreas: Case report with targeted sequencing analysis. Pancreatology. 2015;15(3):302–4.
8. Ahn H, Sim J, Kim H, Yi K, Han H, Chung Y, Rehman A, Paik SS. Lymphoepithelioma-like carcinoma of the renal pelvis: A case report and
9. Suzuki I, Chakkabat P, Goicochea L, Campassi C, Chumsri S. Lymphoepithelioma-like carcinoma of the breast presenting as breast abscess. World J Clin Oncol. 2014;5(5):1107–12.
10. Zukerberg LR, Harris NL, Young RH. Carcinomas of the urinary bladder simulating malignant lymphoma. A report of five cases. Am J Surg Pathol. 1991;15(6):569–76.
11. Lopez-Beltrán A, Luque RJ, Vicioso L, Anglada F, Requena MJ, Quintero A, Montironi R. Lymphoepithelioma-like carcinoma of the urinary bladder: a clinicopathologic study of 13 cases. Virchows Arch. 2001;438(6):552–7.
12. Gulley ML, Amin MB, Nicholls JM, Banks PM, Ayala AG, Srigley JR, Eagan PA, Ro JY. Epstein-Barr virus is detected in undifferentiated nasopharyngeal carcinoma but not in lymphoepithelioma-like carcinoma of the urinary bladder. Hum Pathol. 1995;26(11):1207–14.
13. Amin MB, Ro JY, Lee KM, Ordóñez NG, Dinney CP, Gulley ML, Ayala AG. Lymphoepithelioma-like carcinoma of the urinary bladder. Am J Surg Pathol. 1994;18(5):466–73.
14. Bianchini E, Lisato L, Rimondi AP, Pegoraro V. Lymphoepithelioma-like carcinoma of the urinary bladder. J Urol Pathol. 1996;5:45–9.
15. Cai G, Parwani AV. Cytomorphology of lymphoepithelioma-like carcinoma of the urinary bladder: report of two cases. Diagn Cytopathol. 2008;36(8):600–3.
16. Chen KC, Yeh SD, Fang CL, Chiang HS, Chen YK. Lymphoepithelioma-like carcinoma of the urinary bladder. J Formos Med Assoc. 2003;102(10):722–5.
17. Chikwava KR, Gingrich JR, Parwani AV. Lymphoepithelioma-like carcinoma of the urinary bladder. Pathology. 2008;40(3):310–1.
18. Constantinides C, Giannopoulos A, Kyriakou G, Androulaki A, Ioannou M, Dimopoulos M, Kyroudi A. Lymphoepithelioma-like carcinoma of the bladder. BJU Int. 2001;87(1):121–2.
19. Dinney CP, Ro JY, Babaian RJ, Johnson DE. Lymphoepithelioma of the bladder: a clinicopathological study of 3 cases. J Urol. 1993;149(4):840–1.
20. Fadare O, Renshaw IL, Rubin C. Pleomorphic lymphoepithelioma-like carcinoma of the urinary bladder. Int J Clin Exp Pathol. 2009;2(2):194–9.
21. Guresci S, Doganay L, Altaner S, Atakan HI, Kutlu K. Lymphoepithelioma-like carcinoma of the urinary bladder: a case report and discussion of differential diagnosis. Int Urol Nephrol. 2005;37(1):65–8.
22. Guresci S, Simsek G, Kara C, Tezer A, Bozkurt O, Unsal A. Cytology of lymphoepithelioma-like carcinoma of the urinary bladder. Cytopathology. 2009;20(4):268–9.
23. Holmäng S, Borghede G, Johansson SL. Bladder carcinoma with lymphoepithelioma-like differentiation: a report of 9 cases. J Urol. 1998;159(3):779–82.
24. Izquierdo-García FM, García-Díez F, Fernández I, Pérez-Rosado A, Sáez A, Suárez-Vilela D, Guerreiro-González R, Benéitez-Alvarez M. Lymphoepithelioma-like carcinoma of the bladder: three cases with clinicopathological and p53 protein expression study. Virchows Arch. 2004;444(5):420–5.
25. Kessler ER, Amini A, Wilson SS, Breaker K, Raben D, La Rosa FG. Lymphoepithelioma-like carcinoma of the urinary bladder. Oncology (Williston Park). 2015;29(6):462. C3.
26. Kozyrakis D, Petraki C, Prombonas I, Grigorakis A, Kanellis G, Malovrouvas D. Lymphoepithelioma-like bladder cancer: clinicopathologic study of six cases. Int J Urol. 2011;18(10):731–4.
27. Kushida N, Kushakabe T, Kataoka M, Kumagai S, Aikawa K, Kojima Y. External beam radiotherapy for focal lymphoepithelioma-like carcinoma in the urinary bladder: a case report and literature review. Case Rep Oncol. 2015;8(1):15–20.
28. Mayer EK, Beckley I, Winkler MH. Lymphoepithelioma-like carcinoma of the urinary bladder–diagnostic and clinical implications. Nat Clin Pract Urol. 2007;4(3):167–71.
29. Mina SN, Antonios SN. Lymphoepithelioma-like carcinoma of the urinary bladder associated with schistosomiasis: A case report and review of literature. J Egypt Soc Parasitol. 2015;45(2):385–8.
30. Mori K, Ando T, Nomura T, Sato F, Mimata H. Lymphoepithelioma-like carcinoma of the bladder: A case report and review of the literature. Case Rep Urol. 2013;2013:356576.
31. Nagai T, Naiki T, Kawai N, Iida K, Etani T, Ando R, Hamamoto S, Sugiyama Y, Okada A, Mizuno K, Umemoto Y, Yasui T. Pure lymphoepithelioma-like carcinoma originating from the urinary bladder. Case Rep Oncol. 2016;9(1):188–94.

32. Pantelides NM, Ivaz SL, Falconer A, Hazell S, Winkler M, Hrouda D, Mayer EK. Lymphoepithelioma-like carcinoma of the urinary bladder: A case report and review of systemic treatment options. Urol Ann. 2012;4(1):45–7.

33. Porcaro AB, Gilioli E, Migliorini F, Antoniolli SZ, Iannucci A, Comunale L. Primary lymphoepithelioma-like carcinoma of the urinary bladder: report of one case with review and update of the literature after a pooled analysis of 43 patients. Int Urol Nephrol. 2003;35(1):99–106.

34. Raphael V, Jitani AK, Sailo SL, Vakha M. Lymphoepithelioma-like carcinoma of the urinary bladder: A rare case report. Urology Annals. 2015;7(4):516–9.

35. Singh NG, Mannan AA, Rifaat AA, Kahvic M. Lymphoepithelioma-like carcinoma of the urinary bladder: report of a rare case. Ann Saudi Med. 2009;29(6):478–81.

36. Spinelli GP, Lo Russo G, Pacchiarotti A, Stati V, Prete AA, Tomao F, Sciarretta C, Arduin M, Basso E, Chiotti S, Sinjari M, Venezia M, Zoccoli G, Tomao S. A 68-year-old Caucasian man presenting with urinary bladder lymphoepithelioma: a case report. J Med Case Rep. 2013;7:161.

37. Stamatiou K, Christopoulos G, Tsavari A, Koulia K, Manoloudaki K, Vassilakaki T. Lymphoepithelioma-like carcinoma of the bladder: A case report. Arch Ital Urol Androl. 2016;88(2):147–9.

38. Tamas EF, Nielsen ME, Schoenberg MP, Epstein JI. Lymphoepithelioma-like carcinoma of the urinary tract: a clinicopathological study of 30 pure and mixed cases. Mod Pathol. 2007;20(8):828–34.

39. Trabelsi A, Abdelkrim SB, Rammeh S, Stita W, Sriha B, Mokni M, Korbi S. Lymphoepithelioma-like carcinoma of the bladder in a North African man: A case report. N Am J Med Sci. 2009;1(7):375–6.

40. Ward JN, Dong WF, Pitts Jr WR. Lymphoepithelioma-like carcinoma of the bladder. J Urol. 2002;167(6):2523–4.

41. Williamson SR, Zhang S, Lopez-Beltran A, Shah RB, Montironi R, Tan PH, Wang M, Baldridge LA, MacLennan GT, Cheng L. Lymphoepithelioma-like carcinoma of the urinary bladder: clinicopathologic, immunohistochemical, and molecular features. Am J Surg Pathol. 2011;35(4):474–83.

42. Yaqoob N, Kayani N, Piryani J, Sulaiman MN, Hasan SH. Lymphoepithelioma-like carcinoma of urinary bladder: (LELCA). J Pak Med Assoc. 2005;55(9):402–3.

43. Yoshino T, Ohara S, Moriyama H. Lymphoepithelioma-like carcinoma of the urinary bladder: a case report and review of the literature. BMC Res Notes. 2014;7:779.

44. Young RH, Eble JN. Unusual forms of carcinoma of the urinary bladder. Hum Pathol. 1991;22(10):948–65.

45. Yun HK, Yun SI, Lee YH, Kang KM, Kwak EK, Kim JS, Cho SR, Kwon JB. Lymphoepithelioma-like carcinoma of the urinary bladder. J Korean Med Sci. 2010;25(11):1672–5.

46. Ziouziou I, Karmouni T, El Khader K, Koutani A, Andaloussi AI. Lymphoepithelioma-like carcinoma of the bladder: a case report. J Med Case Rep. 2014;8:424.

47. Moher D, Shamseer L, Clarke M, Ghersi D, Liberati A, Petticrews M, Shekelle P, Stewart LA, and PRISMA-P Group. Preferred reporting items for systematic review and meta-analysis protocols (PRISMA-P) 2015 statement. Syst Rev. 2015;4:1.

12

Silodosin 8 mg improves benign prostatic obstruction in Caucasian patients with lower urinary tract symptoms suggestive of benign prostatic enlargement: results from an explorative clinical study

Ferdinando Fusco[*] ⓘ, Massimiliano Creta, Nicola Longo, Francesco Persico, Marco Franco and Vincenzo Mirone

Abstract

Background: To preliminary investigate the effects of silodosin 8 mg once daily on obstruction urodynamic parameters and subjective symptoms in Caucasian patients with lower urinary tract symptoms suggestive of benign prostatic enlargement.

Methods: We performed a single-center, open-label, single-arm, post-marketing interventional clinical trial. Inclusion criteria were: Caucasian subjects aged ≥50 years waiting to undergo surgery for lower urinary tract symptoms suggestive of benign prostatic enlargement, international prostate symptom total score ≥ 13, international prostate symptom-quality of life score ≥ 3, prostate volume ≥ 30 ml, maximum urine flow rate ≤ 15 mL/s, bladder outlet obstruction index > 40. Eligible subjects received one capsule of silodosin 8 mg once daily for 8 weeks. Invasive urodynamic evaluations were performed at baseline and at 8-weeks follow-up. International prostate symptom questionnaire was administered at baseline, after 4-weeks and 8-weeks of treatment.

Results: Overall, 34 subjects were included. Mean bladder outlet obstruction index significantly decreased from 70.6 to 39.2 and bladder outlet obstruction index class improved in 16 patients (53.3%). Statistically significant improvements of mean total international prostate symptom score, mean storage sub-score, mean voiding sub-score and mean quality of life sub-score were evident after 4-weeks of treatment with further improvements after 8-weeks. At the end of the treatment, all patients declared that their condition improved enough to spare or delay surgery.

Conclusions: Silodosin 8 mg once daily significantly improves benign prostatic obstruction in Caucasian patients with lower urinary tract symptoms suggestive of benign prostatic enlargement waiting for surgery.

Keywords: Benign prostatic enlargement, Benign prostatic obstruction, Lower urinary tract symptoms, Silodosin, Urodynamic

* Correspondence: ferdinando-fusco@libero.it
Department of Neurosciences, Human Reproduction and
Odontostomatology, University of Naples, Federico II - Via Pansini 5, 80131
Naples, Italy

Background

Silodosin is a new, highly selective α1-blocker (AB) approved in Japan in 2006 and recently in more than 50 countries including United States and Europe for the treatment of Lower Urinary Tract Symptoms suggestive of Benign Prostatic Enlargement (LUTS/BPE) [1]. This agent has a very strong affinity for the AR, the predominant α1A Adrenergic Receptor (α1-AR) subtype expressed in human prostate where it mediates smooth muscle contraction and therefore functional obstruction of the lower urinary tract [2–7]. Phase III randomized controlled trials as well as post hoc analyses of these studies performed in Japan, US and Europe demonstrated that silodosin provides clinically relevant benefits in terms of storage and voiding LUTS as well as in terms of Quality of Life (QoL) as assessed by the International Prostate Symptom Score (IPSS) [8–11]. Benign Prostatic Obstruction (BPO) is considered a key pathophysiological link between Benign Prostatic Enlargement (BPE) and LUTS [12, 13]. Moreover, long lasting BPO may activate pathways leading to progressive remodeling of both lower and upper urinary tract with subsequent functional impairments [12]. Therefore, BPO relief represents a major goal of LUTS/BPE treatment. A diagnosis of BPO requires an invasive Pressure/Flow studies (PFS) that allows to calculate the Bladder Outlet Obstruction Index (BOOI) [12]. Clinical studies investigating invasive urodynamic measures of BPO in LUTS/BPE patients receiving silodosin demonstrated that this agent, as other ABs, significantly improves BOOI [11–13]. Based on indirect comparisons, the magnitude of BPO improvement with silodosin appears to be greater if compared to other ABs [12–14]. Until now, however, urodynamic data on silodosin in terms of BPO mainly derive from three major studies involving Japanese LUTS/BPH patients [15–17]. It is widely recognized that ethnic and even population differences exist in the pharmacokinetics and pharmacodynamics of drugs [18]. Moreover, in two of these studies, silodosin was administered at the dosage of 4 mg twice daily whereas the dose of silodosin recommended by both the Food and Drug Administration and EMA is 8 mg once a day [15, 17, 19]. We aimed to preliminary investigate the effects of silodosin 8 mg once daily in Caucasian patients with LUTS/BPE in terms of invasive BPO urodynamic parameters and subjective symptoms.

Methods

We performed a single-center, open-label, single-arm, post-marketing interventional clinical trial (EudraCT n. 2015-002277-38). The local ethics committee approved the study protocol. The study was carried out according to the Declaration of.

Helsinki. All patients enrolled complained with LUTS severe enough to require surgery and reported poor results with previous pharmacological treatments.

Study inclusion criteria were: Caucasian subjects aged ≥50 years waiting to undergo surgical intervention for LUTS/BPH, IPSS total score ≥ 13, IPSS-QoL score ≥ 3, prostate volume ≥ 30 ml, maximum urine flow rate (Q_{max}) ≤ 15 mL/s, BOOI > 40. Exclusion criteria were: pharmacological treatment for LUTS/BPH in the last 4 weeks or 6 months in case of previous assumption of 5alpha-reductase inhibitors, absolute indication for surgery therapy, hypersensitivity to the active substance or to any of the excipients, neurological causes of detrusor overactivity, active urinary tract infections, presence or history of bladder calculi, presence of prostate cancer, Post-Void Residual Volume (PVR) > 300 mL, clinically significant cardiovascular and cerebrovascular disease within 6 months prior to screening, renal or hepatic impairment, patients for whom cataract surgery was scheduled, history of orthostatic hypotension or syncope. After a washout period of 6 months, in patients taking 5-alpha reductase inhibitors, or of 4 weeks in patient taking any other drug or herbal remedy for LUTS/BPH, four visits were foreseen: at screening (Visit 1, week – 1), at baseline (Visit 2) and after 4 (Visit 3) and 8 (Visit 4) weeks of treatment. Screening procedures consisted of: medical history collection, check of prior and concomitant medications, symptom assessment by IPSS questionnaire, physical examination, measurement of vital signs (sitting blood pressure and heart rate), evaluation of prostate volume and PVR by suprapubic ultrasound, measurement of Q_{max}, 12-lead ECG, laboratory tests, including Prostate Specific Antigen value. Each patient signed an informed consent. Inclusion and exclusion criteria were preliminarily evaluated. At baseline, the following evaluations were performed: vital signs, urodynamic study. A final evaluation of inclusion and exclusion criteria was performed at this stage and patients with a BOOI< 40 were excluded. Eligible subjects received one capsule of silodosin 8 mg once daily for 8 weeks. They agreed not to use any other approved or experimental medication for LUTS/BPE or overactive bladder anytime during the study. At the end of the 4-weeks treatment period, patients underwent the following evaluations: IPSS questionnaire and patient-reported Treatment-Emergent Adverse Events (TEAEs) evaluated based on the terminology of the Medical Dictionary for Regulatory Activities. At the end of the 8-weeks treatment period, patients underwent the following evaluations: physical examination, IPSS questionnaire, vital signs, laboratory tests, PVR, urodynamic study. Moreover, TEAEs were evaluated again. All urodynamic studies were performed by the same operator based on standard International Continence Society (ICS) procedure [20]. A 6-F double lumen catheter was inserted transurethrally, and a balloon catheter was inserted from the anus to measure abdominal pressure. The test was done with the patient standing. Physiological saline solution was injected into the bladder at 50 ml per minute after evacuating the bladder. Intravesical pressure, abdominal pressure and detrusor pressure in the storage phase were simultaneously measured and recorded. Detrusor pressure was measured by electrically subtracting the abdominal pressure from the intravesical pressure. Detrusor Overactivity (DO) was defined as involuntary detrusor contractions during the filling phase which may be spontaneous or provoked. At maximum cystometric capacity the pressure/flow study was performed. The BOOI was defined as Detrusor Pressure at Q_{max} ($PdetQ_{max}$) - $2Q_{max}$ [21]. According to BOOI value, subjects were classified as obstructed (BOOI > 40), equivocal (BOOI 20 – 40), or unobstructed (BOOI < 20) [21]. The primary objective of the study was to evaluate BOOI variations with respect to baseline. The followings were considered secondary outcomes: variations of other urodynamic parameters, improvement from baseline in obstruction class on the ICS BOOI nomogram, PVR variations, IPSS variations, percentage of subjects considering their condition improved enough to spare or delay the surgical intervention for LUTS/BPE, safety profile of the drug. Continuous variables were expressed as mean ± standard deviation (SD) and categorical variables as number and percentages. Changes from baseline for continuous data were compared using the paired Student's T test. McNemar's or Bowker's Symmetry tests were used for shift tables assessment P values of less than 0.05 were regarded as statistically significant. Statistical analysis was performed using SAS software (SAS Institute Inc., Cary, N.C.).

Results

Overall, 34 subjects were screened. Of them, 4 were excluded after PFS indicated that they were unobstructed. Demographic and clinical characteristics of the 30 subjects enrolled into the study are summarized in Table 1.

All patients completed the study protocol and were available for follow-up evaluations. Table 2 and Fig. 1 summarizes the variations of main urodynamic parameters from baseline to the end of the study.

Mean BOOI significantly decreased from 70.6 to 39.2 and BOOI class improved in 16 patients (53.3%). Obstruction persisted in 14/30 subjects (46.7%). Statistically significant improvements were observed in terms of Detrusor opening pressure, $PdetQ_{max}$, Maximum Detrusor Pressure ($Pdet_{max}$), Q_{max}, and Bladder Contractility Index. No statistically significant variations in terms of incidence of DO and amplitude of the largest DO contraction were observed. Total IPSS score, IPSS storage and voiding sub-scores as well as IPSS QoL sub-score improved in a statistically significant

Table 1 Baseline patients' characteristics

Demographics	
Age, yr., mean (SD)	63.1 (9.2)
Age category, n (%)	
< 65 yr	16 (53.3)
65–74 yr	10 (33.3)
≥ 75 yr	4 (13.3)
Race, n (%)	
White	30 (100)
Clinical characteristics	
Body Mass Index, kg/m², mean (SD)	24.7 (1.8)
Time elapsed from the diagnosis of LUTS/BPE (yr), mean (SD)	6.0 (3.9)
Prostate volume mL, mean (SD)	58.2 (17.4)
PVR volume, mL, mean (SD)	71.1 (33.1)
Q_{max}, mL/s, mean (SD)	9.0 (2.7)
Prostate Specific Antigen, ng/mL, mean (SD)	2.3 (1.8)
Comorbidities, n (%)	
Hypercholesterolemia	1 (3.3)
Asthma	1 (3.3)
Essential hypertension	4 (13.3)

SD Standard Deviation

manner after 4-weeks of treatment and further improvements were evident after 8-weeks (Table 3).

Mean total IPSS score improved by 6.7 points and by 10.7 points after 4 and 8 weeks of treatment, respectively. Mean IPSS storage sub-score improved by 2.2 points and 4.0 points after 4 and 8 weeks of treatment, respectively. Mean IPSS voiding sub-score improved by 4.5 points and 6.7 points after 4 and 8 weeks of treatment, respectively. Mean IPSS QoL sub-score improved by 1.7 points and 3.0 points after 4 and 8 weeks of treatment, respectively. At the end of the treatment all patients answered "yes" to the question: "After the treatment with silodosin, is your condition improved enough to spare or, delay the surgical intervention for BPH/LUTS?". In total, 11/30 patients (36.7%) experienced TEAEs. All TEAEs were drug related. The most frequently reported TEAE was retrograde ejaculation occurring in 8/30 patients (26.7%). Other TEAEs were asthenia (1/30, 3.3%), fatigue (1/30, 3.3%), and nasal congestion (1/30, 3.3%). There were no serious adverse events and all adverse evets were of mild intensity. There were no TEAEs leading to drug discontinuation. No clinical changes were found in terms of vital signs and laboratory parameters.

Discussion

ABs aim to inhibit the effect of endogenously released noradrenaline on smooth muscle cells in the prostate and thereby reduce prostate tone and BPO [21, 22]. To date,

Table 2 Urodynamic parameters at baseline and after 8 weeks of therapy

	Baseline	8 weeks	P value
Volume at first desire to void, mL, mean (SD)	105.7 (36.6)	130.3 (42.5)	0.004[‡]
Maximum cystometric capacity, mL, mean (SD)	229.7 (70.0)	257.5 (71.2)	0.0717[‡]
Bladder compliance (mL/ cmH_2O), mean (SD)	17.2 (27.7)	26.5 (38.9)	0.2851[‡]
DO, n (%)	4 (13.3)	2 (6.7)	0.3173[†]
Amplitude of the largest DO contraction, cmH_2O, mean (SD)	9.0 (25.0)	4.3 (12.1)	0.3098[‡]
Pdet Q_{max}, cmH_2O, mean (SD)	86.1 (19.7)	58.2 (17.3)	< 0.0001[‡]
Pdet$_{max}$, cmH_2O, mean (SD)	99.6 (23.5)	72.0 (22.4)	< 0.0001[‡]
Detrusor opening pressure, cmH_2O, mean (SD)	72.1 (31.0)	50.3 (23.1)	0.0031[‡]
Qmax, mL/s, mean (SD)	7.8 (3.1)	9.5 (3.8)	0.015[‡]
BOOI, mean (SD)	70.6 (18.9)	39.2 (18.3)	< 0.0001[‡]
BOOI< 20 n, (%)	0 (0)	4 (13.3)	
BOOI 20–40 n, (%)	0 (0)	12 (40.0)	
BOOI> 40 n, (%)	30 (100)	14 (46.7)	
Bladder Contractility Index, mean (SD)	121 (34.7)	105.6 (26.5)	0.0274[‡]
PVR volume, mL, mean (SD)	71.1 (33.1)	52.5 (23.2)	< 0.0001[‡]

BOOI Bladder Outlet Obstruction Index, *DO* Detrusor Overactivity, *Pdet$_{max}$* Maximum Detrusor Pressure, *PdetQ$_{max}$* Detrusor Pressure at Q_{max}, *PFS* Pressure/Flow Study, *PVR* Post-Void Residual Volume, *Q$_{max}$* Maximum urine flow rate, *SD* Standard Deviation
[†]Mc Nemar's Test
[‡]paired T Test

six ABs (terazosin, doxazosin, tamsulosin, naftopidil, alfuzosin, and silodosin) have been approved for the treatment of LUTS/BPE. Although all ABs improve BPO, the magnitude of improvement varies according to the type of AB and is greater after silodosin with values comparable to that obtained after transurethral microwave thermotherapy [12, 13]. To our knowledge, this is the first study investigating the urodynamic efficacy of silodosin 8 mg once a day in terms of BPO in Caucasian patients with LUTS/BPE waiting for surgery. We demonstrated that silodosin significantly improves BOOI in this selected subset of patients characterized by significant subjective and objective impairments. The magnitude of BOOI improvement (31.4 points) was both statistically and clinically significant and in line with published ranges for silodosin (21.2 - 37.6). To date, the rationale behind the urodynamic profile of silodosin is not completely understood. Based on published data, however, the existence of a positive relationship between α-1A/ α-1B receptor affinity ratio and BPO improvement has been hypothesized [12]. Moreover, the magnitude of BOOI improvement with ABs has been reported to increase also with the

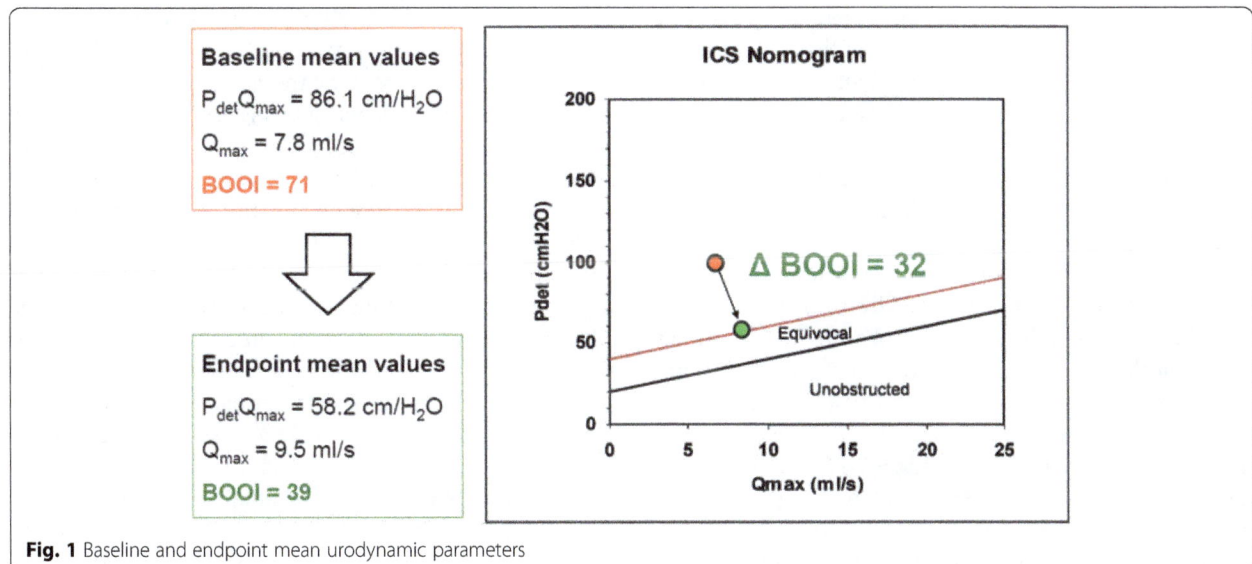

Fig. 1 Baseline and endpoint mean urodynamic parameters

Table 3 IPSS scores at baseline, after 4 weeks and after 8 weeks of treatment

	Baseline	4 weeks		8 weeks	
	Mean (SD)	Mean (SD)	$p^\dagger$	Mean (SD)	$p^\dagger$
Total IPSS score	21.6 (3.1)	14.9 (3.6)	< 0.0001	10.9 (2.2)	< 0.0001
IPSS storage sub-score	8.3 (1.8)	6.2 (1.5)	< 0.0001	4.4 (1.0)	< 0.0001
IPSS voiding subs-core	13.2 (2.2)	8.7 (2.4)	< 0.0001	6.5 (1.5)	< 0.0001
IPSS-QoL sub-score	4.6 (0.8)	2.9 (0.8)	< 0.0001	1.5 (0.7)	< 0.0001

IPSS International Prostate Symptom Score, *SD* Standard Deviation, *QoL* Quality of Life
†with respect to baseline (Paired T Test)

percentage of patients with obstruction at baseline [13]. Nevertheless, direct comparisons among ABs in terms of BPO improvement are lacking thus limiting the value of current evidences. We found that obstruction class improved in 53.3% of patients. This finding is in line with published data. In the study by Yamanishi et al., the obstruction grade was improved in 15 patients (56%) (obstructed to unobstructed in 5, obstructed to equivocal in 8, and equivocal to unobstructed in 2) and unchanged in 12 (44%) (obstructed to obstructed in 9, and equivocal to equivocal in 3) [16]. The BOOI value is obtained from Q_{max} and $PdetQ_{max}$ values. Results from the present study show statistically significant improvements of both $PdetQ_{max}$ and Q_{max}. However, although mean $PdetQ_{max}$ variation was clinically robust, mean Q_{max} improvement was clinically marginal (only 1.8 mL/s). This finding is coherent with published urodynamic data obtained in LUTS/BPE patients treated with ABs in general as well as in the subgroup of Japanese patients treated with silodosin at the dosages of both 4 mg twice daily and 8 mg once a day [13–17]. From a pathophysiological point of view, we can hypothesize that the reduction of detrusor pressure represents a priority with respect to urinary flow improvement and, when the relief of outflow resistances is small as after therapy with ABs, the lower urinary tract mainly adapts by reducing detrusor pressures thus potentially preserving the integrity of the bladder itself and of the upper urinary tract [12]. Therefore, in everyday clinical practice, Q_{max} improvement alone may underestimate the urodynamic benefits deriving from ABs therapy. Unlike some published data, our study did not demonstrate statistically significant variations of urodynamic parameters relative to DO [15–17]. However, the number of patients with DO at baseline in the present study was very low and further studies are needed to specifically address this issue.

In line with published data, we observed a statistically and clinically significant therapeutic effect, including improvements in both obstructive and irritative sub-scores, which was reflected by improvements in QoL. Interestingly, the magnitude of improvement we found in all these domains after 8 weeks of treatment was higher if compared to results from phase III clinical studies on silodosin as well as to results obtained in the urodynamic studies

involving mainly obstructed patients after a 12 weeks treatment period [1, 15–17]. Matsukawa et al. reported mean improvements of total IPSS, voiding IPSS sub-score, storage IPSS sub-score and QoL sub-score of 6.2, 3.6, 2.6, and 1.6 points, respectively [17]. Yamanishi et al. reported mean improvement of total IPSS, voiding IPSS sub-score, storage IPSS sub-score and QoL sub-score were 7.9, 3.8, 2.0, and 1.1 points, respectively [16]. In the study by Chapple et al., mean improvement of total IPSS, voiding IPSS sub-score, storage IPSS sub-score and QoL sub-score were 7.0, 4.5, 2.5, and 1.1 points, respectively [10]. The rationale behind the differences observed between our results and published ones is unknown. Although we can hypothesize that baseline characteristics of subjects may have a role and that subjects with a moderate-to-high compromised baseline level, such that involved into the present study, may have a greater margin of improvement if compared to subjects that are less compromised at baseline, further studies are needed to confirm this hypothesis. At the end of the treatment, all patients declared that their condition had improved enough to spare or delay surgery. Results from the present study have relevant clinical implications. Indeed, therapy with ABs may represent an interesting "rescue treatment" option for patients with BPO waiting for surgical treatment.

Although a timely indication to surgery is crucial to prevent bladder decompensation leading to surgical failure, this treatment may postpone the need to perform a surgical treatment in patients showing an improvement of BPO and LUTS and/or an improvement of their QoL due to LUTS while waiting for surgery. Moreover, this treatment may cause a reduction in the waiting list for the other patients confirming the need to perform surgery. The urodynamic profile of silodosin characterized by the highest level of BOOI improvement with respect to other ABs, makes it a drug of greatest interest in this subset of patients. We confirmed the good safety profile of silodosin. In line with published data, retrograde ejaculation was the more frequently reported adverse event. However, none of subjects interrupted the treatment due to this event. We acknowledge potential limitations of the present study. First, it was a single arm, open-label study using neither a placebo nor a control group. Although a placebo-effect cannot be excluded in terms of changes of both subjective and urodynamic parameters, results from a previous meta-analysis suggested the absence of significant placebo effects on urodynamic parameters of BPO after therapy with ABs [13]. Moreover, our study sample voluntarily included patients with urodynamic proven BPO thus making questionable the generalizability of our results to subjects that in the everyday clinical practice do not routinely undergo invasive urodynamic investigations. However, the combination of the clinical criteria we adopted in the pre-screening procedure (age ≥ 50 years, IPSS total score ≥ 13, prostate volume of ≥ 30 ml, $Q_{max} \leq 15$ mL/s) represented a good proxy of BPO as it allowed us to identify a population of subjects with a high prevalence of urodynamic proven BPO (88.2%, $n = 30/34$). Therefore, in every day clinical practice, findings from the present study can be generalizable to subjects with the aforementioned clinical features even in the absence of urodynamic confirmation of BPO. Overall, results from the present study should be considered as preliminary and confirmatory randomized placebo controlled trials with adequate follow-up are needed. In conclusions, silodosin 8 mg once daily provides statistically and clinically significant improvement of BPO and symptoms in LUTS/BPE Caucasian men with confirmed BPO waiting for surgery.

Conclusions

In conclusions, based on these preliminary data, silodosin 8 mg once daily significantly improves BPO in Caucasian patients with LUTS/BPE waiting for surgery.

Abbreviations

AB: Alpha Blocker; AR: Adrenergic Receptor; BOOI: Bladder Outlet Obstruction Index; BPE: Benign Prostatic Enlargement; BPO: Benign Prostatic Obstruction; DO: Detrusor Overactivity; ICS: International Continence Society; IPSS: International Prostate Symptom Score; LUTS: Lower Urinary Tract Symptoms; PdetQ$_{max}$: Detrusor Pressure at Q$_{max}$; PFS: Pressure/Flow studies; PVR: Post-Void Residual Volume; Q$_{max}$: Maximum Urine Flow Rate; QoL: Quality of Life; SD: Standard Deviation; TEAEs: Treatment-Emergent Adverse Events

Acknowledgements
We have no acknowledgements for this study.

Funding
This work was supported by Recordati S.p.A. Recordati contributed in the study design definition and was involved in the collection and analysis of the data.

Authors' contributions
Conception and design: FF, MC and VM; enrollment of patients and acquisition of data: FF, NL, FP and MF; drafting of the manuscript: FF and MC; statistical analysis: FF, FP; analysis and interpretation of data: MC, MF, NL; supervision: NL, VM. We confirm that all authors read and approved the final manuscript.

Competing interests
Ferdinando Fusco, Massimiliano Creta and Vincenzo Mirone have been consultants for Recordati S.p.A.

References
1. Osman NI, Chapple CR, Cruz F, Desgrandchamps F, Llorente C, Montorsi F. Silodosin: a new subtype selective alpha-1 antagonist for the treatment of lower urinary tract symptoms in patients with benign prostatic hyperplasia. Expert Opin Pharmacother. 2012 Oct;13(14):2085–96.
2. Lepor H, Shapiro E. Characterization of alpha1 adrenergic receptors in human benign prostatic hyperplasia. J Urol. 1984;132(6):1226–9.
3. Lepor H, Tang R, Meretyk S, Shapiro E. Alpha 1 adrenoceptor subtypes in the human prostate. J Urol. 1993;149(3):640–2.
4. Kobayashi S, Tang R, Shapiro E, Lepor H. Characterization and localization of prostatic alpha 1 adrenoceptors using radioligand receptor binding on slide-mounted tissue section. J Urol. 1993;150(6):2002–6.
5. Walden PD, Gerardi C, Lepor H. Localization and expression of the alpha1A-1, alpha1B and alpha1D-adrenoceptors in hyperplastic and non-hyperplastic human prostate. J Urol. 1999;161(2):635–40.
6. Forray C, Bard JA, Wetzel JM, et al. The alpha 1-adrenergic receptor that mediates smooth muscle contraction in human prostate has the pharmacological properties of the cloned human alpha 1c subtype. Mol Pharmacol. 1994;45(4):703–8.
7. Imperatore V, Fusco F, Creta M, et al. Medical expulsive therapy for distal ureteric stones: tamsulosin versus silodosin. Arch Ital Urol Androl. 2014 Jun 30;86(2):103–7.
8. Kawabe K, Yoshida M, Homma Y, Silodosin Clinical Study Group. Silodosin, a new alpha1A-adrenoceptor-selective antagonist for treating benign prostatic hyperplasia: results of a phase III randomized, placebo-controlled, double-blind study in Japanese men. BJU Int. 2006 Nov;98(5):1019–24.
9. Marks LS, Gittelman MC, Hill LA, Volinn W, Hoel G. Silodosin in the treatment of the signs and symptoms of benign prostatic hyperplasia: a 9-month, open-label extension study. Urology. 2009 Dec;74(6):1318–22.
10. Chapple CR, Montorsi F, Tammela TL, et al. Silodosin therapy for lower urinary tract symptoms in men with suspected benign prostatic hyperplasia: results of an international, randomized, double-blind, placebo- and active-controlled clinical trial performed in Europe. Eur Urol. 2011 Mar;59(3):342–52.
11. Osman NI, Chapple CR, Tammela TL, Eisenhardt A, Oelke M. Open-label, 9-month extension study investigating the uro-selective alpha-blocker silodosin in men with LUTS associated with BPH. World J Urol. 2015 May; 33(5):697–706.
12. Fusco F, Creta M, Imperatore V, et al. Benign prostatic obstruction relief in patients with lower urinary tract symptoms suggestive of benign prostatic enlargement undergoing endoscopic surgical procedures or therapy with alpha-blockers: a review of urodynamic studies. Adv Ther. 2017 Apr;34(4):773–83.
13. Fusco F, Palmieri A, Ficarra V, et al. α1-blockers improve benign prostatic obstruction in men with lower urinary tract symptoms: a systematic review and meta-analysis of urodynamic studies. Eur Urol. 2016 Jun;69(6):1091–101.
14. Creta M, Bottone F, Sannino S, et al. Effects of alpha1-blockers on urodynamic parameters of bladder outlet obstruction in patients with lower urinary tract symptoms suggestive of benign prostatic enlargement: a review. Minerva Urol Nefrol. 2016;68(2):209–21.
15. Matsukawa Y, Gotoh M, Komatsu T, Funahashi Y, Sassa N, Hattori R. Efficacy of silodosin for relieving benign prostatic obstruction: prospective pressure flow study. J Urol. 2009;182:2831–5.
16. Yamanishi T, Mizuno T, Tatsumiya K, Watanabe M, Kamai T, Yoshida K. Urodynamic effects of silodosin, a new alpha 1A-adrenoceptor selective antagonist, for the treatment of benign prostatic hyperplasia. Neurourol Urodyn. 2010;29:558–62.
17. Matsukawa Y, Takai S, Funahashi Y, Kato M, Yamamoto T, Gotoh M. Long-term efficacy of a combination therapy with an anticholinergic agent and an α1-blocker for patients with benign prostatic enlargement complaining both voiding and overactive bladder symptoms: a randomized, prospective, comparative trial using a urodynamic study. Neurourol Urodyn. 2017 Mar; 36(3):748–54.
18. Kurose K, Sugiyama E, Saito Y. Population differences in major functional polymorphisms of pharmacokinetics/pharmacodynamics-related genes in Eastern Asians and Europeans: implications in the clinical trials for novel drug development. Drug Metab Pharmacokinet. 2012;27(1):9–54. Epub 2011 Nov 29.

13

Assessment of lower urinary symptom flare with overactive bladder symptom score and International Prostate Symptom Score in patients treated with iodine-125 implant brachytherapy: long-term follow-up experience at a single institute

Makito Miyake[1], Nobumichi Tanaka[1*], Isao Asakawa[2], Shunta Hori[1], Yosuke Morizawa[1], Yoshihiro Tatsumi[1,3], Yasushi Nakai[1], Takeshi Inoue[1], Satoshi Anai[1], Kazumasa Torimoto[1], Katsuya Aoki[1], Masatoshi Hasegawa[2], Tomomi Fujii[3], Noboru Konishi[3] and Kiyohide Fujimoto[1]

Abstract

Background: The aim of this study was to evaluate the combined use of the overactive bladder symptom score (OABSS) and International Prostate Symptom Score (IPSS) as an assessment tool for urinary symptom flare after iodine-125 (^{125}I) implant brachytherapy. The association between urinary symptom flare and prostate-specific antigen (PSA) bounce was investigated.

Methods: Changes in the IPSS and OABSS were prospectively recorded in 355 patients who underwent seed implantation. The percentage distribution of patients according to the difference between the flare peak and post-implant nadir was plotted to define significant increases in the scores. The clinicopathologic characteristics, treatment parameters, and post-implant dosimetric parameters were compared between the non-flare and flare groups. PSA bounce was defined as an elevation of ≥0.1 ng/mL or ≥0.4 ng/mL compared to the previous lowest value, followed by a decrease to a level at or below the pre-bounce value.

Results: A clinically significant increase required an IPSS increase of at least 12 points and an OABSS increase of at least 6 points based on a time-course analysis of total scores and the QOL index. Assessment only by IPSS failed to detect 40 patients (11%) who had urinary symptom flare according to the OABSS. Univariate and multivariate analyses revealed that patients treated with higher biologically effective doses and those without diabetes mellitus had higher risks of urinary flare. There was no statistical correlation between the incidence and time of urinary symptom flare onset and that of a PSA bounce.

(Continued on next page)

* Correspondence: sendo@naramed-u.ac.jp
[1]Department of Urology, Nara Medical University, 840 Shijo-cho, Nara 634-8522, Japan
Full list of author information is available at the end of the article

(Continued from previous page)

Conclusions: To our knowledge, this is the first report to prove the clinical potential of the OABSS as an assessment tool for urinary symptom flare after seed implantation. Our findings showed that persistent lower urinary tract symptoms after seed implantation were attributed to storage rather than to voiding issues. We believe that assessment with the OABSS combined with the IPSS would aid in decision-making in terms of timing, selection of a treatment intervention, and assessment of the outcome.

Keywords: Prostate cancer, Brachytherapy, International Prostate Symptom Score, Overactive bladder symptom score, Biologically effective dose, PSA bounce,

Background

Low-dose rate brachytherapy using iodine-125 (^{125}I) seed implantation with or without supplemental external beam radiotherapy (EBRT) is currently a standard treatment for localized prostate cancer (PCa). According to a nationwide prospective cohort study, the Japanese Prostate Cancer Outcome Study of Permanent Iodine-125 Seed Implant (J-POPS), over 25,000 patients with PCa underwent brachytherapy in Japan as of 2014 [1, 2]. A previous survey investigating the treatment distribution of primary therapy for cT1–2N0M0 PCa at our institute showed a brachy-therapy rate of 38% [3]. While brachytherapy has positive long-term oncological outcomes, there are clinical concerns. These include the incidence of post-treatment adverse effects such as lower urinary tract symptoms (LUTS) and quality of life (QOL) deterioration [2, 4–11].

Worsening LUTSs are one of the most bothersome consequences of brachytherapy; however, acute symptoms tend to mitigate as the baseline is gradually restored within 1 year [4, 5]. During further follow-up, transient relapse of LUTS is observed in some patients, which Cesaretti et al. termed a "urinary symptom flare" [12]. Since then, predictive factors of urinary symptom flares have been explored in large cohorts of patients undergoing brachytherapy [4, 8–11]. In previous reports, chronological changes on International Prostate Symptom Score (IPSS) questionnaires were used to evaluate the urinary symptom flare. The results showed that urinary symptom flare incidence was associated with erectile dysfunction, higher baseline IPSS, maximal post-implant IPSS, age, the biologically effective dose (BED), and implementation of supplementary EBRT [4, 9, 11].

The IPSS has been predominantly utilized as a tool for defining urinary symptom flares, which are termed IPSS flares [4, 8–12]. Bothersome symptoms after radiotherapy seem to mainly be characterized by storage urinary characteristics including frequency, urgency, and nocturia [13]. The overactive bladder symptom score (OABSS) was developed in 2006 as an evaluation tool for patients with overactive bladder syndrome (OAB) and has been validated in Japanese as well as in other populations [14–16]. The OABSS evaluates relevant symptoms with only 4 questions that cover daytime frequency, nocturia, urgency, and urge incontinence. This questionnaire is simple and quick, and it agrees with corresponding diary variables [17] and treatment-related improvement with anticholinergic use [18]. Therefore, the OABSS may be beneficial for evaluating urinary symptom flares after brachytherapy.

To date, no reported studies have investigated urinary symptom flare after ^{125}I brachytherapy in a single cohort by using both the IPSS and the OABSS. In this prospective study, we focused on the predictive factors for urinary symptom flare based on the IPSS and OABSS questionnaires. In addition, we investigated the association between urinary symptom flare and the incidence of prostate-specific antigen (PSA) bounce because research on this issue is limited.

Methods

Patients and data collection

Between April 2004 and September 2010, 355 consecutive patients underwent ^{125}I brachytherapy for localized PCa in the Nara Medical University Hospital. The clinicopathologic characteristics of the patients, the treatments, and the BED are listed in Table 1. The median age was 71 years (range, 48–83). The median initial PSA was 7.11 ng/mL (range, 3.10–32.2). Two pathologists (T. Fujii and N. Konishi) with expertise in Pca diagnosis reviewed the Gleason scores of all biopsy specimens. Tumor stages were identified according to the 2002 Union for International Cancer Control classification. Patients were stratified according to the D'Amico risk classification [19]. The baseline (BL) urinary function was prospectively determined by the IPSS, IPSS-QOL index, OABSS, Sexual Health Inventory for Men (SHIM), and a voiding study before implantation and during the post-implant follow-ups that were conducted at 1, 3, 6, 12, 24, 36, 48, and 60 months after implantation. The voiding symptoms-related IPSS (V-IPSS; the sum of questions 1, 3, 5, and 6) and storage symptoms-related IPSS (S-IPSS; the sum of questions 2, 4, and 7) subscores were calculated separately [13]. PSA level was monitored 1, 3, 6, 12, 18, 24, 30, 36, 48, and 60 months after implantation. In the present study, PSA bounce was defined as an increase of at least 0.1 ng/mL or 0.4 ng/mL (two different cutoffs)

Table 1 Characteristics of 355 patients

Variables	Total ($n = 355$)	%
Age at brachyterapy (years) [a]	71 (48–83)	
Initial PSA (ng/mL) [a]	7.11 (3.10–32.2)	
Clinical T category		
T1c	197	55%
T2a	128	36%
T2b or T2c	30	8%
D'Amico risk classification		
Low	153	43%
Intermidiate	166	47%
High	36	10%
Gleason sum		
6	206	58%
7	131	37%
8 or 9	18	5%
Hypertention		
No	243	68%
Yes	112	32%
Diabetis		
No	318	90%
Yes	37	10%
Pre-use of alpha-1 adrenoceptor antagonist		
No	304	86%
Yes	51	14%
Baseline IPSS (0 to 35)		
Continuous [a]	7 (0–33)	
1 to 7	201	57%
8 to 19	130	37%
20 to 35	23	6%
Baseline OABSS (0 to 15)		
Continuous [a]	3 (0–13)	
0 to 5	289	81%
6 to 11	59	17%
12 to 15	4	1%
Prostate volume at diagnosis (mL) [a]	24.2 (7.8–59.9)	
Prostate volume at implant (mL) [a]	25.7 (7.8–61.9)	
Supplementary EBRT		
No	247	70%
Yes	108	30%
Combined ADT		
No	227	64%
Yes	128	36%

Table 1 Characteristics of 355 patients (Continued)

No of needles [a]	23 (14–36)
No of seeds [a]	60 (30–95)
BED (Gy2)	194.8 (120.3–253.2)

PSA prostate-specific antigen, IPSS International Prostate Symptom Score, OABSS overactive bladder symptom score, SD standard deviation, EBRT external beam radiotherapy, ADT androgen deprivation therapy, BED biologically effective dose
[a] expressed by medians and ranges

more than the previous lowest value (excluding the 1 month PSA value), followed by a decrease to a level at or below the pre-bounce value [20].

Definition of urinary symptom flare

Patients in the study and in previous reports [5] experienced a transient elevation of urinary symptom scores after implantation. After the peak, the scores subsequently returned to the BL. The lowest score after the peak is termed the "urinary symptom nadir." A subgroup of patients experienced a relapse in negative urinary symptoms without any bacterial urinary tract infections, which is called a "urinary symptom flare." Previous studies defined the IPSS of 5 or 8 points greater than the post-implant nadir of the IPSS as urinary symptom flare. However, the optimized cutoff point has not been defined yet. To define the significant increase in the IPSS and OABSS in a Japanese cohort, we plotted the percentage distribution of patients according to the difference between the flare peak and post-implant nadir as previously reported [9, 12]. Two cutoff points for the difference between the flare peak and nadir were established, so that approximately 25 and 50% of patients, respectively, were classified as experiencing urinary symptom flare. To examine significant factors predicting the occurrence of this condition, clinicopathologic variables and post-implant dosimetric parameters were evaluated with univariate and multivariate analyses.

Procedure of the seed implantation, EBRT, and post-implant dosimetry

We performed the implantation procedure as previously described [20, 21]. The prescribed radiation dose was 145 or 160 Gy in the implantation monotherapy group and 110 Gy of radiation combined with 45 Gy of EBRT administered in 25 fractions in the combined group [21]. Of the 355 patients, 108 (30%) were treated with combined androgen depletion therapy (ADT) in which luteinizing hormone-releasing hormone agonist, anti-androgen, or a combination of the two was used. An experienced radiation oncologist (I. Asakawa) performed a computed tomography scan about 1 month after implantation to obtain the post-implant dosimetric parameters. The BED was calculated with the formulas reported by Stock et al., in which the prostate D90,

EBRT dose, and α/β ratio of 2 (Gy2) for the effect-specific parameter were taken into account [22].

Statistical analysis

We evaluated chronological changes by plotting each IPSS and OABSS in line graphs where scores were expressed as the mean ± standard deviation (SD). The Mann-Whitney U-test, chi-square test, and Fisher's exact test were used to analyze the clinicopathologic variables. The independent association was evaluated using the odds ratio (OR) and a 95% confidence interval (CI) derived from standard logistic regression methods. For multivariate analysis, variables were selected on the condition that the P value was less than 0.1 in the univariate analysis. The interrelationship between the time of the urinary symptom flare and the time of the PSA bounce

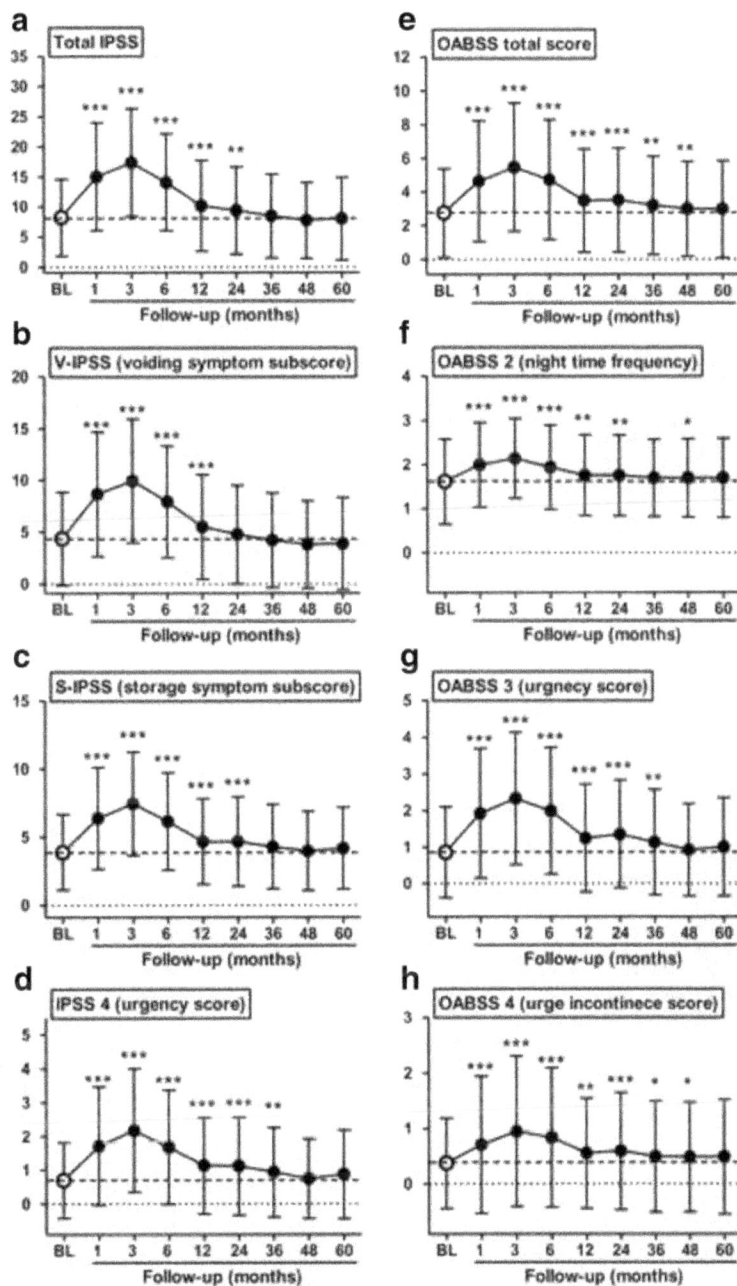

Fig. 1 Changes in representative parameters for lower urinary symptoms during follow-up after seed implant. IPSS (**a–d**) and OABSS (**e–h**) questionnaires were used for evaluation. Scores at each time point (the baseline and 1, 3, 6, 12, 24, 36, 48, and 60 months after implant) were compared with the baseline scores with the Mann-Whitney U-test. Data are expressed by means and standard deviations. Changes in other parameters are shown in Additional file 1: Figure S1. BL, the baseline; * $P < 0.05$, ** $P < 0.01$, *** $P < 0.001$

was examined using Spearman's correlation. IBM SPSS version 21 (SPSS Inc., Chicago, IL, USA) and Prism software 5.00 (GraphPad Software, San Diego, CA, USA) were utilized for statistical analyses and data plotting, respectively. A *P* value of <0.05 was considered statistically significant.

Results
Time-course changes in the IPSS, OABSS, and subscores after seed implantation
The clinicopathologic characteristics, treatment parameters, and BED are listed in Table 1. The median follow-

up after implantation was 72 months (range, 2–126). The changes in the IPSS and OABSS from BL to 60 months after implantation were plotted on line graphs (Fig. 1a-h and Additional file 1: Figure S1). For all analyzed data, the worst symptom scores were observed 3 months after implantation; however, most scores decreased with time. Although the V-IPSS returned to the BL after 24 months (Fig. 1b), the S-IPSS did not (Fig. 1c), resulting in an elevated total IPSS at 24 months (Fig. 1a). The worsening of the urgency score persisted most among the 7 scores of IPSS questionnaire (Fig. 1d and Additional file 1: Figure S1). While the total

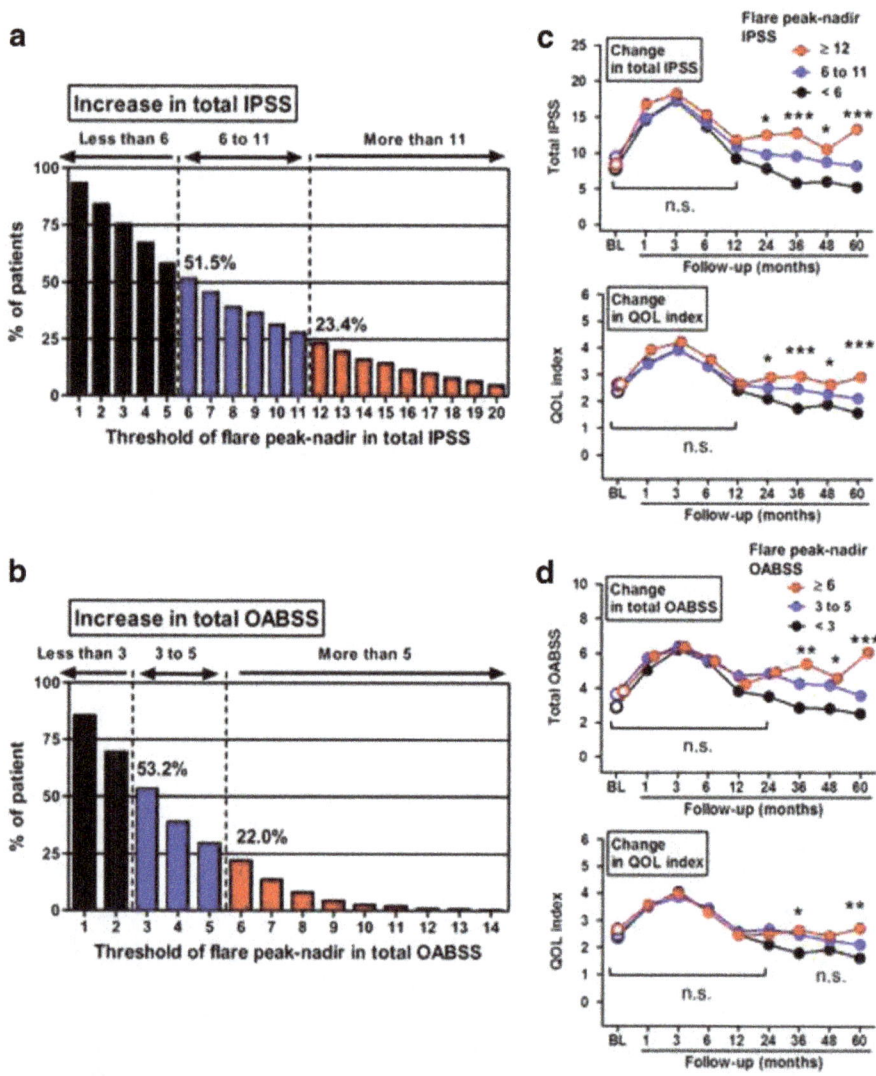

Fig. 2 Percentage distribution of patients for IPSS and OABSS urinary symptom flare after seed implant. Cutoffs for the difference between the flare peak and nadir were established. Two vertical dashed lines delineate approximately 25% and 50% of patients who experienced the urinary symptom flare assessed by the IPSS (**a**) and the OABSS (**b**). Time-course changes in total IPSS (**c**) and QOL (**d**) index scores during follow-up are plotted according to the flare peak-nadir of total IPSS (< 6, 6–10, and ≥ 12). Time-course changes in total OABSS and QOL index scores during follow-up are plotted according to the flare peak-nadir of total OABSS (< 3, 3–5, and ≥ 5). Data are plotted by means. Scores of groups with less than 6 and 6 to 10 point increases and the group with at least a 12-point increase are compared in each time point by the Mann-Whitney *U*-test. n.s, not significant; BL, baseline; * *P* < 0.05, ** *P* < 0.01, *** *P* < 0.001

IPSS returned to the BL after 36 months, the heightened total OABSS, OABSS 2 (night time frequency), and OABSS 3 (urge incontinence) lasted for over 48 months (Fig. 1e, f, and h). OABSS 3 (urgency score) returned to the BL after 48 months, similar to the results of the IPSS 4 (urgency score) (Fig. 1d and g). These findings support the idea that persistent LUTS after implantation are attributed to persistent storage rather than voiding symptoms.

Analysis and definition of the urinary symptom flare in IPSS and OABSS

The second increase in IPSS and OABSS scores and the flare incidence are shown in Fig.s 2a and b, respectively. The mean absolute increases ± the SD of the IPSS and the OABSS were 4.6 ± 4.0 points (median 4; range 0–20) and 3.3 ± 2.7 points (median 3; range 0–14), respectively. In the analysis of IPSS flare, when the cutoff values of an IPSS increase were set at ≥ 6 points and ≥ 12 points, the flare incidences were 51.5 and 23.4%, respectively (Fig. 2a). The time-course line graphs for total IPSS and the QOL index of the three groups divided according to IPSS increases are plotted in Fig. 2c. The patients with an IPSS increase of >11 points had persistent decrease of both types of IPSS even 60 months after implantation, while the other two groups (an IPSS increase of ≤ 11points) returned to the BL with time. The time-course change in the QOL index was almost parallel to that of the IPSS (Fig. 2c, lower panel). The same analysis was performed for the OABSS with similar results (Fig. 2b and d). When the cutoff values of an OABSS increase were set at ≥ 3 and ≥ 6 points, the flare incidence was 51.5 and 23.4%, respectively (Fig. 2a). The distribution of patients based on the time until urinary symptom flare is listed according to the two cutoff values in the IPSS and the OABSS (Additional file 2: Table S1). Approximately 30% of patients developed the flare between the second and third year, while 15–20% had a flare during the fifth year.

Based on these findings, those who had an increase of 12 points or more in the IPSS and an increase of 6 points or more from the nadir in an OABSS were thought to have a clinically significant flare in urinary symptoms after seed implantation. For further analyses, higher cutoff values in the IPSS and OABSS were used to define the urinary symptom flare and divide the patients into a "flare group" and a "non-flare group."

Correlation between IPSS flare and OABSS flare

To evaluate the correlation between IPSS flare and OABSS flare, the number of additional points (peak subtracted by nadir) in total IPSS and total OABSS were plotted and examined using Spearman's correlation (Fig. 3a). There was a moderate correlation between the increased points of total IPSS and total OABSS (ρ = 0.49,

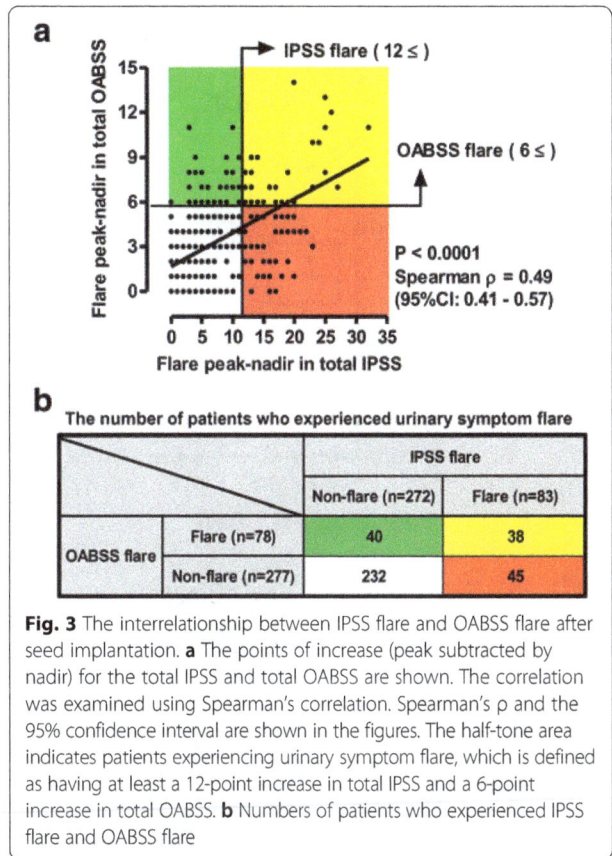

Fig. 3 The interrelationship between IPSS flare and OABSS flare after seed implantation. a The points of increase (peak subtracted by nadir) for the total IPSS and total OABSS are shown. The correlation was examined using Spearman's correlation. Spearman's ρ and the 95% confidence interval are shown in the figures. The half-tone area indicates patients experiencing urinary symptom flare, which is defined as having at least a 12-point increase in total IPSS and a 6-point increase in total OABSS. b Numbers of patients who experienced IPSS flare and OABSS flare

$P < 0.0001$). Of 355 patients, 38 (11%) showed both IPSS flare and OABSS flare, whereas 75 (21%) showed either IPSS flare or OABSS flare (Fig. 3b). A high concordance rate was observed for the assessment of urinary symptom flare by IPSS and OABSS (76%, 270 out of 355 patients). However, our findings revealed that assessment solely with the IPSS questionnaire failed to detect 40 patients (11%) with urinary symptom flare whose predominant complaint was likely to be storage symptoms after seed implantation. In contrast, we found that assessment solely with the OABSS questionnaire failed to detect 45 patients (13%) with urinary symptom flare. Our findings revealed that a certain percentage of people will be independently discovered as flare on OABSS and IPSS, without overlap. The OABSS can be used as a validated patient reported outcome to assess LUTS after brachytherapy in addition to the IPSS.

Comparison of clinicopathologic parameters between the flare group and non-flare group

Of 355 patients, 83 (23.4%) and 78 (22.0%) were categorized as the "flare group" based on the point increase in the IPSS and the OABSS, respectively. The clinicopathologic characteristics, treatment parameters, and post-implant dosimetric parameters were compared between the non-flare group and flare group

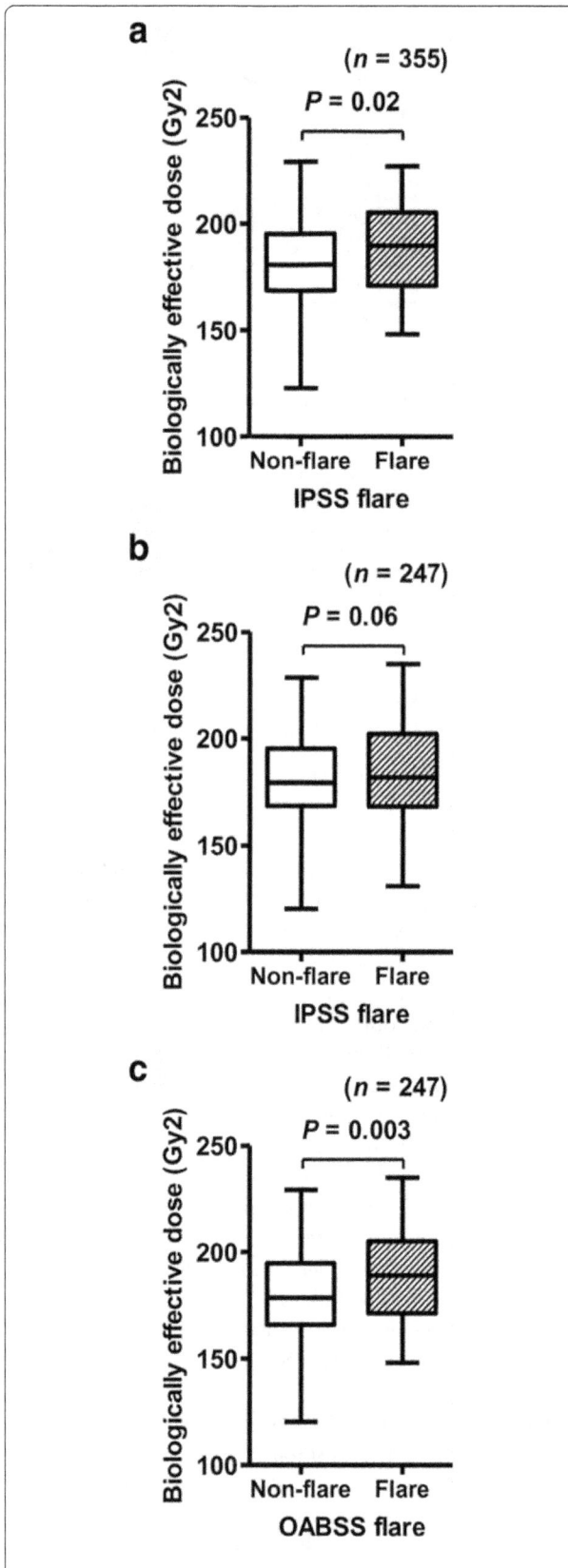

a (*n* = 355)

P = 0.02

Biologically effective dose (Gy2)
Non-flare Flare
IPSS flare

b (*n* = 247)

P = 0.06

Biologically effective dose (Gy2)
Non-flare Flare
IPSS flare

c (*n* = 247)

P = 0.003

Biologically effective dose (Gy2)
Non-flare Flare
OABSS flare

Fig. 4 The association between biologically effective dose (BED) and urinary symptom flare. The BED calculated from post-implant dosimetry is depicted by Tukey box plots. Horizontal lines within boxes indicate median levels. **a**, Comparison of BED between the IPSS non-flare group (*n* = 272) and flare group (*n* = 83) in the 355 total patients. **b** and **c**, Comparison of BED between the IPSS non-flare group (*n* = 190) and flare group (*n* = 57) in the 247 patients who did not undergo supplementary EBRT (**b**) and between the OABSS non-flare group (*n* = 193) and flare group (*n* = 54) (**c**). Significance was tested using the Mann-Whitney *U*-test

(Additional file 3: Table S2). Among the studied variables, a higher BED (*P* = 0.02) was associated with IPSS flare incidence (Fig. 4a). Patients without diabetes mellitus (DM) were more susceptible to an IPSS flare compared to those with DM (*P* = 0.02). Patients with higher Gleason sums had a tendency of having higher incidences of IPSS flares (*P* = 0.09). Independent predictive parameters for IPSS flares were then identified. Based on *P* values of less than 0.1 on the univariate analysis, BED, DM, and the Gleason sum were included in the multivariate analysis. The optimal cut-off values of BED were determined using a dichotomous test. Multivariate logistic regression analysis identified BED (< 200 *v.* ≥ 200; OR = 1.81; *P* = 0.02) and DM (no *v.* yes; OR = 0.26; *P* = 0.03) as being independently associated with the incidence of IPSS flare (Table 2). No significantly different variable was detected in the OABSS non-flare and flare groups, older patients showed a trend of experiencing an OABSS flare more frequently (*P* = 0.06, Additional file 3: Table S2). Contrary to a previous report [4], urinary symptom flare was not associated with baseline erectile dysfunction, as measured with SHIM.

To exclude the effect of supplementary EBRT, a subgroup analysis of the 247 patients who were not administered supplementary EBRT was performed. The clinicopathologic characteristics, treatment parameters, and post-implant dosimetric parameters are listed in Additional file 4: Table S3. Of 247 patients, 57 (23.1%)

Table 2 Multivariate analysis for IPSS flare

Variables	OR	95% CI	P value
Gleason sum			
6	1		
7/8/9	1.43	0.84–2.43	0.18
Diabetes mellitus			
No	1		
Yes	0.26	0.07–0.87	0.03
BED (Gy2)			
< 200	1		
200 ≤	1.81	1.10–2.98	0.02

OR odds ratio, *CI* confidence interval, *BED* biologically effective dose

Assessment of lower urinary symptom flare with overactive bladder symptom score and International...

89

and 54 (21.8%) were determined to be the "flare group" according to an increase in the IPSS and the OABSS, respectively. The clinicopathologic characteristics, treatment parameters, and post-implant dosimetric parameters were compared between the non-flare group and flare group (Additional file 5: Table S4). Patients with higher BED ($P = 0.06$, Fig. 4b), D90 ($P = 0.06$), and V100 ($P = 0.08$) tended to have higher incidences of IPSS flare. Among the studied variables, only higher BED ($P = 0.003$, Fig. 4c) and higher D90 ($P = 0.001$) were associated with OABSS flare incidence (Additional file 5: Table S4).

The association between the urinary symptom flare and PSA bounce

A temporary increase in the PSA level after the post-implant nadir is called PSA bounce, and it occurs during the first 12 to 36 months after radiotherapy in the majority of cases [23]. We hypothesized that there was a clinical association between two phenomena, the urinary symptom flare and PSA bounce. As testosterone recovery and ADT affect the PSA level, patients treated with neoadjuvant and/or adjuvant ADT ($n = 128$) were excluded in order to determine the frequency of true PSA bounce. Of 355 patients, 227 (64%) were included in the analysis. A PSA bounce of 0.1 ng/mL or more was observed in 101 (44%) of the 227 patients. The mean ± SD and the median time until the PSA bounce were 23.5 ± 12.4 months and 20.0 months (range: 7–71), respectively. The mean height and duration of the PSA bounce were 0.45 ng/mL (median: 0.23 ng/mL) and 12.3 months (median: 7.0 months), respectively. On the analysis of IPSS flare, 27 (26.7%) of the 101 patients with PSA bounce experienced the flare, while 32 (25.4%) of the 126 patients without PSA bounce ($P = 0.47$, Additional file 3: Table S2) had a flare. The same analysis was performed for OABSS flare, revealing that 19 (18.8%) of the 101 patients with PSA bounce experienced the flare as compared to 32 (25.4%) of the 126 patients without PSA bounce ($P = 0.15$, Additional file 6: Table S5). Next, we performed a correlation analysis between the time of the urinary symptom flare and the time of the PSA bounce in the patients who experienced both phenomena (Fig. 5). Neither the time of the IPSS flare ($n = 27$) nor the time until the OABSS flare ($n = 19$) correlated with the time of PSA bounce. The results demonstrated no significant clinical association between a urinary symptom flare and PSA bounce. When PSA bounce of 0.4 ng/mL or more was defined as the cutoff, PSA bounce was observed in 29 (12.7%) of the 227 patients. The mean ± SD and the median time to the PSA bounce were 20.7 ± 8.0 months and 19.0 months (range: 8–48), respectively. The mean height and duration of the PSA bounce were 1.08 ng/mL (median: 0.84 ng/mL) and 13.0 months (median:

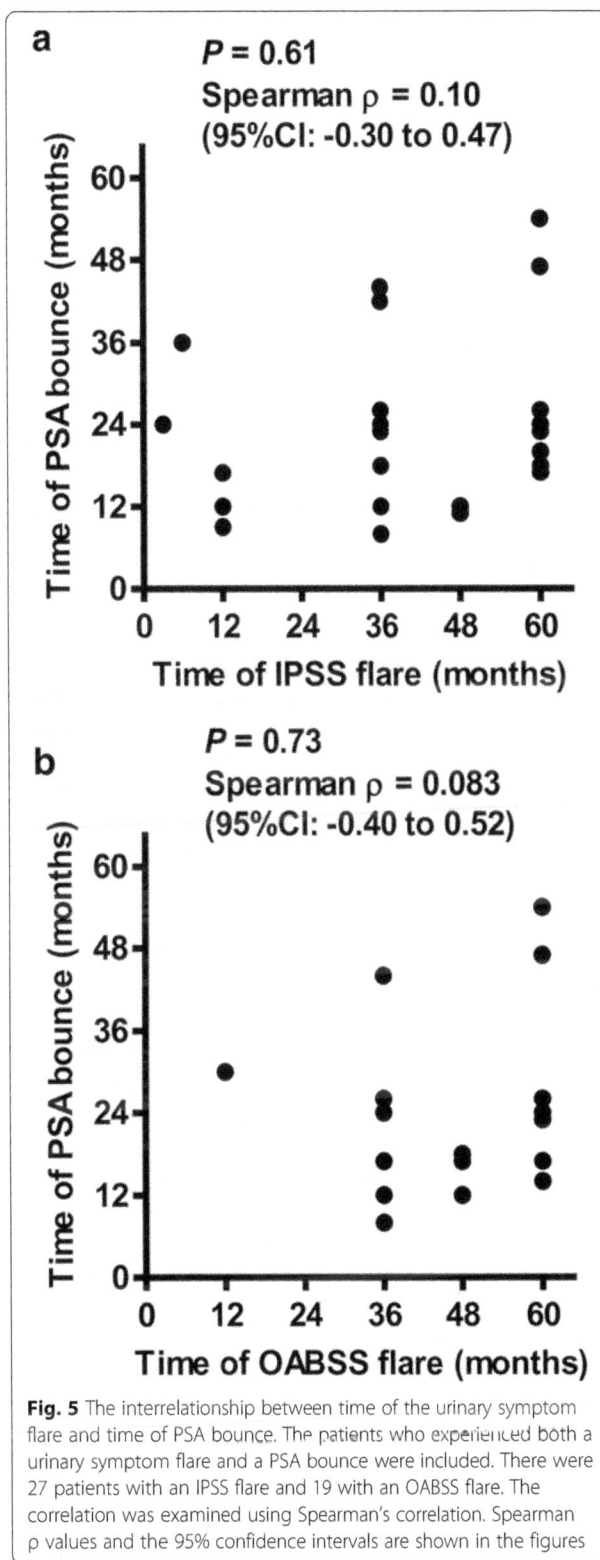

Fig. 5 The interrelationship between time of the urinary symptom flare and time of PSA bounce. The patients who experienced both a urinary symptom flare and a PSA bounce were included. There were 27 patients with an IPSS flare and 19 with an OABSS flare. The correlation was examined using Spearman's correlation. Spearman ρ values and the 95% confidence intervals are shown in the figures

12.0 months), respectively. When the same analysis was performed, no significant clinical association was found between a urinary symptom flare and PSA bounce of 0.4 ng/mL or more (Additional file 7: Table S6).

Discussion

The initial worsening of LUTS after implantation has been thoroughly studied by several groups [2, 5, 8, 10, 11]. We previously reported that the total IPSS and QOL index peak approximately 3 months after implantation and gradually return to the BL scores after 12 months [5]. The etiology of worsening LUTS revealed that the peak IPSS after seed implantation was associated with the total amount implanted and the dose delivered to the prostatic gland, bladder, and urethra [24]. The recurrent LUTS exacerbation after a variable asymptomatic period occurred between 6 and 60 months after seed implantation [12], which is called "urinary symptom flare." The IPSS flare has been utilized predominantly as a tool for determining urinary symptom flare [4, 8–12]. A previous study evaluated the spectrum of pathophysiology underlying persistent LUTS after seed implantation [25]. In their cohort, 79% of the patients had overactive symptoms, and 71% had urinary incontinence, while only 44% had obstructive symptoms. A urodynamic study revealed that men undergoing seed implantation had a much higher incidence of detrusor overactivity. Many urologists and general practitioners currently use the IPSS to evaluate the severity of LUTS, decide upon an intervention, and assess the treatment outcome. Total IPSS was reported as unreliable for correctly diagnosing bladder outlet obstruction and OAB [26]. Additionally, voiding symptoms and storage symptoms do not always directly reflect those dysfunctions [27]. Since persistent LUTS is largely characterized by storage symptoms, it may be reasonable to use the OABSS to evaluate changes in LUTS after implantation. In the present study, the OABSS as well as the IPSS were accurate, useful, and sensitive to changes during a follow-up survey for patients with localized PCa after seed implantation (Fig. 2b).

Although some reports regarding urinary symptoms after seed implantation have been published, an accepted definition of urinary flare does not exist. An increase in urinary symptom score seems to be useful and practical in clinical settings and academic research. In the first detailed evaluation by Cesaretti et al., when an increase in total IPSS of ≥ 5 points was defined as a urinary flare, 36% of patients were determined to experience a flare [12]. In the report by Keyes et al., two different definitions of flare, an increase in total IPSS of ≥ 5 and ≥ 8 points, were determined, and significant predictive factors for flare were explored separately [9]. In this study, an increase in total IPSS of ≥ 12 points and of ≥ 6 points in the OABSS were determined to be clinically significant (Fig. 2). The definition used in this study is thought to be reasonable because it qualifies patients who experience long-lasting LUTS and lower QOL (Fig. 2c and d).

With our definition, approximately 25% of patients were determined to experience urinary symptom flare after the nadir. A multivariate analysis of the possible predictors for the incidence of urinary symptom flare revealed that patients treated by higher BED stratified to <200 Gy2 and ≥200 Gy2 and patients without DM had higher risks of urinary flare (Table 2). A recent paper from Japan demonstrated that high BED was associated with the incidence of IPSS flare (defined as an increase in total IPSS of ≥ 5 points) and urinary toxicity of CTCAE grade 2 or higher, but no significant association was found between BED and the first IPSS resolution [11]. In the present study, the presence of DM was associated with a lower risk of having an IPSS flare, which was a controversial result [9, 11]. One possible explanation is that the urinary symptom flare is masked by the generally worse baseline urinary function and symptoms in those with DM as compared to those without the condition [28]. Neuropathy, which is caused by ischemic change, is known to be a DM-related comorbidity. Insensitivity to inflammation and irritability, which is usually induced by radiotherapy, may be another explanation.

With regards to the PSA bounce after radiotherapy, the predictors of bounce, features that distinguish benign bounce and biochemical failure, and the prognostic impact of bounce have been well studied [29–32]. However, the detailed mechanism underlying PSA bounce remains unclear, as does the mechanism behind a urinary symptom flare. We decided to investigate the association between urinary symptom flare and PSA bounce after implantation because the data are extremely limited [12]. In our cohort, PSA bounce was observed at a similar rate of approximately 20% in the non-flare and flare groups, showing no significant difference (Additional file 2: Table S2). An additional correlation analysis revealed that the two phenomena did not occur with similar timing. Our findings and the data reported by Cesaretti et al. strongly suggested that the etiologies of bounce and urinary flare are distinct.

Limitations of this study include the relatively small sample size, which lowers the ability to obtain significant results and identify other predictors of urinary symptom flare. This was a single-institution nonrandomized study. Moreover, assessment with the IPSS and OABSS questionnaires was only conducted once a year, starting from the second year after seed implantation. More frequent assessments, such as once every 3 to 6 months, may improve the findings.

Conclusions

To our knowledge, the present study is the first to demonstrate the clinical potential of the OABSS as an assessment tool for urinary symptom flare after seed implantation. We also investigated the predictors of IPSS and OABSS flares and the correlation between PSA bounce and urinary symptom flare. Although this single institution study, with only one surgeon, may not be representative of the experiences in the wider community, the data reflect the current status of LUTS management after implantation. Symptom flare is common and occurs in many patients within 5 years. A future prospective multi-center clinical trial will be needed to develop strategies for employing medications such as alpha-1 adrenoceptor antagonist, anti-cholinergic drugs, and phosphodiesterase type 5 inhibitors such as tadarafil (Cialis, Adcirca) to palliate bothersome symptoms. We believe that combined assessment with the OABSS and IPSS is useful when faced with the decision-making process, as it helps with both the timing and selection of treatment intervention, as well as with tracking of the outcome.

Additional files

> **Additional file 1: Figure S1.** Changes in parameters for lower urinary symptoms during follow-up after seed implantation. Scores, which are not shown in Fig. 1, were compared with the baseline scores with the Mann-Whitney U-test. Data are expressed as means and standard deviations. BL, the baseline; * $P < 0.05$, ** $P < 0.01$, *** $P < 0.001$.
>
> **Additional file 2: Table S1.** Time to urinary symptom flare.
>
> **Additional file 3: Table S2.** Comparison of clinicopathologic parameters by IPSS flare and OABSS flare in the 355 patients.
>
> **Additional file 4: Table S3.** Characteristics of 247 patients without supplementary EBRT.
>
> **Additional file 5: Table S4.** Comparison by IPSS flare and OABSS flare in the 247 patients without supplementary EBRT.
>
> **Additional file 6: Table S5.** Comparison of PSA bounce and urinary symptom flare in patients without androgen deprivation therapy. PSA bounce was defined as an elevation of ≥0.1 ng/mL compared to the previous lowest value, followed by a decrease to a level at or below the pre-bounce value.
>
> **Additional file 7: Table S6.** Comparison of PSA bounce and urinary symptom flare in patients without androgen deprivation therapy. PSA bounce was defined as an elevation of ≥0.4 ng/mL compared to the previous lowest value, followed by a decrease to a level at or below the pre-bounce value.

Abbreviations

[125]I: Iodine-125; ADT: Androgen-deprivation therapy; BED: Biologically effective dose; BL: Baseline; CI: Confidence interval; CTCAE: Common Terminology Criteria for Adverse Events; D90: Minimal does (Gy) received by 90% of the prostate gland; DM: Diabetes mellitus; EBRT: External beam radiotherapy; IPSS: International Prostate Symptom Score; J-POPS: Japanese Prostate Cancer Outcome Study; LUTS: Lower urinary tract symptoms; OAB: Overactive bladder; OABSS: Overactive bladder symptom score; OR: Odds ratio; PCa: Prostate cancer; PSA: Prostate-specific antigen; QOL: Quality of life; RP: Radical prostatectomy; SD: Standard deviation; SHIM: Sexual Health Inventory For Men; S-IPSS: Storage symptoms-related IPSS; V-IPSS: Voiding symptoms-related IPSS

Acknowledgments
Authors would like to thank patients for their important contribution to this study.

Funding
This research did not receive any specific grant from funding agencies in the public, commercial, or not-for-profit sectors.

Authors' contributions
MM and NT contributed to conception and design, and acquisition of patients data, and analysis and interpretation of data. IA and MH contributed to acquisition of data and interpretation of data. SH, YM, YN, TI, SA, KT, and KA assisted with acquisition of data and interpretation of data. YT, TF, and NK contributed to conception and design and review of pathologic diagnosis of prostatectomy tissues. KF was involved in the design of study and wrote the manuscript. All authors have been involved in drafting the manuscript and revising it critically for important intellectual content and approved the version to be published. All authors have participated sufficiently in this work to take public responsibility for appropriate portions of the content. All authors read and approved the final manuscript.

Competing interests
The authors declare that they have no competing interests.

Author details
[1]Department of Urology, Nara Medical University, 840 Shijo-cho, Nara 634-8522, Japan. [2]Department of Radiation Oncology, Nara Medical University, Nara, Japan. [3]Department of Pathology, Nara Medical University, Nara, Japan.

References
1. Saito S, Ito K, Yorozu A, Aoki M, Koga H, Satoh T, Ohashi T, Shigematsu N, Maruo S, Kikuchi T, Kojima S, Dokiya T, Fukushima M, Yamanaka H. Nationwide Japanese prostate cancer outcome study of permanent iodine-125 seed implant (J-POPS). Int J Clin Oncol. 2015;20:375–85.
2. Tanaka N, Asakawa I, Hasegawa M, Fujimoto K. Urethral toxicity after LDR brachytherapy: experience in Japan. Brachytherapy. 2015;14:131–5.
3. Tanaka N, Fujimoto K, Hirayama A, Samma S, Momose H, Kaneko Y, Haramoto M, Hayashi Y, Nakagawa Y, Otani T, Watanabe S, Hirao Y. The primary therapy chosen for patients with localized prostate cancer between the university hospital and its affiliated hospitals in Nara Uro-Oncological research group registration. BMC Urol. 2011;11:6.
4. Lehrer S, Cesaretti J, Stone NN, Stock RG. Urinary symptom flare after brachytherapy for prostate cancer is associated with erectile dysfunction and more urinary symptoms before implant. BJU Int. 2006;98:979–81.
5. Tanaka N, Fujimoto K, Hirao Y, Asakawa I, Hasegawa M, Konishi N. Variations in international prostate symptom scores, uroflowmetric parameters, and prostate volume after ^{125}I permanent brachytherapy for localized prostate cancer. Urology. 2009;74:407–11.
6. Tanaka N, Fujimoto K, Asakawa I, Hirayama A, Yoneda T, Yoshida K, Hirao Y, Hasegawa M, Konishi N. Variations in health-related quality of life in Japanese men who underwent iodine-125 permanent brachytherapy for localized prostate cancer. Brachytherapy. 2010;9:300–6.
7. Tanaka N, Asakawa I, Anai S, Hirayama A, Hasegawa M, Konishi N, Fujimoto K. Periodical assessment of genitourinary and gastrointestinal toxicity in patients who underwent prostate low-dose-rate brachytherapy. Radiat Oncol. 2013;8:25.
8. Keyes M, Miller S, Moravan V, Pickles T, McKenzie M, Pai H, Liu M, Kwan W, Agranovich A, Spadinger I, Lapointe V, Halperin R, Morris WJ. Predictive factors for acute and late urinary toxicity after permanent prostate brachytherapy: long-term outcome in 712 consecutive patients. Int J Radiat Oncol Biol Phys. 2009;73:1023–32.
9. Keyes M, Miller S, Moravan V, Pickles T, Liu M, Spadinger I, Lapointe V, Morris WJ. Urinary symptom flare in 712 ^{125}I prostate brachytherapy patients: long-term follow-up. Int J Radiat Oncol Biol Phys. 2009;75:649–55.
10. Crook J, Fleshner N, Roberts C, Pond G. Long-term urinary sequelae following 125iodine prostate brachytherapy. J Urol. 2008;179:141–6.
11. Eriguchi T, Yorozu A, Kuroiwa N, Yagi Y, Nishiyama T, Saito S, Toya K, Hanada T, Shiraishi Y, Ohashi T, Shigematsu N. Predictive factors for urinary toxicity after iodine-125 prostate brachytherapy with or without supplemental external beam radiotherapy. Brachytherapy. 2016;15:288–95.
12. Cesaretti JA, Stone NN, Stock RG. Urinary symptom flare following I-125 prostate brachytherapy. Int J Radiat Oncol Biol Phys. 2003;56:1085–92.
13. Miyake M, Tanaka N, Asakawa I, Tatsumi Y, Nakai Y, Anai S, Torimoto K, Aoki K, Yoneda T, Hasegawa M, Konishi N, Fujimoto K. Changes in lower urinary tract symptoms and quality of life after salvage radiotherapy for biochemical recurrence of prostate cancer. Radiother Oncol. 2015;115:321–6.

14 Homma Y, Yoshida M, Seki N, Yokoyama O, Kakizaki H, Gotoh M, Yamanishi T, Yamaguchi O, Takeda M, Nishizawa O. Symptom assessment tool for overactive bladder syndrome–overactive bladder symptom score. Urology. 2006;68:318–23.

15 Jeong SJ, Homma Y, Oh SJ. Korean version of the overactive bladder symptom score questionnaire: translation and linguistic validation. Int Neurourol J. 2011;15:135–42.

16 Weinberg AC, Brandeis GH, Bruyere J, Tsui JF, Weiss JP, Rutman MP, Blaivas JG. Reliability and validity of the overactive bladder symptom score in Spanish (OABSS-S). Neurourol Urodyn. 2012;31:664–8.

17 Homma Y, Kakizaki H, Yamaguchi O, Yamanishi T, Nishizawa O, Yokoyama O, Takeda M, Seki N, Yoshida M. Assessment of overactive bladder symptoms: comparison of 3-day bladder diary and the overactive bladder symptoms score. Urology. 2011;77:60–4.

18 Tanaka Y, Masumori N, Tsukamoto T. Urodynamic effects of solifenacin in untreated female patients with symptomatic overactive bladder. Int J Urol. 2010;17:796–800.

19 D'Amico AV, Whittington R, Malkowicz SB, Schultz D, Blank K, Broderick GA, Tomaszewski JE, Renshaw AA, Kaplan I, Beard CJ, Wein A. Biochemical outcome after radical prostatectomy, external beam radiation therapy, or interstitial radiation therapy for clinically localized prostate cancer. JAMA. 1998;280:969–74.

20 Tanaka N, Asakawa I, Kondo H, Tanaka M, Fujimoto K, Hasegawa M, Konishi N, Hirao Y. Technical acquisition and dosimetric assessment of iodine-125 permanent brachytherapy in localized prostate cancer: our first series of 100 patients. Int J Urol. 2009;16:70–4.

21 Tanaka N, Torimoto K, Asakawa I, Miyake M, Anai S, Hirayama A, Hasegawa M, Konishi N, Fujimoto K. Use of alpha-1 adrenoceptor antagonists in patients who underwent low-dose-rate brachytherapy for prostate cancer - a randomized controlled trial of silodosin versus naftopidil. Radiat Oncol. 2014;9:302.

22 Stock RG, Stone NN, Cesaretti JA, Rosenstein BS. Biologically effective dose values for prostate brachytherapy: effects on PSA failure and posttreatment biopsy results. Int J Radiat Oncol Biol Phys. 2006;64:527–33.

23 Toledano A, Chauveinc L, Flam T, Thiounn N, Solignac S, Timbert M, Rosenwald JC, Cosset JM. PSA bounce after permanent implant prostate brachytherapy may mimic a biochemical failure: a study of 295 patients with a minimum 3-year followup. Brachytherapy. 2006;5:122–6.

24 Desai J, Stock RG, Stone NN, Iannuzzi C, DeWyngaert JK. Acute urinary morbidity following I-125 interstitial implant of the prostate gland. Radiat Oncol Investig. 1998;6:135–41.

25 Blaivas JG, Weiss JP, Jones M. The pathophysiology of lower urinary tract symptoms after brachytherapy for prostate cancer. BJU Int. 2006;98:1233–7.

26 Oelke M, Baard J, Wijkstra H, de la Rosette JJ, Jonas U, Höfner K. Age and bladder outlet obstruction are independently associated with detrusor overactivity in patients with benign prostatic hyperplasia. Eur Urol. 2008;54:419–26.

27 Madersbacher S, Pycha A, Klingler CH, Schatzl G, Marberger M. The international prostate symptom score in both sexes: a urodynamics-based comparison. Neurourol Urodyn. 1999;18:173–82.

28 Podnar S, Vodušek DB. Lower urinary tract dysfunction in patients with peripheral nervous system lesions. Handb Clin Neurol. 2015;130:203–24.

29 Engeler DS, Schwab C, Thöni AF, Hochreiter W, Prikler L, Suter S, Stucki P, Schiefer J, Plasswilm L, Schmid HP, Putora PM. PSA bounce after ^{125}I-brachytherapy for prostate cancer as a favorable prognosticator. Strahlenther Onkol. 2015;191:787–91.

30 Galego P, Silva FC, Pinheiro LC. Analysis of monotherapy prostate brachytherapy in patients with prostate cancer. Initial PSA and Gleason are important for recurrence? Int Braz J Urol. 2015;41:353–9.

31 Kanzaki H, Kataoka M, Nishikawa A, Uwatsu K, Nagasaki K, Nishijima N, Hashine K. Kinetics differences between PSA bounce and biochemical failure in patients treated with 125I prostate brachytherapy. Jpn J Clin Oncol. 2015;45:688–94.

32 Hackett C, Ghosh S, Sloboda R, Martell K, Lan L, Pervez N, Pedersen J, Yee D, Murtha A, Amanie J, Usmani N. Distinguishing prostate-specific antigen bounces from biochemical failure after low-dose-rate prostate brachytherapy. J Contemp Brachytherapy. 2014;6:247–53.

14

Intraoperative and postoperative feasibility and safety of total tubeless, tubeless, small-bore tube, and standard percutaneous nephrolithotomy: a systematic review and network meta-analysis of 16 randomized controlled trials

Joo Yong Lee[1], Seong Uk Jeh[2], Man Deuk Kim[3], Dong Hyuk Kang[4], Jong Kyou Kwon[5], Won Sik Ham[1], Young Deuk Choi[1] and Kang Su Cho[6*]

Abstract

Background: Percutaneous nephrolithotomy (PCNL) is performed to treat relatively large renal stones. Recent publications indicate that tubeless and total tubeless (stentless) PCNL is safe in selected patients. We performed a systematic review and network meta-analysis to evaluate the feasibility and safety of different PCNL procedures, including total tubeless, tubeless with stent, small-bore tube, and large-bore tube PCNLs.

Methods: PubMed, Cochrane Central Register of Controlled Trials, and EMBASE™ databases were searched to identify randomized controlled trials published before December 30, 2013. One researcher examined all titles and abstracts found by the searches. Two investigators independently evaluated the full-text articles to determine whether those met the inclusion criteria. Qualities of included studies were rated with Cochrane's risk-of-bias assessment tool.

Results: Sixteen studies were included in the final syntheses including pairwise and network meta-analyses. Operation time, pain scores, and transfusion rates were not significantly different between PCNL procedures. Network meta-analyses demonstrated that for hemoglobin changes, total tubeless PCNL may be superior to standard PCNL (mean difference [MD] 0.65, 95% CI 0.14–1.13) and tubeless PCNLs with stent (MD -1.14, 95% CI -1.65--0.62), and small-bore PCNL may be superior to tubeless PCNL with stent (MD 1.30, 95% CI 0.27–2.26). Network meta-analyses also showed that for length of hospital stay, total tubeless (MD 1.33, 95% CI 0.23–2.43) and tubeless PCNLs with stent (MD 0.99, 95% CI 0.19–1.79) may be superior to standard PCNL. In rank probability tests, small-bore tube and total tubeless PCNLs were superior for operation time, pain scores, and hemoglobin changes.

Conclusions: For hemoglobin changes, total tubeless and small-bore PCNLs may be superior to other methods. For hospital stay, total tubeless and tubeless PCNLs with stent may be superior to other procedures.

Keywords: Calculi, Lithotripsy, Nephrostomy, Percutaneous, Meta-analysis, Bayes theorem

---

* Correspondence: kscho99@yuhs.ac
[6]Department of Urology, Gangnam Severance Hospital, Urological Science Institute, Yonsei University College of Medicine, 211 Eonju-ro, Gangnam-gu, Seoul 06273, South Korea
Full list of author information is available at the end of the article

Background

Urinary stone is one of the most prevalent urological disorders. Reports suggest that up to 12% of people will suffer from urinary tract calculi during their lifetime, and the rates of recurrence is close to 50% [1]. There are several treatment modalities for renal stones, including observation expecting spontaneous passage, extracorporeal shock wave lithotripsy (ESWL), percutaneous nephrolithotomy (PCNL), and retrograde intrarenal surgery (RIRS) using flexible ureterorenoscope [2]. PCNL is currently the standard treatment for large renal stones considered too large for or refractory to shock wave lithotripsy [3, 4]. Conventionally, a 20-24 French nephrostomy catheter is placed routinely after PCNL to provide urine drainage, prevent extravasation of urine, and make tamponade against bleeding [5, 6]. In addition, it can be used as a tract for a second-look PCNL [7]. The need for placing a conventional large-bore nephrostomy catheter has been questioned because of its accompanying increase in postoperative discomfort and other morbidity, and the low incidence of second-look operations [8, 9]. In recent years, tubeless or small-bore PCNL has been widely used, and previously reported systematic reviews have demonstrated the safety and efficacy in these techniques.

The recently introduced network meta-analysis is a meta-analysis in which multiple treatments are compared using both direct comparisons of interventions within randomized controlled trials (RCTs), and indirect comparisons across trials based on a common comparator [10–14]. Thus, we performed a systematic review and network meta-analysis based on published relevant studies to evaluate the feasibility and safety of each PCNL procedure, including total tubeless, tubeless with stent, small-bore tube, and large-bore tube PCNLs, for the treatment of renal stones.

Methods

Inclusion and exclusion criteria

Reported RCTs that fitted the following criteria were selected: (i) a design of each study that involved comparing the feasibility and safety for least two PCNL procedures, including total tubeless, tubeless with stent, small-bore tube, and large-bore tube PCNLs; (ii) the study groups were matched for baseline characteristics, including the total number of subjects and the values of each variable; (iii) at least one of the following outcomes was assessed: operation time, hospital stay length, hemoglobin decrease, return to normal activity, and complication rate; and (iv) the full text of each study was accessible and written in English.

The exclusion criteria were as follows: (i) noncomparative studies; (ii) the trial included children; and (iii) the trial did not exclude patients who underwent bilateral simultaneous PCNL or had complete or partial staghorn stones, more than two nephrostomy tracts, anatomical anomalies, or urinary infection. This report was prepared in compliance with the Preferred Reporting Items for Systematic Reviews and Meta-Analyses (PRISMA) statement (accessible at http://www.prisma-statement.org/) [15].

Search strategy

A literature search was performed to identify RCTS published prior to December 30, 2013 in PubMed, the Cochrane Central Register of Controlled Trials, and EMBASE™ online databases. A cross-reference search of eligible articles was performed to identify additional studies not found by the computerized search. Combinations of the following MeSH and key words were used: percutaneous nephrolithotomy or nephrostomy or percutaneous nephrostomy or nephrolithiasis or PCNL or PCN or PNL, and total tubeless or tubeless or nephrostomy free.

Data extraction

One researcher (J.Y.L.) screened the title and abstract of all articles retrieved using the search strategy. The other two investigators (D.H.K. and H.L.) independently assessed the full text of the articles to determine whether they met the inclusion criteria. For each included study, the following data were extracted independently as follows; authors, date, demographics of included patients, PCNL methods, feasibility, efficacy outcomes, complications, and inclusion of a reference standard. Disagreements arising in the study selection and data extraction processes were resolved by discussion until a consensus was reached or by arbitration employing another researcher (K.S.C.).

Study quality assessment

Once the final group of articles was agreed upon, two researchers (J.Y.L. and D.H.K.) independently examined the quality of each article using the Cochrane's risk-of-bias as a quality assessment tool for RCTs. The assessment involves the assignment of a "yes," "no," or "unclear" rating for each domain, designating a low, high, or unclear risk of bias, respectively. If ≤1 domain was rated "unclear" or "no," the study was classified as having a low risk of bias. If ≥4 domains were rated "unclear" or "no," the study was classified as having a high risk of bias. If 2 or 3 domains were rated "unclear" or "no," the study was classified as having a moderate risk of bias. [16]. Quality assessment was performed using Review Manager 5.2 (RevMan 5.2.11, Cochrane Collaboration, Oxford, UK).

Statistical analyses

Each outcome variable at specific time-points was compared by network meta-analysis using the odds ratio (OR) or mean difference (MD) with 95% confidence interval (CI). A random-effect model was used. Each analysis was based on non-informative priors for effect size and precision. Convergence and lack of auto-correlation were checked and confirmed after four chains and a 50,000-simulation burn-in phase, and direct probability statements were based on an additional 100,000-simulation phase. Calculation of the probability that each group had the lowest rate of clinical events was performed using Bayesian Markov Chain Monte Carlo modeling. Sensitivity analyses were performed by repeating the main computations using a fixed-effect method. Model fit was appraised by computing and comparing estimates for deviance and deviance information criterion. Pairwise inconsistency and inconsistency between direct and indirect effect estimates were assessed with the I^2-statistic, with values <25%, 25% to 50%, and >50% representing mild, moderate, and severe inconsistency, respectively. The extent of small study effects/publication bias was assessed by visual inspection of funnel plots for the pairwise meta-analyses. All statistical analyses were performed using Review Manager 5 and R (R version 3.0.3, R Foundation for Statistical Computing, Vienna, Austria; http://www.r-project.org) [17], and its meta, forestplot, gemtc, and R2WinBUGS packages for pairwise and network meta-analyses using Bayesian Markov Chain Monte Carlo modeling.

Results

Eligible studies

Our database search identified 43 studies that could be potentially included in the meta-analysis. Based on the inclusion and exclusion criteria, 18 articles were excluded during screening of the titles and abstracts because they were retrospective studies (11 articles) or case series (7 articles). This left 25 RCTS that evaluated various types of PCNL procedures for renal stones. After reviewing the full-text articles for these studies, 9 were excluded because they reported irrelevant results. Therefore, 16 RCTs were ultimately included in the qualitative analysis, as well as the quantitative synthesis using pairwise and network meta-analyses (Fig. 1).

There were differences in procedures among the included studies. Five studies included comparisons between standard and total tubeless PCNLs, and five RCTs also compared standard and tubeless PCNLs. Four trials reported on various factors in small-bore and tubeless PCNLs. In two studies, the results of three arms—standard, small-bore, and tubeless PCNLs—were published (Table 1). Finally, the included studies covered four different PCNL procedures: total tubeless, tubeless, standard and small-bore PCNLs (Fig. 2).

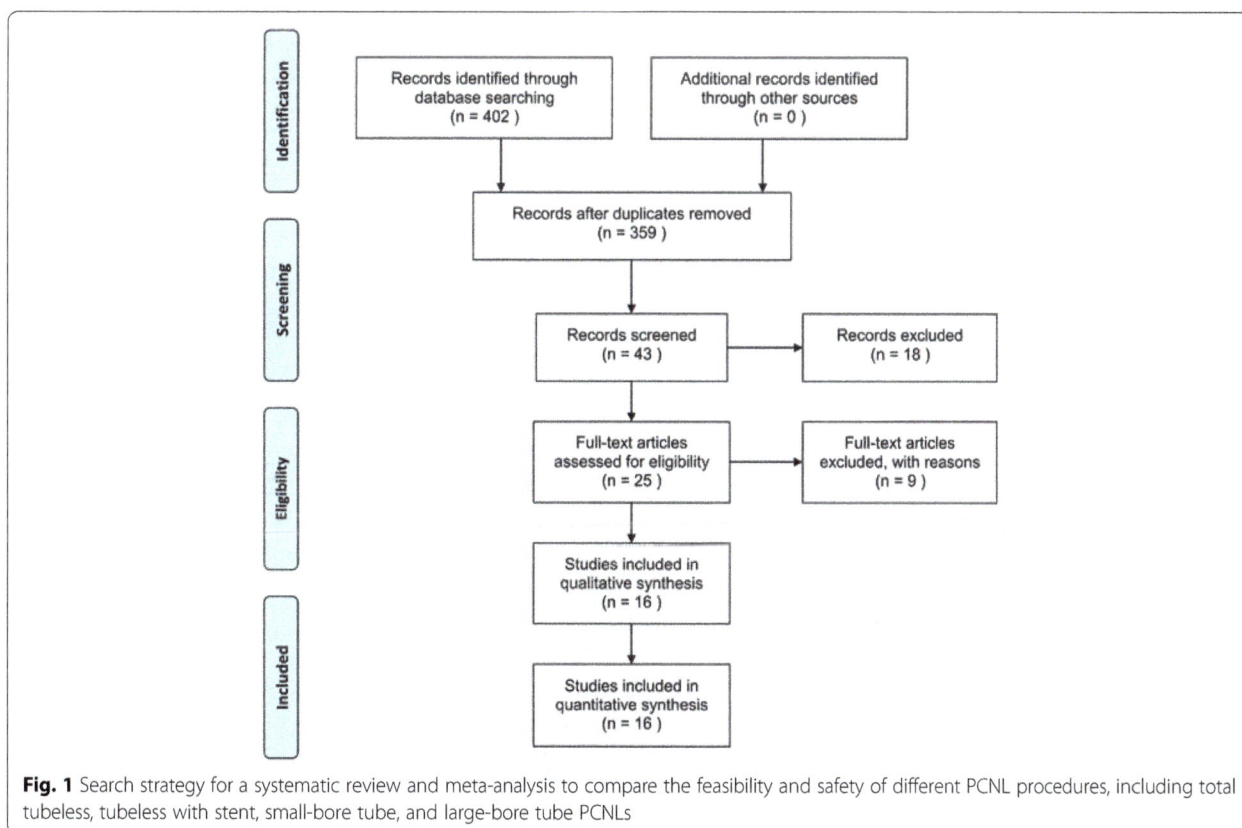

Fig. 1 Search strategy for a systematic review and meta-analysis to compare the feasibility and safety of different PCNL procedures, including total tubeless, tubeless with stent, small-bore tube, and large-bore tube PCNLs

Table 1 Characteristics of included trials

Study	Year	Design	Procedures	Sample size	Age (year)	Stone burden Size	P-value	Tube	Stone-free rate (%)	P-value	Quality assessment
Chang et al. [41].	2011	RCT	Standard	63	58.7	24.86 ± 2.78 mm	0.722	20 Fr (7 Fr)	75%	0.51	Low
			Total tubeless	68	59.2	24.74 ± 2.69 mm		None	74%		
Aghamir et al. [42].	2011	RCT	Standard	35	40	2.87 ± 0.62 cm^2	0.66	NA	83%	NA	Low
			Total tubeless	35	38.4	2.81 ± 0.59 cm^2		None	86%		
Kara et al. [43].	2010	RCT	Standard	30	66.5	25.6 mm	NA	18 Fr	90%	>0.05	Low
			Total tubeless	30	67.7	22.3 mm		None	96%		
Mishra et al. [44].	2010	RCT	Standard	11	42.5	2737 μL	0.18	20 Fr	81.8%	0.14	Low
			Tubeless	11	42.3	2934.2 μL		None (6 Fr)	72.7%		
Istanbulluoglu et al. [45].	2009	RCT	Standard	45	43.9	432.35 ± 195.97 mm^2	0.46	14 Fr	NA	NA	Low
			Total tubeless	45	47.5	448.93 ± 249.13 mm^2		None	NA		
Crook et al. [46].	2008	RCT	Standard	25	53	17.5 mm	NA	26 Fr	84%	NA	Low
			Total tubeless	25	52	21.6 mm		None	96%		
Agrawal et al. [47].	2008	RCT	Standard	101	31	NA	NA	16 Fr	100%	–	Low
			Tubeless	101	33	NA		None (6 Fr)	100%		
Singh et al. [48].	2008	RCT	Standard	30	34	800 mm^2	>0.05	22 Fr	93.3%	0.64	Moderate
			Tubeless	30	31	750 mm^2		None (NA)	90%		
Shah et al. [18].	2008	RCT	Small-bore tube	32	46.7	495.92 mm^2	0.88	8Fr	87.5%	0.96	Low
			Tubeless	33	44.1	535.36 mm^2		None (6 Fr)	87.9%		
Sofikerim et al. [35].	2007	RCT	Standard	24	54.1	425 mm^2	NA	24 Fr or 18 Fr	85% (24 Fr),	0.71	Moderate
			Tubeless	24	47.8	428 mm^2		None (6 Fr)	83% (18 Fr), 79%		
Tefekli et al. [49].	2007	RCT	Standard	18	41.32	3.1 cm	NA	14 Fr	89%	>0.05	Moderate
			Tubeless	17	38.4	2.8 cm		None (NA)	94%		
Weiland et al. [50].	2007	RCT	Small-bore tube	9	65	6.7 cm^2	0.15	8.3 Fr			Moderate
			Tubeless	9	54	3.2 cm^2		None (8.2 Fr)			
Choi et al. [32].	2006	RCT	Small-bore tube	12	47	32.41 mm	0.77	8.2 Fr	91.7%	0.64	High
			Tubeless	12	52.9	28.5 mm		None (6 Fr)	100%		
Desai et al. [51].	2004	RCT	Standard	10	43.4	263.7 mm^2	>0.05	20 Fr	100%	–	Moderate
			Small-bore tube	10	44.8	243 mm^2		9 Fr	100%		
			Tubeless	10	41.1	249.1 mm^2		None (6 Fr)	100%		

Table 1 Characteristics of included trials (*Continued*)

Study	Year	Design	Group	n							
Marcovich et al. [52].	2004	RCT	Standard	20	58	3.6 cm	0.64	24 Fr		0.63	Moderate
			Small-bore tube	20	61	3 cm		8 Fr			
			Tubeless	20	57	3.4 cm		None (NA)			
Feng et al. [53].	2001	RCT	Standard	10	53	8.4 cm³	0.75	22 Fr	31.5%	NA	Moderate
			Tubeless	8	62	4.4 cm³		None (NA)	71.4%		

NA not applicable, *RCT* randomized controlled trial

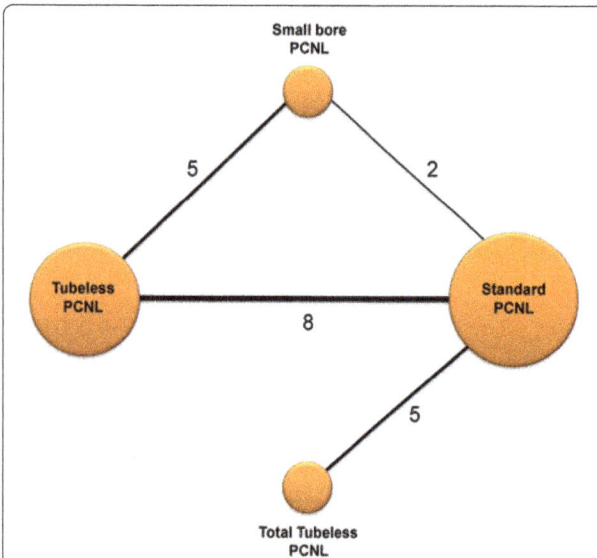

Fig. 2 Comparison network of included randomized controlled trials. Five studies included comparisons between standard and total tubeless PCNLs, and five RCTs also compared standard and tubeless PCNLs. Four trials reported on various factors in small-bore and tubeless PCNLs. In two studies, the results of three arms—standard, small-bore, and tubeless PCNLs—were published

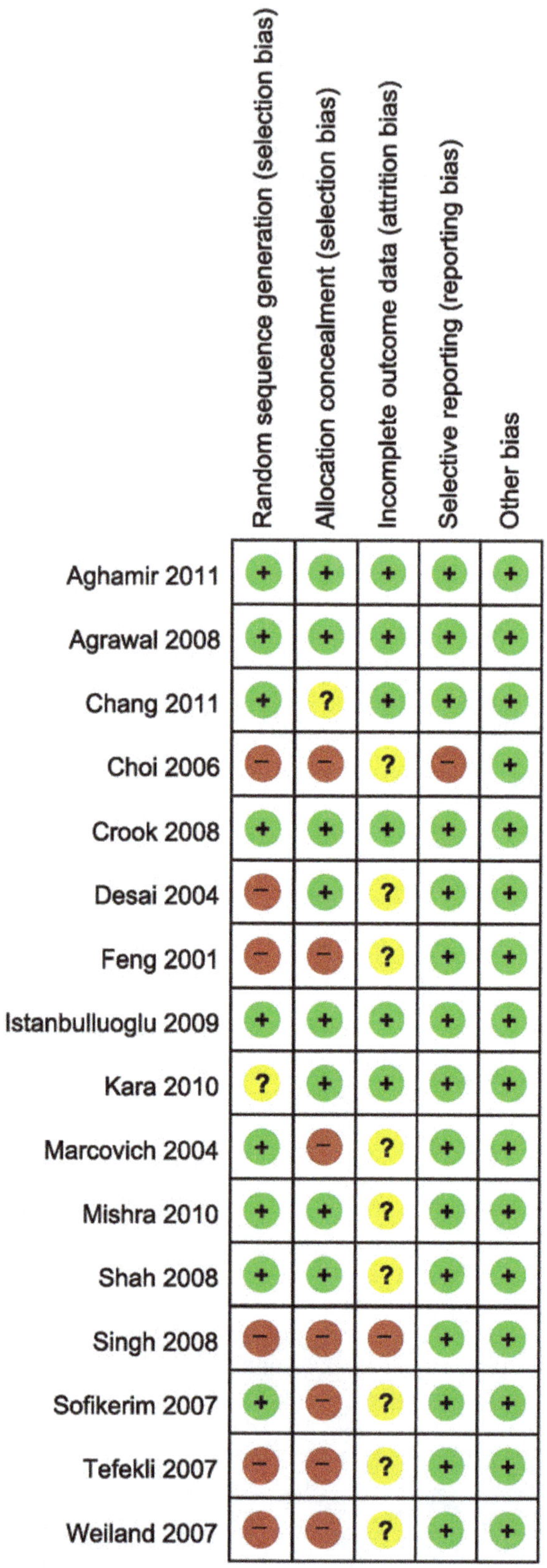

Quality assessment and publication bias

Figures 3 and 4 present the details of quality assessment, as measured by the Cochrane Collaboration risk-of-bias tool. Seven trials exhibited a moderate risk of bias for all quality criteria and only one study was classified as having a high risk of bias (Table 1). For operation time, hemoglobin change, and transfusion rate, little evidence of publication bias was demonstrated on funnel plots; however, for the visual analogue scale (VAS) pain score and hospital stay, moderate evidence of publication bias was demonstrated on these plots (Fig. 5).

Operation time

During the pairwise meta-analysis of operation time between standard and total tubeless PCNLs, there was a significant degree of heterogeneity among these studies, and data were pooled with a random effects model ($P = 0.04$, $I^2 = 69\%$). There was no statistically significant difference in operation time between standard and total tubeless PCNLs, although the MD was 6.19 (95% CI -0.14 to 12.52) (Fig. 6a). Between standard and tubeless PCNLs with stent, the MD also demonstrated no statistical difference (MD 7.43, 95% CI -1.70 to 16.57) (Fig. 6b). Likewise, the MDs did not exhibit statistically significant differences for standard versus small-bore PCNLs (MD -1.0, 95% CI -11.93 to 9.93) or tubeless versus small-bore PCNLs (MD 0.86, 95% CI -7.95 to 9.68) (Fig. 6c). Using network meta-analysis, there were no significant differences among all procedures (Fig. 7a) (Table 2), although total tubeless and small-bore PCNLs had higher rank probabilities than the other procedures (Fig. 8a).

Fig. 3 Risk-of-bias summary: review of the authors' judgments on each risk-of-bias item for each included study

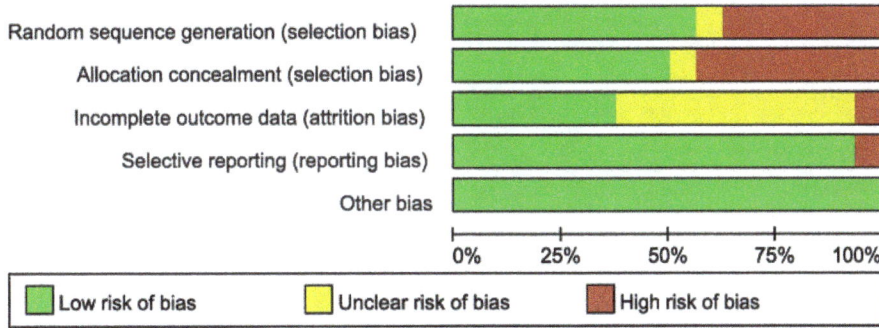

Fig. 4 Risk-of-bias graph: review of the authors' judgments on each risk-of-bias item presented as percentages across all included studies

Visual analogue scale pain score

In the pairwise meta-analysis of VAS pain scores, there was a significant degree of heterogeneity among studies and the data were pooled with a random effects model. There were no statistically significant differences comparing standard versus total tubeless PCNLs with stent (MD 0.06, 95% CI -0.56 to 0.69, $P = 0.84$) (Fig. 9a) or tubeless versus small-bore PCNLs (MD 1.21, 95% CI -0.02 to 2.44, $P = 0.05$) (Fig. 9b). In the network meta-analysis, there were no statistically significant differences among all

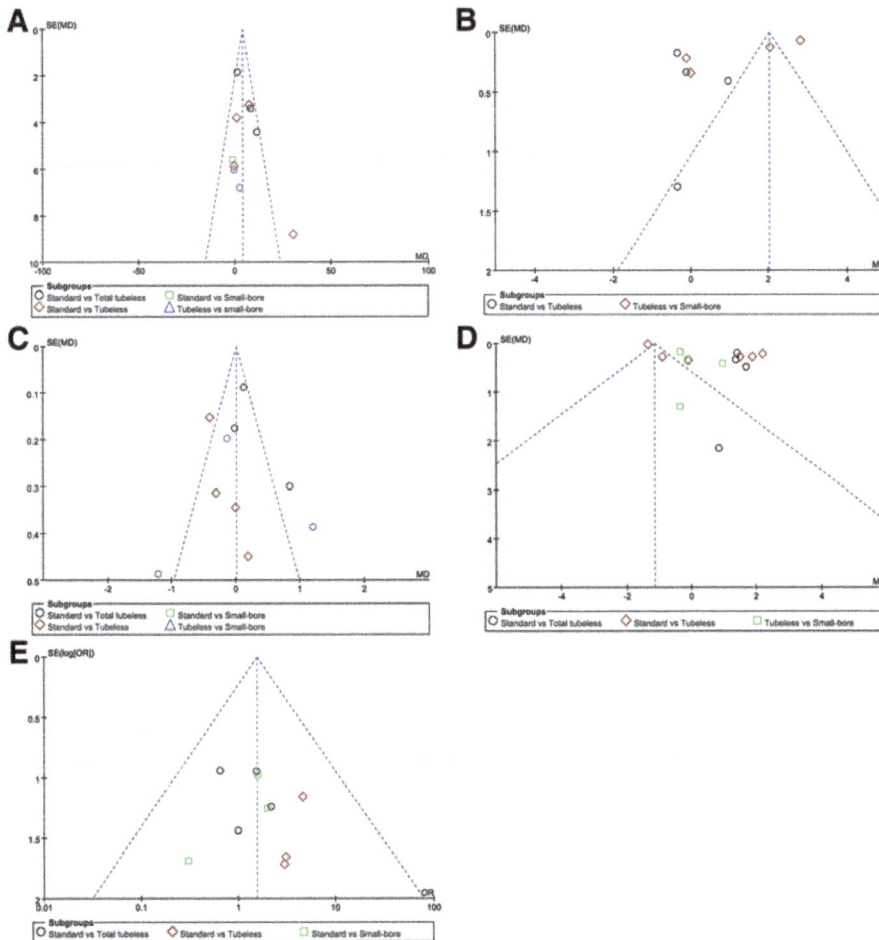

Fig. 5 Funnel plots of each variable. **a** Operation time, **b** visual analogue scale (VAS) pain score, **c** hemoglobin change, **d** length of stay, and **e** transfusion rate. For operation time, hemoglobin change, and transfusion rate, little evidence of publication bias was demonstrated on visual or statistical examination of the funnel plots; however, for VAS scores and hospital stay, moderate evidence of publication bias was demonstrated on visual or statistical examination of the plots

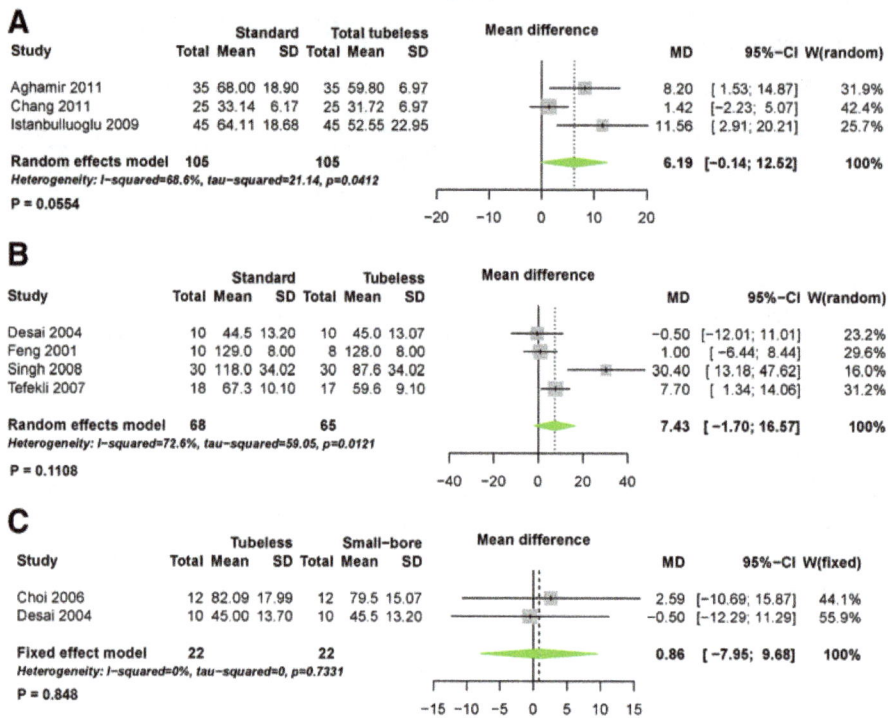

Fig. 6 Forest plots for operation time using pairwise meta-analysis. **a** Standard versus total tubeless PCNLs, **b** standard versus tubeless PCNLs, and **c** tubeless versus small-bore PCNLs. SD, standard deviation; MD, Mean difference; CI, confidence interval; W, Weight

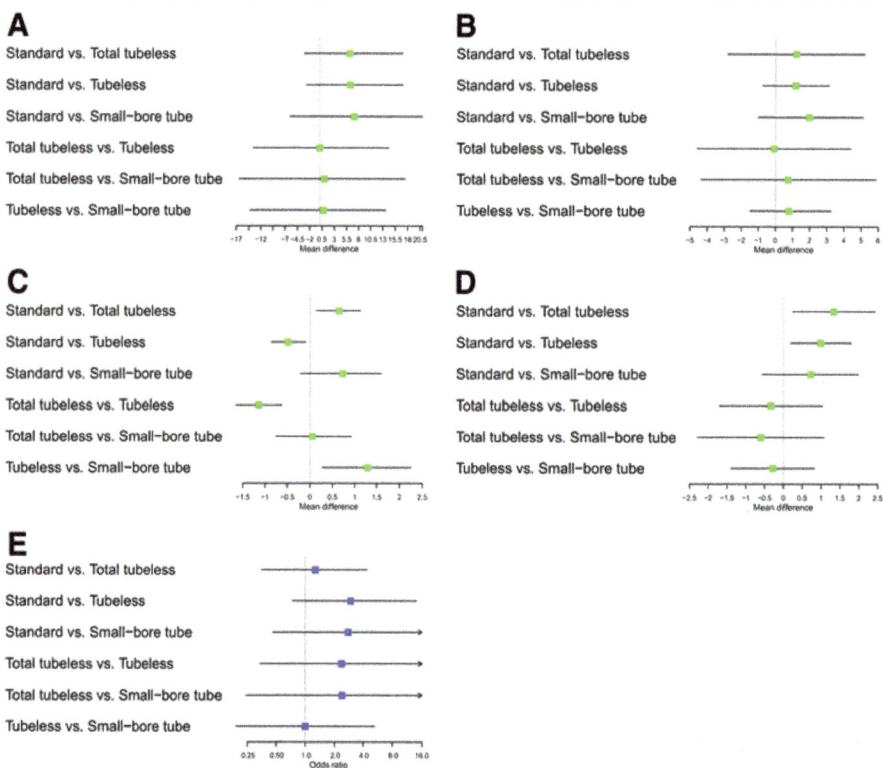

Fig. 7 Forest plots for (**a**) operation time, **b** visual analogue scale, **c** hemoglobin change, **d** hospital stay, and **e** transfusion rate using network meta-analysis

Table 2 Results of network and pairwise meta-analyses comparing procedures for operation time, visual analogue scale pain score, hemoglobin change, and hospital stay

Procedures	Network meta-analysis		Pairwise meta-analysis	
	Mean difference	95% CI	Mean difference	95% CI
Operation time				
Standard				
Total tubeless	6.11	−3.14 – 17.02	6.19[a]	−0.14 – 12.52
Tubeless	6.28	−2.71 – 17.06	7.43[a]	−1.70 – 16.57
Small-bore tube	7.09	−6.03 – 20.95	NA	
Total tubeless				
Tubeless	0.08	−13.60 – 14.27	NA	
Small-bore tube	0.95	−16.46 – 17.52	NA	
Tubeless				
Small-bore tube	0.80	−14.27 – 13.60	0.86[b]	−7.95 – 9.68
Visual analogue scale pain score				
Standard				
Total tubeless	1.25	−2.80 – 5.22	NA	
Tubeless	1.20	−0.75 – 3.14	0.06[a]	−0.56 – 0.69
Small-bore tube	2.00	−1.03 – 5.14	NA	
Total tubeless				
Tubeless	−0.07	−4.58 – 4.41	NA	
Small-bore tube	0.75	−4.37 – 5.89	NA	
Tubeless				
Small-bore tube	0.80	−1.51 – 3.24	1.21[a]	−0.02 – 2.44
Hemoglobin change				
Standard				
Total tubeless	0.65	0.14 – 1.13	0.23[a]	−0.12 – 0.58
Tubeless	−0.48	−0.87 – −0.09	-0.29[a]	−0.53 – −0.05
Small-bore tube	0.73	−0.21 – 1.60	NA	
Total tubeless				
Tubeless	−1.14	−1.65 – −0.62	NA	
Small-bore tube	0.06	−0.76 – 0.92	NA	
Tubeless				
Small-bore tube	1.30	0.27 – 2.26	−0.02[a]	−1.13 – 1.10
Hospital stay				
Standard				
Total tubeless	1.33	0.23 – 2.43	1.42[b]	1.10 – 1.75
Tubeless	0.99	0.19 – 1.79	0.54[a]	−1.03 – 2.11
Small-bore tube	0.73	−0.57 – 1.98	NA	
Total tubeless				
Tubeless	−0.33	−1.71 – 1.04	NA	
Small-bore tube	−0.60	−2.29 – 1.08	NA	
Tubeless				
Small-bore tube	−0.28	−1.39 – 0.83	0.06[a]	−0.56 – 0.69

CI confidence interval, *NA* not applicable

[a]Random-effect model with inverse variance method

[b]Fixed-effect model with inverse variance method

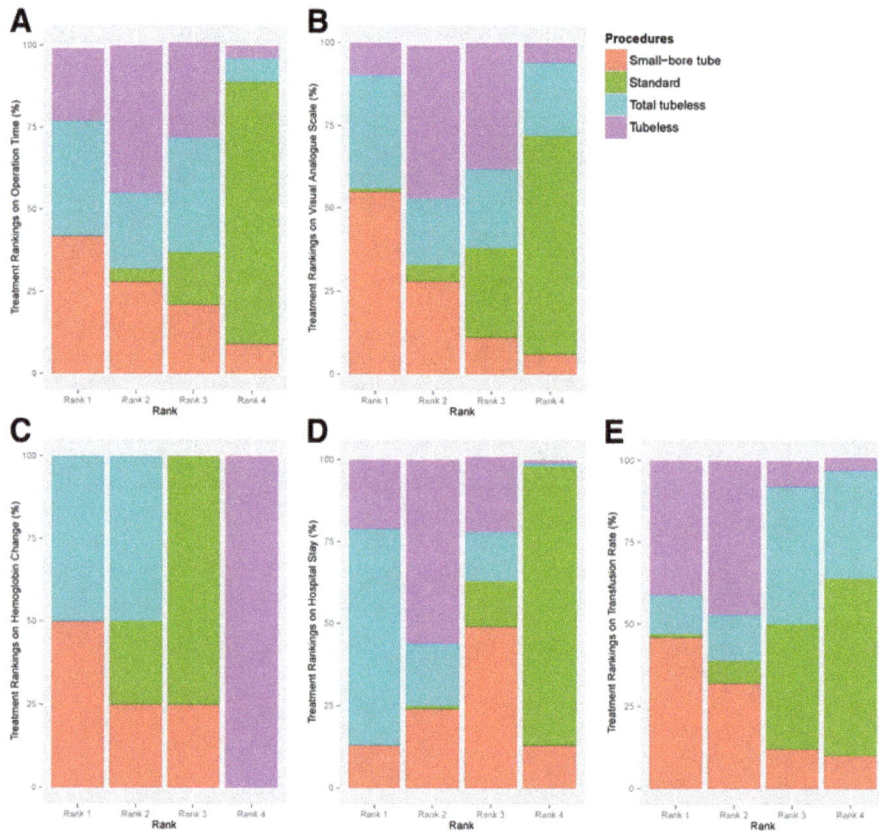

Fig. 8 Rank probability test. **a** Operation time, **b** visual analogue scale, **c** hemoglobin change, **d** hospital stay, and **e** transfusion rate

procedures for VAS pain scores (Fig. 7b) (Table 2), although the rank probabilities demonstrated that small-bore and total tubeless PCNLs may be superior to the other procedures (Fig. 8b).

Hemoglobin change

Using pairwise meta-analysis for hemoglobin change, three comparisons, including standard versus total tubeless PCNLs, standard versus tubeless PCNLs with stent,

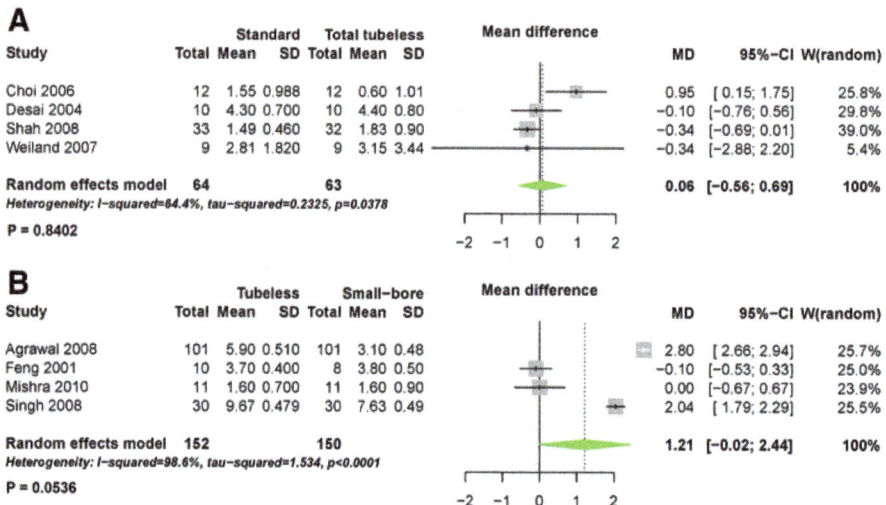

Fig. 9 Forest plots for visual analogue scale pain score using pairwise meta-analysis. **a** Standard versus total tubeless PCNLs, and **b** standard versus tubeless PCNLs, SD, standard deviation; MD, Mean difference; CI, confidence interval; W, Weight

and tubeless versus small-bore PCNLs, were examined (Fig. 10). Only one comparison for standard versus tubeless PCNLs with stent showed a statistically significant difference (MD -0.29, 95% CI -0.53 to -0.05, $P = 0.02$) (Fig. 10b). Network meta-analysis demonstrated that total tubeless PCNL may be superior to standard PCNL (MD 0.65, 95% CI 0.14 to 1.13). Total tubeless (MD -1.14, 95% CI -1.65 to -0.62), and small-bore PCNLs (MD 1.30, 95% CI 0.27 to 2.26) were also superior to tubeless PCNL with stent for hemoglobin change (Fig. 7c) (Table 2). In rank probabilities, total tubeless and small-bore PCNLs were ranked higher than the other procedures (Fig. 8c).

Hospital stay

The length of hospital stay in patients who underwent total tubeless PCNL was shorter than for those who underwent standard PCNL (MD 1.42, 95% CI 1.10 to 1.75, $P < 0.01$) during pairwise meta-analysis (Fig. 11). Network meta-analysis also demonstrated that total tubeless (MD 1.33, 95% CI 0.23 to 2.43) and tubeless PCNLs with stent (MD 0.99, 95% CI 0.19 to 1.79) may be superior to standard PCNL, producing a shorter hospital stay (Fig. 7d). However, there was no significant difference between total tubeless and tubeless PCNLs with stent (MD -0.33, 95% CI -1.71 to 1.04) (Table 2), although total tubeless PCNL showed the highest rank probability of all procedures (Fig. 8d).

Transfusion rate

The transfusion rate did not exhibit significant differences between any of the procedures during both pairwise analysis (Fig. 12) and network meta-analysis (Fig. 7e) (Table 3). Rank probabilities demonstrated that small-bore and tubeless PCNLs with stent may be superior to the other procedures (Fig. 8e).

Discussion

Conventionally, the placement of a nephrostomy tube after PCNL was considered a necessary safety option. However, the use of a nephrostomy tube has been associated with a prolonged hospital stay and more postoperative pain [18]. In 1997, Bellman et al. first reported the use of tubeless PCNL using a double-J ureteral stent and Council catheter [19]. They demonstrated that hospital length of stay, analgesia requirements, time to return to normal activities, and cost were significantly less with this procedure. Although the procedure gained popularity, tubeless PCNL with stent had two important problems: ureteral stent discomfort and loss of the advantages of a nephrostomy tube. Thus, some urologists used the approach of placing the smallest possible nephrostomy tube to minimize patient discomfort while maintaining access to the renal collecting system [20]. With the recent development of a high-density telescope, high-quality lithotripters, and radiological interventional techniques to embolize blood vessels, several investigators reported that tubeless and total

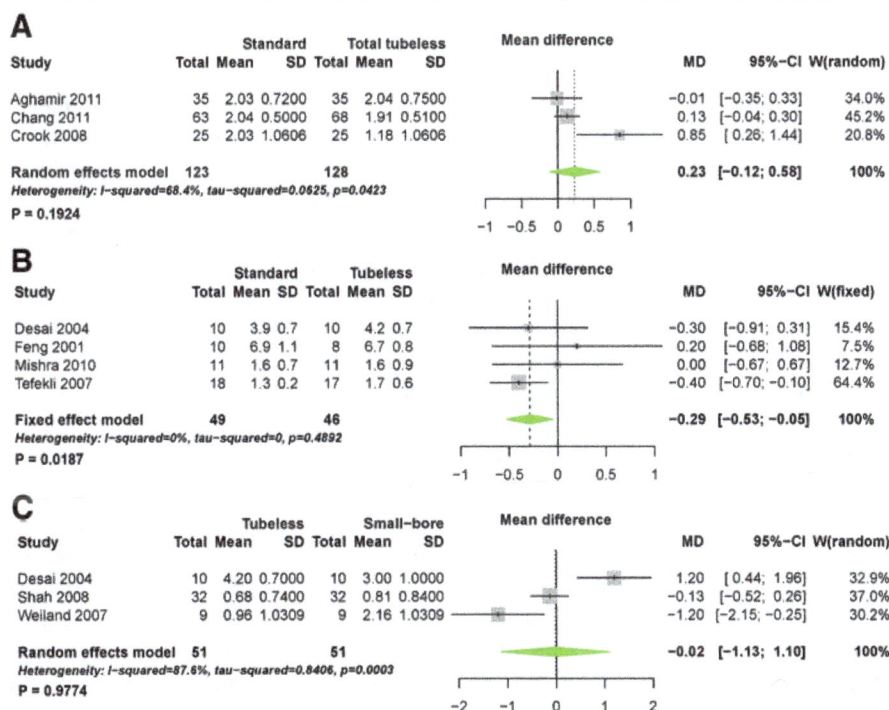

Fig. 10 Forest plots for hemoglobin change using pairwise meta-analysis. **a** Standard versus total tubeless PCNLs, **b** standard versus tubeless PCNLs, and **c** tubeless versus small-bore PCNLs. SD, standard deviation; MD, Mean difference; CI, confidence interval; W, Weight

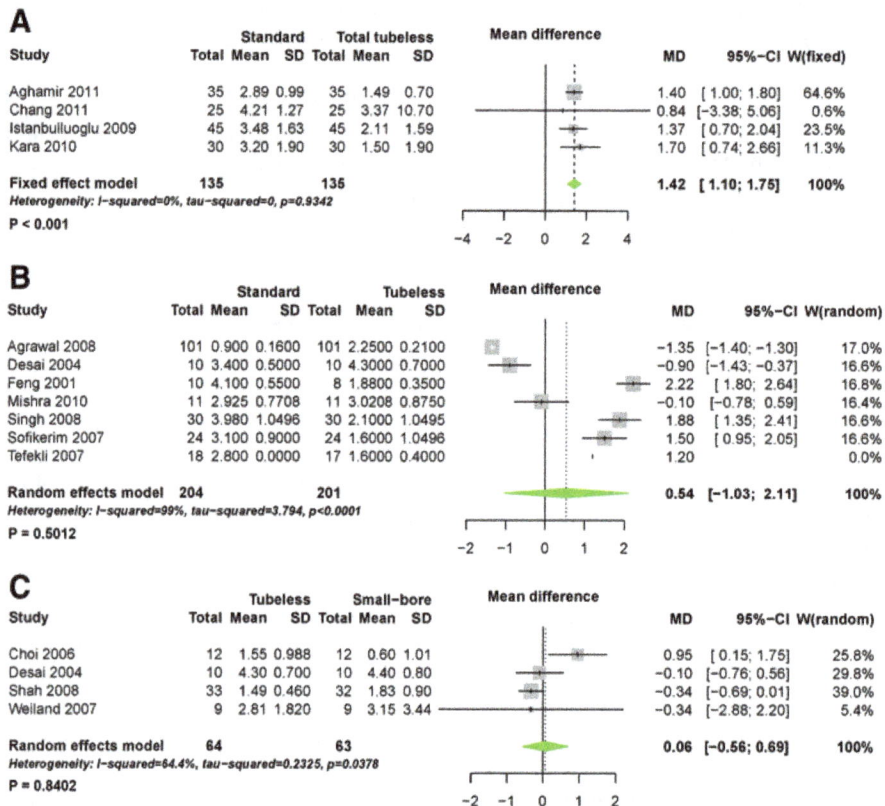

Fig. 11 Forest plots for hospital stay using pairwise meta-analysis. **a** Standard versus total tubeless PCNLs, **b** standard versus tubeless PCNLs, and **c** tubeless versus small-bore PCNLs. SD, standard deviation; MD, Mean difference; CI, confidence interval; W, Weight

tubeless (stentless) PCNL in selected patients was safe and associated with a reduced hospital length of stay and analgesic requirements.

The results of RCTs for each PCNL procedure have been reported, and previous systematic reviews and meta-analyses have been published. However, most of the studies reported in the previous meta-analyses compared standard PCNL versus tubeless PCNL with stent or standard PCNL versus total tubeless PCNL [21–25]. Therefore, an integrated analysis of standard, small-bore tube, tubeless with stent, and total tubeless PCNLs has not yet been published.

In our study, using network meta-analysis, there were no significant differences in operation time for the four procedures. It is known that large stones increase operation time and complication rates [26, 27], and operation times vary depending on the size and characteristics of the stone.

We also detected no statistically significant differences between methods for the VAS pain scores. No significant differences were observed between standard versus total tubeless PCNLs and tubeless versus small-bore tube PCNLs not only during the network meta-analysis, but even during pairwise meta-analyses. Operation-related factors that may prolong pain after PCNL include the

nephrostomy tube size [28] and stent discomfort caused by a double-J stent [29], but statistically significant differences between procedures were not observed. This finding is presumably due to the relatively small sample size (only eight studies reported the VAS pain scores), and the possibility of publication bias, as suggested by the asymmetric funnel plot (Fig. 5b). However, in the rank probability test of pain scores using Bayesian Markov Chain Monte Carlo modeling, small-bore tube PCNL was ranked highest, followed by the total tubeless PCNL and then tubeless PCNL with stent (Fig. 8b). Additional RCTs are necessary in the future to more definitively address this issue.

With regard to the hemoglobin changes, network meta-analysis showed that total tubeless and small-bore tube PCNLs were superior, and tubeless with stent PCNL was the worst. In addition, total tubeless and small-bore PCNLs showed similar superiority in the network meta-analysis and rank probability test (Fig. 8c). Considering that all enrolled studies were RCTs, the possibility of selection bias between patients who had total tubeless or small-bore tube PCNLs and other procedures should be relatively low. For tubeless PCNLs, the possibility of bleeding caused by ureteral stenting should be considered. In previous studies, hematuria

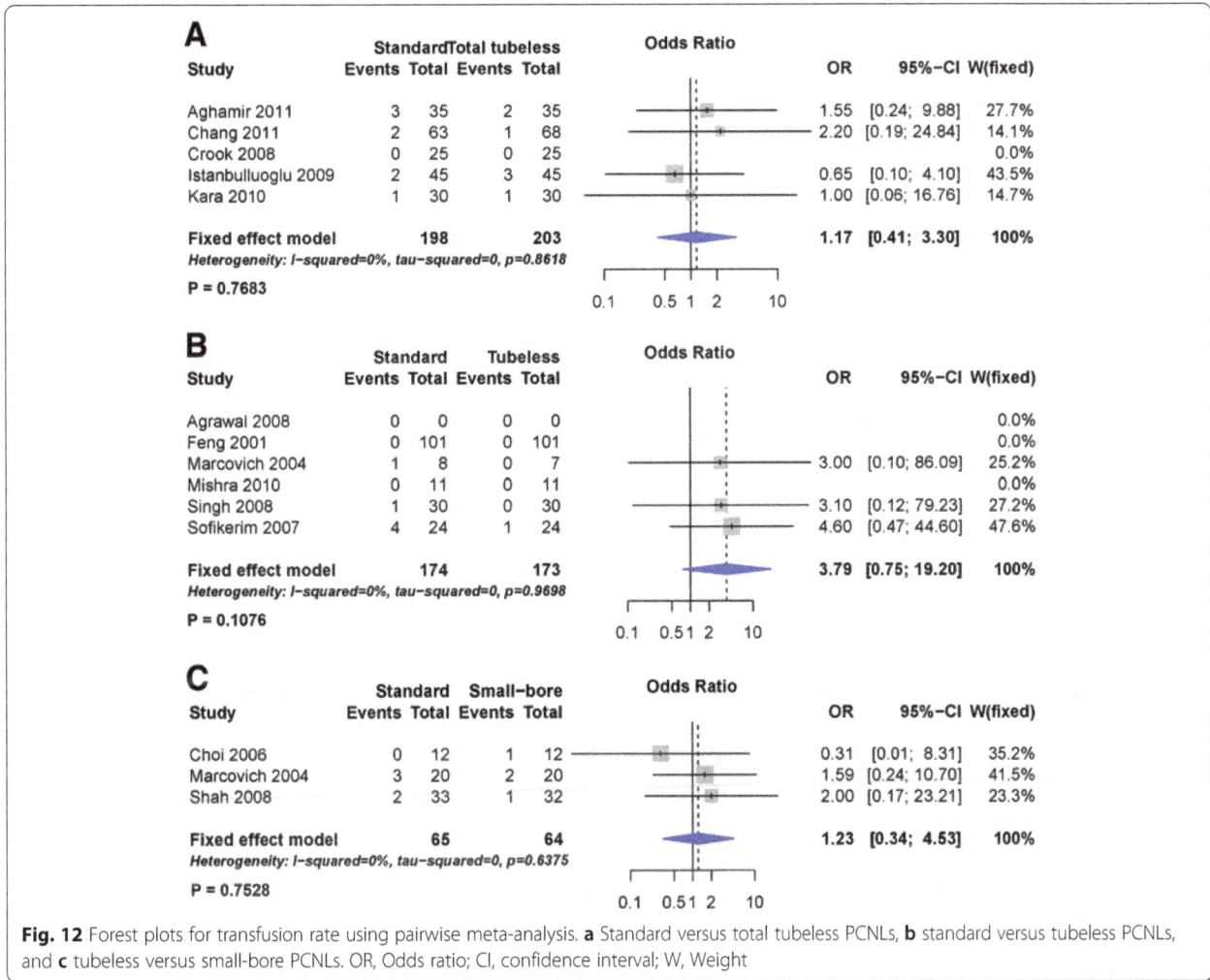

Fig. 12 Forest plots for transfusion rate using pairwise meta-analysis. **a** Standard versus total tubeless PCNLs, **b** standard versus tubeless PCNLs, and **c** tubeless versus small-bore PCNLs. OR, Odds ratio; CI, confidence interval; W, Weight

accounted for 13.6% of early complications and 18.1% of late complications after tubeless PCNL with stent [29]. In contrast to the hemoglobin changes, transfusion rates were not different between the four procedures. This

Table 3 Results of network and pairwise meta-analyses comparing procedures for transfusion rate

Procedures	Network meta-analysis		Pairwise meta-analysis[a]	
	OR	95% CI	OR	95% CI
Standard				
Total tubeless	1.27	0.35–4.40	1.17	0.41–3.30
Tubeless	2.94	0.73–14.06	3.79	0.75–19.20
Small-bore tube	2.76	0.46–24.52	NA	
Total tubeless				
Tubeless	2.37	0.34–18.19	NA	
Small-bore tube	2.39	0.24–22.21	NA	
Tubeless				
Small-bore tube	1.00	0.19–5.30	1.23	0.34–4.53

CI confidence interval, OR odds ratio
[a]Fixed-effect model with Mantel-Haenszel method

lack of difference is likely due to the development of high-quality surgical skills and patient monitoring approaches because of the popularity of PCNL procedures.

For the length of hospital stay, the total tubeless and tubeless PCNLs showed superiority. We assumed that this is because these methods do not require additional procedures, such as nephrostomy tube removal or tract revision.

During the rank probability for each variable, small-bore and tubeless PCNLs were ranked higher for operation time, VAS pain scores, and hemoglobin change. In addition, total tubeless PCNL was ranked highest for hospital stay and transfusion rate. Notably, total tubeless PCNL was ranked highest for each item. However, total tubeless PCNL has not been in widespread use, even considering the potential benefits of this approach, because of concerns that potentially fatal complications, such as massive bleeding without a nephrostomy tube in place, may occur [30]. Because omitting a nephrostomy catheter may potentially increase the risk of bleeding and serious complications, various methods have been used in an attempt to seal the tract. Milkahi and colleagues were the first to describe the instillation of the hemostatic agent Tiseel® into the nephrostomy tract [31]. However, they were unable to determine whether this diminished postoperative bleeding or urinary extravasation following tubeless PCNL. Choi et al. instilled gel matrix thrombin (Floseal®) into the tract whenever persistent bleeding was observed after omitting the nephrostomy catheter [32]. Okeke et al. explored cryoablation of the nephrostomy tract after tubeless PCNL, where they inserted a cryoprobe into the access tract and performed a 10-min freeze-thaw cycle at a temperature -20 °C. This method did not significantly affect the rate of delayed bleeding or urinary extravasation [33]. Recently, a randomized study by Cormio et al. showed that TachoSil® provided better tract control and a shorter hospital stay than nephrostomy tube placement, although it did not reduce pain or analgesic requirements [34].

Total tubeless PCNL is advocated by leading surgeons in the field of endourology. The future role of tubed PCNL will likely reside primarily in cases of severe intraoperative bleeding or major damage to the collecting system, and when there is the possibility of a second-look operation. However, some controversies remain about the feasibility and efficacy of tubeless PCNLs in certain clinical settings. In their prospective randomized study, Shoma et al. suggested that the tubeless approach might not be suitable for patients with chronic kidney disease or those who require a supracostal approach [30]. However, Shah et al. reported the successful use of a tubeless technique in a patient with chronic kidney disease. Likewise, Sofikerim et al. reported that tubeless PCNL is a safe and effective technique, even for supracostal access, and is associated with less postoperative pain and shorter hospital stay [35]. Resorlu et al. maintained that single or no nephrostomy drainage following multitract PCNL offered the potential advantages of decreased postoperative analgesic requirements and shorter hospital stay, without increasing the rate of complications [36].

A limitation of our study was that we did not perform subgroup analyses based on the size of the stone. We also did not compare success rates because the success rates were high in each study. In addition, there was some degree of publication bias. However, in the review of 48 articles from the Cochrane Database of Systematic Reviews performed by Sutton et al., publication or related biases were noted to be common within the sample of assessed meta-analyses, but did not affect the conclusions in most cases [37]. Additionally, the position of the patient during PCNL (prone or supine position) can influence the outcomes of a tubeless or not tubeless procedure. Anesthesiologists prefer the supine position because of better airway control during procedures. Another advantage of the supine position is that there is no need for

position changes when performing additional endoscopic procedures, such as cystoscopic or ureteroscopic operations [38]. Endoscopic combined intrarenal surgery is also a novel way of performing PCNL in the supine position [39]. Better visualization with the procedure allows for correct puncture of the kidney, and thus, can improve the safety and feasibility of a tubeless or total tubeless procedure.

Despite these limitations and shortcomings, our study has the substantial advantage of including larger samples from each study than the previously conducted pairwise meta-analyses [40]. Moreover, this is the first study to use network meta-analysis to compare PCNL methods, which enhances the statistical confidence and overcomes the limitations of pairwise meta-analyses.

Conclusions
In comparing each procedure through network meta-analysis, total tubeless and small-bore PCNLs were superior in terms of hemoglobin change, and total tubeless and tubeless PCNLs were superior with regard to the length of hospital stay. These findings indicate that conventional PCNL can be replaced with other techniques, especially total tubeless PCNL, in selected patients.

Abbreviations
PCNL: Percutaneous nephrolithotomy; RCT: Randomized controlled trial; VAS: Visual analogue scale

Funding
This study was supported by a faculty research grant from the Yonsei University College of Medicine for 2014 (6-2014-0156).

Authors' contributions
Systematic review and meta-analysis JYL, SUJ, MDK, DHK, JKK, WSH, YDC, KSC. Identification of studies, critical evaluation and discussion. JYL, KSC, DHK, WSH, YDC. All authors read and approved the final manuscript.

Competing interests
All the authors declare that they have no competing interests.

Author details
[1]Department of Urology, Severance Hospital, Urological Science Institute, Yonsei University College of Medicine, Seoul, South Korea. [2]Department of Urology, Gyeongsang National University Hospital, Gyeongsang National University School of Medicine, Jinju, South Korea. [3]Department of Radiology, Severance Hospital, Research Institute of Radiological Science, Yonsei University College of Medicine, Seoul, South Korea. [4]Department of Urology, Inha University School of Medicine, Incheon, South Korea. [5]Department of

Urology, Severance Check-Up, Yonsei University Health System, Seoul, South Korea. [6]Department of Urology, Gangnam Severance Hospital, Urological Science Institute, Yonsei University College of Medicine, 211 Eonju-ro, Gangnam-gu, Seoul 06273, South Korea.

References

1. Teichman JM. Clinical practice. Acute renal colic from ureteral calculus. N Engl J Med. 2004;350:684–93.
2. Lee JW, Park J, Lee SB, Son H, Cho SY, Jeong H. Mini-percutaneous Nephrolithotomy vs Retrograde Intrarenal Surgery for Renal Stones Larger Than 10 mm: A Prospective Randomized Controlled Trial. Urology. 2015;86:873–7.
3. Sivalingam S, Al-Essawi T, Hosking D. Percutaneous nephrolithotomy with retrograde nephrostomy access: a forgotten technique revisited. J Urol. 2013;189:1753–6.
4. Jung GH, Jung JH, Ahn TS, Lee JS, Cho SY, Jeong CW, et al. Comparison of retrograde intrarenal surgery versus a single-session percutaneous nephrolithotomy for lower-pole stones with a diameter of 15 to 30 mm: A propensity score-matching study. Korean J Urol. 2015;56:525–32.
5. Istanbulluoglu MO, Cicek T, Ozturk B, Gonen M, Ozkardes H. Percutaneous nephrolithotomy: nephrostomy or tubeless or totally tubeless? Urology. 2010;75:1043–6.
6. Paul EM, Marcovich R, Lee BR, Smith AD. Choosing the ideal nephrostomy tube. BJU Int. 2003;92:672–7.
7. Shah HN, Kausik VB, Hegde SS, Shah JN, Bansal MB. Tubeless percutaneous nephrolithotomy: a prospective feasibility study and review of previous reports. BJU Int. 2005;96:879–83.
8. Akman T, Binbay M, Yuruk E, Sari E, Seyrek M, Kaba M, et al. Tubeless Procedure is Most Important Factor in Reducing Length of Hospitalization After Percutaneous Nephrolithotomy: Results of Univariable and Multivariable Models. Urology. 2011;77:299–304.
9. Li H, Zhang Z, Li H, Xing Y, Zhang G, Kong X. Ultrasonography-guided percutaneous nephrolithotomy for the treatment of urolithiasis in patients with scoliosis. Int Surg. 2012;97:182–8.
10. Caldwell DM, Ades AE, Higgins JP. Simultaneous comparison of multiple treatments: combining direct and indirect evidence. BMJ. 2005;331:897–900.
11. Mills EJ, Thorlund K, Ioannidis JP. Demystifying trial networks and network meta-analysis. BMJ. 2013;346:f2914.
12. Yuan J, Zhang R, Yang Z, Lee J, Liu Y, Tian J, et al. Comparative effectiveness and safety of oral phosphodiesterase type 5 inhibitors for erectile dysfunction: a systematic review and network meta-analysis. Eur Urol. 2013;63:902–12.
13. Kwon JK, Cho KS, Oh CK, Kang DH, Lee H, Ham WS, et al. The beneficial effect of alpha-blockers for ureteral stent-related discomfort: systematic review and network meta-analysis for alfuzosin versus tamsulosin versus placebo. BMC Urol. 2015;15:55.
14. Lee JY, Cho KS, Kang DH, Jung HD, Kwon JK, Oh CK, et al. A network meta-analysis of therapeutic outcomes after new image technology-assisted transurethral resection for non-muscle invasive bladder cancer: 5-aminolaevulinic acid fluorescence vs hexylaminolevulinate fluorescence vs narrow band imaging. BMC Cancer. 2015;15:566.
15. Moher D, Liberati A, Tetzlaff J, Altman DG. Preferred reporting items for systematic reviews and meta-analyses: the PRISMA statement. PLoS Med. 2009;6:e1000097.
16. Chung JH, Lee SW. Assessing the quality of randomized controlled urological trials conducted by korean medical institutions. Korean J Urol. 2013;54:289–96.
17. R Development Core Team. R: A language and environment for statistical computing. Vienna: R Foundation for Statistical Computing; 2011. Accessed at www.R-project.org on 18 Mar 2013
18. Shah HN, Sodha HS, Khandkar AA, Kharodawala S, Hegde SS, Bansal MB. A randomized trial evaluating type of nephrostomy drainage after percutaneous nephrolithotomy: small bore v tubeless. J Endourol. 2008;22:1433–9.
19. Bellman GC, Davidoff R, Candela J, Gerspach J, Kurtz S, Stout L. Tubeless percutaneous renal surgery. J Urol. 1997;157:1578–82.
20. Kim SC, Tinmouth WW, Kuo RL, Paterson RF, Lingeman JE. Using and choosing a nephrostomy tube after percutaneous nephrolithotomy for large or complex stone disease: a treatment strategy. J Endourol. 2005;19:348–52.
21. Zhong Q, Zheng C, Mo J, Piao Y, Zhou Y, Jiang Q. Total tubeless versus standard percutaneous nephrolithotomy: a meta-analysis. J Endourol. 2013;27:420–6.
22. Yuan H, Zheng S, Liu L, Han P, Wang J, Wei Q. The efficacy and safety of tubeless percutaneous nephrolithotomy: a systematic review and meta-analysis. Urol Res. 2011;39:401–10.
23. Wang J, Zhao C, Zhang C, Fan X, Lin Y, Jiang Q. Tubeless vs standard percutaneous nephrolithotomy: a meta-analysis. BJU Int. 2012;109:918–24.
24. Shen P, Liu Y, Wang J. Nephrostomy tube-free versus nephrostomy tube for renal drainage after percutaneous nephrolithotomy: a systematic review and meta-analysis. Urol Int. 2012;88:298–306.
25. Borges CF, Fregonesi A, Silva DC, Sasse AD. Systematic Review and Meta-Analysis of Nephrostomy Placement Versus Tubeless Percutaneous Nephrolithotomy. J Endourol. 2010;24:1739–46.
26. Michel MS, Trojan L, Rassweiler JJ. Complications in percutaneous nephrolithotomy. Eur Urol. 2007;51:899–906. discussion
27. Lee JK, Kim BS, Park YK. Predictive factors for bleeding during percutaneous nephrolithotomy. Korean J Urol. 2013;54:448–53.
28. Pietrow PK, Auge BK, Lallas CD, Santa-Cruz RW, Newman GE, Albala DM, et al. Pain after percutaneous nephrolithotomy: impact of nephrostomy tube size. J Endourol. 2003;17:411–4.
29. Damiano R, Oliva A, Esposito C, De Sio M, Autorino R, D'Armiento M. Early and late complications of double pigtail ureteral stent. Urol Int. 2002;69:136–40.
30. Shoma AM, Elshal AM. Nephrostomy tube placement after percutaneous nephrolithotomy: critical evaluation through a prospective randomized study. Urology. 2012;79:771–6.
31. Mikhail AA, Kaptein JS, Bellman GC. Use of fibrin glue in percutaneous nephrolithotomy. Urology. 2003;61:910–4. discussion 4
32. Choi M, Brusky J, Weaver J, Amantia M, Bellman GC. Randomized trial comparing modified tubeless percutaneous nephrolithotomy with tailed stent with percutaneous nephrostomy with small-bore tube. J Endourol. 2006;20:766–70.
33. Okeke Z, Lee BR. Small renal masses: the case for cryoablation. J Endourol. 2008;22:1921–3.
34. Cormio L, Perrone A, Di Fino G, Ruocco N, De Siati M, de la Rosette J, et al. TachoSil((R)) sealed tubeless percutaneous nephrolithotomy to reduce urine leakage and bleeding: outcome of a randomized controlled study. J Urol. 2012;188:145–50.
35. Sofikerim M, Demirci D, Huri E, Ersekerci E, Karacagil M. Tubeless percutaneous nephrolithotomy: safe even in supracostal access. J Endourol. 2007;21:967–72.
36. Resorlu B, Kara C, Sahin E, Unsal A. Comparison of nephrostomy drainage types following percutaneous nephrolithotomy requiring multiple tracts: single tube versus multiple tubes versus tubeless. Urol Int. 2011;87:23–7.
37. Sutton AJ, Duval SJ, Tweedie RL, Abrams KR, Jones DR. Empirical assessment of effect of publication bias on meta-analyses. BMJ. 2000;320:1574–7.
38. Chung DY, Lee JY, Kim KH, Choi JH, Cho KS. Feasibility and efficacy of intermediate-supine percutaneous nephrolithotomy: initial experience. Chonnam Med J. 2014;50:52–7.
39. Cracco CM, Scoffone CM. ECIRS (Endoscopic Combined Intrarenal Surgery) in the Galdakao-modified supine Valdivia position: a new life for percutaneous surgery? World J Urol. 2011;29:821–7.
40. Li K, Lin T, Zhang C, Fan X, Xu K, Bi L, et al. Optimal frequency of shock wave lithotripsy in urolithiasis treatment: a systematic review and meta-analysis of randomized controlled trials. J Urol. 2013;190:1260–7.
41. Chang CH, Wang CJ, Huang SW. Totally tubeless percutaneous nephrolithotomy: a prospective randomized controlled study. Urol Res. 2011;39:459–65.
42. Aghamir SM, Modaresi SS, Aloosh M, Tajik A. Totally tubeless percutaneous nephrolithotomy for upper pole renal stone using subcostal access. J Endourol. 2011;25:583–6.
43. Kara C, Resorlu B, Bayindir M, Unsal A. A randomized comparison of totally tubeless and standard percutaneous nephrolithotomy in elderly patients. Urology. 2010;76:289–93.
44. Mishra S, Sabnis RB, Kurien A, Ganpule A, Muthu V, Desai M. Questioning the wisdom of tubeless percutaneous nephrolithotomy (PCNL): a prospective randomized controlled study of early tube removal vs tubeless PCNL. BJU Int. 2010;106:1045–8. discussion 8–9
45. Istanbulluoglu MO, Ozturk B, Gonen M, Cicek T, Ozkardes H. Effectiveness of totally tubeless percutaneous nephrolithotomy in selected patients: a prospective randomized study. Int Urol Nephrol. 2009;41:541–5.
46. Crook TJ, Lockyer CR, Keoghane SR, Walmsley BH. A randomized controlled trial of nephrostomy placement versus tubeless percutaneous nephrolithotomy. J Urol. 2008;180:612–4.

47. Agrawal MS, Agrawal M, Gupta A, Bansal S, Yadav A, Goyal J. A randomized comparison of tubeless and standard percutaneous nephrolithotomy. J Endourol. 2008;22:439–42.
48. Singh I, Singh A, Mittal G. Tubeless percutaneous nephrolithotomy: is it really less morbid? J Endourol. 2008;22:427–34.
49. Tefekli A, Altunrende F, Tepeler K, Tas A, Aydin S, Muslumanoglu AY. Tubeless percutaneous nephrolithotomy in selected patients: a prospective randomized comparison. Int Urol Nephrol. 2007;39:57–63.
50. Weiland D, Pedro RN, Anderson JK, Best SL, Lee C, Hendlin K, et al. Randomized prospective evaluation of nephrostomy tube configuration: impact on postoperative pain. Int Braz J Urol. 2007;33:313–8. discussion 9–22
51. Desai MR, Kukreja RA, Desai MM, Mhaskar SS, Wani KA, Patel SH, et al. A prospective randomized comparison of type of nephrostomy drainage following percutaneous nephrostolithotomy: large bore versus small bore versus tubeless. J Urol. 2004;172:565–7.
52. Marcovich R, Jacobson AI, Singh J, Shah D, El-Hakim A, Lee BR, et al. No panacea for drainage after percutaneous nephrolithotomy. J Endourol. 2004;18:743–7.
53. Feng MI, Tamaddon K, Mikhail A, Kaptein JS, Bellman GC. Prospective randomized study of various techniques of percutaneous nephrolithotomy. Urology. 2001;58:345–50.

15

New steps of robot-assisted radical prostatectomy using the extraperitoneal approach: a propensity-score matched comparison between extraperitoneal and transperitoneal approach in Japanese patients

Satoshi Kurokawa[1,2]* iD, Yukihiro Umemoto[2], Kentaro Mizuno[2], Atsushi Okada[2], Akihiro Nakane[2], Hidenori Nishio[2], Shuzo Hamamoto[2], Ryosuke Ando[2], Noriyasu Kawai[2], Keiichi Tozawa[2], Yutaro Hayashi[2] and Takahiro Yasui[2]

Abstract

Background: Robot-assisted radical prostatectomy (RARP) is commonly performed using the transperitoneal (TP) approach with six trocars over an 8-cm distance in the steep Trendelenburg position. In this study, we investigated the feasibility and the benefit of using the extraperitoneal (EP) approach with six trocars over a 4-cm distance in a flat or 5° Trendelenburg position. We also introduced four new steps to the surgical procedure and compared the surgical results and complications between the EP and TP approach using propensity score matching.

Methods: Between August 2012 and August 2016, 200 consecutive patients without any physical restrictions underwent RARP with the EP approach in a less than 5° Trendelenburg position, and 428 consecutive patients underwent RARP with the TP approach in a steep Trendelenburg position. Four new steps to RARP using the EP approach were developed: 1) arranging six trocars; 2) creating the EP space using laparoscopic forceps; 3) holding the separated prostate in the EP space outside the robotic view; and 4) preventing a postoperative inguinal hernia. Clinicopathological results and complications were compared between the EP and TP approaches using propensity score matching. Propensity scores were calculated for each patient using multivariate logistic regression based on the preoperative covariates.

Results: All 200 patients safely underwent RARP using the EP approach. The mean volume of estimated blood loss and duration of indwelling urethral catheter use were significantly lower with the EP approach than the TP approach (139.9 vs 184.9 mL, $p = 0.03$ and 5.6 vs 7.7 days, $p < 0.01$, respectively). No significant differences in the positive surgical margin were observed. None of the patients developed an inguinal hernia postoperatively after we introduced this technique.

(Continued on next page)

* Correspondence: sakun1974@hotmail.com
[1]Department of Urology, Nagoya Tokushukai General Hospital, 2-52, Kouzouji-cho-kita, Kasugai 487-0016, Japan
[2]Department of Nephro-urology, Nagoya City University Graduate School of Medical Sciences, 1, Kawasumi, Mizuho-cho, Mizuho-ku, Nagoya 467-8601, Japan

(Continued from previous page)

Conclusions: The EP approach to RARP was safely performed regardless of patient physique or contraindications to a steep Trendelenburg position. Our method, which involved using the EP approach to perform RARP, can decrease the amount of perioperative blood loss, the duration of indwelling urethral catheter use, and the incidence of postoperative inguinal hernia development.

Keywords: Robot-assisted radical prostatectomy, Extraperitoneal approach, Transperitoneal approach, Small physique, Trendelenburg position, Inguinal hernia, Propensity score

Background

Robot-assisted radical prostatectomy (RARP) has been used worldwide since it was introduced in 2000 [1, 2]. The 4-armed da Vinci® S surgical system (Intuitive Surgical, Sunnyvale, CA, USA), which is responsible for the widespread use of RARP, has 8-cm-wide arms, and the trocars should be spaced at intervals >8 cm to prevent them from colliding with each other [3]. RARP is commonly performed using the transperitoneal (TP) approach because it offers enough arm distance, a larger working space, and familiar laparoscopic intraperitoneal landmarks [2]. The working space is relatively smaller when using the extraperitoneal (EP) approach. However, the procedure can be performed with little effect on patients with previous intraabdominal surgery or severe obesity [4], and it causes minimal intraabdominal complications [2, 5]. Furthermore, because the steep Trendelenburg position is not required, the EP approach is effective in patients with contraindications to this position [6, 7]. However, the EP approach has several limitations including a small working space and collision of the robotic arms with one another. Within a small operating cavity, the separated prostate impedes the operator's visibility, and performing the vesicourethral anastomosis becomes difficult. It is challenging to acquire enough space to keep the removed prostate out of the robotic view and avoid collision of the robotic arms in patients who are physically small in particular. The development of new methods is necessary to overcome these difficulties.

Herein, we introduce four new steps for the surgical procedure and investigate the feasibility of using the EP approach with six trocars over a 4-cm distance in a less than 5° Trendelenburg position. We also compare the surgical results and complications of RARP using the EP and TP approaches.

Methods

The study protocol was approved by the Tokushukai Group Ethical Committee (approval number: TGE00700–016). Clinical data were gathered starting from the beginning of our experience with RARP. The database included preoperative, operative, and postoperative information.

From August 2012 to August 2016, we retrospectively reviewed the data of 200 consecutive patients who underwent RARP with the EP approach in a flat or 5° Trendelenburg position and 428 consecutive patients who underwent RARP with the TP approach in a steep Trendelenburg position. Our surgical team began performing RARP using the TP approach in May 2011. Prior to that, they had experience performing >600 laparoscopic radical prostatectomies using TP and EP approaches [8–11]. After we managed 135 cases of RARP with the TP approach, we began performing RARP with the EP approach.

Preoperative, operative, and postoperative data

Preoperative clinical data pertaining to patient background and prostate cancer such as the prostate-specific antigen (PSA) value, Gleason score, and clinical T stage were collected. Patient background included age, physique (height, weight, and body mass index [BMI]), and medical history. Patients with glaucoma, severe valvular heart disease, or intracranial diseases (e.g., an unruptured cerebral aneurysm) were submitted a priori to RARP using the EP approach in advance to avoid complications from the Trendelenburg position. Operative characteristics including the total operative time, robot console time, vesicourethral anastomosis time, estimated volume of blood loss, weight of the removed prostate, performance of lymph-node dissection, and surgical complications were also studied. Pathological variables included the Gleason score, presence of extension, seminal vesicle invasion, and surgical margin status. Postoperative information including the duration of indwelling urethral catheters and presence of postoperative complications was collected. Functional outcome was assessed based on urinary continence 6 months postoperatively. Continence was defined as using no pads or one safety pad per day.

Surgical procedure

All the surgeries were conducted by the same surgical team using the da Vinci® S surgical system. All surgeons had reached the plateau in the learning curve having had experience with more than 50 cases [12, 13]. RARP using the TP approach was performed as described in previous articles [14, 15]. RARP using the EP approach was performed as follows.

First, we determined the position of the six trocars whose distances were 4 cm apart when performing RARP using the EP approach (Fig. 1). Traditionally, trocars are placed 7–8 cm apart during RARP using the EP approach [16–18]. However, it was difficult to space the trocars >7 cm apart in patients with small physiques. The decision to space the trocars 4 cm apart was based on a recommendation for performing robotic surgery in children [19].

Second, we created the EP space using a balloon dilator, finger assistance, and laparoscopic forceps. Furthermore, we developed a new technique for placing the trocar in a small space. A 4-cm transverse infraumbilical incision was made through the anterior rectus sheath. We intended to dissect the EP space digitally at the position of the trocars of robotic arm no. 1 or no. 2. We inserted a balloon dilator (Pajunk® balloon systems, Pajunk, Germany) and created the EP space using the laparoscopic view. If the EP space was insufficient to insert all six trocars, it was expanded using laparoscopic forceps through the trocar of robotic arm no. 1 or no. 2 as a working port. When placing a trocar in a small adhesive space, there is a risk for the trocar to become lost in the adhesion tissue. Therefore, we used a laparoscopic dissector with a pointed tip to penetrate the abdominal wall from the small space of the EP cavity to the outside of the body (Fig. 2). The shaft of the laparoscopy forceps was placed along the inner cylinder, and it was possible to extracorporeally guide

the outer tube of the 5-mm trocar. When attempting to guide the 12-mm trocar, the tract of the trocar was gradually dilated after the 5-mm trocar was inserted, followed by the insertion of the 8-mm and 12-mm trocars.

Third, we prepared to hold the freed prostate in the right abdominal EP space outside of robotic view. A 14-gauge intravenous indwelling needle was penetrated into the EP space from outside of the abdominal wall between the no. 1 and no. 3 robotic trocars (Fig. 1). After inserting a 14-gauge needle, the plastic cannula (outer cylinder) was left and the inner time (metal needle) removed. The plastic cannula was closed with the lid of the three-way stopcock to prevent carbon dioxide gas from leaking. After the prostate was dissected from the bladder neck in an antegrade manner, the separated prostate was stored in a pouch. Then, the thread of the pouch was pulled outside of the body through a 14-gauge plastic cannula (Fig. 3). The prostate was held on the right side of the abdomen outside of robotic view. After using the Rocco suture method, vesicourethral anastomosis was performed using the single-knot method with Lapra-Ty clips [9, 20].

Fourth, to prevent an indirect inguinal hernia postoperatively, we dissected and peeled the peritoneum from the spermatic cord at the inner inguinal ring. This technique was originally performed during retropubic radical prostatectomy [21], and it was introduced in RARP using the EP approach for all patients after the twenty-first patient. The cord-like structures of the cremaster muscle and fibrous tissue were transected around the spermatic cord, and the testicular vessels and vas deference were separated (Fig. 4).

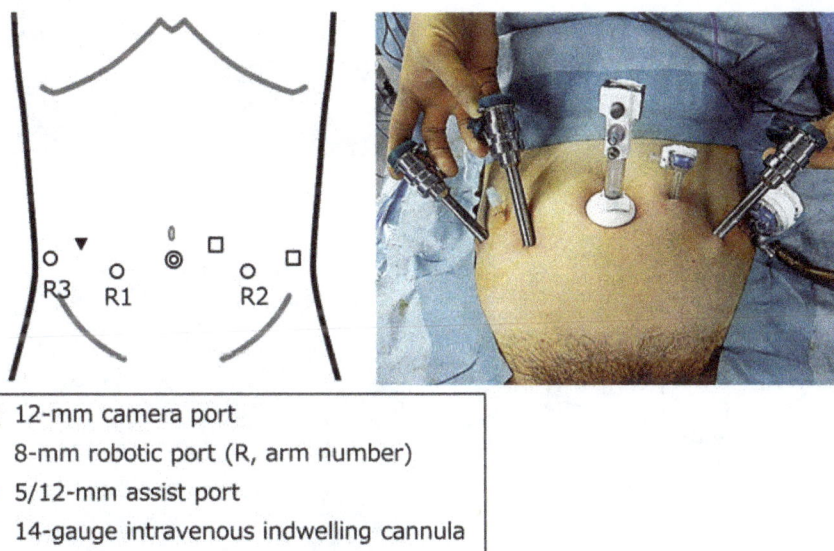

Fig. 1 Placement of ports in the extraperitoneal approach to robot-assisted radical prostatectomy. In addition to six trocars, we place a 14-gauge intravenous indwelling cannula in the right lower abdominal region

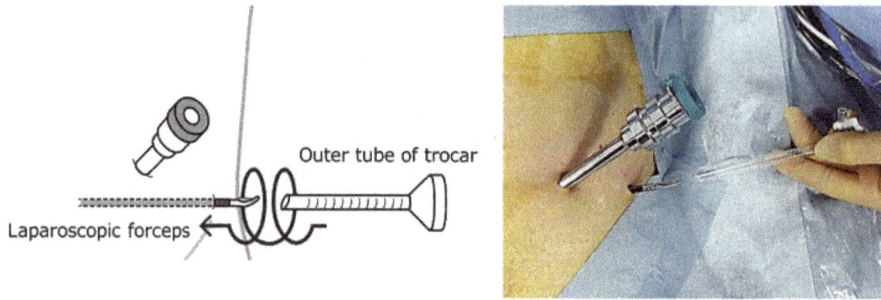

Fig. 2 Method of placing a trocar in a small space (left side, assist port). We use laparoscopic forceps (a curved dissector) to penetrate from the small space of the extraperitoneal cavity to outside the body. Forceps are used instead of the inner cylinder of the trocar and only the outer tube of the trocar guides insertion of the forceps

Finally, the prostate was removed, and a 10-French closed drain was indwelled. The drain was removed on postoperative day 2, and on postoperative days 4–7, the urethral catheter was removed after confirming that there was no leakage using cystourethrography.

In selected patients whose risk of lymph node metastases was >10% according to the preoperative nomogram for Japanese patients or who were classified into the high-risk group according to the D'Amico criteria, pelvic lymph-node dissection was performed after the fourth step of preventing an inguinal hernia [22, 23].

Propensity score matching and statistical analysis
Propensity scores were calculated for each patient using multivariate logistic regression analysis based on the preoperative covariates. The covariates used to compare the EP and TP groups were: follow-up duration, age, height, weight, BMI, prostate-specific antigen value, biopsy Gleason score, and clinical T stage. The covariates of the chronological comparison in the EP group excluded follow-up duration. Subsequently, balance of matching was assessed using statistical comparison. In propensity-score matched groups of the EP and TP approach, we analyzed operative results and postoperative outcomes.

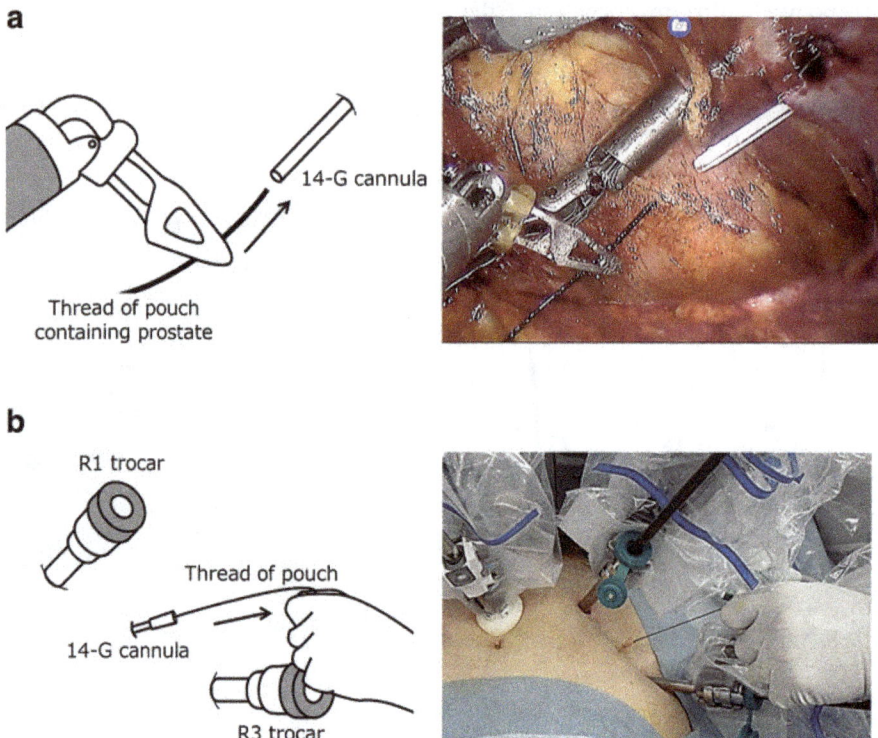

Fig. 3 The prostate is placed in a pouch and retracted to the lower right abdomen. The thread of the pouch containing the prostate is pulled out of the body through the 14-gauge intravenous indwelling cannula (**a-b**) G, gauge

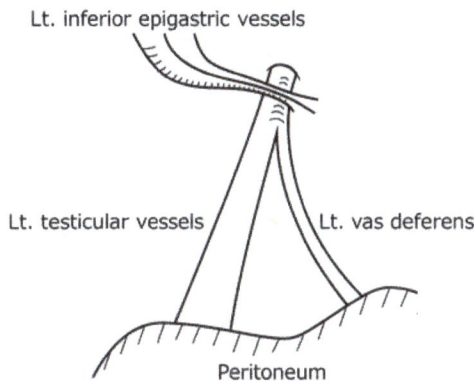

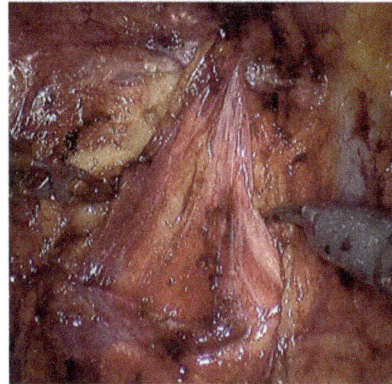

Fig. 4 Technique to prevent postoperative inguinal hernia (Lt side). The peritoneum is dissected and peeled from the spermatic cord on the cranial side of the inner inguinal ring. Cord-like structures between the spermatic cord and peritoneum are transected, and the spermatic cord is separated into the testicular vessels and vas deferens Lt, left

In the two propensity-score matched chronological subgroups in the EP group, operative and postoperative outcomes were also compared. The comparisons were evaluated using an χ^2-test for qualitative variables and the Mann-Whitney U test for quantitative variables. A two-tailed p-value <0.05 was considered significant. Statistical analysis was performed with the JMP 13.0® software (SAS Institute Corp., Cary, NC, USA).

Results

Patients in the EP and TP group were balanced using propensity score matching (Table 1). The patient with the smallest physique in the EP group was 143.6 cm tall and weighed 34.8 kg; he underwent RARP using the EP

approach safely. Patient backgrounds such as follow-up duration, age, height, weight, and BMI were not significantly different between the groups (Table 1). Preoperative clinical characteristics such as the mean PSA level, biopsy Gleason score, clinical stage, and previous abdominal surgery, were also not significantly different between the groups (Table 1).

Table 2 shows the operative and postoperative results, as well as complications in both groups. The mean operative time was significantly longer in the EP group than in the TP group (254.5 vs 225.8 min, $p < 0.01$). The mean robot console time and vesicourethral anastomosis time were not significantly different between the EP and TP group (180.5 vs 175.4 min, $p = 0.07$; and 30.3 vs

Table 1 Patients' preoperative clinical characteristics by surgical procedures

Variables	EP approach	TP approach	p-Value
Patients (n)	190	190	
Follow-up (months)	27.3 ± 13.8 (4–52)	27.8 ± 154.3 (4–52)	0.78
Age (years)	69.4 ± 6.0 (51–82)	69.3 ± 4.7 (51–79)	0.70
Height (cm)	165.2 ± 6.1 (143.6–186.0)	165.4 ± 5.3 (152.5–183.2)	0.70
Weight (kg)	63.7 ± 9.3 (34.8–103.0)	63.6 ± 9.4 (38.0–122.0)	0.89
BMI (kg/m²)	23.3 ± 3.0 (16.9–34.5)	23.2 ± 2.9 (15.8–36.3)	0.73
PSA (ng/mL)	10.7 ± 11.6 (2.2–84.4)	10.8 ± 10.4 (2.3–73.1)	0.24
Biopsy Gleason score (%)			0.12
2–6	36 (19.0)	44 (23.2)	
7	100 (52.6)	80 (42.1)	
8–10	54 (28.4)	66 (34.7)	
Clinical stage (%)			0.15
T1	41 (21.6)	49 (25.8)	
T2	142 (74.7)	126 (66.3)	
T3	7 (3.7)	15 (7.9)	
Previous abdominal surgery (%)	62 (32.3)	65 (35.4)	0.91

EP extraperitoneal, *TP* transperitoneal, *BMI* body mass index, *PSA* prostate-specific antigen

Table 2 Comparison of operative and postoperative results, and complications between the extraperitoneal and transperitoneal approaches

Variables	EP approach	TP approach	p–Value
Patients (n)	190	190	
Operative time (min)	254.5 ± 42.5 (144–464)	225.8 ± 44.0 (131–410)	<0.01
Robot console time (min)	180.5 ± 31.7 (98–304)	175.4 ± 40.9 (98–351)	0.07
Anastomosis time (min)	30.3 ± 11.7 (7–73)	28.0 ± 10.0 (8–66)	0.09
Blood loss (mL)	139.9 ± 118.7 (5–800)	184.9 ± 195.8 (0–1485)	0.03
Prostate weight (g)	46.0 ± 13.1 (22–96)	44.8 ± 16.4 (8–132)	0.13
Indwelling urethral catheter (days)	5.6 ± 1.7 (4–16)	7.7 ± 3.7 (4–33)	<0.01
Pathological Gleason score (%)			0.02
2–6	24 (12.6)	21 (11.1)	
7	118 (62.1)	142 (74.7)	
8–10	54 (28.4)	27 (14.2)	
Pathological stage (%)			<0.01
pT2	121 (63.7)	153 (80.5)	
pT3	69 (36.3)	37 (19.5)	
Positive surgical margin (%)			
pT2	13 (10.7)	30 (19.6)	0.09
pT3	37 (53.6)	21 (56.8)	0.76
Lymphadenectomy (%)	63 (33.2)	71 (37.4)	0.22
Continence (%)	173 (91.1)	170 (89.5)	0.60
Complications (%)			
Anastomosis stenosis	2 (1.1)	5 (2.6)	0.20
Blood transfusion	0 (0.0)	1 (0.5)	0.32
Colorectal injury	0 (0.0)	2 (1.1)	0.16
Conversion to open surgery	0 (0.0)	1 (0.5)	0.32
Ileus	0 (0.0)	2 (1.1)	0.16
Indirect inguinal hernia	2 (1.1)	14 (7.4)	<0.01
Symptomatic lymphocele	0 (0.0)	1 (0.5)	0.32

EP extraperitoneal, TP transperitoneal

28.0 min, $p = 0.09$, respectively). The mean volume of estimated blood loss and duration of indwelling urethral catheters were significantly lower in the EP group than in the TP group (139.9 vs 184.9 mL, $p < 0.01$; and 5.6 vs 7.7 days, $p < 0.01$, respectively). There were no significant differences between the groups in terms of the positive surgical margin, lymph-node dissection rate, and urinary continence. The rate of postoperative inguinal hernia was significantly lower in the EP group than in the TP group (1.1 vs 7.4%, $p < 0.01$). There were no cases of conversion to open surgery in the EP group.

Table 3 compares the surgical and pathological results of the 200 patients in the EP group subdivided into two chronological groups of 100 patients. The mean operative time, robot console time, and vesicourethral anastomosis time were significantly shorter in the latter group (257.9 vs 247.2 min, $p < 0.01$; 184.5 vs 174.1 min,

$p < 0.01$; and 33.4 vs 24.2 min, $p < 0.01$, respectively). None of the patients developed an indirect inguinal hernia postoperatively after our method was introduced.

Discussion

Our method of RARP using the EP approach can be safely implemented, even in patients with small physiques. RARP using the EP approach has the benefit of reducing the amount of blood loss and shortening the duration of indwelling urethral catheter use compared with RARP using the TP approach.

We divided the surgical procedure into four steps. First, we arranged six trocars spaced 4 cm apart. In all 200 patients in the EP group, it was possible to perform surgery without revising the trocar placement. This result suggests that it is possible to perform RARP with the EP approach using six trocars spaced 4 cm apart.

Table 3 Comparison of outcomes of the extraperitoneal approach according to the extent of surgical experience

Variables	EP approach		
	1–100	101–200	p–Value
Patients (n)	82	82	
Operative time (min)	258.6 ± 40.5	244.1 ± 43.2	<0.01
Robot console time (min)	183.5 ± 30.9	169.9 ± 26.2	<0.01
Anastomosis time (min)	33.1 ± 10.5	22.9 ± 7.7	<0.01
Blood loss (mL)	157.3 ± 116.6	104.8 ± 95.7	<0.01
Prostate weight (g)	46.3 ± 11.6	46.7 ± 14.4	0.93
Indwelling urethral catheter (days)	5.2 ± 1.0	5.6 ± 1.6	0.20
Pathological Gleason score (%)			0.04
2–6	14 (17.1)	4 (4.9)	
7	48 (58.5)	55 (67.1)	
8–10	20 (24.4)	23 (28.0)	
Pathological stage (%)			0.34
pT2	53 (64.6)	47 (57.3)	
pT3	29 (35.4)	35 (42.7)	
Positive srgical margin (%)			
pT2	6 (11.3)	2 (4.3)	0.15
pT3	20 (69.0)	12 (34.3)	<0.01
Lymphadenectomy (%)	26 (31.7)	31 (37.8)	0.25
Continence (%)	73 (89.0)	76 (92.7)	0.42
Complications (%)			
Indirect inguinal hernia	2 (2.4)	0 (0.0)	0.16
Anastomosis stenosis	1 (1.2)	1 (1.2)	1.00

EP extraperitoneal

Second, we created the EP space and guided the trocar with a new technique. Normally, the trocar is placed using finger assistance or laparoscopy to confirm the tip of the trocar so that it does not damage the surrounding structures [24]. However, when the location of trocar placement cannot be sufficiently exposed because of adhesions, it is difficult to appropriately confirm the tip of the trocar. Therefore, we used the laparoscopic dissector to penetrate from the EP space to outside of the body, to avoid the adhesive site, and to guide the trocar. This technique is a useful way to place the trocar into a narrow space, and it can be used during robotic surgery as well as any laparoscopic surgery.

Third, we developed a new technique to hold the separated prostate in the EP space. A 14-gauge cannula can serve as a tract for the thread of the pouch. During robotic or laparoscopic pyeloplasty, a 14-gauge cannula is used as a tract for the insertion of a ureteral stent [25, 26]. Thus, using an intravenous indwelling needle as a small tract through the abdominal wall can be helpful during minimally invasive surgery.

Fourth, the technique of preventing a postoperative inguinal hernia was simple and effective. This technique was originally performed during retropubic radical prostatectomy [21]. Before we introduced this technique, a postoperative inguinal hernia developed in 2 (10%) patients. However, none of the patients developed postoperative inguinal hernia after introducing this technique. The average follow-up duration in our study was over 27 months. The average interval between prostatectomy and postoperative inguinal hernia diagnosis was reported to be 10.6 months [21]. Thus, the follow-up duration we used in our study was sufficient to determine the effect of this technique.

Urethral anastomosis stenosis was observed in 1.1% of patients in the EP group and 2.6% of patients in the TP group. The incidence of strictures of the vesico-urethral anastomosis after radical prostatectomy has been reported to range from 0.5 to 32%, with most occurring within 5 months of radical prostatectomy [27–29]. Thus, the rate of anastomosis stenosis in our study was lower than those in the literature and the follow-up duration of our study was sufficient to evaluate the rate of anastomosis stenosis after RARP.

Symptomatic lymphocele occurred in 0% of patients in the EP group and 0.5% of patients in the TP group. We removed drains on postoperative day 2 after confirming a decrease in the drain fluid. The duration of pelvic drainage has been reported to influence the rate of symptomatic lymphocele [30]. The group whose drains were removed on postoperative day 1 exhibited higher rates of symptomatic lymphocele than patients whose drains were removed on postoperative day 7 and patients without drainage [30]. In general, lymphatic fluid cannot be absorbed by the peritoneal surface in the EP approach. Accordingly, the rate of lymphocele in the EP approach is greater than that in the TP approach. During the postoperative course of our study, we removed the pelvic drain after the amount of drain fluid decreased. Thus, the rate of lymphocele was low compared with that in the literature [31].

Our four new steps were demonstrated to be successful for performing RARP using the EP approach safely. The positive surgical margin and the time of operation, robot console, and vesicourethral anastomosis were compatible to those in the literature [32]. In particular, the amount of the blood loss and the incidence of the postoperative complications, such as inguinal hernia, anastomosis stenosis, and lymphocele, were low compared with those in the literature [31, 32].

The robot console time and vesicourethral anastomosis time of the EP approach became shorter after 100 cases, and they became shorter than those of the TP approach. However, the total operative time of the EP approach was still longer after 100 cases than that of the TP approach.

There is a possibility that extra time was needed to create the EP space. As the operative space is relatively smaller in the EP approach, bleeding should be carefully controlled to maintain the robotic view. Vesicourethral anastomosis was performed after completing hemostasis. The values of blood loss and duration of indwelling urethral catheter use were significantly lower from the beginning of the EP approach than those of the TP approach. We first started RARP using the TP approach, and we overcame the learning curve of 50–100 cases before starting to perform the EP approach [12, 13]. However, 100 cases of the EP approach were needed to overcome the learning curve of EP approach.

We acknowledge that our study had strengths and weaknesses. One strength of our study is that we created a propensity-score matched comparison, which had a balanced covariate preoperative factor profiling, reducing the possibility of cofounding. Although our study was retrospectively designed, the propensity-score matched comparison might reduce selection bias. There were a few additional limitations to our study. First, the sample size might be relatively small for a study of this nature. Second, the model for propensity score matching may not include potentially relevant factors that are simply unknown at this time. Third, erectile data evaluation was not performed. Fourth, the operation was performed by the same surgical team but not by a single surgeon, which might have had an impact on the outcomes of the operation and the postoperative course.

Conclusions

RARP with the EP approach using four new steps was safely performed regardless of patient physique and medical history. Our method of RARP with the EP approach can reduce the amount of perioperative blood loss, the duration of indwelling urethral catheters, and the incidence of postoperative inguinal hernia development. In addition to RARP using the TP approach, the EP approach is useful and it should be learned and mastered for all types of patients regardless of their medical history, if possible.

Abbreviations
BMI: Body mass index; DVC: Deep vein complex; EP: Extraperitoneal; PSA: Prostate-specific antigen; RARP: Robot-assisted radical prostatectomy; TP: Transperitoneal

Acknowledgements
None

Funding
None.

Authors' contributions
SK, YU, KM, AO, AN, HN, SH, RA, NK, KT, and TY were members of our surgical team, and SK, YU, KT, and TY were surgeons with experience in over 50

cases, which is the plateau of the learning curve. SK contributed to the conception, design, analyses, and interpretation of the data. In addition, SK also drafted the manuscript, and agreed to be accountable for the accuracy and all other aspects of the work. SK and SH contributed to the data entry and management. YH and TY did the supervision job throughout this study. All authors read and approved the final manuscript.

Competing interests
The authors declare that they have no competing interests.

References
1. Abbou CC, Hoznek A, Salomon L, Lobontiu A, Saint F, Cicco A, et al. Remote laparoscopic radical prostatectomy carried out with a robot. Report of a case. Prog Urol. 2000;10:520–3.
2. Li-Ming S, Scott MG, Joseph AS Jr. Laparoscopic and robotic-assisted laparoscopic radical prostatectomy and pelvic lymphadenectomy. In: Wein AJ, Kavoussi LR, Partin AW, Peters CA, editors. Campbell-Walsh urology. 11th ed. Philadelphia: Elsevier; 2016. p. 2663–8.
3. Joseph AS Jr. Robot-assisted laparoscopic prostatectomy. In: Joseph Jr AS, Stuart SH, Edward JM, Glenn MP, editors. Hinman's atlas of urologic surgery. 3rd ed. Philadelphia: Elsevier; 2012. p. 435–6.
4. Agrawal V, Feng C, Joseph J. Outcomes of extraperitoneal robot-assisted radical prostatectomy in the morbidly obese: a propensity score-matched study. J Endourol. 2015;29:677–82.
5. Akand M, Erdogru T, Avci E, Ates M. Transperitoneal versus extraperitoneal robot-assisted laparoscopic radical prostatectomy: a prospective single surgeon randomized comparative study. Int J Urol. 2015;22:916–21.
6. Ventura LM, Golubev I, Lee W, Nose I, Parel JM, Feuer WJ, et al. Head-down posture induces PERG alterations in early glaucoma. J Glaucoma. 2013;22:255–64.
7. Haas S, Haese A, Goetz AE, Kubitz JC. Haemodynamics and cardiac function during robotic-assisted laparoscopic prostatectomy in steep Trendelenburg position. Int J Med Robot. 2011;7:408–13.
8. Nakane A, Akita H, Okamura T, Nagata D, Kojima Y, Akita H, et al. Feasibility of a novel extraperitoneal two-port laparoendoscopic approach for radical prostatectomy: an initial study. Int J Urol. 2013;20:729–33.
9. Naiki T, Kawai N, Okamura T, Nagata D, Kojima Y, Akita H, et al. Neoadjuvant hormonal therapy is a feasible option in laparoscopic radical prostatectomy. BMC Urol. 2012;12:36.
10. Yasui T, Itoh Y, Maruyama T, Akita H, Hashimoto Y, Tozawa K, et al. The single-knot method with Lapra-Ty clips is useful for training surgeons in vesicourethral anastomosis during laparoscopic radical prostatectomy. Int Urol Nephrol. 2009;41:281–5.
11. Tozawa K, Hashimoto Y, Yasui T, Itoh Y, Nagata D, Akita H, et al. Evaluation of operative complications related to laparoscopic radical prostatectomy. Int J Urol. 2008;15:222–5.
12. Hashimoto T, Yoshioka K, Gondo T, Kamoda N, Satake N, Ozu C, et al. Learning curve and perioperative outcomes of robot-assisted radical prostatectomy in 200 initial Japanese cases by a single surgeon. J Endourol. 2013;27:1218–23.
13. Doumerc N, Yuen C, Savdie R, Rahman MB, Rasiah KK, Pe Benito R, et al. Should experienced open prostatic surgeons convert to robotic surgery? The real learning curve for one surgeon over 3 years. BJU Int. 2010;106:378–84.
14. Yasui T, Tozawa K, Okada A, Kurokawa S, Kubota H, Mizuno K, et al. Outcomes of robot-assisted laparoscopic prostatectomy with a posterior approach to the seminal vesicle in 300 patients. Int Sch Res Notices. 2014;2014:565737.
15. Yasui T, Tozawa K, Kurokawa S, Okada A, Mizuno K, Umemoto Y, et al. Impact of prostate weight on perioperative outcomes of robot-assisted laparoscopic prostatectomy with a posterior approach to the seminal vesicle. BMC Urol. 2014;14:6.
16. Lee JY, Diaz RR, Cho KS, Yu HS, Chung JS, Ham WS, et al. Lymphocele after extraperitoneal robot-assisted radical prostatectomy: a propensity score-matching study. Int J Urol. 2013;20:1169–76.
17. Dogra PN, Saini AK, Singh P, Bora G, Nayak B. Extraperitoneal robot-assisted laparoscopic radical prostatectomy: initial experience. Urol Ann. 2014;6:130–4.
18. Joseph JV, Rosenbaum R, Madeb R, Erturk E, Patel HR. Robotic extraperitoneal radical prostatectomy: an alternative approach. J Urol. 2006;175:945–50.
19. Casale P. Principles of laparoscopic and robotic surgery in children. In: Wein AJ, Kavoussi LR, Partin AW, Peters CA, editors. Campbell-Walsh urology. 11th ed. Philadelphia: Elsevier; 2016. p. 2969–74.

20. Van Velthoven RF, Ahlering TE, Peltier A, Skarecky DW, Clayman RV. Technique for laparoscopic running urethrovesical anastomosis: the single knot method. Urology. 2003;61:699–702.

21. Taguchi K, Yasui T, Kubota H, Fukuta K, Kobayashi D, Naruyama H, et al. Simple method of preventing postoperative inguinal hernia after radical retropubic prostatectomy. Urology. 2010;76:1083–7.

22. Naito S, Kuroiwa K, Kinukawa N, Goto K, Koga H, Ogawa O, et al. Validation of Partin tables and development of a preoperative nomogram for Japanese patients with clinically localized prostate cancer using 2005 International Society of Urological Pathology consensus on Gleason grading: data from the Clinicopathological research Group for Localized Prostate Cancer. J Urol. 2008;180:904–9.

23. D'Amico AV, Whittington R, Malkowicz SB, Schultz D, Blank K, Broderick GA, et al. Biochemical outcome after radical prostatectomy, external beam radiation therapy, or interstitial radiation therapy for clinically localized prostate cancer. JAMA. 1998;280:969–74.

24. Asimakopoulos AD, Mugnier C, Hoepffner JL, Lopez L, Rey D, Gaston R, et al. Laparoscopic treatment of benign prostatic hyperplasia (BPH): overview of the current techniques. BJU Int. 2011;107:1168–82.

25. Mizuno K, Kojima Y, Kurokawa S, Kamisawa H, Nishio H, Moritoki Y, et al. Robot-assisted laparoscopic pyeloplasty for ureteropelvic junction obstruction: comparison between pediatric and adult patients-Japanese series. J Robot Surg. 2016; doi: 10.1007/s11701-016-0633-5.

26. Kojima Y, Umemoto Y, Mizuno K, Tozawa K, Kohri K, Hayashi Y. Comparison of laparoscopic pyeloplasty for ureteropelvic junction obstruction in adults and children: lessons learned. J Urol. 2011;185:1461–7.

27. Song J, Eswara J, Brandes SB. Postprostatectomy anastomosis stenosis: a systematic review. Urology. 2015;86:211–8.

28. Pfalzgraf D, Siegel FP, Kriegmair MC, Wagener N. Bladder neck contracture after radical prostatectomy: what is the reality of care? J Endourol. 2017;31:50–6.

29. Park R, Martin S, Goldberg JD, Lepor H. Anastomotic strictures following radical prostatectomy: insights into incidence, effectiveness of intervention, effect on continence, and factors predisposing to occurrence. Urology. 2001;57:742–8.

30. Danuser H, Di Pierro GB, Stucki P, Mattei A. Extended pelvic lymphadenectomy and various radical prostatectomy techniques: is pelvic drainage necessary? BJU Int. 2013;111:963–9.

31. Chung JS, Kim WT, Ham WS, Yu HS, Chae Y, Chung SH, et al. Comparison of oncological results, functional outcomes, and complications for transperitoneal versus extraperitoneal robot-assisted radical prostatectomy: a single surgeon's experience. J Endourol. 2011;25:787–92.

32. Atug F, Castle EP, Woods M, Srivastav SK, Thomas R, Davis R. Transperitoneal versus extraperitoneal robotic-assisted radical prostatectomy: is one better than the other? Urology. 2006;68:1077–81.

16

Assessment of free-hand transperineal targeted prostate biopsy using multiparametric magnetic resonance imaging-transrectal ultrasound fusion in Chinese men with prior negative biopsy and elevated prostate-specific antigen

Huibo Lian[1,4†], Junlong Zhuang[1,4†], Wei Wang[1,4*], Bing Zhang[2], Jiong Shi[3], Danyan Li[2], Yao Fu[3], Xuping Jiang[5], Weimin Zhou[5] and Hongqian Guo[1,4*]

Abstract

Background: To evaluate the role of free-hand transperineal targeted prostate biopsy using multiparametric magnetic resonance imaging-transrectal ultrasound (mpMRI-TRUS) fusion in Chinese men with repeated biopsy.

Methods: A total of 101 consecutive patients suspicious of prostate cancer (PCa) at the mpMRI scan and with prior negative biopsy and elevated PSA values were prospectively recruited at two urological centers. Suspicious areas on mpMRI were defined and graded using PI-RADS score. Targeted biopsies (TB) were performed for each suspicious lesion and followed a 12-core systematic biopsy (SB). Results of biopsy pathology and whole-gland pathology at prostatectomy were analyzed and compared between TB and SB. The risk for biopsy positivity was assessed by univariate and multivariate logistic regression analysis.

Results: Fusion biopsy revealed PCa in 41 of 101 men (40.6%) and 25 (24.8%) were clinically significant. There was exact agreement between TB and SB in 74 (73.3%) men. TB diagnosed 36% more significant cancer than SB (22 vs 13 cases, $P = 0.012$). When TB were combined with SB, an additional 14 cases (34.1%) of mostly significant PCa (71.4%) were diagnosed ($P = 0.036$). TB had greater sensitivity and accuracy for significant cancer than SB in 26 men with whole-gland pathology after prostatectomy. PI-RADS score on mpMRI was the most powerful predictor of PCa and significant cancer.

Conclusions: Free-hand transperineal TB guided with MRI-TRUS fusion imaging improves detection of clinical significant PCa in Chinese men with previously negative biopsy. PI-RADS score is a reliable predictor of PCa and significant cancer.

Keywords: Magnetic resonance imaging, Prostate cancer, Repeat biopsy, Targeted biopsy, Transrectal ultrasound

* Correspondence: wawe9999@163.com; dr.guohongqian@gmail.com
†Equal contributors
[1]Department of Urology, Drum Tower Hospital, Medical School of Nanjing University, 321 Zhongshan Road, Nanjing 210008, Jiangsu, People's Republic of China
Full list of author information is available at the end of the article

Background

Since the 1980s, transrectal ultrasound (TRUS) guided systematic prostate biopsy is performed on patients with abnormal serum prostate-specific antigen (PSA) or suspicious digital rectal examination [1]. This conventional method has been shown to have limited sensitivity for detecting prostate cancer (PCa), which of the false-negative rate may be as high as 47% [2]. PSA related anxiety and repeated biopsy dilemma consist in many of the men with negative biopsies and persistently elevated serum PSA levels [3]. Approximately 38% of them undergo a repeat biopsy within 5 years with cancer detection only in an additional 13 to 41% [4].

In order to improve biopsy sensitivity, the concept of targeted biopsy (TB) on suspicious areas through magnetic resonance imaging (MRI) guidance was established [5]. Although multiparametric MRI (mpMRI) offered an increased sensitivity and specificity on prostate biopsy guidance, the disadvantage of time-consuming and equipment-specialization made it not widely used [6]. Recently, MRI-TRUS fusion technique has been developed and proposed, because of its combination of the soft tissue resolution of MRI and the practicability of TRUS [7]. The mpMRI-TRUS image fusion biopsy system is a novel fusion technology which not only provides visualization of both recorded multiplanar reconstruction images on that one monitor, but also real-timely makes diagnostic or procedural decisions [8]. Using one such fusion device, we got initial encouraging result for targeted prostate biopsy as reported by other researchers [9–11]. Unfortunately, targeted MRI-TRUS fusion biopsy has not been well evaluated with free-hand transperineal approach, especially in Asian men with previously negative biopsy.

We present double center results to evaluate the impact of using mpMRI-TRUS image fusion technology for free-hand transperineal TB in Chinese men with prior negative biopsy and elevated PSA, and compare biopsy performance between TB and 12-core systematic biopsy (SB) in the cancer detection.

Methods
Study population

After the approval of institutional review board, a prospective study of free-hand transperineal TB guided with MRI-TRUS fusion imaging was performed at two Chinese urological centers from May 2014 to March 2016 (Drum Tower Hospital, Medical School of Nanjing University, and the Affiliated Yixing people's Hospital of Jiangsu University). One hundred and one consecutive patients with at least one prior negative prostate biopsy and persistently elevated serum PSA levels were included. All of them were evaluated with prostate mpMRI and considered having at least one suspicious area in mpMRI images.

Multiparametric MRI

All mpMRI was performed using a 3 Tesla MRI scanner (Achieva; Philips Medical System, The Netherlands) with a 32-channel phased array coil. The protocol of acquisition of different MRI sequences was recently published [12]. Images analyses were performed and supervised by two experienced uroradiologists. Suspicious areas were defined and a likelihood score from 2 to 5 for each lesion was provided according to the Prostate Imaging Reporting and Data System (RI-PADS) [13] based on the European Society of Urogenital Radiology prostate MRI guidelines [14]. We didn't use the PI-PADS Version 2 [15], because the new system had not been well validated and most of the patients' lesions were evaluated before its publication.

Biopsy procedure

All biopsies were performed with an mpMRI-TRUS fusion guided biopsy technique (RVS®, Real-time Virtual Sonography, Hitachi Medical Corporation, Tokyo, Japan) and 18-G automatic biopsy guns with 22 mm specimen size (Bard Magnum; Bard Medical, Covington, GA, USA) as described previously [12]. In brief, morphological MRI data was loaded into the biopsy system and suspicious areas were marked on high resolution transversal T2 W sequences (Fig. 1 a-d). Then, ultrasound probe with magnetic position sensor was used to get the TRUS images. During fusing two kinds of images, the MR images reconstructed from the MRI volume data were corresponded to the ultrasound sagittal images using internal urethral orifice as the fiducial landmark. Thus, mpMRI data with the marked suspicious lesions were real-timely superimposed on the TRUS images at the same monitor.

Then, the biopsy started with TB using the free-hand transperineal technique without the guide of template by one experienced urologist. Cancer-suspicious lesions identified on MRI were semiautomatically displayed on the real-time TRUS image to guide biopsy needle [10]. During free-hand transperineal biopsy procedure, the puncture point was chose to keep away from pubis and adjacent organs, and make the needle correspond to the ultrasound sagittal images (Fig. 1 e). Every targeted lesion was biopsied at least each one core in axial and sagittal planes. Standard 12-core SB using same transperineal approach was carried out afterwards by another experienced urologist who was blinded to the MRI targeted lesions. During the biopsy procedure, all patients with lithotomy position underwent general anesthesia using a larynx mask.

Pathological analysis

All biopsies and prostatectomy whole mount pathology were examined and analyzed by two senior pathologists

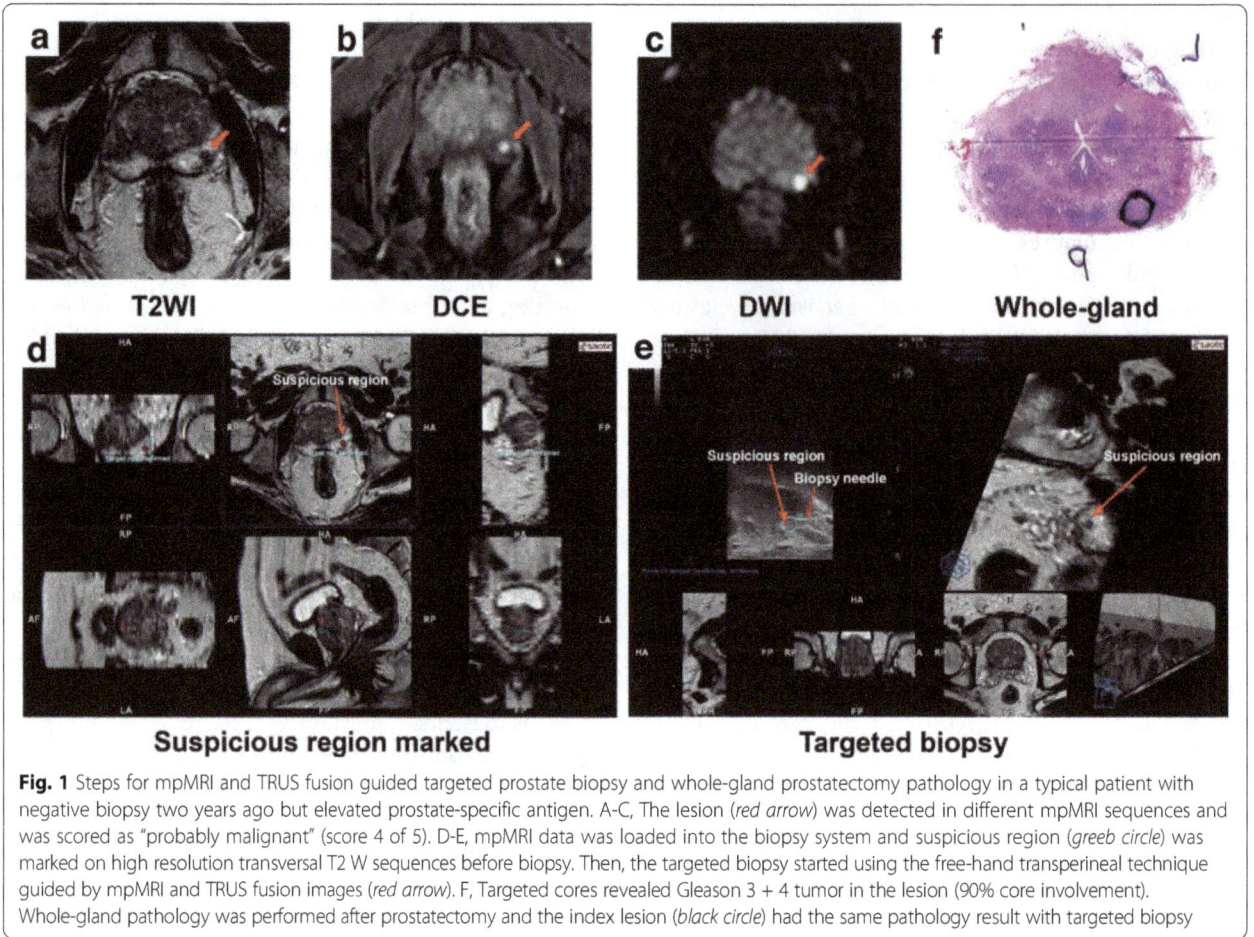

Fig. 1 Steps for mpMRI and TRUS fusion guided targeted prostate biopsy and whole-gland prostatectomy pathology in a typical patient with negative biopsy two years ago but elevated prostate-specific antigen. A-C, The lesion (*red arrow*) was detected in different mpMRI sequences and was scored as "probably malignant" (score 4 of 5). D-E, mpMRI data was loaded into the biopsy system and suspicious region (*greeb circle*) was marked on high resolution transversal T2 W sequences before biopsy. Then, the targeted biopsy started using the free-hand transperineal technique guided by mpMRI and TRUS fusion images (*red arrow*). F, Targeted cores revealed Gleason 3 + 4 tumor in the lesion (90% core involvement). Whole-gland pathology was performed after prostatectomy and the index lesion (*black circle*) had the same pathology result with targeted biopsy

(J.S. and Y.F.). The highest Gleason score from the TB or the standard 12-core SB was determined for each patient. Clinically significant cancer on biopsy was defined as Gleason score 3 + 4 or higher or Gleason score 6 with maximal cancer core length ≥ 4 mm [16, 17]. This definition was selected in an effort to incorporate both grade and volume, and avoid the bias caused by multiple cores from the same tumor.

Each prostatectomy specimen was processed using the modified Stanford technique, with 5 mm transverse step-sectioned samples taken from the apex to the base and the sagittal section of the distal 5–8 mm of the apex and base [18]. The step sectioned specimens were denoted as the apex, middle, or base of the prostate for analyses of three equal trisections of the prostate. Pathologists were blinded to the MRI and TRUS imaging results. The index tumor lesion in prostatectomy specimens was defined as the lesion with extraprostatic extension, the highest Gleason score, or the largest volume if Gleason scores were the same, in order of priority. The pathology slide with the greatest cross-section of the index lesion was used for location matching analysis. The tumor center of the index lesion was defined

as the point of intersection of the lesion height and width dimensions and was registered retrospectively in the 27-ROI schema by urologists [19]. Significant PCa at prostatectomy histology was defined using active surveillance criteria (total tumor volume ≥ 0.7 ml or Gleason score > 3 + 4) [20]. The Steps for mpMRI and TRUS fusion guided targeted prostate biopsy and whole-gland prostatectomy pathology are outlined in Fig. 1.

Data statistics

Statistical analyses were performed using SPSS version 17.0 (SPSS, Inc., Chicago, IL). The Fisher's exact test was used to compare categorical variables. Univariate analysis was applied with one-way ANOVA test. Multivariate logistic regression analysis was performed to identify potential predicted factors for the positive result of biopsy. Data was presented as mean ± SD. A P value <0.05 was considered statistically significant.

Results

Patient demographics and summary of fusion-guided biopsy findings are shown in Table 1. A total of 101 patients with prior negative biopsy and elevated PSA

Table 1 Patient demographics and summary of fusion-guided biopsy findings

	All patients	Men with PCa	Prostatectomy cohort
Men, no.	101	41 (40.6)	26 (25.7)
Age, year	68.9 ± 8.1	67.8 ± 8.0	65.2 ± 7.2
PSA, ng/ml	10.8 ± 6.1	11.3 ± 6.3	11.2 ± 6.3
Prostate volume, ml	42.1 ± 15.3	39.4 ± 13.6	35.1 ± 11.8
Prior negative biopsy, no.	1.5 ± 0.7	1.4 ± 0.6	1.4 ± 0.6
MRI lesions per patient, no.	1.9 ± 1.0	2.1 ± 1.1	2.4 ± 1.0
PI-RAD score, no. (%)			
2	13 (12.9)	1 (1.0)	0 (0)
3	31 (30.7)	3 (3.0)	0 (0)
4	36 (35.6)	19 (18.8)	12 (11.9)
5	21 (20.8)	18 (17.8)	14 (13.9)
TB cores per patiens	4.2 ± 1.5	4.8 ± 1.6	4.9 ± 1.8
Insignificant PCa	-	16 (15.8)	6 (5.9)
Significant PCa	-	25 (24.8)	20 (19.8)
Gleason score, no. (%)			
Gleason 6	-	17 (16.8)	6 (5.9)
Gleason 7 (3 + 4)	-	9 (8.9)	8 (7.9)
Gleason 7 (4 + 3)	-	7 (6.9)	5 (5.0)
Gleason ≥8	-	8 (7.9)	7 (6.9)

Continuous variables reported as mean ± standard deviation

PSA prostate-specific antigen, MRI magnetic resonance imaging, PCa prostate cancer, SB systematic biopsy, TB targeted biopsy

were suspected to have PCa with a PI-RADS score between 2 and 5 according to mpMRI examination. The mean age of the patient population was 68.9 years (SD 8.1) and mean number of MRI lesions was 1.9 (SD 1.0). The mean pre-fusion-guided biopsy PSA level was 10.8 ng/ml (SD 6.1) and prostate volume was 42.1 ml (SD 15.3). The mean number of targeted biopsy cores per patient was 4.2 (SD 1.5). Of 101 suspected patients, 41 (40.6%) were diagnosed PCa, including 16 (15.8%) insignificant and 25 (24.8%) significant cancers. Twenty-six patients who ultimately underwent prostatectomy were analyzed as a subgroup. Compared with all biopsy populaiton, patients who underwent prostatectomy were younger (65.2 vs 68.9 years, $P = 0.028$), had smaller prostate volumes (35.1 vs 42.1 ml, $P = 0.015$), had more MRI lesions (2.4 vs 1.9, $P = 0.029$), and had more TB cores (4.9 vs 4.2, $P = 0.040$).

The comparative pathologic outcomes of prostate systemic biopsy and targeted biopsy are shown in Table 2 and Additional file 1: Table S1. Seventy-four patients (60 + 4 + 10) of the total population (73.3%) demonstrated exact agreement between TB and SB. TB diagnosed a similar PCa number (31 cases) to SB (27 cases). However, TB diagnosed 36% more significant cancers than SB (22 vs 13 cases, $P = 0.012$). Among the 16 cases (4 + 10 + 2, 15.8%) in which TB revealed a higher risk category from SB group, 12

(10 + 2, 75%) were upgraded to significant cancers; whereas in 11 cases (8 + 2 + 1, 10.9%) which SB demonstrated a higher risk category from TB group, only 3 (2 + 1, 27.3%) were upgraded to significant cancers ($P = 0.022$). In addition, the utility of TB alone lead to 10 less cases of cancer (24.4%), only 2 (20%) of these were significant. However, SB alone missed 14 cases of cancer (34.1%) and 10 (71.4%) were significant ($P = 0.036$). In other words, when TB were combined with SB, an additional 14 cases of mostly significant PCa (10 cases) were diagnosed.

The subgroup of 26 patients who underwent prostatectomy was also analyzed because pathology results

Table 2 Comparison of pathology from systematic biopsy and targeted biopsy for prostate cancer

	SB			
	No cancer	Insignificant cancer	Significant cancer	Totals
TB				
No cancer.	60	8	2	70
Insignificant cancer	4	4	1	9
Significant cancer	10	2	10	22
Totals	74	14	13	101

SB systematic biopsy, TB targeted biopsy

from TB and SB could be compared against the whole-gland prostatectomy pathology (Table 3 and Additional file 1: Table S1). Within this subcohort, nine patients (the sum of all "no cancer" values for SB, 1 + 1 + 1 + 6) were diagnosed with PCa preoperatively only by TB, of whom 6 (66.7%) were significant cancer on whole-gland pathology. By contrast, 4 patients were diagnosed with PCa only by SB, only 1 (25%) were significant cancer on whole-gland pathology. When assessing the ability of preoperative biopsy to predict whole-gland pathology significance, the sensitivity of TB were 85% versus 45% for SB ($P = 0.019$), while the specificities were same (83.3%). The total accuracy of TB were 84.6% versus 53.8% for SB ($P = 0.034$).

In order to identify any potential predictor associated with detection of PCa and significant cancer, univariate and multivariate analysis were performed (Table 4). PI-RADS score was significantly correlated with both the PCa and significant PCa (both $P < 0.001$). Age, MRI lesions and PSA value of patients was only correlated with PCa ($P = 0.028$, $P < 0.001$ and $P = 0.03$). The further multivariate analysis revealed that PSA value and PI-RADS score were independent predictive factors of the positive biopsy of PCa ($P = 0.004$, OR = 1.22; $P = 0.001$, OR = 3.64). Moreover, patients with high PI-RADS scores (4, 5) had an over 10-fold higher risk of positive biopsy compared to those with low PI-RADS scores (2, 3). Additional file 2: Figure S1 also showed a strong relationship between PI-RADS score and biopsy results.

Discussion

Imaging techniques, mainly mpMRI, have developed as an accurate modality in PCa detection. Lesions identified

Table 3 Comparison of whole-mount prostatectomy outcome with target biopsy and systematic biopsy pathology for prostate cancer

	Whole-Mount Pathology (Prostatectomy)				
	Insig cancer		Sig cancer		Totals
TB	SB		SB		
No cancer	No cancer	0	No cancer	0	4
	Insig cancer	2	Insig cancer	1	
	Sig cancer	1	Sig cancer	0	
Insig cancer	No cancer	1	No cancer	1	4
	Insig cancer	1	Insig cancer	1	
	Sig cancer	0	Sig cancer	0	
Sig cancer	No cancer	1	No cancer	6	18
	Insig cancer	0	Insig cancer	2	
	Sig cancer	0	Sig cancer	9	
Totals	6		20		26

SB systematic biopsy, TB targeted biopsy, Insig Insignificant, Sig significant

Table 4 Univariate and multivariate analysis (logistic regression) predicting prostate cancer and clinically significant cancer

	Diagnosed with PCa			Sig PCa
	Univariate	Multivariate		Univariate
	P value	P value	OR (95% CI)	P value
Age	0.028	0.847	1.01 (0.93–1.10)	0.812
PSA	<0.001	0.004	1.22 (1.07–1.39)	0.070
Prostate volume	0.114	-	-	0.397
Prior negative biopsy	0.541	-	-	0.483
MRI lesions per patient	0.030	0.193	1.67 (0.77–3.59)	0.953
Biopsy cores	0.165	-	-	0.587
PI-RAD score	<0.001	0.001	3.64 (1.74–7.63)	<0.001
4 + 5 vs 2 + 3	<0.001	<0.001	10.94 (3.0–40.1)	<0.001

PCa prostate cancer, Sig significant, PSA prostate-specific antigen, MRI magnetic resonance imaging

on mpMRI correlate with tumor location on radical prostatectomy specimens [21]. Real-time fusion of mpMRI and TRUS images of the prostate is feasible and potentially able to identify cancerous regions for subsequent biopsy. This kind of biopsy can be performed using MRI localization information without requiring the cost, difficulties, or inconvenience of an MRI suite or MRI-compatible equipment. This double center prospective study evaluated the impact of real time free-hand transperineal targeted prostate biopsy guided by MRI-TRUS fusion imaging and made comparisons of biopsy performance between TB and traditional 12-core SB in Chinese men with prior negative biopsy sessions.

Our study indicated that PCa detection rate of TB and SB was 30.7 and 26.7% respectively, while the overall rate increased to 40.6% when combined the two approaches. With a mean of only 16.2 biopsies, we achieved a comparable overall detection rate to the others. Taira et al. reported a cancer yield ranging from 34.4 to 55.5% for men with 1, 2, and ≥3 prior negative biopsies [2]. They used transperineal template guided mapping biopsy approach with an average of 54 cores. Walz et al. showed a cancer detection rate of 41% by using a 24-core transrectal saturation biopsy in men with at least two prior negative 8-core biopsies [4]. It indicated that MRI-TRUS fusion guided free-hand transperineal biopsy with lower cores obtained higher or almost cancer detection rate compared to transperineal template mapping biopsy or transrectal saturation approach. Our result was similar to Brock's, with a TB detection rate of 26.7% and overall rate of 40.6% by using transrectal MRI/real-time elastography fusion biopsy [22]. Besides, our overall cancer detection rate seemed higher than Sonn's result of 34% [23], who used transrectal MRI-TRUS fusion biopsy in men with one or more previously negative biopsies and elevated PSA levels. We considered that the inconsistent result was because of the different biopsy pathway and patient demography, with older mean age and higher average PSA level in our cohort.

Current evidence demonstrates the improved sensitivity for detecting high grade or clinically significant PCa using MRI-TRUS fusion guided TB than with 12-core SB [9, 10, 24]. In this study, TB significantly increased the detection of significant PCa while decreasing the detection of insignificant cancer compared with SB in a repeat biopsy setting. When using the whole-gland pathology significance as the "gold standard", TB had a greater accuracy than SB for significant cancer on prostatectomy and a higher sensitivity of 85% versus 45%. Thus, our results demonstrated that TB could significantly change the distribution of clinical significance in repeated biopsy patients diagnosed with PCa toward diagnosis of more significant disease.

The European Society of Urogenital Radiology (ESUR) published the PI-RADS to standardize the MRI scoring system in 2012 [14], which had been validated in primary and repeat biopsy cohorts [7, 25]. Portalez, D et al. considered that ESUR scoring system provided a clinically relevant stratification of the risk of showing PCa in the challenging situation of repeat biopsies [25]. Brock M et al. reported that the prediction of PCa and significant cancer was calculated with an AUC of 0.79 and 0.81 for PI-RADS score in lesion of repeat biopsies. Sonn GA et al. showed that image grade [26] of suspicion on MRI was the most powerful predictor of significant cancer on multivariate analysis [23]. In our cohort, using univariate and multivariate analysis, PI-RADS score was proven to be the strongest predictor of PCa or significant cancer as well (Table 4). Moreover, a strong relationship existed between PI-RADS score and biopsy results (Additional file 2: Figure S1). Patients with high PI-RADS scores (4, 5) had an over 10-fold higher risk of biopsy positivity compared to those with low PI-RADS scores (2, 3).

It is well known that the incidence of infectious complications following TRUS guided transrectal prostate biopsy is steadily increased. In a European randomized trial of 10,474 prostate needle biopsies, the febrile complication rate was as high as 4.2% [27]. In the patients of repeated transrectal biopsies, there was a higher chance of acquiring sepsis with organisms resistant to standard antibiotics, such as multiresistant *Escherichia coli* [28]. Recently, there was an increased interest in the use of a transperineal approach for prostate biopsy [28, 29]. Transperineal prostate biopsy has the advantage of avoiding penetration of rectal mucosa and thus minimizing inoculation of the prostate with bowel flora. Many published series of transperineal prostate biopsy reported their incidence of febrile complication with either zero or close to zero [28–30]. In this series, we use the

prostate biopsy methodology of free-hand transperineal approach with general anesthesia, and no peri-procedure complication including infectious and anaesthetic complications was noted.

Several limitations of the present study needed to be mentioned. The study population consisted of patients referred to Chinese men in Eastern China, which could have induced selection bias. Second, patients with no lesion on mpMRI were excluded from the study, which could influence cancer detection rate of SB. Third, the sample size was small, which might have an effect on the results of the study.

Conclusions

This clinical study showed encouraging results for free-hand transperineal targeted prostate biopsy guided with MRI-TRUS fusion imaging in Chinese men with previously negative biopsies and elevated PSA levels. MRI-TRUS fusion guided TB improves detection of clinical significant PCa in a repeat biopsy setting. Combination of TB and SB can maximize the PCa detection rate. PI-RADS score is the strongest predictor of PCa and significant cancer.

Abbreviations
ESUR: European Society of Urogenital Radiology; mp: Multiparametric; MRI: Magnetic resonance imaging; PCa: Prostate cancer; PI-RADS: Prostate Imaging Reporting and Data System; PSA: Prostate-specific antigen; SB: Systematic biopsy; TB: Targeted biopsy; TRUS: Transrectal ultrasound

Acknowledgements
None.

Funding
No funding was obtained for this study.

Authors' contributions
HL conception and design, acquisition of data, analysis and interpretation of data; drafting of manuscript. JZ conception and design, acquisition of data, or analysis and interpretation of data; drafting of manuscript. WW conception and design, acquisition of data, analysis and interpretation of data; drafting of manuscript. BZ acquisition of data, analysis and interpretation of data. JS acquisition of data, analysis and interpretation of data. DL analysis and interpretation of data. YF analysis and interpretation of data. XJ acquisition of data, analysis and interpretation of data. WZ acquisition of data, analysis and interpretation of data, supervision. HG conception and design, analysis and interpretation of data; drafting of manuscript, supervision. All authors have read and approved the final version of this manuscript.

Competing interests
The authors declare that they have no competing interests.

Author details
[1]Department of Urology, Drum Tower Hospital, Medical School of Nanjing University, 321 Zhongshan Road, Nanjing 210008, Jiangsu, People's Republic of China. [2]Department of Radiology, Drum Tower Hospital, Medical School of Nanjing University, 321 Zhongshan Road, Nanjing 210008, Jiangsu, People's

Republic of China. [3]Department of Pathology, Drum Tower Hospital, Medical School of Nanjing University, 321 Zhongshan Road, Nanjing 210008, Jiangsu, People's Republic of China. [4]Institute of Urology, Nanjing University, Nanjing 210008, Jiangsu, People's Republic of China. [5]Department of Urology, the Affiliated Yixing people's Hospital of Jiangsu University, Yixing, Jiangsu 212000, China.

References

1. Pinsky PF, Black A, Parnes HL, et al. Prostate cancer specific survival in the prostate, lung, colorectal, and ovarian (PLCO) cancer screening trial. Cancer Epidemiol. 2012;36:e401–6.
2. Taira AV, Merrick GS, Galbreath RW, et al. Performance of transperineal template-guided mapping biopsy in detecting prostate cancer in the initial and repeat biopsy setting. Prostate Cancer Prostatic Dis. 2010;13:71–7.
3. Puppo P. Repeated negative prostate biopsies with persistently elevated or rising PSA: a modern urologic dilemma. Eur Urol. 2007;52:639–41.
4. Walz J, Graefen M, Chun FK, et al. High incidence of prostate cancer detected by saturation biopsy after previous negative biopsy series. Eur Urol. 2006;50:498–505.
5. D'Amico AV, Tempany CM, Cormack R, et al. Transperineal magnetic resonance image guided prostate biopsy. J Urol. 2000;164:385–7.
6. Sartor AO, Hricak H, Wheeler TM, et al. Evaluating localized prostate cancer and identifying candidates for focal therapy. Urology. 2008;72:S12–24.
7. Rais-Bahrami S, Siddiqui MM, Turkbey B, et al. Utility of multiparametric magnetic resonance imaging suspicion levels for detecting prostate cancer. J Urol. 2013;190:1721–7.
8. Miyagawa T, Ishikawa S, Kimura T, et al. Real-time virtual Sonography for navigation during targeted prostate biopsy using magnetic resonance imaging data. Int J Urol. 2010;17:855–60.
9. Wysock JS, Rosenkrantz AB, Huang WC, et al. A prospective, blinded comparison of magnetic resonance (MR) imaging-ultrasound fusion and visual estimation in the performance of MR-targeted prostate biopsy: the PROFUS trial. Eur Urol. 2014;66:343–51.
10. Siddiqui MM, Rais-Bahrami S, Truong H, et al. Magnetic resonance imaging/ultrasound-fusion biopsy significantly upgrades prostate cancer versus systematic 12-core transrectal ultrasound biopsy. Eur Urol. 2013;64:713–9.
11. Siddiqui MM, Rais-Bahrami S, Turkbey B, et al. Comparison of MR/ultrasound fusion-guided biopsy with ultrasound-guided biopsy for the diagnosis of prostate cancer. JAMA. 2015;313:390–7.
12. Zhang Q, Wang W, Yang R, et al. Free-hand transperineal targeted prostate biopsy with real-time fusion imaging of multiparametric magnetic resonance imaging and transrectal ultrasound: single-center experience in China. Int Urol Nephrol. 2015;47:727–33.
13. Rosenkrantz AB, Kim S, Lim RP, et al. Prostate cancer localization using multiparametric MR imaging: comparison of prostate imaging Reporting and data system (PI-RADS) and Likert scales. Radiology. 2013;269:482–92.
14. Barentsz JO, Richenberg J, Clements R, et al. ESUR prostate MR guidelines 2012. Eur Radiol. 2012;22:746–57.
15. Weinreb JC, Barentsz JO, Choyke PL, et al. PI-RADS prostate imaging - Reporting and data system: 2015, version 2. Eur Urol. 2016;69:16–40.
16. Harnden P, Naylor B, Shelley MD, Clements H, Coles B, Mason MD. The clinical management of patients with a small volume of prostatic cancer on biopsy: what are the risks of progression? A systematic review and meta-analysis. Cancer. 2008;112:971–81.
17. Ahmed HU, Hu Y, Carter T, et al. Characterizing clinically significant prostate cancer using template prostate mapping biopsy. J Urol. 2011;186:458–64.
18. Stamey TA, Freiha FS, McNeal JE, Redwine EA, Whittemore AS, Schmid HP. Localized prostate cancer. Relationship of tumor volume to clinical significance for treatment of prostate cancer. Cancer. 1993;71:933–8.
19. Dickinson L, Ahmed HU, Allen C, et al. Magnetic resonance imaging for the detection, localisation, and characterisation of prostate cancer: recommendations from a European consensus meeting. Eur Urol. 2011;59:477–94.
20. Wolters T, Roobol MJ, van Leeuwen PJ, et al. A critical analysis of the tumor volume threshold for clinically insignificant prostate cancer using a data set of a randomized screening trial. J Urol. 2011;185:121–5.
21. Radtke JP, Schwab C, Wolf MB, et al. Multiparametric Magnetic Resonance Imaging (MRI) and MRI-Transrectal Ultrasound Fusion Biopsy for Index Tumor Detection: Correlation with Radical Prostatectomy Specimen. Eur Urol. 2016;70(5):846-53.
22. Brock M, Loppenberg B, Roghmann F, et al. Impact of real-time elastography on magnetic resonance imaging/ultrasound fusion guided biopsy in patients with prior negative prostate biopsies. J Urol. 2015;193:1191–7.
23. Sonn GA, Chang E, Natarajan S, et al. Value of targeted prostate biopsy using magnetic resonance-ultrasound fusion in men with prior negative biopsy and elevated prostate-specific antigen. Eur Urol. 2014;65:809–15.
24. Borkowetz A, Platzek I, Toma M, et al. Comparison of systematic transrectal biopsy to transperineal magnetic resonance imaging/ultrasound-fusion biopsy for the diagnosis of prostate cancer. BJU Int. 2015;116:873–9.
25. Portalez D, Mozer P, Cornud F, et al. Validation of the European Society of Urogenital Radiology scoring system for prostate cancer diagnosis on multiparametric magnetic resonance imaging in a cohort of repeat biopsy patients. Eur Urol. 2012;62:986–96.
26. Sonn GA, Natarajan S, Margolis DJ, et al. Targeted biopsy in the detection of prostate cancer using an office based magnetic resonance ultrasound fusion device. J Urol. 2013;189:86–91.
27. Loeb S, van den Heuvel S, Zhu X, Bangma CH, Schroder FH, Roobol MJ. Infectious complications and hospital admissions after prostate biopsy in a European randomized trial. Eur Urol. 2012;61:1110–4.
28. Chang DT, Challacombe B, Lawrentschuk N. Transperineal biopsy of the prostate–is this the future? Nat Rev Urol. 2013;10:690–702.
29. Vyas L, Acher P, Kinsella J, et al. Indications, results and safety profile of transperineal sector biopsies (TPSB) of the prostate: a single centre experience of 634 cases. BJU Int. 2014;114:32–7.
30. Pepe P, Aragona F. Morbidity after transperineal prostate biopsy in 3000 patients undergoing 12 vs 18 vs more than 24 needle cores. Urology. 2013;81:1142–6.

17

Comparison of clinicopathologic characteristics, epigenetic biomarkers and prognosis between renal pelvic and ureteral tumors in upper tract urothelial carcinoma

Dong Fang[1†]●, Shiming He[1†], Gengyan Xiong[1], Nirmish Singla[2], Zhenpeng Cao[1], Lei Zhang[1], Xuesong Li[1*] and Liqun Zhou[1*]

Abstract

Background: There's no consensus about the difference between renal pelvic and ureteral tumors in terms of clinical features, pathological outcomes, epigenetic biomarkers and prognosis.

Methods: The data of 341 patients with renal pelvic tumors and 271 patients with ureteral tumors who underwent radical nephroureterectomy between 1999 and 2011 were retrospectively reviewed. The clinicopathologic features, gene promoters methylation status and oncologic outcomes were compared. Regression analysis was performed to identify oncologic prognosticators.

Results: Patients with ureteral tumors were relatively older ($p = 0.002$), and had higher likelihood of pre-operative renal insufficiency ($p < 0.001$), hypertension ($p = 0.038$) and hydronephrosis ($P < 0.001$), while in patients with renal pelvic tumors gross hematuria was more prevalent ($p < 0.001$). Renal pelvic tumors tended to exhibit non-organ-confined disease ($p = 0.004$) and larger tumor diameter ($p = 0.001$), while ureteral tumors had a higher likelihood of exhibiting high grade ($p < 0.001$) and sessile architecture ($p = 0.023$). Hypermethylated gene promoters were significantly more prevalent in renal pelvic tumors ($p < 0.001$), specifically for TMEFF2, GDF15, RASSF1A, SALL3 and ABCC6 (all $p < 0.05$). Tumor location failed to independently predict cancer-specific survival, overall survival, intravesical or contralateral recurrence (all $p > 0.05$), while gene methylation status was demonstrated to be an independent prognostic factor.

Conclusion: Renal pelvic tumors and ureteral tumors exhibited significant differences in clinicopathologic characteristics and epigenetic biomarkers. Gene promoter methylation might be an important mechanism in explaining distinct tumor patterns and behaviors in UTUC.

Keywords: Methylation, Prognosis, Radical nephroureterectomy (RNU), Renal pelvis, Upper tract urothelial carcinomas (UTUC), Ureter

* Correspondence: pineneedle@sina.com; zhoulqmail@sina.com
†Equal contributors
[1]Department of Urology, Peking University First Hospital, Institute of Urology, Peking University, National Urological Cancer Centre, No. 8 Xishiku St, Xicheng District, Beijing 100034, China
Full list of author information is available at the end of the article

Background

Urothelial carcinomas could be located anywhere throughout the whole urinary tract, e.g. renal pelvis, ureter, bladder and urethra [1]. Upper tract urothelial carcinoma refers to renal pelvic and ureteral tumors [2], with radical nephroureterectomy (RNU) and excision of the bladder cuff as the standard treatment [3].

Since both ureteral tumors and renal pelvic tumors originate from the urothelium, they have been traditionally classified as a single entity (UTUC) and managed in a relatively similar fashion, barring nephron-sparing approaches for more distally located tumors. In recent years there have been studies focusing on the impact of tumor location on prognosis [4–7], though evidence concerning clinical, pathological and genetic differences between renal pelvic and ureteral tumors remains scarce [8].

Microsatellite instability and hypermethylation have been proposed as key genetic differences between bladder cancer and UTUC [9–11], and we recently found gene promoter methylation status to hold biologic and prognostic significance in UTUC [12]. In the present study based on a large cohort of Chinese UTUC patients, we investigated the difference between renal pelvic and ureteral tumors in terms of clinical features, pathological outcomes, epigenetic biomarkers and prognosis.

Methods
Patient selection

Review board approve from Peking University First Hospital was acquired and all patients signed the informed consent to participate into the study. We evaluated consecutive Chinese UTUC patients who underwent RNU from 1999 to 2011 at Peking University First Hospital. We excluded patients with synchronous bilateral UTUC, distant metastasis prior to surgery or without complete follow-up data. Patients without available DNA from the surgical specimen for analysis of gene promoter methylation status were also excluded. Six hundred and-twelve patients were finally enrolled for analysis.

RNU including an extravesical excision of distal ureter by open Gibson incision was performed in all patients. No patients received neoadjuvant chemotherapy or prophylactic post-operative intravesical instillation (MMC or THP), while adjuvant chemotherapy for high-risk patients was administered at the treating physician's discretion.

Patient evaluation

Computed tomography (CT) or magnetic resonance imaging (MRI), urological ultrasound, and cystoscopy were performed in all patients before surgery. Urinary cytology and ureteroscopy were used to help diagnosis.

Renal function was assessed by estimated glomerular filtration rate (eGFR) calculated by Chinese population-specific equation: $eGFR(ml/min/1.73m^2) = 175 \times Scr^{-1.234} \times age^{-0.179}$ ($\times 0.79$ if female) [13]. Ipsilateral hydronephrosis was determined pre-operatively.

Patients were categorized into 2 groups (renal pelvis versus ureter) in the current analysis based on the location of the main lesion on pathological specimen (e.g. the highest tumor stage). Pathological examination was performed according to standard procedures by a dedicated pathologist. Tumors were staged per the 2002 Union for International Cancer Control (UICC) TNM classification, and grading was evaluated per the World Health Organization (WHO) classification of 1973.

DNA extraction and methylation analysis

The procedure of DNA extraction and methylation analysis has been reported in a previous publication by our research group [12]. Based on the formalin-fixed paraffin-embedded tumor samples stored in our center, DNA samples were obtained and were treated for bisulfite transformation. Methylation-sensitive polymerase chain reaction (MSP) was used to analyze the gene promoters methylation status [14]. We used methylated human genomic DNA (Qiagen, Hilden, Germany) as positive control and water blanks with polymerase chain reaction mixtures as negative control. Based on previous literatures we did not detect the methylation status of the gene promoters in matched paracarcinoma tissues due to the limited methylation rates [15–20].

Follow-up schedule

Follow-up consisted of cystoscopy, chest X-ray, urine cytology, and serum creatinine every 3 months for the first 3 years and then once per year thereafter. Abdominal ultrasound or CT/MRI was performed to examine the contralateral upper urinary tract. Overall survival (OS), cancer specific survival (CSS), bladder recurrence and contralateral recurrence were documented and compared by tumor location. Bladder recurrence was defined as subsequent bladder tumor detected by cystoscopy and confirmed by pathologic examination, and contralateral recurrence was defined as urothelial carcinoma found in the contralateral upper urinary tract. Cause of death was determined by death certificates, by medical notes or by the patients' responsible physicians.

Statistical analysis

Statistical analysis was carried by using R software i386 2.15.3 (R Foundation for Statistical Computing, http://www.r-project.org) and SPSS 20.0 (IBM Corp, Armonk, NY, USA). Categorical variables were tested by the Pearson's test and Chi-square test, while variables with a continuous distribution were evaluated by the Mann-

Table 1 Clinical and pathological characteristics of all UTUC patients stratified by tumor location

	All	Tumor location		Univariate analysis	
		Renal pelvis	Ureter	Chi-square or Z	p value
Patients, no. (%)	612 (100)	341 (55.7)	271 (44.3)		
Pre-operative characteristic					
Gender, no. (%)				0.160	0.743
Male	340 (55.6)	187 (54.8)	153 (56.5)		
Female	272 (44.4)	154 (45.2)	118 (43.5)		
Age, no. (%)				4.929	0.027*
<70	340 (55.6)	203 (59.5)	137 (50.6)		
≥ 70	272 (44.4)	138 (40.5)	134 (49.4)		
Age, mean ± SD		65.29 ± 11.11	68.07 ± 10.20	−3.173	0.002*
Previous or concomitant bladder cancer, no. (%)				1.931	0.193
Absent	545 (89.1)	309 (90.6)	236 (87.1)		
Present	67 (10.9)	32 (9.4)	35 (12.9)		
Initial complaint, no. (%)				24.205	< 0.001*
Absent	84 (13.7)	26 (7.6)	58 (21.4)		
Present	528 (86.3)	315 (92.4)	213 (78.6)		
Gross hematuria, no. (%)				65.132	< 0.001*
Absent	148 (24.2)	40 (11.7)	108 (39.9)		
Present	464 (75.8)	301 (88.3)	163 (60.1)		
Preoperative renal function, no. (%)				23.703	< 0.001*
End-stage CKD (eGFR<15)	34 (5.6)	24 (7.0)	10 (3.7)		
Moderate CKD (60>eGFR≥15)	198 (32.4)	83 (24.3)	115 (42.4)		
Early CKD (eGFR≥60)	378 (61.8)	233 (68.3)	145 (53.5)		
eGFR, mean ± SD		69.69 ± 30.11	62.43 ± 22.32	−4.329	< 0.001*
Side, no. (%)				1.115	0.329
Left	315 (51.5)	182 (53.4)	133 (49.1)		
Right	297 (48.5)	159 (46.6)	138 (50.9)		
Hydronephrosis, no. (%)				134.680	< 0.001*
Absent	273 (44.6)	223 (65.4)	50 (18.5)		
Present	339 (55.4)	118 (34.6)	221 (81.5)		
Multifocality, no. (%)				0.339	0.563
Single	472 (77.1)	266 (78.0)	206 (76.0)		
Multiple	140 (22.9)	75 (22.0)	65 (24.0)		
Smoking, no. (%)				0.050	0.836
No	497 (81.2)	278 (81.5)	219 (80.8)		
Yes	115 (18.8)	63 (18.5)	52 (19.2)		
Alcohol, no. (%)				0.697	0.452
No	539 (88.1)	297 (87.1)	242 (89.3)		
Yes	73 (11.9)	44 (12.9)	29 (10.7)		
Diabetes, no. (%)				0.249	0.661
No	511 (83.5)	287 (84.2)	224 (82.7)		
Yes	101 (16.5)	54 (15.8)	47 (17.3)		

Table 1 Clinical and pathological characteristics of all UTUC patients stratified by tumor location *(Continued)*

		Tumor location		Univariate analysis	
	All	Renal pelvis	Ureter	Chi-square or Z	p value
Hypertension, no. (%)				4.454	0.038*
No	363 (59.3)	215 (63.0)	148 (54.6)		
Yes	249 (40.7)	126 (37.0)	123 (45.4)		
Pre-RNU ureteroscopy, no. (%)				20.495	< 0.001*
No	536 (87.6)	317 (93.0)	219 (80.8)		
Yes	76 (12.4)	24 (7.0)	52 (19.2)		
Pathological outcomes					
Architecture, no. (%)				40.135	< 0.001*
Papillary	479 (78.3)	299 (87.7)	180 (66.4)		
Sessile	133 (21.7)	42 (12.3)	91 (33.6)		
Tumor stage, no. (%)				0.094	0.796
Ta-T1	206 (33.7)	113 (33.1)	93 (34.3)		
T2–4	406 (66.3)	228 (66.9)	178 (65.7)		
Tumor grade, no. (%)				31.628	< 0.001*
G1	19 (3.1)	4 (1.2)	15 (5.5)		
G2	334 (54.6)	218 (63.9)	116 (42.8)		
G3	259 (42.3)	119 (34.9)	140 (51.7)		
Lymph node status, no. (%)				4.014	0.051
N0 or Nx	571 (93.3)	312 (91.5)	259 (95.6)		
N+	41 (6.7)	29 (8.5)	12 (4.4)		
Non-organ-confined disease, no. (%)				8.257	0.004*
No	412 (67.3)	213 (62.5)	199 (73.4)		
Yes	200 (32.7)	128 (37.5)	72 (26.6)		
Tumor size, mean ± SD		3.58 ± 2.15	3.27 ± 2.41	−3.342	0.001*
Histologic Subtype					
Tumor necrosis, no. (%)				0.038	0.901
No	537 (87.7)	300 (88.0)	237 (87.5)		
Yes	75 (12.3)	41 (12.0)	34 (12.5)		
Squamous metaplasia, no. (%)				0.038	0.878
No	566 (92.5)	316 (92.7)	250 (92.3)		
Yes	46 (7.5)	25 (7.3)	21 (7.7)		
Sarcomatoid metaplasia, no. (%)				0.039	0.843
No	586 (95.8)	327 (95.9)	259 (95.6)		
Yes	26 (4.2)	14 (4.1)	12 (4.4)		
Gland-like differentiation, no. (%)				2.738	0.119
No	591 (96.6)	333 (97.7)	258 (95.2)		
Yes	21 (3.4)	8 (2.3)	13 (4.8)		
Presence of CIS, no. (%)				3.987	0.071
No	596 (97.4)	336 (98.5)	260 (95.9)		
Yes	16 (2.6)	5 (1.5)	11 (4.1)		

UTUC upper tract urothelial carcinoma, CKD chronic kidney disease, eGFR estimated glomerular filtration rate, RNU radical nephroureterectomy, CIS carcinoma in situ, SD standard deviation, HR Hazard Ratio, CI confidence interval
*Statistically significant

Table 2 Molecular biomarkers

	All	Renal pelvis	Ureter	Chi-square or Z	p value
Patients, no. (%)	612 (100)	341 (55.7)	271 (44.3)		
TMEFF2, no. (%)				6.717	0.011*
Unmethylated	346 (56.5)	177 (51.9)	169 (62.4)		
Methylated	266 (43.5)	164 (48.1)	102 (37.6)		
HSPA2, no. (%)				3.172	0.083
Unmethylated	355 (58.0)	187 (54.8)	168 (62.0)		
Methylated	257 (42.0)	154 (45.2)	103 (38.0)		
GDF15, no. (%)				57.000	< 0.001*
Unmethylated	304 (49.7)	123 (36.1)	181 (66.8)		
Methylated	308 (50.3)	218 (63.9)	90 (33.2)		
RASSF1A, no. (%)				20.465	< 0.001*
Unmethylated	448 (73.2)	225 (66.0)	223 (82.3)		
Methylated	164 (26.8)	116 (34.0)	48 (17.7)		
SALL3, no. (%)				7.119	0.008*
Unmethylated	403 (65.8)	209 (61.3)	194 (71.6)		
Methylated	209 (34.2)	132 (38.7)	77 (28.4)		
VIM, no. (%)				2.347	0.128
Unmethylated	219 (35.8)	113 (33.1)	106 (39.1)		
Methylated	393 (64.2)	228 (66.9)	165 (60.9)		
ABCC6, no. (%)				4.719	0.037*
Unmethylated	523 (85.5)	282 (82.7)	241 (88.9)		
Methylated	89 (14.5)	59 (17.3)	30 (11.1)		
CDH1, no. (%)				0.208	0.728
Unmethylated	524 (85.6)	290 (85.0)	234 (86.3)		
Methylated	88 (14.4)	51 (15.0)	37 (13.7)		
THBS1, no. (%)				0.005	1.000
Unmethylated	457 (74.7)	255 (74.8)	202 (74.5)		
Methylated	155 (25.3)	86 (25.2)	69 (25.5)		
BRCA1, no. (%)				0.460	0.523
Unmethylated	504 (82.4)	284 (83.3)	220 (81.2)		
Methylated	108 (17.6)	57 (16.7)	51 (18.8)		
Presence of hypermethylation in any gene, no. (%)				9.420	0.003*
Unmethylated	70 (11.4)	27 (7.9)	43 (15.9)		
Methylated	542 (88.6)	314 (92.1)	228 (84.1)		
Mean methylated genes		3.71 ± 2.33	2.85 ± 2.19	−4.503	< 0.001*
Number of methylated genes, no. (%)				17.202	< 0.001*
0–2	254 (41.5)	118 (34.6)	136 (50.2)		
3–5	243 (39.7)	145 (42.5)	98 (36.2)		
6–10	115 (18.8)	78 (22.9)	37 (13.7)		
Number of methylated genes, no. (%) in Ta-1				11.251	0.004*
All	206 (100)	113 (54.9)	93 (45.1)		
0–2	95 (46.1)	41 (36.3)	54 (58.1)		
3–5	80 (38.8)	49 (43.4)	31 (33.3)		

Table 2 Molecular biomarkers *(Continued)*

	All	Renal pelvis	Ureter	Chi-square or Z	p value
6–10	31 (15.0)	23 (20.4)	8 (8.6)		
Number of methylated genes, no. (%) in T2–4				7.318	0.026*
All	406 (100)	228 (56.2)	178 (43.8)		
0–2	159 (39.2)	77 (33.8)	82 (46.1)		
3–5	163 (40.1)	96 (42.1)	67 (37.6)		
6–10	84 (20.7)	55 (24.1)	29 (16.3)		
Number of methylated genes, no. (%) in G1–2				18.433	< 0.001*
All	353 (100)	222 (62.9)	131 (37.1)		
0–2	156 (44.2)	80 (36.0)	76 (58.0)		
3–5	141 (39.9)	97 (43.7)	44 (33.6)		
6–10	56 (15.9)	45 (20.3)	11 (8.4)		
Number of methylated genes, no. (%) in G3				4.449	0.108
All	259 (100)	119 (45.9)	140 (54.1)		
0–2	98 (37.8)	38 (31.9)	60 (42.9)		
3–5	102 (39.4)	48 (40.3)	54 (38.6)		
6–10	59 (22.8)	33 (27.7)	26 (18.6)		

*Statistically significant
UTUC upper tract urothelial carcinoma

Whitney U test. Cox regression model was used for survival analysis, and Kaplan-Meier curves including log-rank test was employed. A single-sided p value of lower than 0.05 was regarded as statistical significance.

Results

Clinical characteristics

Overall, 612 patients with either renal pelvic tumor (n = 341; 55.7%) or ureteral tumor (n = 271; 44.3%) were included. The median age of the entire cohort of patients was 68 (interquartile range, IQR: 60–74) years, and 272 (44.4%) were female, with a male:female ratio of 1.25:1. Previous or concomitant bladder cancer was present in 67 patients (10.9%).

The clinical features are exhibited in Table 1, grouped by tumor location. Patients with ureteral tumors were relatively older (p = 0.002), and suffered from high likelihood of pre-operative renal insufficiency (p < 0.001), hypertension (p = 0.038) and hydronephrosis (P < 0.001), while in patients with renal pelvic tumors gross hematuria was more prevalent (p < 0.001).

Pathological outcomes

The frequencies of muscle-invasive disease (≥pT2) and lymph node metastasis were comparable between groups; however, non-organ-confined tumors (≥pT3) were more prevalent in patients with renal pelvic tumors versus the ureteral tumor counterparts (p = 0.004). In concordance with this observation, sessile architecture and larger tumor size were more prevalent in patients

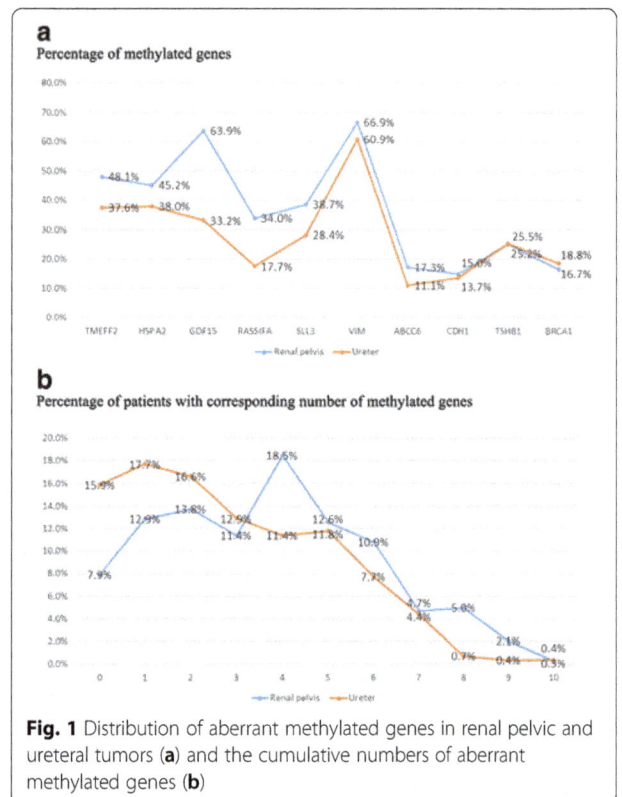

Fig. 1 Distribution of aberrant methylated genes in renal pelvic and ureteral tumors (**a**) and the cumulative numbers of aberrant methylated genes (**b**)

with renal pelvic tumors as well ($p < 0.001$). G3 tumor grade, however, was present more often in ureteral tumors ($p < 0.001$). There were no differences in terms of squamous and glandular differentiation.

Molecular biomarkers

In 542 patients (88.6%) at least one methylated gene promoter was found, with a mean methylated genes number of 3.33 ± 2.31. Methylation was present significantly more frequently in renal pelvic tumors (Table 2), particularly with a higher rate of methylated TMEFF2, GDF15, RASSF1A, SALL3 and ABCC6 (all $p < 0.05$) (Fig. 1a). The mean number methylated genes in renal pelvic tumors was 3.71 ± 2.33, while in ureteral tumors was only 2.85 ± 2.19 ($p < 0.001$). Besides many patients

with ureteral tumors presented with only very few methylated genes. (Fig. 1b).

In subgroup analysis based on tumor stage, renal pelvic tumors exhibited more methylated genes both in non-muscle-invasive and muscle-invasive diseases, while in subgroup analysis based on tumor grade, the difference was significant only in lower tumor stages (G1–2).

Oncologic outcomes

The median follow-up duration was 64 months. In all 210 (34.3%) patients died and 187 (30.6%) died secondary to urothelial cancer. The cumulative 5-year OS and CSS rates were 69.1% and 71.4%, respectively. Bladder recurrence was found in 174 (28.4%) patients, and 32 (5.2%) patients experienced contralateral recurrence.

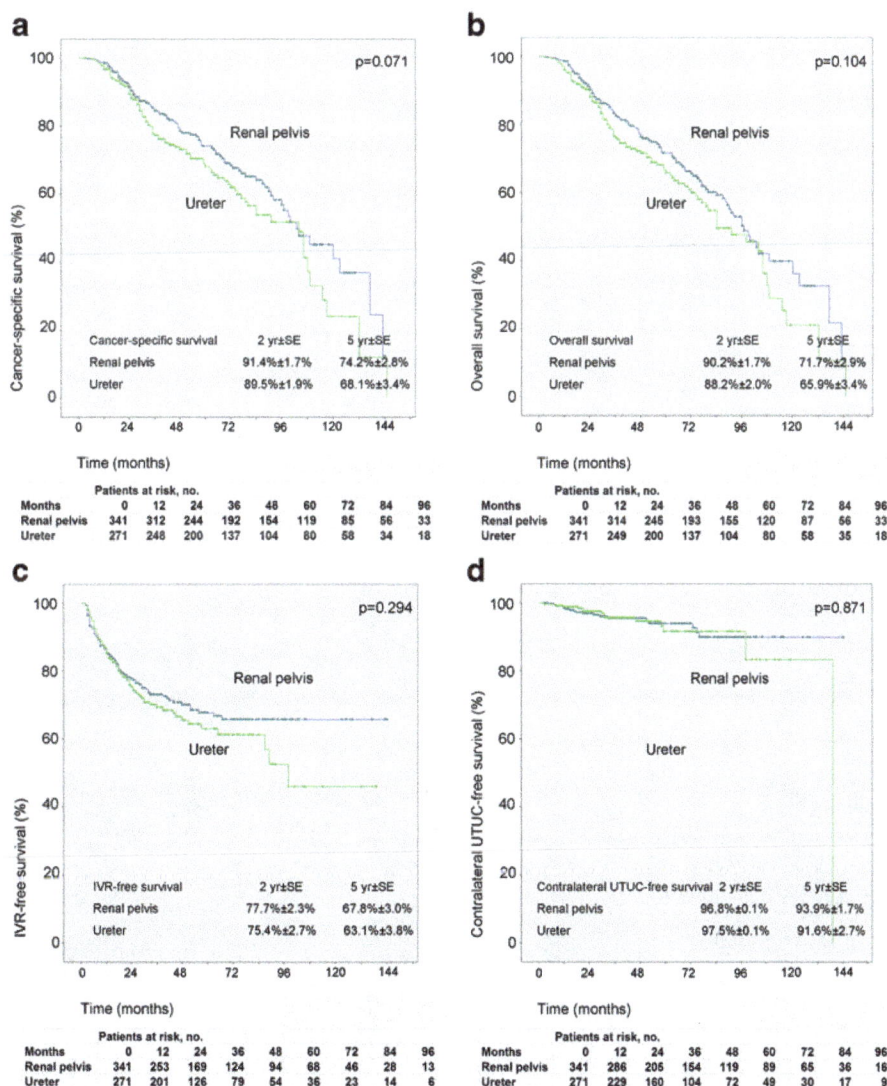

Fig. 2 Estimated Kaplan-Meier overall survival (**a**) ($p = 0.104$), cancer specific survival (**b**) ($p = 0.071$), bladder recurrence-free survival (**c**) ($p = 0.294$) and contralateral carcinoma-free survival (**d**) ($p = 0.871$) curves stratified by tumor location

Table 3 Prognostic factors for cancer-specific survival in the entire cohort of UTUC patients and stratified by tumor location

Variables	All patients (n = 612)						Renal pelvis (n = 341)						Ureter (n = 271)					
	UVA			MVA			UVA			MVA			UVA			MVA		
	HR	95%CI	p value	HR	95%CI	p value	HR	95%CI	p value	HR	95%CI	p value	HR	95%CI	p value	HR	95%CI	p value
Location (ureter vs renal pelvis)	1.302	0.976–1.738	0.073															
Gender (men vs women)	1.611	1.206–2.152	0.001*	1.45	1.07–1.96	0.016*	1.680	1.117–2.527	0.013*	1.46	0.94–2.27	0.091	1.574	1.039–2.383	0.032*	1.43	0.93–2.21	0.103
Age (continuous)	1.020	1.005–1.035	0.009*	1.32	1.07–1.64	0.010*	1.008	0.988–1.028	0.422				1.032	1.008–1.056	0.008*	1.09	0.78–1.52	0.628
Preoperative hydronephosis	1.595	1.183–2.151	0.002*	1.77	1.28–2.45	0.001*	1.766	1.168–2.671	0.007*	1.89	1.20–2.98	0.006*	1.191	0.691–2.053	0.529			
Multifocality (presence of multiple foci vs absence)	1.414	1.028–1.943	0.033*	1.57	1.10–2.24	0.014*	1.675	1.088–2.578	0.019*	1.70	1.03–2.82	0.040*	1.145	0.711–1.845	0.577			
Preoperative renal function(eGFR, continuous)	0.996	0.991–1.001	0.119				1.000	0.993–1.007	0.993				0.989	0.979–0.998	0.021*	0.77	0.55–1.06	0.106
Previous or concomitant BT (presence vs absence)	1.544	1.019–2.339	0.041*	1.53	0.97–2.41	0.070	1.980	1.099–3.568	0.023*	2.03	1.04–3.94	0.037*	1.183	0.657–2.132	0.575			
Gross hematuria (presence vs absence)	0.913	0.650–1.282	0.599				0.625	0.353–1.104	0.105				1.329	0.845–2.090	0.218			
Smoke (presence vs absence)	1.102	0.765–1.588	0.601				1.242	0.757–2.037	0.391				0.985	0.572–1.698	0.958			
Alcohol (presence vs absence)	1.108	0.726–1.690	0.634				1.546	0.912–2.619	0.105				0.713	0.344–1.477	0.363			
Diabetes (presence vs absence)	0.891	0.592–1.340	0.579				0.994	0.563–1.756	0.984				0.797	0.442–1.437	0.451			
Hypertension (presence vs absence)	1.180	0.879–1.584	0.270				1.056	0.689–1.618	0.802				1.230	0.810–1.868	0.332			
Preoperative ureteroscopy	0.616	0.383–0.992	0.046*	0.72	0.44–1.18	0.194	0.234	0.058–0.951	0.042*	0.24	0.06–1.03	0.055	0.663	0.387–1.137	0.135			
Tumor stage^ (T4 vs T3 vs T2 vs T1 vs Ta)	1.725	1.443–2.061	<0.001*	2.42	1.56–3.76	<0.001*	1.514	1.197–1.915	0.001*	1.83	1.04–3.21	0.035*	2.288	1.716–3.050	<0.001*	2.53	1.46–4.38	0.001*
Tumor grade^ (G3 vs G2 vs G1)	1.593	1.222–2.075	0.001*	0.69	0.36–1.34	0.274	1.284	0.868–1.900	0.211				1.856	1.271–2.710	0.001*	1.30	0.47–3.61	0.611
Lymph node status (N+ vs Nx vs N-)	2.524	1.583–4.023	<0.001*	1.82	1.08–3.07	0.024*	2.863	1.615–5.074	<0.001*	2.49	1.26–4.92	0.009*	2.356	1.024–5.417	0.044*	1.18	0.49–2.84	0.713
Architecture (presence of sessile vs absence)	1.974	1.437–2.713	<0.001*	1.38	0.92–2.07	0.125	2.105	1.242–3.566	0.006*	1.20	0.63–2.28	0.584	1.811	1.186–2.766	0.006*	0.98	0.55–1.75	0.951
CIS (presence of sessile vs absence)	1.027	0.480–2.202	0.994				1.386	0.424–4.535	0.590				0.808	0.296–2.210	0.678			

Table 3 Prognostic factors for cancer-specific survival in the entire cohort of UTUC patients and stratified by tumor location (Continued)

Variables	All patients (n = 612)						Renal pelvis (n = 341)						Ureter (n = 271)					
	UVA			MVA			UVA			MVA			UVA			MVA		
	HR	95%CI	p value	HR	95%CI	p value	HR	95%CI	p value	HR	95%CI	p value	HR	95%CI	p value	HR	95%CI	p value
Necrosis(presence vs absence)	1.925	1.302–2.846	0.001*	1.36	0.84–2.18	0.207	1.606	0.905–2.850	0.105				2.352	1.375–4.025	0.002*	1.36	0.69–2.70	0.376
Squamous metaplasia (presence vs absence)	1.783	1.081–2.943	0.024*	1.45	0.85–2.48	0.171	2.123	1.063–4.241	0.033*	2.31	1.06–5.02	0.034*	1.485	0.716–3.079	0.288			
Sarcomatoid metaplasia (presence vs absence)	2.595	1.526–4.413	<0.001*	0.79	0.40–1.56	0.493	2.541	1.171–5.513	0.018*	1.03	0.40–2.62	0.955	2.629	1.266–5.459	0.010*	1.00	0.41–2.45	0.993
Gland-like differentiation (presence vs absence)	1.963	0.965–3.995	0.063				3.394	1.239–9.296	0.017*	2.08	0.68–6.34	0.197	1.229	0.449–3.362	0.688			
Tumor size (continuous)	1.172	1.112–1.236	<0.001*	1.17	1.04–1.32	0.010*	1.163	1.070–1.264	<0.001*	1.16	0.93–1.44	0.188	1.184	1.110–1.264	<0.001*	1.26	1.06–1.49	0.008*
TMEFF2 (methylated vs unmethylated)	1.812	1.353–2.427	<0.001*	1.67	1.12–2.50	0.012*	1.634	1.085–2.459	0.019*	1.16	0.70–1.92	0.562	2.189	1.434–3.340	<0.001*	1.84	0.97–3.50	0.061
HSPA2 (methylated vs unmethylated)	1.815	1.349–2.442	<0.001*	1.52	1.03–2.24	0.036*	2.064	1.365–3.119	0.001*	1.40	0.86–2.28	0.180	1.698	1.097–2.626	0.017*	1.08	0.60–1.97	0.793
GDF15 (methylated vs unmethylated)	1.242	0.930–1.660	0.142				1.575	1.025–2.421	0.038*	1.24	0.73–2.12	0.426	1.152	0.741–1.793	0.530			
RASSF1A (methylated vs unmethylated)	1.383	1.002–1.908	0.049*	1.15	0.78–1.70	0.477	1.271	0.824–1.961	0.279				1.796	1.102–2.929	0.019*	1.57	0.87–2.82	0.135
SALL3 (methylated vs unmethylated)	1.214	0.887–1.662	0.226				0.887	0.565–1.392	0.602				1.853	1.190–2.885	0.006*	1.58	0.93–2.68	0.094
VIM (methylated vs unmethylated)	1.360	1.002–1.847	0.049*	0.99	0.68–1.44	0.941	1.630	1.041–2.550	0.033*	1.37	0.81–2.32	0.243	1.208	0.786–1.857	0.388			
ABCC6 (methylated vs unmethylated)	1.430	0.928–2.203	0.105				1.206	0.682–2.134	0.519				2.283	1.165–4.476	0.016*	1.51	0.67–3.38	0.317
CDH1 (methylated vs unmethylated)	1.178	0.766–1.812	0.456				1.112	0.618–2.001	0.724				1.401	0.741–2.649	0.300			
THBS1 (methylated vs unmethylated)	1.131	0.811–1.577	0.468				0.877	0.534–1.439	0.603				1.415	0.899–2.227	0.133			
BRCA1 (methylated vs unmethylated)	0.851	0.565–1.280	0.438				0.678	0.361–1.272	0.226				1.026	0.596–1.765	0.927			
No. methylated genes (continuous)	1.348	1.107–1.641	0.003*	0.62	0.30–1.28	0.193	1.225	0.930–1.613	0.149				1.646	1.234–2.196	0.001*	0.58	0.18–1.82	0.351

UVA univariate analysis, MVA multivariate analysis, eGFR estimated glomerular filtration rate, UTUC upper tract urothelial carcinoma, BT bladder tumor, CIS carcinoma in situ, HR Hazard Ratio, CI confidence interval
*Statistically significant

By univariate analysis, there's no relationship between tumor location (renal pelvis versus ureter) OS ($p = 0.104$), CSS ($p = 0.071$), bladder recurrence ($p = 0.294$) or contralateral recurrence ($p = 0.871$). (Fig. 2).

Other factors, including tumor stage, presence of hydronephrosis, and the methylation status of several genes were proved to be important predictive factors for survival. (Table 3). On Kaplan-Meier analysis, less cumulative number of methylated genes was correlated with better CSS, with mean CSS time of 101 months, 79 months and 77 months for patients with 0–2, 3–5 and 6–10 methylated genes, respectively (Fig. 3a). Though not statistically significant, a trend to higher risk for bladder recurrence in patients with less number of methylated genes ($p = 0.081$, Fig. 3b) was found. Besides the number of methylated genes (as continuous) was found to affect CSS (HR = 1.348, $p = 0.003$) and bladder recurrence (HR = 0.787, $p = 0.026$) in univariate analysis (Table 3 and 4).

Sub-group analysis demonstrated differences in oncologic prognosticators for CSS and bladder recurrence based on tumor location (Table 3 and 4). Rerunning the dataset by dividing patients into renal pelvic tumors only ($n = 304$), ureteral tumors only ($n = 267$) and both renal pelvic and ureteral tumors ($n = 41$) did not change the results (Table 5).

Discussions

In a meta-analysis which included 17 studies with 12,094 patients, Wu et al. demonstrated that ureteral tumors exhibited worse CSS and recurrence-free survival than renal pelvic tumors based on adjusted HRs; however, no such results were noticed in subgroup analysis of pT3/4 and pN1 tumors, though the authors observed significant heterogeneity among reported articles [4]. The only corresponding study that additionally included molecular work was published in 2013, in which Krabbe et al. found no difference in the expression of p21, p27, p53, cyclin E, and Ki-67 [8].

Regarding the relatively higher stages of renal pelvic tumors, Raman et al. suggested that ureteral tumors tend to be diagnosed earlier due to ureteric obstruction, and thus were likely to be detected at a lower stage [5]. In the current cohort of patients, more patients with renal pelvic tumors were diagnosed due to gross hematuria, while the prevalent presence of hydronephrosis could help the detection of ureteral tumors by ultrasound in annual regular physical examination in many patients.

It's interesting that the presence of sessile architecture and higher tumor grade was more common in ureteral tumors, which indicated the higher aggressiveness of ureteral tumors, as demonstrated in prior studies [4]. The change of DNA methylation status is regarded to be a key event in transcriptionally repressed regions of the genome [12]. Hypermethylation is a mechanism for repression of gene transcription in cancer [9]. Prior studies on bladder cancer demonstrated aberrant methylation status of some specific gene promoter as a sign of higher aggressiveness and worse prognosis [11, 15–19]. We similarly found that increased number of methylated genes appeared to correlate with worse CSS.

Our results demonstrate that renal pelvic and ureteral tumors, though both belong to UTUC, are not totally

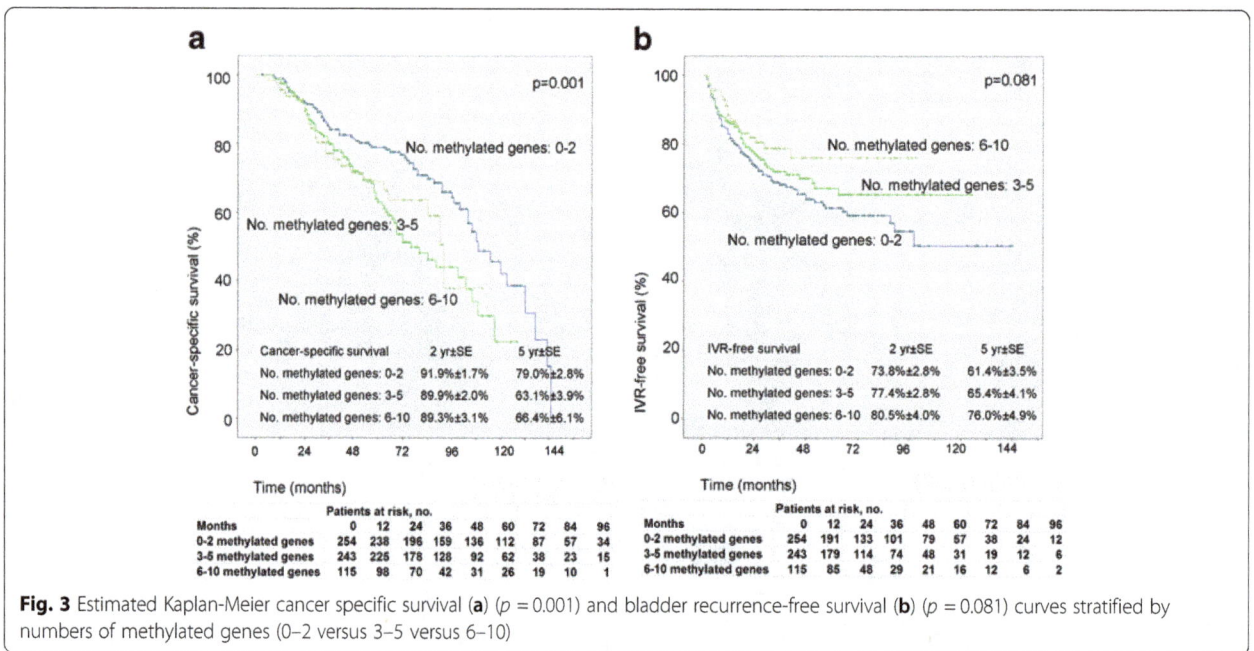

Fig. 3 Estimated Kaplan-Meier cancer specific survival (**a**) ($p = 0.001$) and bladder recurrence-free survival (**b**) ($p = 0.081$) curves stratified by numbers of methylated genes (0–2 versus 3–5 versus 6–10)

Table 4 Prognostic factors for bladder recurrence in the entire cohort of UTUC patients and stratified by tumor location

Variables	All patients (n = 612)						Renal pelvis (n = 341)						Ureter (n = 271)					
	UVA			MVA			UVA			MVA			UVA			MVA		
	HR	95%CI	p value	HR	95%CI	p value	HR	95%CI	p value	HR	95%CI	p value	HR	95%CI	p value	HR	95%CI	p value
Location (ureter vs renal pelvis)	1.172	0.870–1.579	0.297															
Gender (men vs women)	1.150	0.854–1.550	0.357				1.279	0.850–1.924	0.239				1.035	0.668–1.606	0.876			
Age (continuous)	0.987	0.974–1.000	0.050				0.983	0.966–1.000	0.055				0.989	0.970–1.010	0.989			
Preoperative hydronephosis	1.173	0.868–1.585	0.298				1.141	0.745–1.748	0.545				1.050	0.608–1.815	0.861			
Multifocality (presence of multiple foci vs absence)	1.732	1.260–2.381	0.001*	1.42	1.01–2.01	0.045*	1.833	1.185–2.835	0.006*				1.610	1.011–2.566	0.045*	1.44	0.86–2.43	0.167
Preoperative renal function(eGFR, continuous)	0.999	0.993–1.004	0.671				0.999	0.993–1.006	0.876				0.999	0.989–1.009	0.887			
Previous or concomitant BT (presence vs absence)	1.900	1.267–2.850	0.002*	1.47	0.95–2.28	0.081	1.710	0.931–3.138	0.084				2.034	1.176–3.517	0.011*	1.39	0.75–2.58	0.293
Gross hematuria (presence vs absence)	1.108	0.773–1.588	0.577				1.102	0.572–2.125	0.772				1.268	0.802–2.005	0.310			
Smoke (presence vs absence)	0.946	0.644–1.388	0.775				1.097	0.655–1.836	0.726				0.784	0.441–1.394	0.407			
Alcohol (presence vs absence)	0.771	0.473–1.257	0.297				0.901	0.480–1.692	0.746				0.622	0.286–1.351	0.230			
Diabetes (presence vs absence)	1.086	0.736–1.601	0.679				0.842	0.469–1.515	0.567				1.414	0.837–2.388	0.196			
Hypertension (presence vs absence)	0.774	0.566–1.059	0.109				0.916	0.595–1.412	0.692				0.614	0.391–0.967	0.035*	0.71	0.44–1.15	0.163
Preoperative ureteroscopy	1.631	1.111–2.395	0.012*	1.25	0.83–1.87	0.285	2.087	1.137–3.829	0.018*	1.62	0.87–3.02	0.126	1.319	0.794–2.189	0.285			
Tumor stage^ (T4 vs T3 vs T2 vs T1 vs Ta)	0.861	0.731–1.014	0.074				0.956	0.772–1.185	0.683				0.744	0.574–0.965	0.026*	0.81	0.54–1.20	0.292
Tumor grade^ (G3 vs G2 vs G1)	0.655	0.504–0.851	0.002*	0.54	0.31–0.93	0.027*	0.515	0.336–0.789	0.002*	0.30	0.13–0.71	0.006*	0.777	0.555–1.089	0.143			
Lymph node status (N+ vs Nx vs N-)	0.326	0.121–0.879	0.027*	0.45	0.17–1.23	0.120	0.491	0.180–1.338	0.164				0.046	0.000–5.017	0.199			
Architecture (presence of sessile vs absence)	0.718	0.479–1.075	0.108				0.721	0.349–1.490	0.377				0.644	0.389–1.067	0.087			
CIS (presence of sessile vs absence)	1.604	0.789–3.262	0.192				1.498	0.369–6.086	0.572				1.555	0.676–3.573	0.299			

Table 4 Prognostic factors for bladder recurrence in the entire cohort of UTUC patients and stratified by tumor location (Continued)

Variables	All patients (n = 612)						Renal pelvis (n = 341)						Ureter (n = 271)					
	UVA			MVA			UVA			MVA			UVA			MVA		
	HR	95%CI	p value	HR	95%CI	p value	HR	95%CI	p value	HR	95%CI	p value	HR	95%CI	p value	HR	95%CI	p value
Necrosis(presence vs absence)	1.164	0.750–1.806	0.498				1.532	0.881–2.664	0.131				0.810	0.390–1.682	0.572			
Squamous metaplasia(presence vs absence)	0.626	0.308–1.274	0.196				0.630	0.231–1.720	0.367				0.609	0.223–1.665	0.334			
Sarcomatoid metaplasia (presence vs absence)	0.490	0.182–1.321	0.159				0.465	0.114–1.887	0.284				0.541	0.133–2.204	0.392			
Gland-like differentiation (presence vs absence)	0.576	0.184–1.806	0.344				0.619	0.086–4.452	0.634				0.509	0.125–2.073	0.346			
Tumor size (continuous)	0.920	0.850–0.996	0.039*	0.91	0.78–1.06	0.213	0.967	0.872–1.072	0.520				0.875	0.771–0.991	0.036*	0.83	0.64–1.08	0.170
TMEFF2 (methylated vs unmethylated)	0.714	0.521–0.978	0.036*	0.91	0.60–1.38	0.657	0.839	0.554–1.268	0.404				0.593	0.358–0.984	0.043*	1.00	0.50–2.00	0.999
HSPA2 (methylated vs unmethylated)	0.704	0.511–0.968	0.031*	0.82	0.55–1.24	0.348	0.792	0.519–1.207	0.278				0.626	0.380–1.033	0.067			
GDF15 (methylated vs unmethylated)	0.823	0.611–1.110	0.203				0.936	0.616–1.421	0.755				0.738	0.456–1.196	0.217			
RASSF1A (methylated vs unmethylated)	0.598	0.407–0.878	0.009*	0.69	0.45–1.07	0.095	0.786	0.499–1.237	0.298				0.318	0.138–0.731	0.007*	0.41	0.17–0.97	0.042*
SALL3 (methylated vs unmethylated)	0.725	0.519–1.013	0.059				0.669	0.427–1.048	0.079				0.837	0.505–1.386	0.489			
VIM (methylated vs unmethylated)	0.862	0.636–1.167	0.336				1.302	0.831–2.041	0.249				0.567	0.367–0.875	0.010*	0.64	0.38–1.06	0.081
ABCC6 (methylated vs unmethylated)	0.805	0.499–1.297	0.373				1.007	0.578–1.752	0.981				0.508	0.185–1.392	0.188			
CDH1 (methylated vs unmethylated)	0.681	0.413–1.124	0.133				0.870	0.474–1.597	0.654				0.466	0.188–1.155	0.099			
THBS1 (methylated vs unmethylated)	0.960	0.678–1.359	0.818				1.044	0.651–1.675	0.858				0.872	0.522–1.457	0.601			
BRCA1 (methylated vs unmethylated)	0.977	0.659–1.448	0.908				0.858	0.485–1.515	0.597				1.131	0.655–1.955	0.659			
No. methylated genes(continuous)	0.787	0.637–0.972	0.026*	1.14	0.56–2.34	0.718	0.906	0.688–1.193	0.483				0.656	0.460–0.935	0.020*	0.96	0.34–2.72	0.934

*Statistically significant

UVA univariate analysis, MVA multivariate analysis, eGFR estimated glomerular filtration rate, UTUC upper tract urothelial carcinoma, BT bladder tumor, CIS carcinoma in situ, HR Hazard Ratio, CI confidence interval

Table 5 Comparison in patients with renal pelvis tumor only and with ureteral tumor only

	Location				Comparison between three groups		Comparison after excluding cases in both locations	
	All	Renal pelvis only	Ureter only	Both locations	Chi-square or Z	p value	Chi-square or Z	p value
Patients, no. (%)	612 (100)	304 (49.7)	267 (43.6)	41 (6.7)				
Pre-operative characteristic								
Gender, no. (%)					1.595	0.450	0.495	0.501
Male	340 (55.6)	163 (53.6)	151 (56.6)	26 (63.4)				
Female	272 (44.4)	141 (46.4)	116 (43.4)	15 (36.6)				
Age, no. (%)					5.554	0.062	5.391	0.023*
<70	340 (55.6)	182 (59.9)	134 (50.2)	24 (58.5)				
≥ 70	272 (44.4)	122 (40.1)	133 (49.8)	17 (41.5)				
Age, mean ± SD		65.09 ± 11.32	68.12 ± 10.22	66.52 ± 10.79	11.059	0.004*	−3.298	0.001*
Previous or concomitant bladder cancer, no. (%)					31.791	< 0.001*	8.721	0.004*
Absent	545 (89.1)	286 (94.1)	232 (86.9)	27 (65.9)				
Present	67 (10.9)	18 (5.9)	35 (13.1)	14 (34.1)				
Initial complaint, no. (%)					23.992	< 0.001*	23.745	< 0.001*
Absent	84 (13.7)	22 (7.2)	57 (21.3)	5 (12.2)				
Present	528 (86.3)	282 (92.8)	210 (78.7)	36 (87.8)				
Gross hematuria, no. (%)					66.717	< 0.001*	65.579	< 0.001*
Absent	148 (24.2)	33 (10.9)	107 (40.1)	8 (19.5)				
Present	464 (75.8)	271 (89.1)	160 (59.9)	33 (80.5)				
Preoperative renal function, no. (%)					39.081	< 0.001*	29.841	< 0.001*
End-stage CKD (eGFR<15)	34 (5.6)	21 (6.9)	10 (3.7)	3 (7.3)				
Moderate CKD (60>eGFR≥15)	198 (32.4)	64 (21.1)	112 (41.9)	22 (53.7)				
Early CKD (eGFR≥60)	378 (61.8)	218 (71.7)	144 (53.9)	16 (39.0)				
eGFR, mean ± SD		71.30 ± 29.38	62.63 ± 22.32	55.80 ± 31.99	34.160	< 0.001*	−5.108	< 0.001*
Hydronephrosis, no. (%)					156.085	< 0.001*	151.247	< 0.001*
Absent	273 (44.6)	212 (69.7)	49 (18.4)	12 (29.3)				
Present	339 (55.4)	92 (30.3)	218 (81.6)	29 (70.7)				
Multifocality, no. (%)					156.779	< 0.001*	10.618	< 0.001*
Single	472 (77.1)	266 (87.5)	206 (77.2)	0				
Multiple	140 (22.9)	38 (12.5)	61 (22.8)	41 (100)				
Pathological outcomes								
Architecture, no. (%)					39.792	< 0.001*	39.811	< 0.001*
Papillary	479 (78.3)	269 (88.5)	178 (66.7)	32 (78.0)				
Sessile	133 (21.7)	35 (12.5)	89 (33.3)	9 (22.0)				
Tumor stage, no. (%)					0.160	0.923	0.155	0.723
Ta-T1	206 (33.7)	100 (32.9)	92 (34.5)	14 (34.1)				
T2–4	406 (66.3)	204 (67.1)	175 (65.5)	27 (65.9)				
Tumor grade, no. (%)					30.572	< 0.001*	28.242	< 0.001*
G1	19 (3.1)	4 (1.3)	15 (5.6)	0				
G2	334 (54.6)	214 (70.4)	115 (43.1)	25 (61.0)				
G3	259 (42.3)	106 (34.9)	137 (51.3)	16 (39.0)				

Table 5 Comparison in patients with renal pelvis tumor only and with ureteral tumor only *(Continued)*

	Location				Comparison between three groups		Comparison after excluding cases in both locations	
	All	Renal pelvis only	Ureter only	Both locations	Chi-square or Z	*p* value	Chi-square or Z	*p* value
Lymph node status, no. (%)					3.772	0.152	3.769	0.064
N0 or Nx	571 (93.3)	278 (91.4)	255 (95.5)	38 (92.7)				
N+	41 (6.7)	26 (8.6)	12 (4.5)	3 (7.3)				
Non-organ-confined disease, no. (%)					10.339	0.006*	9.592	0.002*
No	412 (67.3)	186 (61.2)	196 (73.4)	30 (73.2)				
Yes	200 (32.7)	118 (38.8)	71 (26.6)	11 (26.8)				
Tumor size, mean ± SD		3.56 ± 1.94	3.25 ± 2.40	3.89 ± 3.39	13.014	0.001*	−3.695	< 0.001*
Methylation status								
TMEFF2, no. (%)					6.972	0.031*	6.481	0.011*
Unmethylated	346 (56.5)	158 (52.0)	167 (62.5)	21 (51.2)				
Methylated	266 (43.5)	146 (48.0)	100 (37.5)	20 (48.8)				
HSPA2, no. (%)					3.398	0.183	3.064	0.089
Unmethylated	355 (58.0)	167 (54.9)	166 (62.2)	22 (53.7)				
Methylated	257 (42.0)	137 (45.1)	101 (37.8)	19 (46.3)				
GDF15, no. (%)					56.507	< 0.001*	56.310	< 0.001*
Unmethylated	304 (49.7)	107 (35.2)	178 (66.7)	19 (46.3)				
Methylated	308 (50.3)	197 (64.8)	89 (33.3)	22 (53.7)				
RASSF1A, no. (%)					22.562	< 0.001*	22.341	< 0.001*
Unmethylated	448 (73.2)	197 (64.8)	220 (82.4)	31 (75.6)				
Methylated	164 (26.8)	107 (35.2)	47 (17.6)	10 (24.4)				
SALL3, no. (%)					9.797	0.007*	6.982	0.010*
Unmethylated	403 (65.8)	188 (61.8)	193 (72.3)	22 (53.7)				
Methylated	209 (34.2)	116 (38.2)	74 (27.7)	19 (46.3)				
VIM, no. (%)					3.367	0.186	1.819	0.192
Unmethylated	219 (35.8)	103 (33.9)	105 (39.3)	11 (26.8)				
Methylated	393 (64.2)	201 (66.1)	162 (60.7)	30 (73.2)				
ABCC6, no. (%)					6.282	0.043*	6.119	0.016*
Unmethylated	523 (85.5)	250 (82.2)	239 (89.5)	34 (82.9)				
Methylated	89 (14.5)	54 (17.8)	28 (10.5)	7 (17.1)				
CDH1, no. (%)					1.054	0.590	0.116	0.809
Unmethylated	524 (85.6)	260 (85.5)	231 (86.5)	33 (80.5)				
Methylated	88 (14.4)	44 (14.5)	36 (13.5)	8 (19.5)				
THBS1, no. (%)					1.041	0.594	0.096	0.772
Unmethylated	457 (74.7)	230 (75.7)	199 (74.5)	28 (68.3)				
Methylated	155 (25.3)	74 (24.3)	68 (25.5)	13 (31.7)				
BRCA1, no. (%)					2.219	0.330	0.863	0.375
Unmethylated	504 (82.4)	256 (84.2)	217 (81.3)	31 (75.6)				
Methylated	108 (17.6)	48 (15.8)	50 (18.7)	10 (24.4)				
Presence of hypermethylation in any gene, no. (%)					8.739	0.013*	8.537	0.004*
Unmethylated	70 (11.4)	24 (7.9)	42 (15.7)	4 (9.8)				

Table 5 Comparison in patients with renal pelvis tumor only and with ureteral tumor only *(Continued)*

	Location				Comparison between three groups		Comparison after excluding cases in both locations	
	All	Renal pelvis only	Ureter only	Both locations	Chi-square or Z	p value	Chi-square or Z	p value
Methylated	542 (88.6)	28 (92.1)	225 (84.3)	37 (90.2)				
Mean methylated genes		3.70 ± 2.33	2.83 ± 2.18	3.85 ± 2.35	21.900	< 0.001*	−4.431	< 0.001*
Number of methylated genes, no. (%)					20.046	< 0.001*	16.108	< 0.001*
0–2	254 (41.5)	108 (35.5)	135 (50.6)	11 (26.8)				
3–5	243 (39.7)	126 (41.4)	97 (36.3)	20 (48.8)				
6–10	115 (18.8)	70 (23.0)	35 (13.1)	10 (24.4)				
Prognostic outcomes								
[a]Overall mortality, no. (%)					0.059	0.011*	4.547	0.033*
Survive	379 (66.4)	210 (69.1)	169 (63.3)	23 (56.1)				
Death	192	94 (30.9)	98 (36.7)	18 (43.9)				
[a]Cancer-specific mortality, no. (%)					0.059	0.011*	4.547	0.033*
Survive	425 (69.4)	223 (73.4)	178 (66.7)	34 (58.5)				
Death	187 (30.6)	81 (26.6)	89 (33.3)	17 (41.5)				
[a]Intravesical recurrence, no. (%)					6.131	0.047*	2.879	0.090
No recurrence	438 (71.6)	228 (75.0)	185 (69.3)	25 (61.0)				
Recurrence	174 (28.4)	76 (25.0)	82 (30.7)	16 (39.0)				
[a]Contralateral recurrence, no. (%)					6.668	0.036*	0.610	0.435
No recurrence	580 (94.8)	291 (95.7)	253 (94.8)	41 (87.8)				
Recurrence	32 (5.2)	13 (4.3)	14 (5.2)	5 (12.2)				

CKD chronic kidney disease, *eGFR* estimated glomerular filtration rate, *SD* standard deviation
*Statistically significant
[a]Log-rank test was used

biologically homogenous and might behave differently. It's interesting that the rate of hypermethylation was much more higher in renal pelvis tumors than in the ureter, but the ureteral tumors exhibited higher aggressiveness and relatively worse prognosis. What's more, it's notable that on sub-analysis, the number of methylated genes was a stronger driver for oncologic outcomes in ureteral tumors. This being said, however, each gene must also be viewed separately, as the prognostic effect of gene hypermethylation appeared to differ by location, further implicating differences in underlying biology between the two groups.

In a published Meta-analysis ureteral location was related to higher risk of bladder recurrence [21]. Although no statistical difference was found in our study, a more distally located tumor within the ureter could conceivably affect bladder recurrence as seen in our previous publication [22].The analysis with gene methylation status didn't seem to be very informative for this phenomenon. In a Japanese multi-institutional study, Tanaka et al. found that the patterns of tumor spread was related to primary location of the

urothelial carcinoma: patients with ureteral tumors (especially at middle and lower part) tended to suffer from local recurrence in the pelvic cavity, while renal pelvic tumors were associated with higher risk of lung metastasis [7]. The underlying biological mechanisms about the differences in the patterns of tumor metastasis corresponding to tumor location remain to be elucidated in the future.

Our study has several limitations related to the retrospective design, and there might be some selection and recall bias, especially considering some patients were excluded due to the unavailable extracted DNA for test. The exact rate and site of distant metastasis and local recurrence were also incompletely available, which precluded further analysis concerning difference patterns of disease recurrence.

Despite these limitations, our study was the first comparative study that integrated epigenetic information with UTUC tumor location, and to our knowledge, the first study that demonstrated the higher prevalence of gene promoter hyper-methylation in renal pelvic tumors. Indeed, future research is warranted to further elucidate the role that gene methylation plays in the development and biology of renal pelvic and ureteral tumors.

Conclusion

Renal pelvic tumors and ureteral tumors exhibited significant differences in clinicopathologic characteristics and epigenetic biomarkers. Gene promoter methylation might be an important mechanism in explaining distinct tumor patterns and behaviors in UTUC.

Abbreviations

CSS: Cancer specific survival; CT: Computed tomography; eGFR: Estimated glomerular filtration rate; HR: Hazard ratio; MRI: Magnetic resonance imaging; MSP: Methylation-sensitive polymerase chain reaction; OS: Overall survival; RNU: Radical nephroureterectomy; UICC: Union for International Cancer Control; UTUC: Upper tract urothelial carcinoma; WHO: World Health Organization

Acknowledgements

The author thank the entire staff of Department of Urology, Peking University First Hospital Structured data processing occurred partially using Medbanks' approach [Medbanks (Beijing) Network Technology CO, Ltd].

Funding

This study was funded by Collaborative Research Foundation of Peking University Health Science Center and National Taiwan University, the College of Medicine (BMU20120318), the Natural Science Foundation of Beijing (7152146), the Clinical Features Research of Capital (No. Z151100004015173), the Capital Health Research and Development of Special (2016–1-4077) and Fund for Fostering Young Scholars of Peking University Health Science Center (BMU2017PY009).

Authors' contributions

DF, SH, XL, LZ (Zhou): Protocol/project development; DF, SH, ZC, GX, LZ (Zhang), XL: Data collection or management; DF, SH GX: Data analysis; DF, SH, NS: Manuscript writing/editing; XL, LZ (Zhou): Critical revision of the manuscript. All authors read and approved the final manuscript.

Competing interests

The authors declare that they have no competing interests.

Author details

[1]Department of Urology, Peking University First Hospital, Institute of Urology, Peking University, National Urological Cancer Centre, No. 8 Xishiku St, Xicheng District, Beijing 100034, China. [2]Department of Urology, University of Texas Southwestern Medical Center, Dallas, TX, USA.

References

1. Perez-Utrilla Perez M, Aguilera Bazan A, Alonso Dorrego JM, Viton Herrero R, Cisneros Ledo J, de la Pena Barthel J. Simultaneous cystectomy and Nephroureterectomy due to synchronous upper urinary tract tumors and invasive bladder Cancer: open and laparoscopic approaches. Currt Urol. 2012;6(2):76–81.
2. Siegel R, Naishadham D, Jemal A. Cancer statistics, 2012. CA Cancer J Clin. 2012;62(1):10–29.
3. Cummings KB. Nephroureterectomy: rationale in the management of transitional cell carcinoma of the upper urinary tract. Urol Clin North Am. 1980;7(3):569–78.
4. Wu Y, Dong Q, Liu L, Han P, Wei Q. The impact of tumor location and multifocality on prognosis for patients with upper tract urothelial carcinoma: a meta-analysis. Sci Rep. 2014;4:6361.
5. Raman JD, Ng CK, Scherr DS, Margulis V, Lotan Y, Bensalah K, Patard JJ, Kikuchi E, Montorsi F, Zigeuner R, Weizer A, Bolenz C, Koppie TM, Isbarn H, Jeldres C, Kabbani W, Remzi M, Waldert M, Wood CG, Roscigno M, Oya M, Langner C, Wolf JS, Strobel P, Fernandez M, Karakiewcz P, Shariat SF. Impact of tumor location on prognosis for patients with upper tract urothelial carcinoma managed by radical nephroureterectomy. Eur Urol. 2010;57(6):1072–9.
6. Isbarn H, Jeldres C, Shariat SF, Liberman D, Sun M, Lughezzani G, Widmer H, Arjane P, Pharand D, Fisch M, Graefen M, Montorsi F, Perrotte P, Karakiewicz PI. Location of the primary tumor is not an independent predictor of cancer specific mortality in patients with upper urinary tract urothelial carcinoma. J Urol. 2009;182(5):2177–81.
7. Tanaka N, Kikuchi E, Kanao K, Matsumoto K, Kobayashi H, Ide H, Miyazaki Y, Obata J, Hoshino K, Shirotake S, Akita H, Kosaka T, Miyajima A, Momma T, Nakagawa K, Hasegawa S, Nakajima Y, Jinzaki M, Oya M. Metastatic behavior of upper tract urothelial carcinoma after radical nephroureterectomy: association with primary tumor location. Ann Surg Oncol. 2014;21(3):1038–45.
8. Krabbe LM, Bagrodia A, Westerman ME, Gayed BA, Haddad AQ, Sagalowsky AI, Shariat SF, Kapur P, Lotan Y, Margulis V. Molecular profile of urothelial carcinoma of the upper urinary tract: are pelvicalyceal and ureteral tumors different? World J Urol. 2016;34(1):105–12.
9. Yates DR, Catto JW. Distinct patterns and behaviour of urothelial carcinoma with respect to anatomical location: how molecular biomarkers can augment clinico-pathological predictors in upper urinary tract tumours. World J Urol. 2013;31(1):21–9.
10. Catto JW, Azzouzi AR, Amira N, Rehman I, Feeley KM, Cross SS, Fromont G, Sibony M, Hamdy FC, Cussenot O, Meuth M. Distinct patterns of microsatellite instability are seen in tumours of the urinary tract. Oncogene. 2003;22(54):8699–706.
11. Catto JW, Azzouzi AR, Rehman I, Feeley KM, Cross SS, Amira N, Fromont G, Sibony M, Cussenot O, Meuth M, Hamdy FC. Promoter hypermethylation is associated with tumor location, stage, and subsequent progression in transitional cell carcinoma. J Clin Oncol. 2005;23(13):2903–10.
12. Xiong G, Liu J, Tang Q, Fan Y, Fang D, Yang K, Xie F, Zhang M, Zhang L, Liu L, Zhang C, Yao L, Yang L, Ci W, Zhao W, Gong Y, He Q, Gong K, He Z, Wang G, Li X, Guo Y, Zhou L. Prognostic and predictive value of epigenetic biomarkers and clinical factors in upper tract urothelial carcinoma. Epigenomics. 2015;7(5):733–44.
13. Ma YC, Zuo L, Chen JH, Luo Q, Yu XQ, Li Y, Xu JS, Huang SM, Wang LN, Huang W, Wang M, Xu GB, Wang HY. Modified glomerular filtration rate estimating equation for Chinese patients with chronic kidney disease. J Am Soc Nephrol. 2006;17(10):2937–44.
14. Herman JG, Graff JR, Myohanen S, Nelkin BD, Baylin SB. Methylation-specific PCR: a novel PCR assay for methylation status of CpG islands. Proc Natl Acad Sci U S A. 1996;93(18):9821–6.
15. Yu J, Zhu T, Wang Z, Zhang H, Qian Z, Xu H, Gao B, Wang W, Gu L, Meng J, Wang J, Feng X, Li Y, Yao X, Zhu J. A novel set of DNA methylation markers in urine sediments for sensitive/specific detection of bladder cancer. Clin Cancer Res. 2007;13(24):7296–304.
16. Maruyama R, Toyooka S, Toyooka KO, Harada K, Virmani AK, Zochbauer-Muller S, Farinas AJ, Vakar-Lopez F, Minna JD, Sagalowsky A, Czerniak B, Gazdar AF. Aberrant promoter methylation profile of bladder cancer and its relationship to clinicopathological features. Cancer Res. 2001; 61(24):8659–63.
17. Costa VL, Henrique R, Danielsen SA, Duarte-Pereira S, Eknaes M, Skotheim RI, Rodrigues A, Magalhaes JS, Oliveira J, Lothe RA, Teixeira MR, Jeronimo C, Lind GE. Three epigenetic biomarkers, GDF15, TMEFF2, and VIM, accurately predict bladder cancer from DNA-based analyses of urine samples. Clin Cancer Res. 2010;16(23):5842–51.
18. Lee MG, Kim HY, Byun DS, Lee SJ, Lee CH, Kim JI, Chang SG, Chi SG. Frequent epigenetic inactivation of RASSF1A in human bladder carcinoma. Cancer Res. 2001;61(18):6688–92.
19. Casadio V, Molinari C, Calistri D, Tebaldi M, Gunelli R, Serra L, Falcini F, Zingaretti C, Silvestrini R, Amadori D, Zoli W. DNA Methylation profiles as predictors of recurrence in non muscle invasive bladder cancer: an MS-MLPA approach. J Exp Clin Cancer Res. 2013;32:94.
20. Kang GH, Shim YH, Jung HY, Kim WH, Ro JY, Rhyu MG. CpG island methylation in premalignant stages of gastric carcinoma. Cancer Res. 2001; 61(7):2847–51.

18

Continuous saline bladder irrigation for two hours following transurethral resection of bladder tumors in patients with non-muscle invasive bladder cancer does not prevent recurrence or progression compared with intravesical Mitomycin-C

Andrew T. Lenis[1,2,3] ⑩, Kian Asanad[1], Maher Blaibel[4], Nicholas M. Donin[1,2,3] and Karim Chamie[1,2,3*]

Abstract

Background: Intravesical Mitomycin-C (MMC) following transurethral resection of bladder tumor (TURBT), while efficacious, is associated with side effects and poor utilization. Continuous saline bladder irrigation (CSBI) has been examined as an alternative. In this study we sought to compare the rates of recurrence and/or progression in patients with NMIBC who were treated with either MMC or CSBI after TURBT.

Methods: We retrospectively reviewed records of patients with NMIBC at our institution in 2012–2015. Perioperative use of MMC (40 mg in 20 mL), CSBI (two hours), or neither were recorded. Primary outcome was time to recurrence or progression. Descriptive statistics, chi-squared analysis, Kaplan-Meier survival analysis, and Cox multivariable regression analyses were performed.

Results: 205 patients met inclusion criteria. Forty-five (22.0%) patients received CSBI, 71 (34.6%) received MMC, and 89 (43.4%) received no perioperative therapy. On survival analysis, MMC was associated with improved DFS compared with CSBI ($p = 0.001$) and no treatment ($p = 0.0009$). On multivariable analysis, high risk disease was associated with increased risk of recurrence or progression (HR 2.77, 95% CI: 1.28–6.01), whereas adjuvant therapy (HR 0.35, 95% CI: 0.20–0.59) and MMC (HR 0.43, 95% CI: 0.25–0.75) were associated with decreased risk.

Conclusions: Postoperative MMC was associated with improved DFS compared with CSBI and no treatment. The DFS benefit seen with CSBI in other studies may be limited to patients receiving prolonged irrigation. New intravesical agents being evaluated may consider saline as a control given our data demonstrating that short-term CSBI is not superior to TURBT alone.

Keywords: Bladder cancer, Therapeutic irrigation, Mitomycin-C, Recurrence, Outcome assessment

* Correspondence: kchamie@mednet.ucla.edu
[1]David Geffen School of Medicine at the University of California Los Angeles, 300 Stein Plaza, Suite 348, Los Angeles, California 90095, USA
[2]Department of Urology, Health Services Research Group, David Geffen School of Medicine at UCLA, Los Angeles, California, USA
Full list of author information is available at the end of the article

Background

Non-muscle invasive bladder cancer (NMIBC) accounts for approximately 70% of new cases of urothelial carcinoma of the bladder. [1] NMIBC has been considered a chronic disease due to its high risk of future complications, including recurrence, which necessitates frequent monitoring and surveillance. The lifelong risk of recurrence and repeated interventions contributes to poor physician and patient compliance with published guidelines, and it significantly burdens the healthcare system from a financial standpoint. [2, 3] Therefore, strategies to prevent recurrence and future complications are paramount to reducing long-term morbidity and mortality.

The standard adjuvant therapy following transurethral resection of bladder tumor (TURBT) for NMIBC is intravesical instillation of Mitomycin-C (MMC), which has been shown to decrease rates of recurrence by approximately 11%, although this is variable depending on the number of and time from prior recurrences. [4, 5] The posited mechanism of action is to prevent free-floating tumor cells in the urine following TURBT from re-implanting onto the bladder wall. Although rare, MMC can potentially cause several significant side effects, including severe lower urinary tract symptoms, persistent chronic bladder pain, and even bladder necrosis in case reports. [6] Furthermore, MMC is contraindicated when there is a concern for bladder perforation and when there is significant post-operative gross hematuria. Considering these limitations, there is an urgent need for alternative strategies to prevent the re-implantation of tumor cells following TURBT, to reduce recurrence and minimize the morbidity of the disease. A 2012 Cochrane review of intravesical gemcitabine yielded conflicting results. [7] Apaziquone is a novel intravesical alkylating agent that has demonstrated safety and tolerability in patients as a post-TURBT instillation and is being evaluated in Phase 3 clinical trials (NCT02563561). [8] Alternatively, several groups have utilized sterile water and saline irrigation over 18–24 h as a strategy to lyse floating tumors cells and prevent the re-implantation of cells into the bladder wall. [9, 10] In our current study, we sought to evaluate continuous bladder irrigation with isotonic (0.9% NaCl) normal saline (CBSI) for two hours following TURBT as a strategy to reduce recurrence or progression in patients with NMIBC.

Methods

Patient cohort

Patients undergoing endoscopic resection of bladder tumors at our institution between March 2012 and July 2015 were identified from the medical record by Current Procedure Terminology (CPT)-4 codes for transurethral biopsy and resection (52204, 52214, 52224, 52234, 52235, 52240). Pathologic and clinical reports were reviewed, and patients with NMIBC were selected for inclusion in the cohort. We excluded all patients with variant histology, including small cell, squamous cell, adenocarcinoma, lymphepithelioid, sarcomatoid, and micropapillary disease. We also excluded patients with a diagnosis of upper tract urothelial carcinoma within one year, unresectable volume of tumor, known metastatic disease, less than three months of follow-up, or patients who underwent cystectomy within three months of diagnosis. Patients were categorized based on a modified AUA Risk Stratification for NMIBC. [11] Low risk was defined as a solitary LG lesion < 2 cm. Intermediate risk was defined as any LG T1, solitary LG Ta > 2 cm, multiple LG Ta, solitary HG Ta < 2 cm, or a history of LG NMIBC. High risk was defined as any CIS, HG T1, HG Ta > 2 cm, multiple HG Ta, or any history of HG Ta lesions or BCG recurrence. Modification of the AUA risk groups was made in order to conform to the size criteria used in the current procedural terminology codes for TURBT. Follow-up was calculated based on the time of the last cystoscopy. All study conduct was approved by the Institutional Review Board at our institution.

Independent variables

All patients received adjuvant CSBI, adjuvant MMC, or no adjuvant treatment at the discretion of the operating surgeon. Typically, patients for whom there was a concern for bladder perforation were not given CSBI or MMC. MMC was given as an instillation of 40 mg in 20 mL of saline. Following a dwell time of 60–90 min, the MMC was drained from the bladder and the catheter was left in place if deemed necessary by the surgeon. CSBI was performed by placement of a three-way Foley catheter at the conclusion of the case and was left running for approximately two hours post-operatively. The rate was kept at maximum flow without titration for this time. Patients did not require an overnight stay specifically for CSBI.

Dependent variables

Our dependent variable of interest was time to recurrence or progression. Recurrence was defined as the presence of pathologically confirmed urothelial carcinoma on biopsy or repeat resection. Patients who were found to have a lesion visible on cystoscopy that warranted intervention in the office (e.g. fulguration) were also classified as having disease recurrence. Cytology results obtained at the time of office fulguration were recorded. Progression was defined as any increase in grade or stage of disease.

Statistical analysis

Comparisons between categorical variables were tested using Chi-squared analysis and Fisher's exact test when appropriate. The two-sample Student's t-test was used to test for differences between continuous variables. Differences in disease-free survival (DFS) were analyzed using the Kaplan-Meier method. Cox proportional hazards models were used to estimate hazards ratios for covariates of interest. All statistical analyses were performed with Stata statistical software version 14 (StataCorp, College Station, TX).

Results

A total of 205 patients underwent TURBT for NMIBC during the study period and met all inclusion criteria. Mean age was 71.9 (SD = 11.4) years and 81.5% were male. Low grade (LG) and high grade (HG) were the primary grades in 105 (51.2%) and 100 (48.8%) patients, respectively. Stage was Ta without CIS, Ta with CIS, T1 without CIS, T1 with CIS, and CIS alone in 126 (61.5%), 12 (5.9%), 36 (17.6%), 13 (6.3%), and 18 (8.8%) patients, respectively. Tumor size was < 0.5 cm, 0.5–2 cm, 2–5 cm, and > 5 cm in 20 (9.8%), 90 (43.9%), 45 (21.9%), and 50 (24.4%) patients, respectively. Multiple tumors were present in 105 (51.2%) patients and 75 (36.6%) had a history of NMIBC. A modified AUA risk stratification as discussed in the methods resulted in 23 (11.2%) low risk patients, 80 (39%) intermediate risk patients, and 102 (49.8%) high risk patients. As immediate perioperative therapy, a total of 45 (22.0%) patients had CSBI, 71 (34.6%) had MMC, and 89 (43.4%) had no perioperative therapy. Only 36 (19.8%) of patients with intermediate or high risk disease underwent a restaging TURBT. Eighty-six (42.0%) patients received adjuvant intravesical therapy, most commonly with bacillus Calmette-Guérin (BCG $n = 76$), BCG + interferon ($n = 6$), Gemcitabine ($n = 2$), or MMC (n = 2). Table 1 and Table 2 summarize the cohort characteristics stratified by perioperative treatment and recurrence and progression, respectively.

Median follow-up time for the entire cohort was 16 [Interquartile range (IQR): 8–28] months. A total of 74 (36.1%) patients recurred at a median of 9.5 [IQR: 4–14] months and 16 (7.8%) progressed at a median of 16 [IQR: 6–31.5] months. The median DFS was 25 months for those who received no perioperative treatment, 55 months for those receiving MMC, and 16 months for those receiving CSBI. The Kaplan-Meier survival curve is presented in Fig. 1 and demonstrates a significant DFS advantage of MMC compared with either CSBI or no perioperative treatment (log rank test: $p < 0.01$). Kaplan-Meier curves for patients with a combination of low and intermediate risk NMIBC (log rank test: $p = 0.02$) and high risk NMIBC (log rank test: $p = 0.04$), and are presented in Figs. 2 and 3, respectively.

Lastly, we created a multivariable model incorporating age, AUA risk stratification, use of additional adjuvant therapy, and type of perioperative therapy (None, MMC, or CSBI). On Cox multivariable modeling, high risk was

associated with increased risk of recurrence or progression (HR 2.77, 95% CI: 1.28–6.01), whereas adjuvant therapy (HR 0.35, 95% CI: 0.20–0.59) and MMC (HR 0.43, 95% CI: 0.25–0.75) were associated with decreased risk of recurrence or progression (Table 3).

Discussion

The burden of NMIBC includes high financial costs to the healthcare system, significant risk of recurrence that necessitates life-long invasive surveillance, and uncertainty of possible progression that would prompt future radical operative intervention, especially in the highest-risk patients. Strategies to reduce the risk of recurrence and progression, including intravesical chemotherapy and immunotherapy, have been shown to be effective. [4, 12] However, none of these are without risk of potential significant side effects. In our current study we sought to utilize postoperative CSBI in a fashion similar to MMC, as an immediate, one-time postoperative treatment following surgery. This strategy avoids the toxicity of intravesical chemotherapy, as well as the inconvenience of an overnight hospital stay for prolonged CSBI.

In our cohort, however, post-operative CSBI for two hours was not equivalent to a single dose of perioperative MMC. Given the small numbers of patients in the low risk subgroup, we combined patients from low risk and intermediate risk groups for analysis. In the low and intermediate risk patients, there was a significant improvement in DFS with MMC compared with CSBI. In fact, CSBI performed no better than no perioperative treatment. In the high risk subgroup, a similar trend was observed. In our study the absolute risk reduction of postoperative MMC compared with no treatment at one year was 12.3%, which is similar to what is reported in the literature (11.7%). [4, 13] This benefit of MMC holds true even in our Cox multivariable model.

With respect to the efficacy of CSBI, our data stands in contrast to results published by others, albeit with some important differences in study design. Onishi et al. performed a non-randomized study comparing 18–22 h of post-operative CSBI to a full year of induction and maintenance MMC in patients with European Organization for Research and Treatment of Cancer (EORTC) intermediate risk NMIBC and showed no difference in several outcomes, including recurrence-free rates, time to first recurrence, and frequency of recurrences. [10] In this manuscript, the authors alluded to a planned prospective study that was recently published. [14] In their follow-up study, 227 patients with primary EORTC low- to intermediate-risk (all LG) NMIBC were randomized 1:1 to receive CSBI for 18 h or a single dose of 30 mg of MMC in 30 mL of saline. After a median follow-up of 37 months, 29% of patients experienced a recurrence. Recurrence-free rates at 1, 3, and 5 years were similar between the CSBI

Table 1 Cohort characteristics stratified by perioperative treatment

Variable	No treatment	MMC	CSBI	p-value
Total no. of patients	89	71	45	–
Age, mean (SD)	73.2 (11.2)	68.2 (12.3)	75.3 (8.9)	< 0.002+
Gender, n (%)				0.54
Male	75 (84.3)	55 (77.5)	37 (83.2)	
Female	14 (15.7)	16 (22.5)	8 (17.8)	
Grade, n (%)				0.9
High	45 (50.6)	34 (47.9)	21 (46.7)	
Low	44 (49.4)	37 (52.1)	24 (53.3)	
Stage, n (%)				0.03*
Ta without CIS	55 (61.8)	41 (57.8)	30 (66.7)	
Ta with CIS	3 (3.4)	4 (5.6)	5 (11.1)	
T1 without CIS	13 (14.6)	18 (25.4)	5 (11.1)	
T1 with CIS	4 (4.5)	6 (8.5)	3 (6.7)	
CIS only	14 (15.7)	2 (2.8)	2 (4.4)	
Tumor size, n (%)				0.12*
< 0.5 cm	11 (12.36)	3 (4.2)	6 (13.3)	
0.5–2.0 cm	33 (37.1)	41 (57.8)	16 (35.6)	
2.0–5.0 cm	22 (24.7)	13 (18.3)	10 (22.2)	
> 5.0 cm	23 (25.8)	14 (19.7)	13 (28.9)	
Multiple tumors, n (%)	47 (52.8)	36 (50.7)	22 (48.9)	0.91
Recurrent disease, n (%)	40 (45.0)	23 (32.4)	12 (26.7)	0.08
AUA Risk Stratification				0.72
Low risk	10 (11.2)	6 (8.5)	7 (15.6)	
Intermediate risk	34 (38.2)	31 (43.7)	15 (33.3)	
High risk	45 (50.6)	34 (47.9)	23 (51.1)	
Restaging resection, n (%)	8 (9.0)	18 (25.4)	10 (22.2)	0.02
Adjuvant therapy, n (%)	35 (39.3)	35 (49.3)	16 (35.6)	0.28
Follow-up in months, median [IQR]	14 [6–28]	23 [11–32]	13 [9–19]	< 0.01§

MMC Mitomycin-C, *CSBI* continuous saline bladder irrigation, *SD* standard deviation, *CIS* carcinoma in situ. +One-way ANOVA. *Fisher's exact test. §non-parametric equality of medians test

and MMC groups on Kaplan-Meier analysis. Subgroup analysis showed no difference when stratified between the low- and intermediate-risk tumors. Adverse events were also compared and the MMC group was found to have significantly higher rates of gross hematuria, irritative bladder symptoms, and dysuria (including retention). While the equivalence of CSBI and MMC demonstrated by Onishi et al. could be explained in part by patient selection (all LG patients), we did not replicate this result even in the low and intermediate risk subgroups of our cohort. One important difference in our protocols is the dose of MMC, which was the standard 40 mg in our study and 30 mg in the study by Onishi et al. The most striking difference between our studies, however, is in the duration of CSBI. We intentionally restricted CSBI to two hours to limit the need for overnight hospital stays. While similarly

efficacious to one instillation of MMC, CSBI used by Onishi et al. was titrated over 18 h, and it was not reported how many of these patients required an overnight stay. While the authors debate the cost advantages of saline compared with MMC, we question whether this may be offset by even a small fraction of patients requiring overnight admissions for CSBI. Nevertheless, this data demonstrates that in addition to a standard dose of 40 mg of MMC, duration may be an important component of the efficacy of CSBI in preventing tumor cell reimplantation.

Our results also appear to conflict with the results of a recent meta-analysis utilizing individual patient data from randomized trials comparing immediate intravesical instillation of various chemotherapy agents to TURBT alone or instillation of control solution (saline

Table 2 Cohort characteristics stratified by Recurrence or Progression

Variable	Recurrence or Progression	No Recurrence or Progression	p-value
Total no. of patients	90	115	–
Age, mean (SD)	73.6 (10.8)	70.6 (11.8)	0.07+
Gender, n (%)			0.81
Male	74 (82.2)	93 (80.9)	
Female	16 (17.8)	22 (19.1)	
Grade, n (%)			0.38
High	47 (52.2)	53 (46.1)	
Low	43 (47.8)	62 (53.9)	
Stage, n (%)			0.09*
Ta without CIS	55 (61.1)	71 (61.7)	
Ta with CIS	3 (3.3)	9 (7.8)	
T1 without CIS	14 (15.6)	22 (19.1)	
T1 with CIS	5 (5.6)	8 (7.0)	
CIS	13 (14.4)	5 (4.4)	
Tumor size, n (%)			0.09
< 0.5 cm	14 (15.6)	6 (5.2)	
0.5–2.0 cm	37 (41.1)	53 (46.1)	
2.0–5.0 cm	17 (18.9)	28 (24.4)	
> 5.0 cm	22 (24.4)	28 (24.3)	
Multiplicity of tumor, n (%)	56 (62.2)	49 (42.6)	< 0.01
Recurrent disease, n (%)	42 (46.7)	33 (28.7)	< 0.01
AUA Risk Stratification			0.07
Low risk	9 (10.0)	14 (12.2)	
Intermediate risk	28 (31.1)	52 (45.2)	
High risk	53 (58.9)	49 (42.6)	
Restaging resection, n (%)	12 (13.3)	24 (20.9)	0.16
Adjuvant therapy, n (%)	32 (35.6)	54 (47.0)	0.10
Perioperative treatment, n (%)			0.004
None	47 (52.2)	42 (36.5)	
MMC	20 (22.2)	51 (44.4)	
CSBI	23 (25.6)	22 (19.1)	

MMC Mitomycin-C, *CSBI* continuous saline bladder irrigation, *SD* standard deviation, *CIS* carcinoma in situ. +One-way ANOVA. *Fisher's exact test

or water). [5] Upon closer examination, however, we are unable to compare the protocols included as published in the meta-analysis or in the original manuscripts to our brief post-operative irrigation protocol. Of the 13 included studies, the use of post-operative irrigation was only documented as consistently used in four of these studies. Irrigation protocols were not detailed in the meta-analysis and review of the original data could not identify specific protocols. Furthermore, at least one study utilized distilled water for irrigation, which has the theoretical advantage of an osmotic cytotoxic effect but the disadvantages of being hypotonic. Therefore, despite a 21% relative reduction in recurrences found in this

meta-analysis with use of post-operative irrigation alone, we can only cautiously compare this result with our data without more detailed information about the irrigation protocols used.

The concept of utilizing irrigation for eradication of residual tumor cells following surgery for cancer is not a new concept, nor is it limited to urology or even endoscopic surgery. Surgeons have traditionally irrigated surgical sites to mechanically wash away debris, dilution of bacterial loads, and as a method of tumor cell lysis, depending on the tonicity of the fluid. A survey in England found that 74% of general surgeons perform intraoperative peritoneal lavage during cancer operations (36%

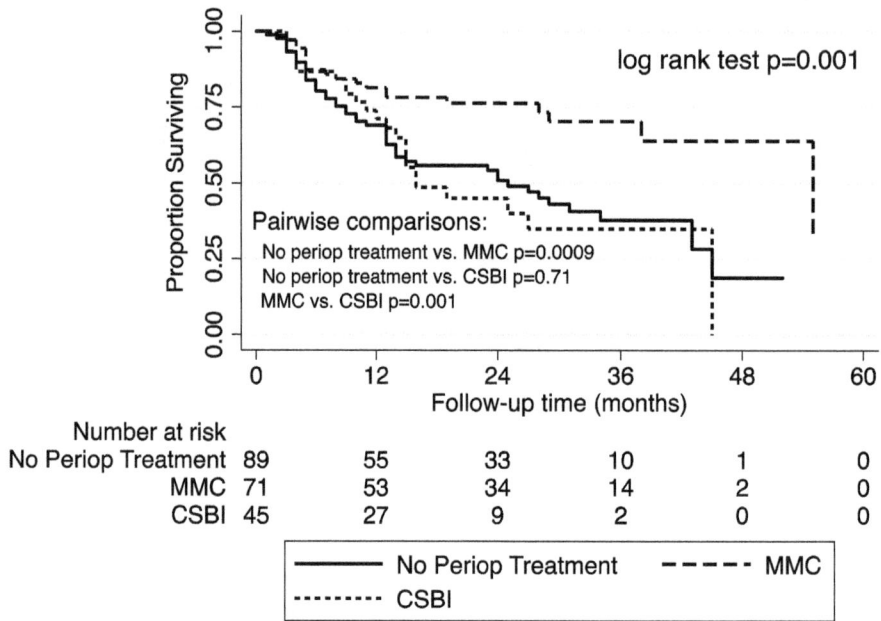

Fig. 1 "DFS in Patients with NMIBC". Kaplan-Meier survival curve for all patients with NMIBC stratified by perioperative treatment. MMC, Mitomycin-C. CSBI, continuous saline bladder irrigation

with water, 21% with saline, and 17% with betadine). [15] However, efficacy data on irrigation type is conflicting. Sweitzer et al. designed an experiment in mice to evaluate whether distilled water or sterile saline irrigation could reduce the burden of orthotopically implanted melanoma tumor cells. [16] Unfortunately, they found that neither the mechanical process of irrigation nor the hypotonicity of water reduced the tumor burden. In contrast, Fumito et al. demonstrated the superiority of water irrigation to saline irrigation following laparotomy in a mouse model of colorectal cancer tumor spillage. [17] In head and neck cancer models, both the type of irrigation and type of cancer cell line contributed to efficacy. [18, 19] These and other conflicting data suggest that multiple

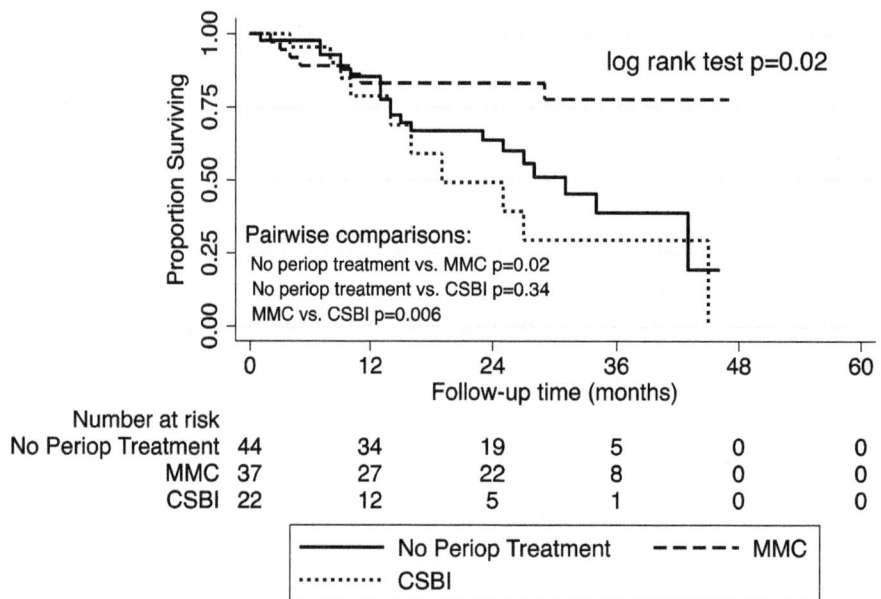

Fig. 2 "DFS in Patients with Low and Intermediate Risk". Kaplan-Meier survival curve for patients with low and intermediate risk disease stratified by perioperative treatment. MMC, Mitomycin-C. CSBI, continuous saline bladder irrigation

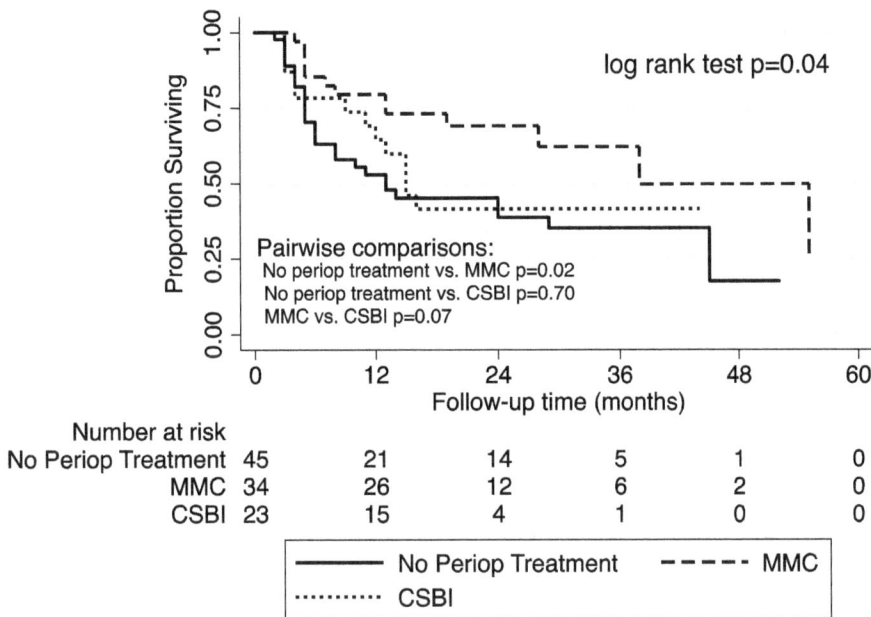

Fig. 3 "DFS in Patients with High Risk". Kaplan-Meier survival curve for patients with high risk disease stratified by perioperative treatment. MMC, Mitomycin-C. CSBI, continuous saline bladder irrigation

factors play a role with respect to the eradication of residual tumor burden, potentially related to the microenvironment and tumor cell-specific factors, such as cell adhesion properties and degree of de-differentiation.

The literature does strongly support irrigation following intra-luminal surgery in other surgical fields. For example, Zhou et al. performed a meta-analysis of studies evaluating intra-luminal washout following anterior resection for rectal cancer and concluded that washout leads to reduced rates of local recurrence. [20] In the urologic literature, Moskovitz et al. first postulated in

1987 that intravesical irrigation with distilled water during and after TURBT would lead to fewer recurrences. [21] While several small studies have demonstrated conflicting results regarding the use of water irrigation compared with no perioperative treatment, no studies have compared CSBI to MMC until the aforementioned studies by Onishi et al. [10, 14, 22, 23] Our study is the first to compare a shorter, perioperative duration of CSBI to both MMC and no perioperative treatment, and to evaluate this strategy in a heterogeneous patient population with low, intermediate, and high risk disease.

Table 3 Cox multivariable model for Recurrence or Progression

Variable	Hazard Ratio	95% Confidence Interval	p-value
Age (per year of age)	1.00	0.98–1.02	0.92
AUA Risk Stratification			
Low Risk	Reference	Reference	
Intermediate Risk	0.84	0.39–1.80	0.66
High Risk	2.77	1.28–6.01	0.01
Adjuvant therapy			
No	Reference	Reference	
Yes	0.35	0.20–0.59	< 0.001
Perioperative treatment			
No perioperative treatment	Reference	Reference	
MMC	0.43	0.25–0.75	0.003
CSBI	0.96	0.58–1.60	0.89

LG low grade, HG high grade, CIS carcinoma in situ, MMC Mitomycin-C, CSBI continuous saline bladder irrigation

Our results, however, should be considered within the context of several limitations. Although this was a hypothesis-based study driven by pre-clinical and clinical data, it was not a randomized controlled study, and was limited to the data available in medical records. Furthermore, the study is underpowered and longer term follow-up is required to fully realize the potential differences between treatment groups. It is possible that a larger cohort with longer term follow up could confirm the null hypothesis, suggesting that no difference exists between treatment groups. However, at our institution we are mainly utilizing intravesical gemcitabine based on recently published data that suggests efficacy at a fraction of the cost and with reduced side effects compared with MMC. [24] Consequently, in combination with the current data that suggests inefficacy of 2 h of CSBI, we are unlikely to treat more patients with adjuvant CSBI. Primarily one surgeon (KC) performed CSBI during the study period while most other surgeons in the department utilized either MMC or no additional perioperative therapy. Therefore, referral patterns may have contributed to patient heterogeneity between groups. Despite some baseline differences between treatment groups described in our results, the data remains consistent when controlling for factors such as tumor grade, stage, and recurrence disease, among others, in a multivariable model. A consistent surveillance cystoscopy protocol was not used for all patients and could have helped standardize follow-up and limit detection bias. Finally, we utilized a clinical definition of recurrence that included any suspicious lesion during office cystoscopy that warranted an intervention (usually fulguration), which may have artificially increased our recurrence rates.

Nevertheless, our study comparing perioperative CSBI, perioperative MMC, and no perioperative treatment answers important questions regarding CSBI as prophylaxis following endoscopic resection for NMIBC. While CSBI for two hours postoperatively should not replace current guideline-recommended perioperative MMC, it does appear that longer duration of CSBI may increase its efficacy. [10, 14] Research is needed to determine whether the duration can be reduced to limit the number of additional hospital stays and whether other, novel perioperative instillations may reduce recurrences and limit side effects.

Conclusions

Our data demonstrates that perioperative CSBI for two hours following TURBT is not equivalent to postoperative MMC in terms of rates of recurrence or progression. CSBI for two hours appears to be equivalent to no perioperative treatment, regardless of tumor grade. It is possible that CSBI may be required for a longer duration to reduce tumor cell re-implantation and, in turn, decrease rates of recurrence or progression.

Acknowledgements

This work was supported by the National Institutes of Health Loan Repayment Program (L30 CA154326 (Principal Investigator: KC)), the STOP Cancer Foundation (Principal Investigator: KC), the H & H Lee Surgical Resident Research Award (Recipient: ATL), and the Short Term Training Program (STTP) at the David Geffen School of Medicine at UCLA (Recipient: KA).

Authors' contributions

ATL was primarily involved in protocol/project development, data collection/management, data analysis, manuscript writing/editing. KA was involved in data collection/management and manuscript writing. MB was involved in data collection/management and manuscript writing. NMD was involved in protocol/project development, data collection/management, data analysis, manuscript writing/editing. KC supervised and was responsible for all study oversight. All authors read and approved the final manuscript.

Competing interests

The authors declare that they have no competing interests.

Author details

[1]David Geffen School of Medicine at the University of California Los Angeles, 300 Stein Plaza, Suite 348, Los Angeles, California 90095, USA. [2]Department of Urology, Health Services Research Group, David Geffen School of Medicine at UCLA, Los Angeles, California, USA. [3]Jonsson Comprehensive Cancer Center, David Geffen School of Medicine at UCLA, Los Angeles, California, USA. [4]Riverside School of Medicine, University of California, Riverside, California, USA.

References

1. Clark PE, Agarwal N, Biagioli MC, Eisenberger MA, Greenberg RE, Herr HW, et al. Bladder cancer J Natl Compr Canc Netw. 2013:446–75.
2. James AC, Gore JL. The costs of non-muscle invasive bladder cancer. Urol. Clin. North Am. 2013;40:261–9 Available from: http://www.ncbi.nlm.nih.gov/pubmed/23540783.
3. Chamie K, Saigal CS, Lai J, Hanley JM, Setodji CM, Konety BR, et al. Compliance with guidelines for patients with bladder cancer: variation in the delivery of care. Cancer. 2011;117:5392–401 Available from: http://www.pubmedcentral.nih.gov/articlerender.fcgi?artid=3206145&tool=pmcentrez&rendertype=abstract.
4. Sylvester RJ, Oosterlinck W, van der Meijden APM. A single immediate postoperative instillation of chemotherapy decreases the risk of recurrence in patients with stage ta T1 bladder cancer: a meta-analysis of published results of randomized clinical trials. J Urol. 2004;171:2186–90 quiz2435.
5. Sylvester RJ, Oosterlinck W, Holmäng S, Sydes MR, Birtle A, Gudjonsson S, et al. Systematic review and individual patient data meta-analysis of randomized trials comparing a single immediate instillation of chemotherapy after transurethral resection with transurethral resection alone in patients with stage pTa-pT1 urothelial carcinoma of the bladder: which patients benefit from the instillation? Eur Urol. 2016;69:231–44.
6. Doherty AP, Trendell-Smith N, Stirling R, Rogers H, Bellringer J. Perivesical fat necrosis after adjuvant intravesical chemotherapy. BJU Int. 1999;83:420–3.
7. Jones G, Cleves A, Wilt TJ, Mason M, Kynaston HG, Shelley M. Intravesical gemcitabine for non-muscle invasive bladder cancer. Cochrane Database Syst Rev John Wiley & Sons, Ltd. 2012;1:CD009294.
8. Hendricksen K, Cornel EB, de Reijke TM, Arentsen HC, Chawla S, Witjes JA. Phase 2 study of adjuvant intravesical instillations of apaziquone for high risk nonmuscle invasive bladder cancer. J Urol. 2012;187:1195–1199.
9. Taoka R, Williams SB, Ho PL, Kamat AM. In-vitro cytocidal effect of water on bladder cancer cells: the potential role for intraperitoneal lavage during radical cystectomy. CUAJ. 2015;9:E109–13.
10. Onishi T, Sasaki T, Hoshina A, Yabana T. Continuous saline bladder irrigation after transurethral resection is a prophylactic treatment choice for non-muscle invasive bladder tumor. Anticancer Res. 2011;31:1471–4.
11. Chang SS, Boorjian SA, Chou R, Clark PE, Daneshmand S, Konety BR, et al. Diagnosis and treatment of non-muscle invasive bladder Cancer: AUA/SUO guideline. J Urol. 2016;196:1021–9.

12. Sylvester RJ, van der Meijden APM, Lamm DL. Intravesical bacillus Calmette-Guerin reduces the risk of progression in patients with superficial bladder cancer: a meta-analysis of the published results of randomized clinical trials. J Urol. 2002;168:1964–70 Available from: http://www.ncbi.nlm.nih.gov/pubmed/12394686.

13. Abern MR, Owusu RA, Anderson MR, Rampersaud EN, Inman BA. Perioperative intravesical chemotherapy in non-muscle-invasive bladder cancer: a systematic review and meta-analysis. J Natl Compr Cancer Netw. 2013;11:477–84.

14. Onishi T, Sugino Y, Shibahara T, Masui S, Yabana T, Sasaki T Randomized controlled study of the efficacy and safety of continuous saline bladder irrigation after transurethral resection for the treatment of n... - PubMed - NCBI. BJU international. 2016.

15. Whiteside OJH, Tytherleigh MG, Thrush S, Farouk R, Galland RB. Intra-operative peritoneal lavage--who does it and why? Ann R Coll Surg Engl. 2005;87:255–8.

16. Sweitzer KL, Nathanson SD, Nelson LT, Zachary C. Irrigation does not dislodge or destroy tumor cells adherent to the tumor bed. J Surg Oncol. 1993;53:184–90.

17. Ito F, Camoriano M, Seshadri M, Evans SS, Kane JM, Skitzki JJ. Water: a simple solution for tumor spillage. Ann Surg Oncol Springer-Verlag. 2011;18:2357–63.

18. Lodhia KA, Dale OT, Winter SC. Irrigation solutions in head and neck cancer surgery: a preclinical efficacy study. Ann Otol Rhinol Laryngol SAGE Publications. 2015;124:68–71.

19. Hah JH, Roh DH, Jung YH, Kim KH, Sung M-W. Selection of irrigation fluid to eradicate free cancer cells during head and neck cancer surgery. Head neck. Wiley subscription services, Inc. A Wiley Company. 2012;34:546–50.

20. Zhou C, Ren Y, Li J, Li X, He J, Liu P. Systematic review and meta-analysis of rectal washout on risk of local recurrence for cancer. - PubMed - NCBI. J Surg Res. 2014;189:7–16.

21. Moskovitz B, Levin DR. Intravesical irrigation with distilled water during and immediately after transurethral resection and later for superficial bladder cancer. Eur Urol. 1987;13:7–9.

22. Sakai Y, Fujii Y, Hyochi N, Masuda H, Kawakami S, Kobayashi T, et al. A large amount of distilled water ineffective for prevention of bladder cancer cell implantation at the time of transurethral resection. Hinyokika Kiyo. 2006;52:173–5.

23. Amos S, Gofrit ON. Prevention of bladder tumor recurrence. Evolving trends in urology. In: Sashi S Kommu, editor. 1st ed. Rijeka, Croatia: InTech; 2012. pp. 69–76. https://doi.org/10.5772/38495.

24. Messing EM, Tangen CM, Lerner SP, Sahasrabudhe DM, Koppie TM, Wood DP, et al. Effect of Intravesical instillation of gemcitabine vs saline immediately following resection of suspected low-grade non-muscle-invasive bladder Cancer on tumor recurrence: SWOG S0337 randomized clinical trial. JAMA. 2018;319:1880–8.

19

Preoperative neutrophil-to-lymphocyte ratio predicts the surgical outcome of Xp11.2 translocation/TFE3 renal cell carcinoma patients

Sezim Agizamhan[1†], Feng Qu[1†], Ning Liu[1], Jing Sun[2], Wei Xu[3], Lihua Zhang[4], Hongqian Guo[1] and Weidong Gan[1*]

Abstract

Background: The preoperative neutrophil-to-lymphocyte ratio (NLR), C-reactive protein/albumin ratio (CRP/Alb ratio) and platelet-to-lymphocyte ratio (PLR) have been demonstrated to predict the clinical outcome of various human cancer, including renal cell carcinoma(RCC). The aim of our study was to explore the prognostic values of these ratios in patients with Xp11.2 translocation/TFE3 gene fusions renal cell carcinoma (Xp11.2 tRCC).

Methods: A retrospective multicentre study was performed in 82 Xp11.2 tRCC patients who underwent radical or partial nephrectomy. The optimal cutoff values of the NLR, CRP/Alb ratio and PLR were determined by the receiver operating characteristic (ROC) analysis. The impact of the NLR, CRP/Alb ratio and PLR, as well as other clinicopathological characteristics, on disease-free survival (DFS) and overall survival (OS) were evaluated using the univariate and multivariate Cox regression analyses.

Results: The optimal cutoff values of the NLR, CRP/Alb ratio and PLR were set at 2.45, 140 and 0.08, respectively, according to the ROC analysis. Univariate analyses showed that the NLR, CRP/Alb ratio and PLR all were associated with DFS of Xp11.2 tRCC patients ($P < 0.001$, $P = 0.005$ and $P = 0.001$, respectively) and OS of Xp11.2 tRCC patients ($P = 0.016$, $P = 0.003$ and $P = 0.014$, respectively). Multivariate analysis indicated that the NLR was independently associated with DFS of Xp11.2 tRCC patients (hazard ratio [HR]: 4.25; 95% confidence interval [95% CI]: 1.19–15.18; $P = 0.026$) along with age ($P = 0.004$), the pT status ($P < 0.001$) and the pN status ($P < 0.019$), and the NLR (HR: 26.26; 95% CI: 1.44–480.3; $P = 0.028$) also was independently associated with OS in patients with Xp11.2 tRCC, along with age ($P = 0.016$) and a tumour thrombus ($P = 0.007$).

Conclusion: Overall, relatively high NLRs, CRP/Alb ratios and PLRs were associated with a poor prognosis of Xp11.2 tRCC patients; among of them, only the NLR independently predicted the progression of Xp11.2 tRCC, and the NLR may help to identify patients with high metastasis or relapse risk.

Keywords: Neutrophil-to-lymphocyte ratio, C-reactive protein/albumin ratio, Platelet-to-lymphocyte ratio, Renal cell carcinoma, Xp11.2 translocation

* Correspondence: gwd@nju.edu.cn
†Sezim Agizamhan and Feng Qu contributed equally to this work.
[1]Department of Urology, Nanjing Drum Tower Hospital, The Affiliated Hospital of Nanjing University Medical School, No. 321 Zhongshan Road, Nanjing 210008, Jiangsu Province, China
Full list of author information is available at the end of the article

Background

Xp11.2 translocation/TFE3 gene fusions renal cell carcinoma (Xp11.2 tRCC) was first listed as a new type of renal cell carcinoma (RCC) in the 2004 by the World Health Organization (WHO). Since then, it has received wide attention [1–5]. Xp11.2 tRCC is characterized by various translocations of the transcription factor E3(TFE3) on chromosome Xp11.2, resulting in overexpression of the TFE3 protein [6]. Xp11.2 tRCC is a kind of relatively rare tumour that predominantly occurs in children and young adults [7]. Regardless of its low incidence, Xp11.2 RCC is more aggressive than conventional RCC because most adult present at advanced stages and invasive clinical courses [3, 4]. Therefore, it is crucial to identify new preoperative prognostic factors to provide additional prognostic information for Xp11.2 tRCC patients. In addition, in regard to the risk of disease recurrence, is important to obtain prognostic information in the preoperative phase for the postoperative surveillance and possible adjuvant therapy.

It is recognized that the inflammatory processes in the tumour microenvironment play a significant role in promoting the proliferation, invasion and metastasis of the malignant cells [8, 9]. Inflammatory markers, such as the neutrophil count(NC), lymphocyte count(LC), platelet count (PLT), neutrophil-to-lymphocyte ratio (NLR), C-reactive protein (CRP), albumin (Alb), C-reactive protein/ albumin ratio (CRP/Alb ratio) and platelet-to-

lymphocyte ratio (PLR), have been shown to predict the clinical outcome of various human cancers [10–13]. For renal cell carcinoma, several publications demonstrated that high NLR, CRP/Alb ratios and PLRs were associated with a poor prognosis in RCC, respectively [14–17].

To our knowledge, the prognostic value of inflammatory markers has never been investigated in the Xp11.2 tRCC patients. Additionally, compared with conventional RCC, Xp11.2 tRCC involves different genetic characteristics and biological pathways and is associated with a more worse prognosis [3, 5, 18]. In addition, inflammatory markers are more easily accessible than other prognostic factors before surgery. Therefore, there is a need to identify new preoperative prognostic markers to predict the clinical outcomes of surgical Xp11.2 tRCC patients. The aims of the present study were to examine the prognostic values of the NLR, CRP/Alb ratio and PLR in patients with Xp11.2 tRCC.

Methods

Patients

Institutional review board approval was obtained at Nanjing Drum Tower Hospital, Jiangsu Province Hospital, Jiangsu Cancer Hospital and Zhongda Hospital Southeast University for this multicentre retrospective study. All the patients have provided informed written consents to have their medical record data used in research. Between January 2007 and July 2017, 89 consecutive patients from the 4

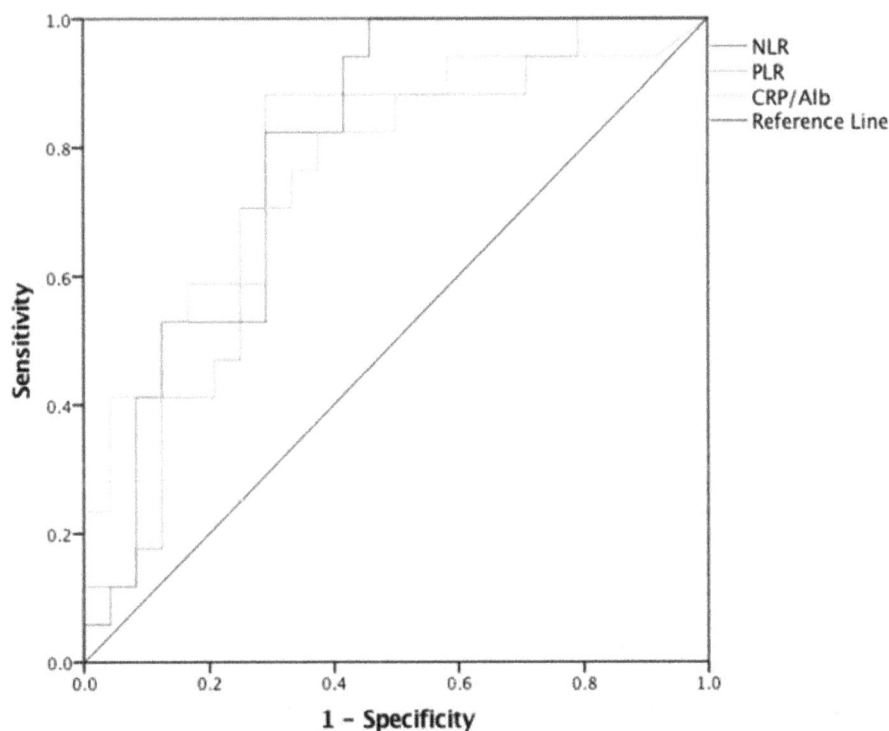

Fig. 1 The predictive abilities of the preoperative NLR, CRP/Alb ratio and PLR were compared using ROC curves

institutions described above who were diagnosed with Xp11.2 tRCC after radical or partial nephrectomy for a renal mass were reviewed for the present study. All clinicopathological data were retrieved from medical records from the department of urology as well as from pathology reports from the Institute of Pathology at each institution. The inclusion criteria included the following: 1) patients who were histologically and immunohistochemically (using the TFE3 protein nuclear stain) diagnosed with Xp11.2 tRCC; 2) the data on complete blood laboratory tests included the serum neutrophil count(NC), lymphocyte count(LC), platelet count (PLT), C-reactive protein (CRP) level and albumin (Alb) level within one week before performing radical or partial nephrectomy; and (3) patients without blood laboratory tests before surgery, patients with active inflammatory disease and patients with other tumours were excluded from the study. Finally, a total of 82 patients were enrolled in this study.

Clinical and pathological evaluation

The baseline clinical characteristics and pathologic information, including data on the age at the time of surgery, gender, tumour location, tumour size, symptoms at presentation, surgical treatment, pathological features, immunohistochemistry results, NC, LC, PLT, CRP level, Alb level, lactate dehydrogenase (LDH) level, urine protein, tumour stage, and nuclear grade, were all collected. Tumour stage was determined according to the seventh edition of the TNM-UICC/AJCC classification system, and the nuclear grade was defined based on the Fuhrman Grading System. The NLR was defined as the ratio of the NC to LC. The PLR was defined as the ratio of the PLT to LC. The CRP/Alb ratio was defined as the ratio of the serum CRP level to the serum albumin (Alb) level. Elevated LDH was defined as serum LDH > 245 U/L. The association between inflammatory parameters (LN, NC, PLT, CRP, NLR, PLR, CRP/Alb) and DFS was explored, and the ROC curves of the NLR, CRP/Alb ratio and PLR are shown in Fig. 1.

Patients follow-up

All patients enrolled in this study were followed-up every 3 months during the first 2 years, every 6 months for 3–5 years and every 12 months after 5 years until July 2017 or until death. A physical examination, laboratory tests, and dynamic computed tomography were performed at every visit. Overall survival (OS) was defined as the time interval between the date of surgery and the date of death or the last follow-up. Disease-free survival (DFS) was defined as the time interval between the date of surgery and date of disease recurrence or metastasis or the last follow-up in localized Xp11.2 tRCC patients who underwent radical or partial nephrectomy.

Statistical analyses

Statistical analyses were performed using SPSS version 24.0 software (SPSS, Chicago, IL, USA). The descriptive data (i.e., tumour size) were presented as the means ± standard deviation or medians, and Student's t-test was used for these variables. A comparison between groups was performed using the Chi-squared test. Receiver operating characteristic (ROC) analysis was used for the selection of effective inflammatory parameters and corresponding optimal cut-off values, and the area under the curve (AUC), sensitivity, specificity and P value

Table 1 Baseline characteristics of 82 Xp11.2 tRCC patients

Characteristic	Case ($n = 82$)
Age in years	
> 45	21
≤ 45	61
Sex	
Male	33
Female	49
Tumour size, cm	5.94 ± 2.65
Location	
Left	31
Right	51
Symptoms	
Asymptomatic	48
Symptomatic	34
Fuhrman grade	
1 to 2	32
3 to 4	50
TNM stage	
I to II	49
III to IV	33
pT status	
T1 to T2	64
T3 to T4	18
pN status	
N0	59
N1	23
pM status	
M0	78
M1	4
Surgical treatment	
Radical	55
Partial	27
Tumour thrombus	
Negative	72
Positive	10

Table 2 Clinicopathological features of Xp11.2 tRCC patients stratified by the cut-off value of the NLR

Characteristic	N (%)	NLR > 2.45 (n = 40)	NLR ≤ 2.45 (n = 42)	P
Age in years				0.004
> 45	21 (25.6%)	16 (40.0%)	5 (11.9%)	
≤ 45	61 (74.4%)	24 (60.0%)	37 (88.1%)	
Sex				0.345
Male	33 (40.2%)	14 (35.0%)	19 (45.2%)	
Female	49 (59.8%)	26 (65.0%)	23 (54.8%)	
Tumour size	5.94 ± 2.65	7.0 ± 3.0	4.0 ± 1.1	< 0.001
Location				0.377
Left	31 (37.8%)	18 (45.0%)	23 (54.8%)	
Right	51 (62.2%)	22 (55.0%)	19 (45.2%)	
Symptoms				0.477
Asymptomatic	48 (58.5%)	25 (62.5%)	23 (54.8%)	
Symptomatic	34 (41.5)	15 (37.5%)	19 (45.2%)	
Fuhrman grade				0.011
1 to 2	32 (39.0%)	10 (25%)	22 (52.4%)	
3 to 4	50 (61.0%)	30 (75%)	20 (47.6%)	
TNM stage				< 0.001
I-II	49 (59.8%)	14 (35.0%)	35 (83.3%)	
III-IV	33 (40.2%)	26 (65.0%)	7 (16.7%)	
pT status				0.001
T1-T2	64 (78.0%)	25 (62.5%)	39 (92.9%)	
T3-T4	18 (22.0%)	15 (37.5%)	3 (7.1%)	
pN status				< 0.001
N0	59 (72.0%)	21 (52.5%)	38 (90.5%)	
N1	23 (28.0%)	19 (47.5%)	4 (9.5%)	
pM status				0.112
M0	78 (95.1%)	36 (90.0%)	42 (100.0%)	
M1	4 (4.9%)	4 (10.0%)	0 (0.0%)	
Surgical treatment				0.307
Radical	55 (67.1%)	29 (72.5%)	26 (61.9%)	
Partial	27 (32.9)	11 (27.5)	16 (38.1%)	
Tumour thrombus				0.014
Negative	72 (87.8%)	31 (77.5%)	41 (97.6%)	
Positive	10 (12.2%)	9 (22.5%)	1 (2.4%)	
CRP/Alb				< 0.001
≤ 0.083	44 (53.7%)	13 (32.5%)	31 (73.8%)	
> 0.083	38 (46.3%)	27 (67.5%)	11 (26.2%)	
PLR				0.001
≤ 140	46 (56.1%)	15 (37.5%)	31 (73.8%)	
> 140	36 (43.9%)	25 (62.5%)	11 (26.2%)	
LDH				0.014
Normal	68 (82.9%)	29 (72.5%)	39 (92.9%)	

Table 2 Clinicopathological features of Xp11.2 tRCC patients stratified by the cut-off value of the NLR (Continued)

Characteristic	N (%)	NLR > 2.45 (n = 40)	NLR ≤ 2.45 (n = 42)	P
Elevated	14 (17.1%)	11 (27.5%)	3 (7.1%)	
Proteinuria				0.013
No	63 (76.8%)	26 (65.0%)	37 (88.1%)	
Yes	19 (23.2%)	14 (35.0%)	5 (11.9%)	

were calculated accordingly. Survival analyses of OS and DFS were performed using the Kaplan-Meier method, and the log-rank test was performed for the significance comparison. A Cox proportional-hazard model was applied for univariate and multivariate analyses, and hazard ratios (HR) with 95% confidence intervals (95% CI) and P values are presented. If variables were significantly associated with other variables, they were excluded from the final multivariable analysis. A P value < 0.05 was considered statistically significant in all statistical analyses.

Results

Patient and tumour characteristics

The clinicopathological characteristics of 82 Xp11.2 tRCC patients are shown in Table 1. Among them, 78 (95.1%) were diagnosed with a localized mass (T1–3 N0/+ M0), while 4 (4.9%) had distant metastasis before surgery. After a median follow-up time of 31 months (range: 2 to 108 months), 14 (17%) died and 34 (41%) developed recurrence or distant metastasis. Their mean age at surgery was 37 years (range: 2 to 71 months). The 5-year overall survival (OS) was 82.9% (68/82), 5-year-cancer-specific survival (CSS) was 86.6% (71/82), and 5-year disease-free survival (DFS) was 61.5% (48/78).

Optimal cut-off values of inflammatory parameters based on ROC analysis

Based on ROC analysis, the area under ROC curve (AUC) values of the NLR, CRP/Alb ratio, and PLR were 0.797 (P = 0.001), 0.772 (P = 0.003), and 0.755 (P = 0.006), respectively, for DFS and the optimal cut-off values for the NLR, CRP/Alb, and PLR were 2.45, 0.83, and 140, respectively. The corresponding sensitivity and specificity values for DFS were, respectively, 82.4 and 72.8% for NLR, 70.6 and 72.8% for CRP/Alb, and 80.0 and 65.9% for PLR.

Association of the preoperative NLR and clinicopathological characteristics

Stratified by the cut-off value, the association between the preoperative NLR and clinicopathological characteristics is summarized in Table 2. An elevated NLR was significantly associated with the tumour size (P < 0.001), Fuhrman-grade (P = 0.011), TNM stage (P < 0.001), pT status (P = 0.001), pN status (P < 0.001), tumour thrombus

Table 3 Clinical-pathological features of Xp11.2 tRCC patients stratified by the cut-off values of the CRP/Alb ratio and PLR

Characteristic	N (%)	CRP/Alb> 0.083 (n = 39)	CRP/Alb≤0.083 (n = 43)	P	PLR > 140 (n = 36)	PLR ≤ 140 (n = 46)	P
Age in years				0.011			0.015
> 45	21 (25.6%)	15 (38.5%)	6 (14.0%)		14 (38.9%)	7 (15.2%)	
≤ 45	61 (74.4%)	24 (61.5%)	37 (86.0%)		22 (61.1%)	39 (84.8%)	
Sex				0.224			0.113
Male	33(40.2%)	13(33.3%)	20(46.5%)		11 (30.6%)	22 (47.8%)	
Female	49(59.8%)	26(66.7%)	23(53.5%)		25 (69.4%)	24 (52.2%)	
Tumor size	5.94 ± 2.65	6.7 ± 3.0	4.8 ± 2.1	0.035	7.4 ± 3.1	4.1 ± 1.2	< 0.001
Location				0.052			0.858
Left	31(37.8%)	19 (48.7%)	12 (27.9%)		14 (38.9%)	17 (37.0%)	
Right	51(62.2%)	20 (51.3%)	31 (72.1%)		22 (61.1%)	29 (63.0%)	
Symptoms				0.412			0.165
Asymptomatic	48 (58.5%)	21 (53.8%)	27 (62.8%)		18 (50.0%)	30 (65.2%)	
Symptomatic	34 (41.5%)	18 (46.2%)	16 (37.2%)		18 (50.0%)	16 (34.8%)	
Fuhrman grade				0.018			0.006
1 to 2	32 (39.0%)	10 (25.6%)	22 (51.2%)		8 (22.2%)	24 (52.2%)	
3 to 4	50 (61.0%)	29 (74.4%)	21 (48.8%)		28 (77.8%)	22 (47.8%)	
TNM stage				0.004			< 0.001
I-II	49 (59.8%)	17 (43.6%)	32 (74.4%)		12 (33.3%)	37 (80.4%)	
III-IV	33 (40.2%)	22 (56.4%)	11 (25.6%)		24 (66.7%)	9 (19.6%)	
pT status				0.018			0.006
T1-T2	64 (78.0%)	26 (66.7%)	38 (88.4%)		22 (61.1%)	42 (91.3%)	
T3-T4	18 (22.0%)	13 (33.3%)	5 (11.6%)		14 (38.9%)	4 (8.7%)	
pN status				0.003			0.003
N0	59 (72.0%)	22 (56.4%)	37 (86.0%)		20 (55.6%)	39 (84.8%)	
N1	23 (28.0%)	17 (43.6%)	6 (14.0%)		16 (44.4%)	7 (15.2%)	
pM status				0.101			0.199
M0	78 (95.1%)	35 (89.7%)	43 (100.0%)		33 (91.7%)	45 (97.8%)	
M1	4 (4.9%)	4 (10.3%)	0 (0.0%)		3 (8.3%)	1 (2.2%)	
Surgical treatment				0.502			0.686
Radical	55 (67.1%)	23 (59.0%)	22 (51.2%)		25 (69.4%)	30 (65.2%)	
Partial	27 (32.9)	16 (41.0%)	11 (48.8%)		11 (30.6%)	16 (34.8%)	
Tumour thrombus				0.011			0.001
Negative	72 (87.8%)	30 (76.9%)	42 (97.7%)		26 (72.2%)	46 (100.0%)	
Positive	10 (12.2%)	9 (23.1%)	1 (2.3%)		10 (27.8%)	0 (0.0%)	
CRP/Alb				–			< 0.001
≤ 0.083	44 (53.7%)	–	–		11 (30.6%)	33 (71.7%)	
> 0.083	38 (46.3%)	–	–		25 (69.4%)	13 (28.3%)	
PLR				0.009			–
≤ 140	46(56.1%)	16 (41.0%)	30 (69.8%)		–	–	
> 140	36(43.9%)	23 (59.0%)	13 (30.2%)		–	–	
LDH				0.011			0.023
Normal	68(82.9%)	28 (71.8%)	40 (93.0%)		26 (72.2%)	42 (91.3%)	

Table 3 Clinical-pathological features of Xp11.2 tRCC patients stratified by the cut-off values of the CRP/Alb ratio and PLR *(Continued)*

Characteristic	N (%)	CRP/Alb> 0.083 (n = 39)	CRP/Alb≤0.083 (n = 43)	P	PLR > 140 (n = 36)	PLR ≤ 140 (n = 46)	P
Elevated	14(17.1%)	11 (28.2%)	3 (7.0%)		10 (27.8%)	4 (8.7%)	
Proteinuria				< 0.001			< 0.001
No	63(76.8%)	22 (56.4%)	41 (95.3%)		20 (55.6%)	43 (93.5%)	
Yes	19 (23.2%)	17 (43.6%)	2 (4.7%)		16 (44.4%)	3 (6.5%)	

($P = 0.014$), CRP/Alb ($P < 0.001$), PLR ($P = 0.001$), LDH ($P = 0.014$) and proteinuria ($P < 0.013$). For patients in the high NLR group, only 35.0% of patients were at stage I/II and 65.0% of patients were at stage III-IV ($P < 0.001$), 62.5% of patients were at stage T1/T2, and 37.5% of patients were at stage T3/T4 ($P = 0.001$). However, for patients in the low NLR group, 83.3% of patients were at stage I/II, 16.7% were at stage III-IV ($P < 0.001$), 92.9% of patients were at stage T1/T2, and 7.1% of patients were at stage T3/T4 ($P = 0.001$). Meanwhile, the percentage values of patients at stage N0/N1 were 52.5% / 47.2%, and the percentage values of patients negative/positive tumour thrombus were 77.5%/22.5% in the high NLR group. By comparison, the percentage values of patients at stage N0/N1 were 90.5%/9.5%, and the percentage values of patients with negative/positive tumour thrombus were 97.6%/2.4% in the low NLR group. These results revealed that a high NLR was associated with tumour progression and a low NLR was associated with early-stage of Xp11.2 tRCC. Similarly, Clinicopathological features of Xp11.2 RCC patients stratified by the cut-off value of the CRP/Alb ratio, PLR are summarized in the Table 3.

Univariate and multivariate analyses for both DFS and OS

The results of univariate and multivariate analyses for both DFS and OS are shown in Tables 4 and 5. Univariate

analysis demonstrated that age, the Fuhrman grade, pT status, pN status, tumour thrombus, the NLR, the CRP/Alb and the PLR were significant predictors for both DFS and OS in Xp11.2 tRCC patients. Multivariable analysis showed that the NLR (HR: 4.25, 95%, CI 1.19–15.18, $P = 0.026$) was an independent predictor of DFS in patients with Xp11.2 tRCC, along with pT status ($P < 0.001$), pT status ($P = 0.019$) and age ($P = 0.004$), and the NLR (HR: 26.26; 95% CI: 1.44–480.3; $P = 0.028$) also was an independent predictor of OS in patients with Xp11.2 tRCC, along with age ($P = 0.016$) and a tumour thrombus ($P = 0.007$).

The relationships of the preoperative NLR, pT status, pN status, age and tumour thrombus with survival

The relationships of the independent predictors in multivariate analyses for DFS and OS, such as the preoperative NLR, pT status, pN status, age and tumour thrombus with survival (OS: $n = 82$; DFS: $n = 78$) were investigated, and the results are shown in Fig. 2. Patients with a preoperative higher NLR had a significantly worse rate of survival than those with a lower NLR ratio with regarding both OS and DFS (Mean OS 49.0 months vs 99.7 months, respectively, log-rank $P = 0.009$; Mean DFS 24.5 months vs 90.2 months, respectively, log-rank $P < 0.001$). Patients age > 45 years had a significantly worse rate of survival than those with age ≤ 45 years with regarding both OS

Table 4 Univariate and multivariate analyses for variables considered for disease-free survival (DFS) (Cox proportional hazard regression model) (n = 78)

Variables	Univariate analysis		Multivariate analysis	
	HR (95% CI)	P	HR (95% CI)	P
Age (> 45)	2.34 (1.03 to 5.30)	0.043	6.25 (1.78 to 21.97)	0.004
Symptoms (yes)	1.06 (0.51 to 2.19)	0.885		
Gender (male)	0.76 (0.36 to 1.64)	0.490		
Fuhrman Grade (G3–G4)	5.24 (2.12 to 12.96)	< 0.001	1.83 (0.64 to 5.24)	0.261
pT status (T3-T4)	6.48 (2.96 to 14.19)	< 0.001	6.84 (2.35 to 19.90)	< 0.001
pN status (N1)	5.21 (2.52 to 10.77)	< 0.001	3.40 (1.22 to 9.43)	0.019
Tumour thrombus (yes)	12.47 (4.81 to 32.34)	< 0.001	2.90 (0.73 to 11.48)	0.129
NLR (> 2.45)	4.98 (2.12 to 11.66)	< 0.001	4.25 (1.19 to 15.18)	0.026
CRP/Alb (> 0.083)	2.90 (1.37 to 6.13)	0.005	1.40 (0.43 to 4.54)	0.574
PLR (> 140)	3.76 (1.74 to 8.13)	0.001	1.36 (0.47 to 3.72)	0.598

Italicized *P* values are statistically significant

Table 5 Univariate and multivariate analyses for variables considered for overall survival (OS) (Cox proportional hazard regression model) ($n = 82$)

Variables	Univariate analysis			Multivariate analysis		
	HR (95% CI)		P	HR (95% CI)		P
Age (> 45 years)	4.90(1.44 to 16.69)		*0.011*	26.56 (1.85 to 380.7)		*0.016*
Symptoms (yes)	2.04 (0.70 to 5.93)		0.189			
Gender (male)	2.14 (0.48 to 9.63)		0.320			
Fuhrman Grade (G3–G4)	1.92 (1.04 to 3.55)		*0.037*	0.30 (0.07 to 1.28)		0.103
pT status (T3-T4)	2.21 (1.24 to 3.95)		*0.007*	1.82 (0.70 to 4.70)		0.217
pN status (N1)	6.22 (2.06 to 18.82)		*0.001*	2.03 (0.20 to 20.45)		0.547
Tumour thrombus (yes)	22.32 (6.76 to 73.72)		*< 0.001*	47.40 (2.92 to 769.9)		*0.007*
NLR (> 2.45)	4.46 (1.33 to 14.97)		*0.016*	26.26 (1.44 to 480.3)		*0.028*
CRP/Alb (> 0.083)	23.51(2.90 to 190.51)		*0.003*	6.65 (0.35 to 127.0)		0.208
PLR (> 140)	4.30 (1.34 to 13.82)		*0.014*	0.14 (0.01 to 1.67)		0.120

Italicized *P* values are statistically significant

and DFS (mean DFS 12.1 months vs 75.0 months, respectively, log-rank $P = 0.005$; mean OS 30.5 months vs 67.8 months, respectively, log-rank $P = 0.035$). Patients at T3-T4 stage and N1 stage had a significantly worse rate of survival than those with at stage T1-T2 and N0 stage regarding DFS (mean DFS 24.5 months vs 90.2 months, respectively, log-rank $P < 0.001$; mean DFS 20.4 months vs 81.9 months, respectively, log-rank $P < 0.001$). Patients positive for a tumour thrombus had a significantly worse rate of survival than those who were negative for a tumour thrombus regarding OS (mean DFS 24.5 months vs 90.2 months, respectively, log-rank $P < 0.001$).

Discussion

In this multicentre retrospective study, we investigated the prognostic values of the NLR, CRP/Alb ratio, and PLR in 82 Xp11.2 tRCC patients who underwent radical or partial nephrectomy. The results demonstrated that the NLR, CRP/Alb ratio and PLR were all significant predictors and that the NLR was an independent prognostic marker for patients with Xp11.2 tRCC.

Increasing evidence has revealed the involvement of systemic inflammation in cancer development and progression. Neutrophils were shown to produce pro-angiogenic factors such as vascular endothelial growth factor to stimulate tumour development and progression [19]. Moreover, the cytokines involved in cancer-related inflammation, IL-6 and TNFα, may induce neutrophilia [20, 21]. Additionally, relative lymphocytopenia may reflect a lower count of CD4+ T-helper lymphocytes, resulting in a suboptimal lymphocyte-mediated immune response to malignancy [22]. Therefore, an NLR may reflect the combined prognostic information of these two inflammatory factors, and a high NLR has been validated as a poor prognostic factor for several different human cancers [10], including clear cell RCC and non-clear cell RCC [14, 17, 22–24].

C-reactive protein (CRP) is a prototype acute phase protein that was demonstrated to be produced in hepatocytes and regulated by growth factors in the malignant tumors such as IL-6 [25]. An elevated CRP level was reported to be associated with a poorer prognosis in various types of human cancers [25–27]. A study conducted by Guo et al. [16] summarized the potential mechanisms regarding how CRP is associated with cancer in follow several aspects:(1). An increased CRP level is created by the tissue inflammation, which is caused by the tumour growth; (2). Tumour antigens activate the immune responses, leading to increased CRP level; (3). Tumour cells increase CRP expression by producing inflammatory proteins, including CRP or by enhancing the role of inflammatory cytokines such as IL-6 and IL-8, which could indirectly increase the CRP level. More recently, several publications demonstrated that the CRP/Alb ratio could be used to predict the prognosis of several cancers [11, 28, 29], and two additional studies confirmed the prognostic value of the CRP/Alb ratio in RCC patients [16, 30].

Since the possible association between an increased platelet level and cancer metastasis was first described in 1968 [31], an increased PLT level was confirmed to be a prognostic marker for several cancers, including RCC [32, 33]. Furthermore, Emerging evidence has shown that the platelet-to-lymphocyte ratio (PLR) can be used to assess the response to systemic inflammation and RCC prognosis [12, 15, 16].

In this study, we explored the relationships of the NLR, CRP/Alb ratio and PLR with survival in Xp11.2 tRCC patients. Compared with the other systemic inflammatory markers, the NLR, CRP/Alb ratio and PLR had better predictive value for DFS (Fig. 1, Tables 2 and 3). Among of them, the NLR had the highest AUC value ($P = 0.001$). The optimal cut-off value of the NLR was 2.45, which is little lower than the cut-off values of two other studies,

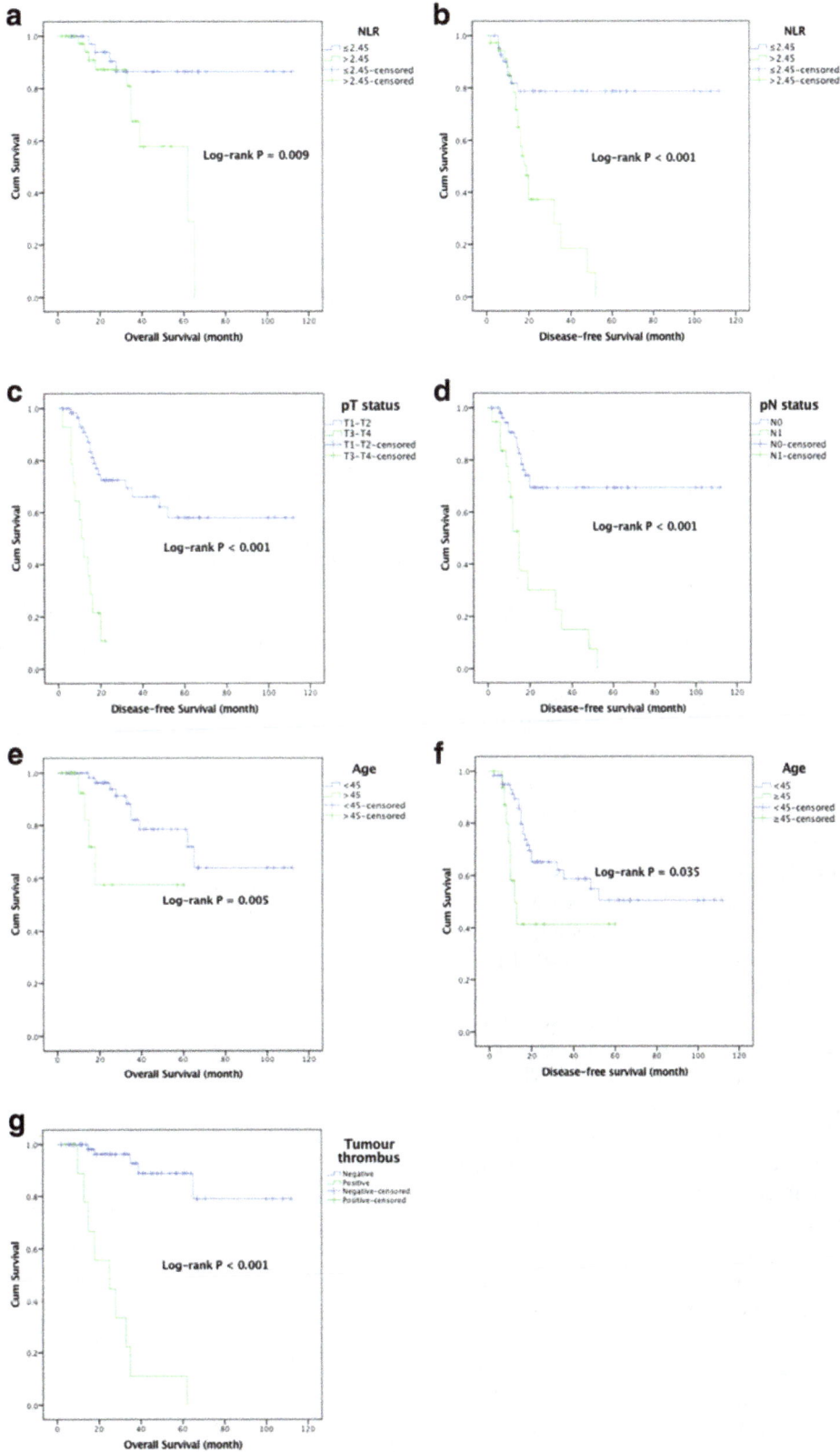

Fig. 2 Kaplan–Meier curves for independent predictors in multivariate analysis regarding DFS (n = 78) and OS (n = 82). **a**: OS stratified by the NLR; **b**: DFS stratified by the NLR; **c**: DFS stratified by pT status; **d**: DFS stratified by pN status; **e**: OS stratified by age; **f**: DFS stratified by age; **g**: OS stratified by tumour thrombus

whose cut-off values were 2.7 and 3.3, respectively [14, 24]. We consider these differences to be due to the small size of our patients and uniqueness of this tumour. Regarding the CRP/Alb ratio and PLR, the optimal cut-off values were 0.083 and 140, respectively, similar to those reported in previous studies on RCC [15, 16]. Univariate analyses for both DFS and OS showed that a higher NLR, CRP/Alb ratio and PLR were all associated with a poorer prognosis of Xp11.2 tRCC patients (Tables 4 and 5), and multivariate analyses showed that only the NLR independently predicted the DFS of patients with Xp11.2 tRCC (HR: 4.25; 95% CI: 1.19–15.18; $P = 0.026$) along with the pT status ($P < 0.001$), pN status ($P = 0.019$) and age (0.014) (Table 4), and the NLR (HR: 26.26; 95% CI: 1.44–480.3; $P = 0.028$) as well as independently predicted the OS of patients with Xp11.2 tRCC, along with age ($P = 0.016$) and tumour thrombus ($P = 0.007$) (Table 5). Our previous studies on Xp11.2 tRCC confirmed that advanced TNM stage and tumour thrombus are the most significant factors that predict a poor prognosis in Xp11 tRCC [4, 34], and we believe that pT status and N status contribute to the advanced TNM stage in the present study. In addition, Kaplan–Meier survival analysis suggested that the patients with a preoperative higher NLR, T3-T4 stage, N1 stage and age > 45 years had a significantly shorter DFS than those with a lower NLR, T1-T2 stage, N0 stage and age ≤ 45 years, individually. The patients with a higher NLR, age > 45 years and positive for tumour thrombus had a significantly shorter OS than those with a lower NLR, age ≤ 45 years and negative for tumour thrombus. Therefore, a low NLR is associated with the early-stage Xp11.2 tRCC and a high NLR indicates advanced-stage Xp11.2 tRCC, suggesting that the NLR could be a new prognostic indicator related to the progression of Xp11.2 tRCC.

Our findings demonstrate that the NLR, CRP/Alb ratio and PLR were all associated with a poor prognosis in Xp11.2 tRCC patients. Among them, only the NLR independently predicted surgical outcomes of Xp11.2 tRCC patients. These results are important for clinicians to make clinical decisions. According to these preoperative inflammatory markers, patients at high risk can be selected for further treatment and management. With these prognostic factors, more suitable preoperative therapies and more frequent follow-up strategies can be considered for certain high-risk patients with Xp11.2 tRCC.

In addition, the prognostic value of inflammatory markers has never been reported with Xp11.2 tRCC patients. We may, for the first time, predict the surgical outcomes of Xp11.2 tRCC patients using the NLR, CRP/Alb ratio and PLR. Moreover, the sample size of this study was the largest among studies of this tumour worldwide.

To the best of our knowledge, this is the first study that focused on the prognostic values of the NLR, CRP/Alb ratio and PLR in patients with Xp11.2 tRCC. However, this study possesses several limitations. First, our study is a retrospective study, which may limit the prognostic values of the NLR, CRP/Alb ratio and PLR. Therefore, a large-scale prospective study is needed to validate our results. Second, due to the low incidence of Xp11.2 tRCC, our sample size was relatively small, warranting a large-scale study. Third, several other factors that are influential to inflammation such as smoking habits and life styles were not included in the study.

Conclusions

In summary, we found that the NLR, CRP/Alb ratio and PLR were all potential markers for the survival of Xp11.2 tRCC; thus, they could be considered for clinical decision-making. Among them, the NLR is an independent predictor of both DFS and OS for patients with Xp11.2 tRCC and can be used to predict the surgical outcomes of Xp11.2 tRCC patients who underwent full resection.

Abbreviations

Alb: Albumin; CRP: C-reactive protein; CRP/Alb: C-reactive protein/albumin; DFS: Disease-free survival; HR: Hazard ratio; LC: Lymphocyte count; LDH: Lactate dehydrogenase level; NC: Neutrophil count; NLR: Neutrophil count to lymphocyte count ratio; OS: Overall survival; PLR: Platelet count to lymphocyte count ratio; PLT: Platelet count; RCC: Renal cell carcinoma; ROC: Receive operating characteristic; TFE3: Transcription factor E3; Xp11.2 tRCC: Xp11.2 translocation/TFE3 gene fusions Renal Cell Carcinoma

Acknowledgements

We thank Gutian Zhang, Xiaogong Li, Linfeng Xu and Xiaozhi Zhao (Nanjing Drum Tower Hospital) for providing patient information, and Jie Gao, Zhen Wang and Wenliang Ma (Nanjing Drum Tower Hospital) for providing technical assistance.

Funding

This research was supported by the National Natural Science Foundation of China (ID: 81572512, 81772710 and 81572519) and Nanjing Medical Science and Technique Development Foundation (ID: QRX17049). The funders played no roles in the design of the study and collection, analysis, and interpretation of data and in writing the manuscript.

Authors' contributions

SA: Project development, Data collection, Data analysis, Manuscript writing and editing. FQ: Project development, Data collection, Data analysis, Manuscript editing. NL: Data analysis, Results interpretation, Manuscript editing. JS: Data collection, Data analysis, Results interpretation. WX: Data collection, Data analysis, Results interpretation. LHZ: Data collection, Data analysis, Results interpretation. HQG: Data collection, Results interpretation, Manuscript editing. WDG: Project development, Data analysis, Manuscript writing and editing. All authors read and approved the final manuscript.

Competing interests
The authors declare that they have no competing interests.

Author details
[1]Department of Urology, Nanjing Drum Tower Hospital, The Affiliated Hospital of Nanjing University Medical School, No. 321 Zhongshan Road, Nanjing 210008, Jiangsu Province, China. [2]Department of Oncology, Jiangsu Province Hospital, The First Affiliated Hospital of Nanjing Medical University, Nanjing, Jiangsu, China. [3]Department of Pathology, Jiangsu Cancer Hospital, The Affiliated Cancer Hospital of Nanjing Medical University, Nanjing, Jiangsu, China. [4]Department of Pathology, Zhongda Hospital Southeast University, Nanjing, Jiangsu, China.

References
1. Ellis CL, Eble JN, Subhawong AP, Martignoni G, Zhon M, Ladanyi M, Epstein JI, Netto GJ, Argani P. Clinical heterogeneity of Xp11 translocation renal cell carcinoma: impact of fusion subtype, age, and stage. Mod Pathol. 2014; 27(6):875–86.
2. Qu Y, Gu C, Wang H, Chang K, Yang X, Zhou X, Dai B, Zhu Y, Shi G, Zhang H, et al. Diagnosis of adults Xp11.2 translocation renal cell carcinoma by immunohistochemistry and FISH assays: clinicopathological data from ethnic Chinese population. Sci Rep. 2016;6:21677.
3. Sukov WR, Hodge JC, Lohse CM, Leibovich BC, Thompson RH, Pearce KE, Wiktor AE, Cheville JC. TFE3 rearrangements in adult renal cell carcinoma: clinical and pathologic features with outcome in a large series of consecutively treated patients. Am J Surg Pathol. 2012;36(5):663–70.
4. Liu N, Wang Z, Gan W, Xiong L, Miao B, Chen X, Guo H, Li D. Renal cell carcinoma associated with Xp11.2 translocation/TFE3 gene fusions: clinical features, treatments and prognosis. PLoS One. 2016;11(11):e0166897.
5. Choo MS, Jeong CW, Song C, Jeon HG, Seo SI, Hong SK, Byun SS, Chung JS, Hong SH, Hwang EC, et al. Clinicopathologic characteristics and prognosis of Xp11.2 translocation renal cell carcinoma: multicenter, propensity score matching analysis. Clin Genitourin Cancer. 2017;15(5):e819–e825.
6. Argani P, Antonescu CR, Illei PB, Lui MY, Timmons CF, Newbury R, Reuter VE, Garvin AJ, Perez-Atayde AR, Fletcher JA, et al. Primary renal neoplasms with the ASPL-TFE3 gene fusion of alveolar soft part sarcoma: a distinctive tumor entity previously included among renal cell carcinomas of children and adolescents. Am J Pathol. 2001;159(1):179–92.
7. Malouf GG, Camparo P, Molinie V, Dedet G, Oudard S, Schleiermacher G, Theodore C, Dutcher J, Billemont B, Bompas E, et al. Transcription factor E3 and transcription factor EB renal cell carcinomas: clinical features, biological behavior and prognostic factors. J Urol. 2011;185(1):24–9.
8. Mantovani A, Allavena P, Sica A, Balkwill F. Cancer-related inflammation. Nature. 2008;454(7203):436–44.
9. Coussens LM, Werb Z. Inflammation and cancer. Nature. 2002;420(6917):860–7.
10. Roxburgh CS, McMillan DC. Role of systemic inflammatory response in predicting survival in patients with primary operable cancer. Future Oncol. 2010;6(1):149–63.
11. Kinoshita A, Onoda H, Imai N, Iwaku A, Oishi M, Tanaka K, Fushiya N, Koike K, Nishino H, Matsushima M. The C-reactive protein/albumin ratio, a novel inflammation-based prognostic score, predicts outcomes in patients with hepatocellular carcinoma. Ann Surg Oncol. 2015;22(3):803–10.
12. Smith RA, Bosonnet L, Raraty M, Sutton R, Neoptolemos JP, Campbell F, Ghaneh P. Preoperative platelet-lymphocyte ratio is an independent significant prognostic marker in resected pancreatic ductal adenocarcinoma. Am J Surg. 2009;197(4):466–72.
13. Walsh SR, Cook EJ, Goulder F, Justin TA, Keeling NJ. Neutrophil-lymphocyte ratio as a prognostic factor in colorectal cancer. J Surg Oncol. 2005;91(3):181–4.
14. Ohno Y, Nakashima J, Ohori M, Hatano T, Tachibana M. Pretreatment neutrophil-to-lymphocyte ratio as an independent predictor of recurrence in patients with nonmetastatic renal cell carcinoma. J Urology. 2010;184(3):873–8.
15. Keskin S, Keskin Z, Taskapu HH, Kalkan H, Kaynar M, Poyraz N, Toy H. Prognostic value of preoperative neutrophil-to-lymphocyte and platelet-to-lymphocyte ratios, and multiphasic renal tomography findings in histological subtypes of renal cell carcinoma. BMC Urol. 2014;14:95.
16. Guo SJ, He XB, Chen Q, Yang GW, Yao K, Dong P, Ye YL, Chen D, Zhang ZL, Qin ZK, et al. The C-reactive protein/albumin ratio, a validated prognostic score, predicts outcome of surgical renal cell carcinoma patients. BMC Cancer. 2017;17:171.
17. de Martino M, Pantuck AJ, Hofbauer S, Waldert M, Shariat SF, Belldegrun AS, Klatte T. Prognostic impact of preoperative neutrophil-to-lymphocyte ratio in localized nonclear cell renal cell carcinoma. J Urol. 2013;190(6):1999–2004.
18. Rao Q, Guan B, Zhou XJ. Xp11.2 translocation renal cell carcinomas have a poorer prognosis than non-Xp11.2 translocation carcinomas in children and young adults: a meta-analysis. Int J Surg Pathol. 2010;18(6):458–64.
19. Kusumanto YH, Dam WA, Hospers GA, Meijer C, Mulder NH. Platelets and granulocytes, in particular the neutrophils, form important compartments for circulating vascular endothelial growth factor. Angiogenesis. 2003;6(4):283–7.
20. Ulich TR, del Castillo J, Guo KZ. In vivo hematologic effects of recombinant interleukin-6 on hematopoiesis and circulating numbers of RBCs and WBCs. Blood. 1989;73(1):108–10.
21. Ulich TR, Delcastillo J, Keys M, Granger GA, Ni PX. Kinetics and mechanisms of recombinant human Interleukin-1 and tumor necrosis factor-alpha-induced changes in circulating numbers of neutrophils and lymphocytes. J Immunol. 1987;139(10):3406–15.
22. Viers BR, Thompson RH, Boorjian SA, Lohse CM, Leibovich BC, Tollefson MK. Preoperative neutrophil-lymphocyte ratio predicts death among patients with localized clear cell renal carcinoma undergoing nephrectomy. Urol Oncol-Semin Ori. 2014;32(8):1277–84.
23. Pichler M, Hutterer GC, Stoeckigt C, Chromecki TF, Stojakovic T, Golbeck S, Eberhard K, Gerger A, Mannweiler S, Pummer K, et al. Validation of the pre-treatment neutrophil lymphocyte ratio as a prognostic factor in a large European cohort of renal cell carcinoma patients. Brit J Cancer. 2013;108(4):901–7.
24. Ayala AG, Srigley JR, Ro JY, Abdul-Karim FW, Johnson DE. Clear cell cribriform hyperplasia of prostate. Report of 10 cases. Am J Surg Pathol. 1986;10(10):665–71.
25. Nozoe T, Korenaga D, Futatsugi M, Saeki H, Maehara Y, Sugimachi K. Immunohistochemical expression of C-reactive protein in squamous cell carcinoma of the esophagus - significance as a tumor marker. Cancer Lett. 2003;192(1):89–95.
26. Deichmann M, Benner A, Waldmann V, Bock M, Jackel A, Naher H. Interleukin-6 and its surrogate C-reactive protein are useful serum markers for monitoring metastasized malignant melanoma. J Exp Clin Cancer Res. 2000;19(3):301–7.
27. Wieland A, Kerbl R, Berghold A, Schwinger W, Mann G, Urban C. C-reactive protein (CRP) as tumor marker in pediatric and adolescent patients with Hodgkin disease. Med Pediatr Oncol. 2003;41(1):21–5.
28. Liu XC, Sun XW, Liu JJ, Kong PF, Chen SX, Zhan YQ, Xu DZ. Preoperative C-reactive protein/albumin ratio predicts prognosis of patients after curative resection for gastric Cancer. Transl Oncol. 2015;8(4):339–45.
29. Zhou T, Zhan JH, Hong SD, Hu ZH, Fang WF, Qin T, Ma YX, Yang YP, He XB, Zhao YY, et al. Ratio of C-reactive protein/albumin is an inflammatory prognostic score for predicting overall survival of patients with small-cell lung Cancer. Sci Rep-Uk. 2015;5:10481.
30. Chen Z, Shao YJ, Fan M, Zhuang QF, Wang K, Cao W, Xu XL, He XZ. Prognostic significance of preoperative C-reactive protein: albumin ratio in patients with clear cell renal cell carcinoma. Int J Clin Exp Patho. 2015;8(11):14893–900.
31. Gasic GJ, Gasic TB, Stewart CC. Antimetastatic effects associated with platelet reduction. P Natl Acad Sci USA. 1968;61(1):46.
32. Long Y, Wang T, Gao Q, Zhou C. Prognostic significance of pretreatment elevated platelet count in patients with colorectal cancer: a meta-analysis. Oncotarget. 2016;7(49):81849–61.
33. Brookman-May S, May M, Ficarra V, Kainz MC, Kampel-Kettner K, Kohlschreiber S, Wenzl V, Schneider M, Burger M, Wieland WF, et al. Does preoperative platelet count and thrombocytosis play a prognostic role in patients undergoing nephrectomy for renal cell carcinoma? Results of a comprehensive retrospective series. World J Urol. 2013;31(5):1309–16.
34. Xu L, Yang R, Gan W, Chen X, Qiu X, Fu K, Huang J, Zhu G, Guo H. Xp11.2 translocation renal cell carcinomas in young adults. BMC Urol. 2015;15:57.

20

Number-needed-to-treat analysis of clinical progression in patients with metastatic castration-resistant prostate cancer in the STRIVE and TERRAIN trials

Neil M. Schultz[1]*, Neal D. Shore[2], Simon Chowdhury[3], Laurence H. Klotz[4], Raoul S. Concepcion[5], David F. Penson[6], Lawrence I. Karsh[7], Hongbo Yang[8], Bruce A. Brown[1], Arie Barlev[9,10] and Scott C. Flanders[1]

Abstract

Background: This analysis estimated the number needed to treat with enzalutamide versus bicalutamide to achieve one additional patient with chemotherapy-naïve metastatic castration-resistant prostate cancer who would obtain clinical benefit regarding progression-free survival, radiographic progression-free survival, or no prostate-specific antigen progression at 1 and 2 years following treatment initiation.

Methods: Clinical event rates were obtained from the STRIVE (NCT01664923) and TERRAIN (NCT01288911) trials, and the number needed to treat was the inverse of the absolute rate difference between the event rates of enzalutamide and bicalutamide. The 95% Confidence Interval of the number needed to treat was derived from the 95% Confidence Interval of the event rate difference.

Results: Using STRIVE data (patients with metastatic disease: $n = 128$ enzalutamide; $n = 129$ bicalutamide) comparing enzalutamide with bicalutamide at 1 and 2 years, the numbers needed to treat to achieve one additional patient with chemotherapy-naïve metastatic castration-resistant prostate cancer with progression-free survival were 2.0 and 2.8, respectively; with radiographic progression-free survival, 2.6 and 3.0, respectively; and without prostate-specific antigen progression, 1.8 and 2.4, respectively. Using TERRAIN data ($n = 184$ enzalutamide; $n = 191$ bicalutamide) comparing enzalutamide with bicalutamide at 1 and 2 years, the numbers needed to treat to achieve one additional patient with progression-free survival were 4.3 and 3.7, respectively; with radiographic progression-free survival, 10.0 and 2.8, respectively; and without prostate-specific antigen progression, 2.1 and 3.2, respectively.

Conclusions: The combined data from TERRAIN and STRIVE demonstrated that treating chemotherapy-naïve metastatic castration-resistant prostate cancer with enzalutamide leads to more patients without clinical progression at 1 and 2 years than with bicalutamide.

Keywords: Enzalutamide, Bicalutamide, Metastatic castration-resistant prostate cancer, Number needed to treat

* Correspondence: neil.schultz@astellas.com
[1]Astellas Pharma, Inc., 1 Astellas Way, Northbrook, IL 60062, USA
Full list of author information is available at the end of the article

Background

Prostate cancer (PC) is the second leading cause of cancer-related deaths and the most commonly diagnosed cancer among men worldwide [1, 2]. Castration-resistant prostate cancer (CRPC) is characterized by a castrate level of testosterone and either rising prostate-specific antigen (PSA) or radiographic disease progression [3]. CRPC may account for approximately 10–20% of PC cases, with over 84% of these cases demonstrating radiographic findings of metastatic CRPC (mCRPC) [4].

Until 2010, treatment for mCRPC was largely limited to taxane chemotherapy (docetaxel) or the oral non-steroidal antiandrogen bicalutamide plus luteinizing hormone-releasing hormone (LHRH) analogs [5]. Bicalutamide is a partial androgen receptor (AR) antagonist approved by the United States Food and Drug Administration (FDA) in 1995 as a 50 mg daily tablet for the treatment of metastatic androgen-sensitive PC, in combination with an LHRH analog [5, 6]. However, bicalutamide has been frequently used to treat various stages of mCRPC as monotherapy or as combination therapy with androgen-deprivation therapy despite a void of Category 1 evidence for its use in this patient population [7]. Until recently, median overall survival, depending on symptomatology and tumor burden, was estimated to be 9–18 months for those with mCRPC [4]. However, since 2010, the approval of new treatments for mCRPC has resulted in increases in median overall survival ranging from 16 to 35 months [7, 8].

One of these new therapies is the AR antagonist enzalutamide (Xtandi®; Astellas Pharma, Inc., IL, and Medivation, Inc., CA, which was acquired by Pfizer, Inc. in September 2016), which was approved by the FDA in 2012 [9]. Enzalutamide, with an approved dose of 160 mg daily for the treatment of mCRPC [9], is shown to have a five- to eight-fold higher AR binding affinity compared to bicalutamide in a preclinical test [10]. Enzalutamide targets three aspects of the AR signaling pathway: blocking androgen binding to ARs; inhibiting nuclear translocation of ARs; and inhibiting binding of ARs to DNA [11]. In contrast to bicalutamide, enzalutamide has received a Category 1 evidence recommendation for mCRPC in multiple US clinical guidelines [7, 12, 13].

Enzalutamide and bicalutamide have been directly compared in patients with chemotherapy-naïve CRPC in two randomized clinical trials: STRIVE and TERRAIN [14, 15]. In TERRAIN, enzalutamide and bicalutamide were compared in patients with chemotherapy-naïve asymptomatic or minimally symptomatic mCRPC [15]. The primary outcome of the TERRAIN trial was significantly improved progression-free survival (PFS) in patients receiving enzalutamide compared to patients receiving bicalutamide (15.7 months vs. 5.8 months,

respectively). Median radiographic PFS (rPFS) was not reached for enzalutamide and was 16.4 months for bicalutamide, and median time to PSA progression was 19.4 months and 5.8 months, respectively. The STRIVE trial compared these two therapies in chemotherapy-naïve non-metastatic CRPC patients and mCRPC patients [14]. In patients with mCRPC, the trial reported a longer median PFS with enzalutamide than with bicalutamide (16.5 months vs. 5.5 months, respectively), and median rPFS was not reached with enzalutamide and was 8.3 months with bicalutamide. Median time to PSA progression was 24.9 months with enzalutamide and 5.7 months with bicalutamide. With respect to the incidence of serious adverse events, in the TERRAIN trial, patients treated with enzalutamide were more likely to experience a serious adverse event than patients treated with bicalutamide (31% vs. 23%, respectively); however, in the STRIVE trial, the rates were similar between the two treatment groups (29% vs. 28%, respectively) [14, 15].

The outcomes data from TERRAIN and STRIVE can be used to generate additional comparative efficacy evidence for enzalutamide versus bicalutamide that is applicable to mCRPC clinical practice and treatment decision-making. A useful and broadly used measure of treatment effect is the number needed to treat (NNT) to avoid a clinical progression event. The NNT is defined as the inverse of the absolute risk reduction [16] and reports the number of patients who need to be treated with one therapy versus an alternative therapy to achieve one additional clinical response or outcome. This approach has been previously used by the FDA to aid benefit-risk treatment comparisons [17] and is widely used in medical literature for its ease of interpretation. Thus, this analysis used outcomes data from the STRIVE and TERRAIN trials to calculate the NNT to avoid a clinical progression event (PFS, rPFS, or PSA progression) in patients with chemotherapy-naïve mCRPC receiving enzalutamide versus bicalutamide at 1 and 2 years.

Methods
Study population

This analysis reviewed data from patients with chemotherapy-naïve mCRPC in the STRIVE [14] (NCT01664923) and TERRAIN [15] (NCT01288911) trials. The definition of mCRPC was confirmed adenocarcinoma of the prostate, serum testosterone level less than 50 ng/dL, disease progression on androgen-deprivation therapy, and bone or soft tissue metastases in both trials [14, 15]. Approximately 65% of patients in the STRIVE trial had radiographic documentation of metastatic disease and all patients in the TERRAIN trial had mCRPC.

Baseline patient characteristics

Baseline demographic categories of the study populations (age, race, weight, and body mass index) were reported. Clinical characteristics including Eastern Cooperative Oncology Group (ECOG) performance status score [18] and serum PSA levels were also summarized [14, 15].

Clinical progression outcomes

Clinical progression events have been previously reported and included PFS, rPFS, and PSA progression at 1 and 2 years. These events were evaluated using end points defined in the STRIVE [14] and TERRAIN [15] trials that were similar but not identical (Table 1).

NNT analysis

The NNT to achieve one additional patient free from clinical progression was calculated as the reciprocal of the rate difference between enzalutamide and bicalutamide at 1 and 2 years. The 95% Confidence Interval (CI) of the NNT was calculated as the inverse of the 95% CI of the rate difference when comparing enzalutamide with bicalutamide. In this analysis, the NNT value represents the number of patients who needed to be treated with enzalutamide versus bicalutamide to achieve one additional patient with PFS, rPFS, or no PSA progression. Lower NNT values indicate greater benefit of enzalutamide over bicalutamide. The time points at 1 and 2 years were selected because the median follow-up was 17 months for both the enzalutamide and bicalutamide arms in the STRIVE trial and 20 and 17 months for the enzalutamide and bicalutamide arms, respectively, in the TER-RAIN trial. In the TERRAIN trial at 2 years, the median time to events was reached for the majority of the evaluated clinical progression events (except rPFS).

NNT analyses were conducted separately from the STRIVE and TERRAIN trial data. For STRIVE, one- and two-year rates and standard errors of PFS, rPFS, and freedom from PSA progression with enzalutamide

and bicalutamide were derived from the available clinical study report [11]. For TERRAIN, one- and two-year rates of PFS, rPFS, and no PSA progression with enzalutamide and bicalutamide were derived from the digitized Kaplan-Meier curves. Pseudo-individual patient data were generated from the digitized Kaplan-Meier curves according to the algorithm described in Guyot et al. [15, 19] were used to estimate the standard errors of the one- and two-year rates of the end point outcomes using Greenwood's formula [20]. The 95% CIs of the rate difference were estimated based on the point estimate and standard error of each individual rate.

Results

Baseline characteristics

A total of 257 (128 enzalutamide, 129 bicalutamide) patients with chemotherapy-naïve mCRPC in STRIVE [14] and 375 (184 enzalutamide, 191 bicalutamide) patients in TERRAIN [15] were included in the analysis. At baseline, the median ages of the STRIVE patients receiving enzalutamide or bicalutamide were 71 and 72 years, respectively; in TERRAIN, the median age of patients receiving either treatment was 71 years. The majority of patients in both trials were white. The distribution of ECOG scores was similar in both trials for patients receiving enzalutamide or bicalutamide, and median serum PSA levels were higher in TERRAIN than in STRIVE (Table 2).

Rates of clinical progression in STRIVE

At 1 year, PFS rates were 59.5% for enzalutamide patients and 9.4% for bicalutamide patients in STRIVE, a difference of 50.1% (95% CI 39.5–60.7) [Table 3]. rPFS rates at 1 year were 74.0 and 35.1% for enzalutamide and bicalutamide patients, respectively, a difference of 38.9% (95% CI 24.7–53.1). At 1 year, 69.4 and 12.9% of enzalutamide and bicalutamide patients, respectively, were free from PSA progression, a difference of 56.5% (95% CI 45.4–67.7).

Table 1 Clinical outcome definitions used in the STRIVE and TERRAIN trials

Outcomes	STRIVE	TERRAIN
PFS	Time from randomization to the earliest objective evidence of PSA progression, radiographic disease progression, or death, whichever occurred first	Time from randomization to the first progression event (i.e. the earliest incidence of centrally determined radiographic disease progression, a skeletal-related event, or initiation of a new antineoplastic therapy) or death, whichever occurred first
rPFS	Time from randomization to the first objective evidence of radiographic disease progression or death, whichever occurred first	Time from randomization to the first objective evidence of radiographic disease progression or death, whichever occurred first. Radiographic progression in bone at or after Week 13 required a confirmatory bone scan
Freedom from PSA progression	Time from randomization to the earliest evidence of PSA progression, as per PCWG2 guidelines. PSA progression was defined as a > 25% increase in PSA with an absolute increase of > 2 ng/mL above the nadir	Time from randomization to the earliest evidence of a confirmed PSA progression, as per PCWG2 guidelines. PSA progression needs to be confirmed by a second consecutive value obtained ≥3 weeks later

PCWG2 Prostate Cancer Working Group 2, *PFS* progression-free survival, *PSA* prostate-specific antigen, *rPFS* radiographic progression-free survival

Table 2 Baseline characteristics of chemotherapy-naïve mCRPC patients in the STRIVE and TERRAIN trials

Baseline characteristics	STRIVE		TERRAIN	
	Enzalutamide (*n* = 128)	Bicalutamide (*n* = 129)	Enzalutamide (*n* = 184)	Bicalutamide (*n* = 191)
Age, years				
Median	71	72	71	71
Range	46–87	50–90	50–96	48–91
Race, *n* (%)				
Black or African-American	14 (10.9)	15 (11.6)	8 (4.3)	10 (5.2)
White	107 (83.6)	111 (86.0)	172 (93.4)	176 (92.1)
Other	7 (5.5)	3 (2.3)	4 (2.2)	5 (2.6)
Baseline weight, kg				
Median	91.6	88.3	88.2	86.8
Range	58.5–166.6	52.7–181.8	57.0–184.1	56.0–143.5
Body mass index, kg/m^2				
Median	30	29	28	28
Range	20–49	16–62	18–51	18–44
ECOG performance status, *n* (%)				
0	92 (71.9)	92 (71.3)	130 (70.7)	146 (76.4)
1	36 (28.1)	37 (28.7)	54 (29.3)	45 (23.6)
Serum PSA, μg/L				
Median	15.1	18.3	21	22
Range	0.0–1499.7	0.2–2849.7	0.6–5000	0.1–4681

ECOG Eastern Cooperative Oncology Group, *mCRPC* metastatic castration-resistant prostate cancer, *PSA* prostate-specific antigen

Similar to the 1-year results in STRIVE, enzalutamide resulted in superior outcomes relative to bicalutamide at 2 years (Table 3). At 2 years, PFS rates were 40.0% for enzalutamide patients and 4.1% for bicalutamide patients, a difference of 35.9% (95% CI 23.4–48.4). rPFS rates at 2 years were 56.4 and 23.2% for enzalutamide and bicalutamide patients, respectively, a difference of 33.1% (95% CI 13.9–52.4). At 2 years, 50.3 and 8.1% of enzalutamide and bicalutamide patients, respectively, were free from PSA progression, a difference of 42.2% (95% CI 27.0–57.4).

NNT in STRIVE

For STRIVE, the NNT for PFS was 2.0 (upper, lower limits: 1.6, 2.5) when comparing enzalutamide and bicalutamide; thus, treating two patients with enzalutamide resulted in one additional patient with PFS at

Table 3 Rates of PFS, rPFS, and freedom from PSA progression in the STRIVE and TERRAIN trials

Outcome	STRIVE			TERRAIN		
	Enzalutamide, %	Bicalutamide, %	Enzalutamide versus bicalutamide difference, % (95% CI)	Enzalutamide, %	Bicalutamide, %	Enzalutamide versus bicalutamide difference, % (95% CI)
PFS						
One year	59.5	9.4	50.1 (39.5–60.7)	55.0	31.7	23.3 (12.6–34.0)
Two years	40.0	4.1	35.9 (23.4–48.4)	37.8	11.0	26.8 (15.0–38.7)
rPFS						
One year	74.0	35.1	38.9 (24.7–53.1)	68.2	58.1	10.1 (−2.6–22.7)
Two years	56.4	23.2	33.1 (13.9–52.4)	61.3	25.6	35.7 (18.3–53.0)
Freedom from PSA progression						
One year	69.4	12.9	56.5 (45.4–67.7)	65.1	18.6	46.5 (34.6–58.5)
Two years	50.3	8.1	42.2 (27.0–57.4)	41.3	10.3	31.0 (16.9–45.1)

CI Confidence Interval, *PFS* progression-free survival, *PSA* prostate-specific antigen, *rPFS* radiographic progression-free survival

1 year versus treating with bicalutamide (Fig. 1). At 2 years, the NNT for PFS was 2.8 (upper, lower limits: 2.1, 4.3) when comparing enzalutamide and bicalutamide. The NNT for rPFS at 2 year was 2.6 (upper, lower limits: 1.9, 4.0) and at 2 years was 3.0 (1.9, 7.2) when comparing enzalutamide and bicalutamide. Lastly, the NNT for freedom from PSA progression was 1.8 (upper, lower limits: 1.5, 2.2) at 1 year and 2.4 (1.7, 3.7) at 2 years when comparing enzalutamide and bicalutamide.

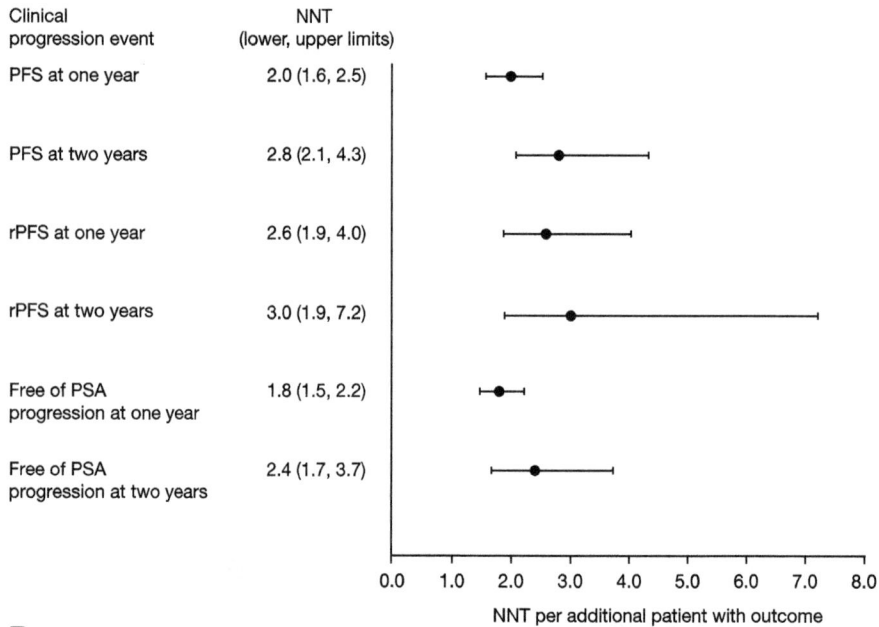

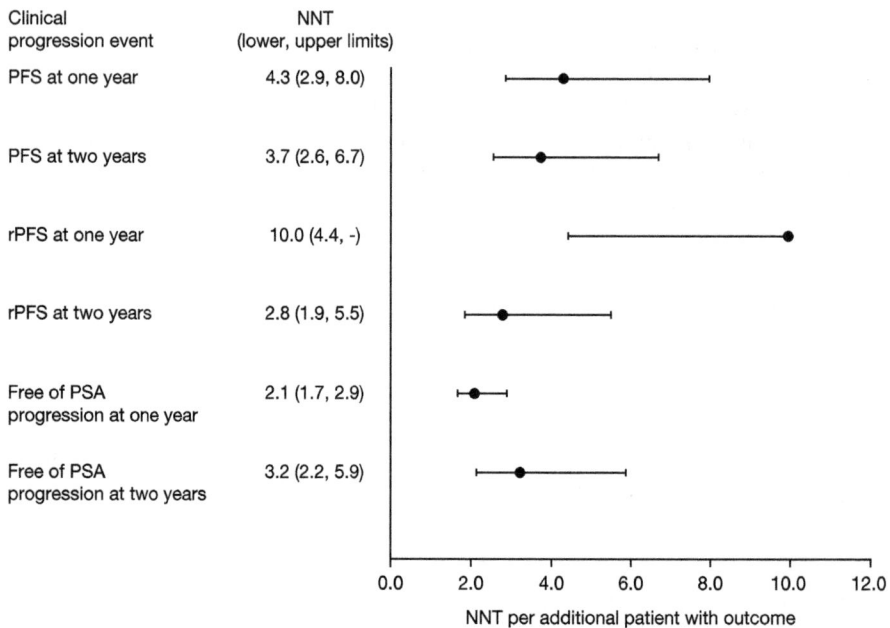

Fig. 1 NNT for PFS, rPFS, and freedom from PSA progression comparing enzalutamide with bicalutamide. NNT for the STRIVE (**a**) and TERRAIN (**b**) trials at 1 and 2 years. The lower limit of NNT for rPFS at 1 year was not reported, as the rate difference between enzalutamide with bicalutamide covers the 0, and it is not meaningful to report a negative NNT value. *NNT* number needed to treat, *PFS* progression-free survival, *PSA* prostate-specific antigen, *rPFS* radiographic progression-free survival

Rates of clinical progression in TERRAIN

At 1 year, PFS rates were 55.0% for enzalutamide patients and 31.7% for bicalutamide patients in TERRAIN, a difference of 23.3% (95% CI 12.6–34.0) [Table 3]. rPFS rates at 1 year were 68.2 and 58.1% for enzalutamide and bicalutamide patients, respectively, a difference of 10.1% (95% CI – 2.6-22.7). At 1 year, 65.1 and 18.6% of enzalutamide and bicalutamide patients, respectively, were free from PSA progression, a difference of 46.5% (95% CI 34.6–58.5).

Similar to the one-year results in TERRAIN, enzalutamide also resulted in superior outcomes relative to bicalutamide at 2 years (Table 3). At 2 years, PFS rates were 37.8% for enzalutamide patients and 11.0% for bicalutamide patients, a difference of 26.8% (95% CI 15.0–38.7). rPFS rates at 2 years were 61.3 and 25.6% for enzalutamide and bicalutamide patients, respectively, a difference of 35.7% (95% CI 18.3–53.0). Lastly, 41.3% and 10.3% of enzalutamide and bicalutamide patients, respectively, were free from PSA progression at 2 years, a difference of 31.0% (95% CI 16.9–45.1).

NNT in TERRAIN

For TERRAIN, the NNT for PFS at 1 year was 4.3 (upper, lower limits: 2.9, 8.0) and at 2 years was 3.7 (2.6, 6.7) when comparing enzalutamide with bicalutamide (Fig. 1). The NNT for rPFS at 1 year was 10.0 (upper, lower limits: 4.4, not evaluable) and at 2 years was 2.8 (1.9, 5.5) when comparing enzalutamide with bicalutamide. The NNT for freedom from PSA progression was 2.1 (upper, lower limits: 1.7, 2.9) at 1 year and 3.2 (2.2, 5.9) at 2 years when comparing enzalutamide with bicalutamide.

Discussion

This analysis used data from the STRIVE [14] and TERRAIN [15] clinical trials comparing two AR inhibitor therapies – enzalutamide and bicalutamide – for the treatment of chemotherapy-naïve patients with mCRPC to calculate NNT to avoid clinical progression. The outcomes reported in the trials were translated into NNTs, a metric of comparative efficacy that can be utilized to inform decision-making in clinical practice. The results show that at 1 year, the NNTs when comparing enzalutamide with bicalutamide in STRIVE and TERRAIN were 2.0 and 4.3, respectively for PFS; 2.6 and 10.0, respectively, for rPFS; and 1.8 and 2.1, respectively, for no PSA progression. At 2 years, the NNTs comparing enzalutamide with bicalutamide in STRIVE and TERRAIN were 2.8 and 3.7, respectively, for PFS; 3.0 and 2.8, respectively, for rPFS; and 2.4 and 3.2, respectively, for no PSA progression.

It is important to consider that NNT values estimated from the STRIVE and TERRAIN trials are generally consistent across time points and across the different clinical trial populations, with the exception of rPFS at 1 year. The NNT of rPFS at 1 year estimated from the TERRAIN trial was 10.0 and the CI of the rPFS rate difference crossed 0; however, the respective NNT value estimated from the STRIVE trial was 2.6. At 2 years, the NNTs for rPFS were similar across the trials, with the values estimated at 3.0 (upper, lower limits: 1.9, 7.2) and 2.8 (upper, lower limits: 1.9, 5.5) for STRIVE and TERRAIN, respectively. This difference indicates that the uncertainties associated with the benefit of enzalutamide versus bicalutamide decreased over the long term. Thus, the numerically lower NNT values for enzalutamide versus those for bicalutamide demonstrate that enzalutamide for mCRPC leads to more patients free from disease progression or death (i.e. PFS), radiographic disease progression, and PSA progression compared with bicalutamide at 1 and 2 years.

NNT analysis was selected to compare enzalutamide with bicalutamide for the treatment of mCRPC because it is an established and interpretable measure that can be used in clinical practice to illustrate treatment effectiveness. This approach has been previously applied in evaluating treatments in PC [21, 22]. For example, Massoudi et al. [22] compared enzalutamide with abiraterone plus prednisone using data from the PREVAIL [23] and COU-AA-302 [24, 25] clinical trials. They reported an NNT of 14 for rPFS, indicating that treating 14 patients with enzalutamide instead of abiraterone plus prednisone would yield one extra patient free of radiographic progression or death at 1 year. When comparing therapies on efficacy outcomes, in general, lower NNTs indicate treatment superiority. The smallest possible NNT is 1; a value that translates for every patient treated with a therapy, there would be a benefit that would not be reached with the comparative treatment. However, values can range widely across NNT comparisons and there is no established threshold for an NNT value to be considered clinically meaningful.

Hildebrandt et al. [26] conducted a literature review of the use of NNT calculations alongside randomized controlled trials (2003 to 2005) and noted that 62 of 734 eligible trials reported NNTs with values ranging from 2 to 325.7. Therefore, each individual NNT measure needs to be evaluated for its clinical interpretation based on the disease and outcomes used for the evaluation. That being said, the value of NNT is evident based on the emerging number of recent publications using this methodology when evaluating oncology treatment options [27–31]. In addition, the 2018 National Comprehensive Cancer Network (NCCN) guidelines for prostate cancer cite studies that report NNT estimates in the discussion of active surveillance and radical prostatectomy [7]. Furthermore, the NNT methodology provides a transparent interpretation of the relative risk for a particular outcome that can be utilized in clinical practice decision-making.

The value of the present analysis is to translate the statistically significant outcome rate differences reported in STRIVE and TERRAIN into a clear effect-size measure relevant to real-world clinical practice and treatment choice when considering enzalutamide versus bicalutamide. With the exception of the NNT for rPFS at 1 year in TERRAIN, all of the NNTs were similar and demonstrated a robust effect size and clinical benefit of enzalutamide over bicalutamide and overall agreement among the robust Phase II trials.

Historically, bicalutamide has been commonly used in the treatment of various stages of PC due to its global accessibility, relatively low cost, once-daily dosing formulation, well-established safety profile, and ability to reduce PSA levels [5, 32, 33]. Bicalutamide can be used as monotherapy or combination therapy (approved in the United States at 50 mg once daily), and its efficacy in PC has been reported in several studies. For example, a 1996 randomized, double-blind, multicenter study compared 50 mg once-daily bicalutamide plus LHRH with 250 mg (3 times a day) flutamide plus LHRH in patients with untreated metastatic PC and reported that bicalutamide was better tolerated than flutamide, although efficacy was similar [33]. Additionally, Klotz et al. [32] reported a 20% reduction in risk of death in metastatic PC patients receiving 50 mg once-daily bicalutamide compared with castration alone.

However, the recent availability of several new therapies for chemotherapy-naïve mCRPC presents opportunities for physicians and patients to optimize treatment decision-making in consideration of all approved therapeutic options and current association guidelines. In particular, among the FDA-approved treatments for chemotherapy-naïve mCRPC, enzalutamide has received recommendations in the NCCN guidelines based on Category 1 evidence, and these recommendations have been adopted in clinical practice [7, 34]. The pivotal trial of enzalutamide (PREVAIL) [23] compared the drug with placebo among chemotherapy-naïve patients and observed improved overall survival (median survival of 32.4 months vs. 30.2 months, respectively) and rPFS (65% vs. 14% at 12 months). The AFFIRM trial [35] assessed patients previously treated with docetaxel-based chemotherapy and also found improved overall survival for enzalutamide versus placebo (median survival of 18.4 months vs. 13.6 months, respectively) and improved rPFS (median of 8.3 months vs. 2.9 months, respectively). As currently discussed, both STRIVE and TERRAIN reinforced the superiority of enzalutamide over bicalutamide for chemotherapy-naïve mCRPC [14, 15]. In addition, in comparison with the PREVAIL and AFFIRM trials which allowed progression on previous bicalutamide, progression on prior bicalutamide was not allowed in the STRIVE and TERRAIN trials [14, 15, 23, 35]. Therefore, these four clinical trials showed clinical efficacy for enzalutamide among patient populations with diverse treatment history (e.g. chemotherapy-naïve, post chemotherapy, bicalutamide-naïve, and bicalutamide-experienced).

The availability of evidence from STRIVE and TERRAIN, as well as this NNT comparison, help establish optimal treatment strategies for mCRPC and may result in a change in the use of enzalutamide and bicalutamide in clinical practice. Future studies could use similar NNT methodology to indirectly compare enzalutamide with other existing and emerging hormonal therapies for the treatment of chemotherapy-naïve mCRPC. In addition, NNT analyses based on follow-up data beyond 2 years from STRIVE and TERRAIN would provide additional value.

Limitations

In addition to the previous comments regarding NNT analyses, this research is subject to the following limitations. First, patients enrolled in clinical trials might not be representative of the overall mCRPC population in real-world clinical practice. Trial-specific events and case report forms may assess outcomes more rigorously than real-world practice. Second, overall survival was not evaluated in the current analysis because the STRIVE and TERRAIN trials did not include it as a standalone end point; therefore the overall survival rate was not reported in the publications [14, 15]. Third, in this analysis, evaluations of clinical progression outcomes were limited to 1 and 2 years due to the availability of the data; however, NNT can be evaluated at additional time points. Fourth, the current NNT analysis focused on clinical efficacy; NNTs related to safety or quality-of-life outcomes were not examined, although future studies evaluating this topic would be valuable. Lastly, while this study focused on NNT comparing these two treatments, future studies should also consider evaluating the cost and cost-efficacy of these two therapies in the mCRPC population.

Conclusions

The results from the current NNT analysis of chemotherapy-naïve mCRPC patients in STRIVE and TERRAIN indicate that treatment with enzalutamide will lead to more patients free from disease progression or death (i.e. PFS), radiographic disease progression, and PSA progression compared with bicalutamide at 1 and 2 years. In addition to the results of STRIVE and TERRAIN, this analysis may assist physicians and patients in choosing the optimal treatment for mCRPC.

Abbreviations

AR: Androgen receptor; CI: Confidence Interval; CRPC: Castration-resistant prostate cancer; ECOG: Eastern Cooperative Oncology Group; FDA: United States Food and Drug Administration; LHRH: Luteinizing hormone-releasing hormone; mCRPC: Metastatic castration-resistant prostate cancer; NCCN: National Comprehensive Cancer Network; NNT: Number needed to treat; PC: Prostate cancer; PFS: Progression-free survival; PSA: Prostate-specific antigen; rPFS: Radiographic progression-free survival

Acknowledgments

Medical writing assistance was provided by Shelley Batts, PhD, an employee of Analysis Group, Inc. Editorial assistance was provided by Lauren Smith, from Complete HealthVizion, and funded by the study sponsors.

Funding

This research was funded by Astellas Pharma, Inc. and Medivation, Inc., which was acquired by Pfizer, Inc. in September 2016, the co-developers of enzalutamide. Medical writing and editing were funded by the study sponsors.

Authors' contributions

The study sponsor was involved in all stages of the study research and manuscript preparation, but all authors participated in the design of the study, contributed to manuscript development, and made the decision to submit the work for publication. Data were extracted from the STRIVE and TERRAIN trial publications by Analysis Group, Inc. and analyzed and interpreted in collaboration with all other authors. Manuscript drafts were prepared by the authors, with editorial assistance from a professional medical writer. All the authors vouch for the accuracy and completeness of the data reported.

Competing interests

NMS, SCF and BAB are employees of Astellas and own stock/stock options at the time of this manuscript, however, SCF and BAB are no longer employees presently of Astellas. AB was an employee of Medivation at the time of the study and owns stock/stock options. NDS has been a consultant/advisor for Amgen, Astellas, Bayer, Dendreon, Ferring, Janssen, Medivation, Sanofi, Takeda, and Inovio and has participated in speaker bureaus for Janssen, Bayer, and Dendreon. SC has acted as a consultant/advisor for Astellas and Janssen and has participated in speaker bureaus for Janssen, Sanofi, Clovis Oncology, and Astellas. LHK reports honoraria for advisory board participation from Astellas, Medivation, Janssen, Amgen, Genomic Health, and AbbVie, outside the submitted work. RSC has been a consultant/advisor for CUSP, Integra Connect, and Dendreon and reports honoraria for participation in speaker bureaus for Astellas, Medivation, Janssen, Bayer, and Sanofi. DFP has been a consultant for Astellas, Medivation, and Dendreon. LIK has been a consultant for 3DBiopsy, Argos, Tokai, Takeda, Heat Biologics, Augmenix, Dendreon, Astellas, Bayer, Janssen, Medivation, and Sanofi, has participated in speaker bureaus for Astellas, Bayer, Janssen, Medivation, Amgen, and Dendreon, has received research funding from Astellas, Bayer, Janssen, Medivation, Sanofi, Spectrum, Ferring, Precision Biopsy, 3DBiopsy, Argos, Tokai, Takeda, Heat Biologics, Augmenix, and Dendreon through his institution, and owns stock options with Swan Valley Medical. HY is an employee of Analysis Group Inc., which has received consultancy fees from Astellas and Medivation.

Author details

[1]Astellas Pharma, Inc., 1 Astellas Way, Northbrook, IL 60062, USA. [2]Carolina Urologic Research Center, Myrtle Beach, SC, USA. [3]Guy's, King's, and St. Thomas' Hospitals, London, UK. [4]Sunnybrook Health Sciences Centre, University of Toronto, Toronto, ON, Canada. [5]Urology Associates, P.C., Nashville, TN, USA. [6]Vanderbilt University Medical Center, Nashville, TN, USA. [7]The Urology Center of Colorado, Denver, CO, USA. [8]Analysis Group, Inc., Boston, MA, USA. [9]Medivation, Inc., San Francisco, TN, USA. [10]Pfizer, Inc., New York, NY, USA.

References

1. Ferlay J, Soerjomataram I, Ervik M, Dikshit R, Eser S, Mathers C, et al. GLOBOCAN 2012 v1.0, Cancer Incidence and Mortality Worldwide: IARC CancerBase No. 11. 2014. http://globocan.iarc.fr. Accessed 22 Mar 2018.
2. Siegel RL, Miller KD, Jemal A. Cancer statistics, 2016. CA Cancer J Clin. 2016; 66(1):7–30.
3. Cornford P, Bellmunt J, Bolla M, Briers E, De Santis M, Gross T, et al. EAU-ESTRO-SIOG guidelines on prostate cancer. Part II: treatment of relapsing, metastatic, and castration-resistant prostate cancer. Eur Urol. 2017;71(4):630–42.
4. Kirby M, Hirst C, Crawford ED. Characterising the castration-resistant prostate cancer population: a systematic review. Int J Clin Pract. 2011;65(11):1180–92.
5. Schellhammer PF, Sharifi R, Block NL, Soloway MS, Venner PM, Patterson AL, et al. Clinical benefits of bicalutamide compared with flutamide in combined androgen blockade for patients with advanced prostatic carcinoma: final report of a double-blind, randomized, multicenter trial. Urology. 1997;50(3):330–6.
6. Food and Drug Administration. Highlights of prescribing information: bicalutamide tablets. 2009. http://www.accessdata.fda.gov/drugsatfda_docs/label/2009/076932s000lbl.pdf. Accessed 11 Apr 2017.
7. National Comprehensive Cancer Network. NCCN clinical practice guidelines in oncology (NCCN guidelines®). Prostate Cancer 2018. https://www.nccn.org/professionals/physician_gls/pdf/prostate.pdf. Accessed 19 Mar 2018.
8. Roviello G, Sigala S, Sandhu S, Bonetta A, Cappelletti MR, Zanotti L, et al. Role of the novel generation of androgen receptor pathway targeted agents in the management of castration-resistant prostate cancer: a literature based meta-analysis of randomized trials. Eur J Cancer. 2016;61: 111–21.
9. Food and Drug Administration. Xtandi [package insert]. 2015. http://www.accessdata.fda.gov/drugsatfda_docs/label/2015/203415s007lbl.pdf. Accessed 11 Apr 2017.
10. Rathkopf D, Scher HI. Androgen receptor antagonists in castration-resistant prostate cancer. Cancer J. 2013;19(1):43–9.
11. Schalken J, Fitzpatrick JM. Enzalutamide: targeting the androgen signalling pathway in metastatic castration-resistant prostate cancer. BJU Int. 2016; 117(2):215–25.
12. Basch E, Loblaw DA, Oliver TK, Carducci M, Chen RC, Frame JN, et al. Systemic therapy in men with metastatic castration-resistant prostate cancer: American Society of Clinical Oncology and Cancer Care Ontario clinical practice guideline. J Clin Oncol. 2014;32(30):3436–48.
13. Cookson MS, Roth BJ, Dahm P, Engstrom C, Freedland SJ, Hussain M, et al. Castration-resistant prostate cancer: AUA guideline. 2015. http://www.auanet.org/common/pdf/education/clinical-guidance/Castration-Resistant-Prostate-Cancer.pdf. Accessed 11 Apr 2017.
14. Penson DF, Armstrong AJ, Concepcion R, Agarwal N, Olsson C, Karsh L, et al. Enzalutamide versus bicalutamide in castration-resistant prostate cancer: the STRIVE trial. J Clin Oncol. 2016;34(18):2098–106.
15. Shore N, Chowdhury S, Villers A, Klotz L, Siemens DR, Phung D, et al. Efficacy and safety of enzalutamide versus bicalutamide for patients with metastatic prostate cancer (TERRAIN): a randomised, double-blind, phase 2 study. Lancet Oncol. 2016;17(2):153–63.
16. Laupacis A, Sackett DL, Roberts RS. An assessment of clinically useful measures of the consequences of treatment. N Engl J Med. 1988;318(26): 1728–33.
17. Center for Drug Evaluation and Research Office of Translational Sciences. Manual of Policies and Procedures. Good Review Practice: Statistical Review Template. 2012. http://www.fda.gov/downloads/aboutfda/centersoffices/officeofmedicalproductsandtobacco/cder/manualofpoliciesprocedures/ucm313814.pdf. Accessed 23 Mar 2017.
18. Oken MM, Creech RH, Tormey DC, Horton J, Davis TE, McFadden ET, et al. Toxicity and response criteria of the Eastern Cooperative Oncology Group. Am J Clin Oncol. 1982;5(6):649–55.
19. Guyot P, Ades AE, Ouwens MJ, Welton NJ. Enhanced secondary analysis of survival data: reconstructing the data from published Kaplan-Meier survival curves. BMC Med Res Methodol. 2012;12:9.
20. Greenwood M. A report on the natural duration of cancer. London: HMSO; 1926.
21. Dranitsaris G, Hatzimichael E. Interpreting results from oncology clinical trials: a comparison of denosumab to zoledronic acid for the prevention of skeletal-related events in cancer patients. Support Care Cancer. 2012;20(7): 1353–60.
22. Massoudi M, Balk M, Yang H, Bui CN, Pandya BJ, Guo J, et al. Number needed to treat and associated incremental costs of treatment with enzalutamide versus abiraterone acetate plus prednisone in chemotherapy-

naïve patients with metastatic castration-resistant prostate cancer. J Med Econ. 2017;20(2):121–8.

23. Beer TM, Armstrong AJ, Rathkopf DE, Loriot Y, Sternberg CN, Higano CS, et al. Enzalutamide in metastatic prostate cancer before chemotherapy. N Engl J Med. 2014;371(5):424–33.

24. Ryan CJ, Smith MR, de Bono JS, Molina A, Logothetis CJ, de Souza P, et al. Abiraterone in metastatic prostate cancer without previous chemotherapy. N Engl J Med. 2013;368(2):138–48.

25. Ryan CJ, Smith MR, Fizazi K, Saad F, Mulders PFA, Sternberg CN, et al. Abiraterone acetate plus prednisone versus placebo plus prednisone in chemotherapy-naive men with metastatic castration-resistant prostate cancer (COU-AA-302): final overall survival analysis of a randomised, double-blind, placebo-controlled phase 3 study. Lancet Oncol. 2015;16(2):152–60.

26. Hildebrandt M, Vervölgyi E, Bender R. Calculation of NNTs in RCTs with time-to-event outcomes: a literature review. BMC Med Res Methodol. 2009;9:21.

27. Anderson D, Lehmann J, Ecker T, Vosgerau S, Donatz V. Cost effectiveness of GnRH antagonists in patients with prostate cancer and cardiovascular risk: comparative analysis against Leuprorelin by the number needed to treat. Urologe A. 2017;56(7):917–24.

28. de Carvalho TM, Heijnsdijk EAM, de Koning HJ. Estimating the individual benefit of immediate treatment or active surveillance for prostate cancer after screen-detection in older (65+) men. Int J Cancer. 2016;138(10):2522–8.

29. Frandsen J, Orton A, Shrieve D, Tward J. Risk of death from prostate cancer with and without definitive local therapy when Gleason pattern 5 is present: a surveillance, epidemiology, and end results analysis. Cureus. 2017; 9(7):e1453.

30. Ho R, Rufino C, Simões J, Alves M. Number Needed to Treat (NNT) and Cost of Preventing an Event (COPE) comparison between the Association of Cobimetinib and Vemurafenib among other treatment options for metastatic melanoma with BRAF V600 mutation. Value Health. 2017;20(9):A875.

31. Löppenberg B, Dalela D, Karabon P, Sood A, Sammon JD, Meyer CP, et al. The impact of local treatment on overall survival in patients with metastatic prostate cancer on diagnosis: a national cancer data base analysis. Eur Urol. 2017;72(1):14–9.

32. Klotz L, Schellhammer P, Carroll K. A re-assessment of the role of combined androgen blockade for advanced prostate cancer. BJU Int. 2004;93(9):1177–82.

33. Schellhammer P, Sharifi R, Block N, Soloway M, Venner P, Patterson AL, et al. Maximal androgen blockade for patients with metastatic prostate cancer: outcome of a controlled trial of bicalutamide versus flutamide, each in combination with luteinizing hormone-releasing hormone analogue therapy. Urology. 1996;47(1A Suppl 1):54–60.

34. Ellis LA, Lafeuille MH, Gozalo L, Pilon D, Lefebvre P, McKenzie S. Treatment sequences and pharmacy costs of 2 new therapies for metastatic castration-resistant prostate cancer. Am Health Drug Benefits. 2015;8(4):185–95.

35. Scher HI, Fizazi K, Saad F, Taplin ME, Sternberg CN, Miller K, et al. Increased survival with enzalutamide in prostate cancer after chemotherapy. N Engl J Med. 2012;367(13):1187–97.

21

The Terry Fox Research Institute Canadian Prostate Cancer Biomarker Network: an analysis of a pan-Canadian multi-center cohort for biomarker validation

Véronique Ouellet[1], Armen Aprikian[2], Alain Bergeron[3], Fadi Brimo[4], Robert G. Bristow[5,6], Simone Chevalier[2], Darrel Drachenberg[7], Ladan Fazli[8], Neil E. Fleshner[6,9], Martin Gleave[8,10], Pierre Karakiewicz[11,12], Laurence Klotz[13], Louis Lacombe[3], Jean-Baptiste Lattouf[1,12], Theodorus van der Kwast[6], Jeremy A. Squire[14,17], Mathieu Latour[1,15], Dominique Trudel[1,15], Anne-Marie Mes-Masson[1,16] and Fred Saad[1,12]*

Abstract

Background: Refinement of parameters defining prostate cancer (PC) prognosis are urgently needed to identify patients with indolent versus aggressive disease. The Canadian Prostate Cancer Biomaker Network (CPCBN) consists of researchers from four Canadian provinces to create a validation cohort to address issues dealing with PC diagnosis and management.

Methods: A total of 1512 radical prostatectomy (RP) specimens from five different biorepositories affiliated with teaching hospitals were selected to constitute the cohort. Tumoral and adjacent benign tissues were arrayed on tissue microarrays (TMAs). A patient clinical database was developed and includes data on diagnosis, treatment and clinical outcome.

Results: Mean age at diagnosis of patients in the cohort was 61 years. Of these patients, 31% had a low grade (≤6) Gleason score (GS), 55% had GS 7 (40% of 3 + 4 and 15% of 4 + 3) and 14% had high GS (≥8) PC. The median follow-up of the cohort was 113 months. A total of 34% had a biochemical relapse, 4% developed bone metastasis and 3% of patients died from PC while 9% died of other causes. Pathological review of the TMAs confirmed the presence of tumor and benign tissue cores for > 94% of patients. Immunohistochemistry and FISH analyses, performed on a small set of specimens, showed high quality results and no biorepository-specific bias.

Conclusions: The CPCBN RP cohort is representative of real world PC disease observed in the Canadian population. The frequency of biochemical relapse and bone metastasis as events allows for a precise assessment of the prognostic value of biomarkers. This resource is available, in a step-wise manner, for researchers who intend to validate prognostic biomarkers in PC. Combining multiple biomarkers with clinical and pathologic parameters that are predictive of outcome will aid in clinical decision-making for patients treated for PC.

Keywords: Prostate cancer, Tissue microarray, Biomarker validation, Immunohistochemistry, Patient prognosis

* Correspondence: fredsaad@videotron.ca
[1]Institut du cancer de Montréal and Centre de recherche du Centre hospitalier de l'Université de Montréal, 900, St-Denis St, room R10-464, Montréal, Québec H2X 0A9, Canada
[12]Department of Surgery, Université de Montréal, Montréal, Québec, Canada
Full list of author information is available at the end of the article

Background

The inability to clearly distinguish indolent versus aggressive disease is a major challenge for physicians caring for patients with prostate cancer (PC) [1]. Patients are stratified into groups ranging from very low to very high risk based on prostate-specific antigen (PSA) levels at time of diagnosis, tumor Gleason score (GS) in biopsies, and tumor stage at clinical presentation [2–4]. However, the biology of PC reflects a multifocal and multiclonal nature of tumors that is far more complex than initial predictions from current clinical parameters [5–7].

Foremost, the prognostic ability of new biomarkers should determine the risk for lethal PC and track disease progression in order for the therapy to be modified [2]. Several emerging biomarker candidates have been described; none so far have been fully validated or robust enough to be added to clinical parameters used in practice. Tissue microarrays (TMAs) represent a high-throughput platform to apply protein- and nucleotide-based assays enabling biomarker testing within a single tumor core [3] of hundreds of patient samples simultaneously [8]. Current strategies aspire to multiplex approaches combining current clinical parameters with a comprehensive panel of biomarkers to improve diagnostic accuracy of disease status and resolve the heterogeneity that confounds risk stratification in PC [2].

The Canadian Prostate Cancer Biomarker Network (CPCBN) represents a community of clinicians and researchers that is committed to improving the clinical management of PC. The CPCBN initiative is a validation rather than discovery platform and invites biomarker proposals from all researchers with preliminary evidence demonstrating their utility in PC management. An application to access the TMA platform is available on the CPCBN website, along with details on the CPCBN program and affiliated partners http://www.tfri.ca/en/research/translational-research/cpcbn.aspx). A compilation of potential biomarkers has already been reviewed and studies are underway using the radical prostatectomy (RP) cohort. Data for well-known PC biomarkers such as ERG, PTEN, Ki67 and AR will be available to researchers upon request. This platform serves as an invaluable resource for the entire PC research community, accelerating breakthroughs in PC research, and supporting the establishment of nomograms to predict patient progression.

In this study, we report a TMA-based validation process which includes assembly of a retrospective multi-center RP cohort to build TMAs that will evaluate both biomarkers and their utility in identifying patients at high risk for biochemical recurrence (BCR) and the development of metastases or PC-specific mortality. To ensure homogeneity across sites, we used the Canadian Tumor Repository Network (CTRNet, www.ctrnet.ca) standards for quality assurance and developed standard operating procedures (SOPs). We also report on the quality control of this RP TMA series with quality assessments and controls, focusing on the TMA suitability for immunohistochemistry (IHC) and fluorescence in situ hybridization (FISH) techniques.

Methods

Patient cohort and participating centers

RP specimens were selected from five different biobanks affiliated with academic health care centers across Canada: Centre hospitalier de l'Université de Montréal (CHUM), CHU de Québec-Université Laval (CHUdeQ-UL), McGill University Health Centre (MUHC), Vancouver Prostate Centre (VPC), and University Health Network (UHN). The selected specimens were biobanked between 1990 and 2011. All patients signed an informed consent to participate within one of the above listed biobanks and agreed to the use of their specimens and data for research purposes. Inclusion criteria included: RP specimens archived as formalin-fixed paraffin-embedded (FFPE) blocks, treatment (hormone or chemotherapy) naïve patients with a minimum follow-up of 24 months. Patients with severe comorbidity were naturally excluded as they are not candidates for RP surgery. Each center received ethical approval from their Institutional Review Board (IRB) for biobanking activity and for their contributions to the CPCBN. CTRNet standards were followed for quality assurance and ensured appropriate handling of human tissue.

Clinical data management

Clinical data for each patient were collated into an Advanced Tissue Management (ATiM) database developed by the CTRNet and customized for the CPCBN. Complete clinical data provided the month and year of diagnosis and surgery, age, pretreatment PSA level, pathologic stage, Gleason grade, margin status, date of BCR, PSA progression, development of metastasis, and treatments received following RP when applicable. BCR endpoints were based on serum PSA measurement in three different conditions: PSA levels of 0.2 ng/mL and rising, a PSA level followed by salvage/adjuvant treatment and finally, when initial post-operative PSA levels were greater than 0.2 ng/mL and rising following surgery (failed RP). Appearance of bone metastasis and PC mortality were considered ultimate endpoints.

TMA construction

TMA construction was performed at each site: CHUM, UHN, and VPC used the TMArrayer (Pathology Devices, Inc., Westminster, MD, USA), while the CHUdeQ-UL and MUHC used the manual tissue arrayer, MTA-1

(Beecher Instruments, WI, USA). A pathologist selected the FFPE block, and the area of interest (tumor or adjacent benign) was circled directly onto the hematoxylin and eosin (H&E) stained slide. Cores of 0.6 mm were extracted from the corresponding FFPE block and arrayed on a receiver paraffin block. A SOP was developed and guided the construction of the different TMA series.

TMA design

To build the quality control TMA (QC-TMA), a TMA block was circulated across four sites where three tumor cores from 10 PC specimens were arrayed to evaluate the feasibility of the multi-center resource. Due to specific institution requirements, one site arrayed their specimens on a separate TMA, resulting in two QC-TMA blocks. However, sections were combined onto the same glass slide for subsequent analyses. The optimization TMA (OPT-TMA) was constructed at the CHUM and included banked tissues from 15 RP, 5 breast cancer and 5 ovarian cancer cases along with mouse xenograft tissues derived from human PC cell lines 22RV1, LNCaP, DU145 and PC3. The Test-TMA series was composed of 250 RP specimens selected from four biobanks: CHUM, MUHC, CHUdeQ-UL (50 RP specimens each), and VPC (100 RP specimens). Each TMA block contained three cores of tumor and two cores of adjacent benign tissues from 50 RP cases. The Validation-TMA series contain prostate tissues from 1262 specimens across five centers. Three to four cores of tumor and one to two cores of adjacent benign tissues were arrayed on receiver blocks. Validation-TMAs also contained 50 RP cases per block with a few exceptions. On each TMA block composing the test or the validation series, two cores of the 4 PC cell line-derived xenografts used for the OPT-TMA were also included. After a first pathology review, cores were repunched as necessary and resulted in a total of seven TMA blocks for the Test-TMA and 31 TMA blocks for the Validation-TMA series.

IHC staining and analysis

Tissue quality was assessed with the following markers: PSMA, PSA, p63, P504s, P501s, Ki67, AR, CK18, and HMW-CK. Details about antibody sources, dilutions, antigen retrieval and incubation conditions are described in Additional file 1. QC-TMA slides were stained at the coordinating center (CHUM) using the BenchMark XT automated stainer (Ventana Medical System Inc.). TMA slides were scanned and assessed visually for analysis (OlyVIA, Olympus, ON, Canada). Two independent observers blindly scored the percentage of stained cells for all markers except for PSA and CK18 where the intensity of staining was also evaluated.

FISH analysis

The *PTEN* FISH probe consisting in a four-color probe combination detecting *PTEN, WAPAL, FAS* and *CEP 10*, was obtained from CymoGenDx/Biocare Medical (Concord, CA) and was used as previously described [9]. The pathologist selected areas of TMA sections stained with DAPI, which were analyzed against immediately adjacent sections stained with H&E. *PTEN* copy number was determined by counting signals of all four markers in 50–100 distinct and intact interphase nuclei per tumor core using SemRock filters selected for excitation/emission spectra of each probe. Cores that showed visible deletions were scored by reviewing 50 cells per core. Hemizygous (single copy) *PTEN* deletion denoted cores with 50% of nuclei exhibiting clonal loss of *PTEN* whereas homozygous *PTEN* deletion was assigned to cores with loss of both *PTEN* loci in 30% of nuclei.

Central pathology review

Central pathology review assessed RP specimens of the QC-TMA, Test-TMA and Validation-TMA series. Scoring criteria included GS, the amount of glandular tissue present, and specificity of the core nature in terms of adjacent benign, cancer, prostatic intraepithelial neoplasia (PIN), intraductal carcinoma (IDC), atypical small acinar proliferation (ASAP), stroma, muscle or inflammation [10]. Upon review, cores were qualified as informative if the specific tissue of interest (adjacent benign or cancer) was present in at least 5 to 10% of the core area. Additional cores were requested for replacement if less than two cores for either tumor or adjacent benign tissues did not meet established criteria. Replacement cores were reviewed and added to a new or existing array, and if tissue samples were depleted, additional cores or patients were included to complete the full cohort.

Statistical analyses

Hierarchical clustering analysis of markers assessed in the QC-TMA was performed with Genespring software (Agilent Genomics, CA, USA) using Pearson correlation as a similarity measure and an average linkage-clustering algorithm. Survival analyses (Cox regression and Kaplan-Meier curves) were performed using the IBM SPSS Statistics (Version 23) software.

Results

Feasibility of the multi-center TMA-based resource

A quality control TMA (QC-TMA) was constructed (Fig. 1, left column) using three cores from 10 PC specimens with GS 7 from each of the five biorepositories. The 150 cores composing this array were evaluated for tissue integrity, antigenicity, and performance in protein and nucleic acid-based assays. These cores were tumors of expected Gleason grade (in at least 2/3 cores) in 94% (47/50)

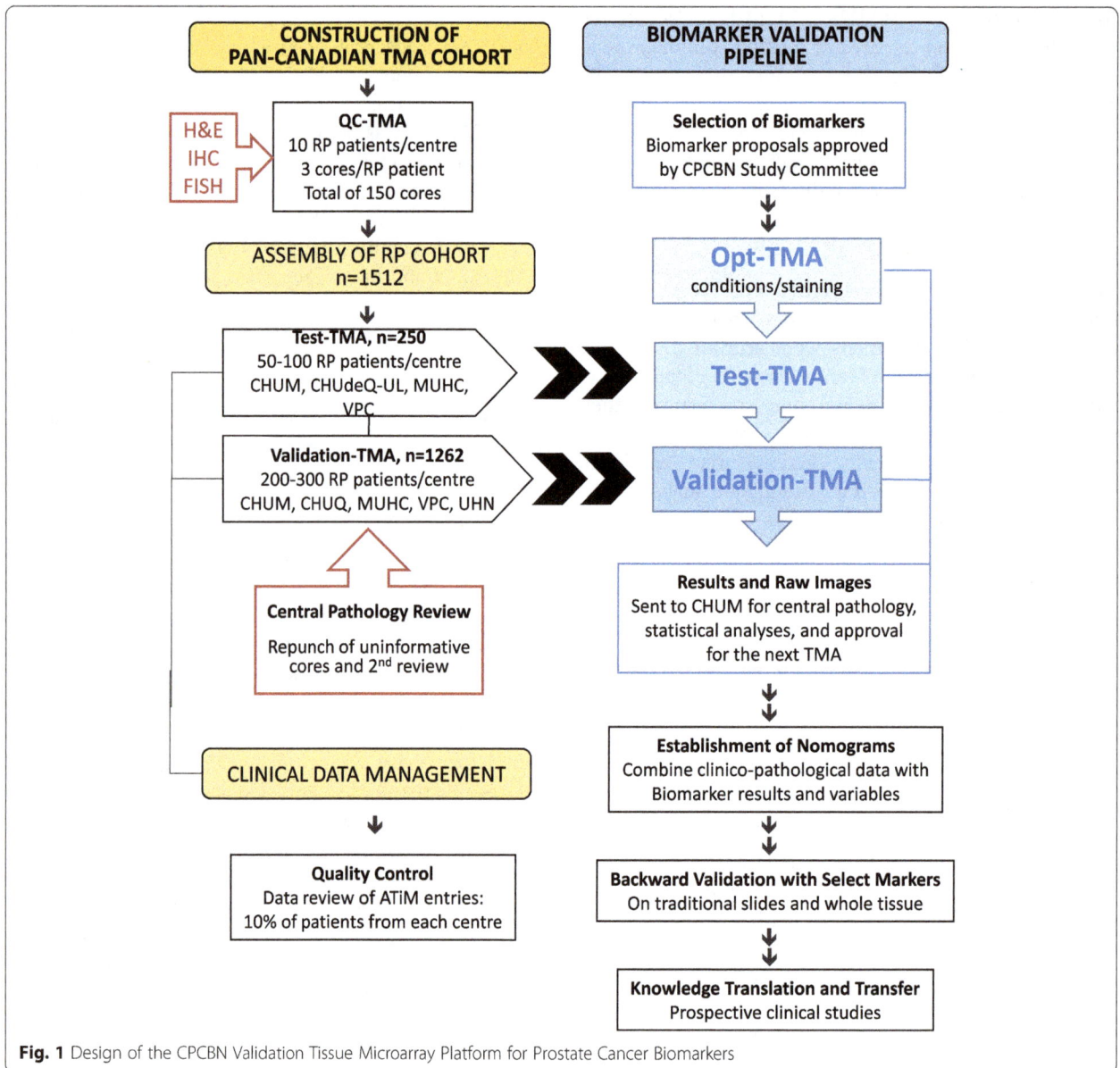

Fig. 1 Design of the CPCBN Validation Tissue Microarray Platform for Prostate Cancer Biomarkers

of samples. Tissue integrity and antigenicity was determined by evaluation of the expression of nine different markers with nuclear and/or cytoplasmic localization (Ki67, AR, CK18) in addition to markers that distinguish tumor vs. benign glands (HMW-CK, p63, and P504S/AMACR) or proteins usually expressed by prostate cells (PSA, P501S and PSMA) (Fig. 2a). Hierarchal clustering using a Pearson centered distance metric was based on the detection of these nine markers. Hierarchal clustering demonstrated that there was no site-specific bias (Fig. 2b).

Analysis of FISH data using the four-probe FISH assay, showed that *PTEN* deletions were hemizygous or homozygous at 15.5% each, whereas the majority of cores

displayed no *PTEN* deletions (69%) (Fig. 3a-d). The FISH results reflected the quality of the cores, reported as very good, intermediate or poor (Fig. 3e). Approximately 13% of cores were considered of poor quality because the core was either absent due to mechanical processing/sectioning, over-digested, or else, yielded a poor signal (Additional file 2). These results highlighted the need for potential modifications for TMA FISH protocols to optimize digestion and reduce background signal. Nonetheless, PTEN status was assessed for 87% of the cores. Overall, the QC-TMA demonstrated the feasibility of co-ordinating a large multi-institutional cohort with specimens of acceptable quality on which protein and DNA markers could be assessed.

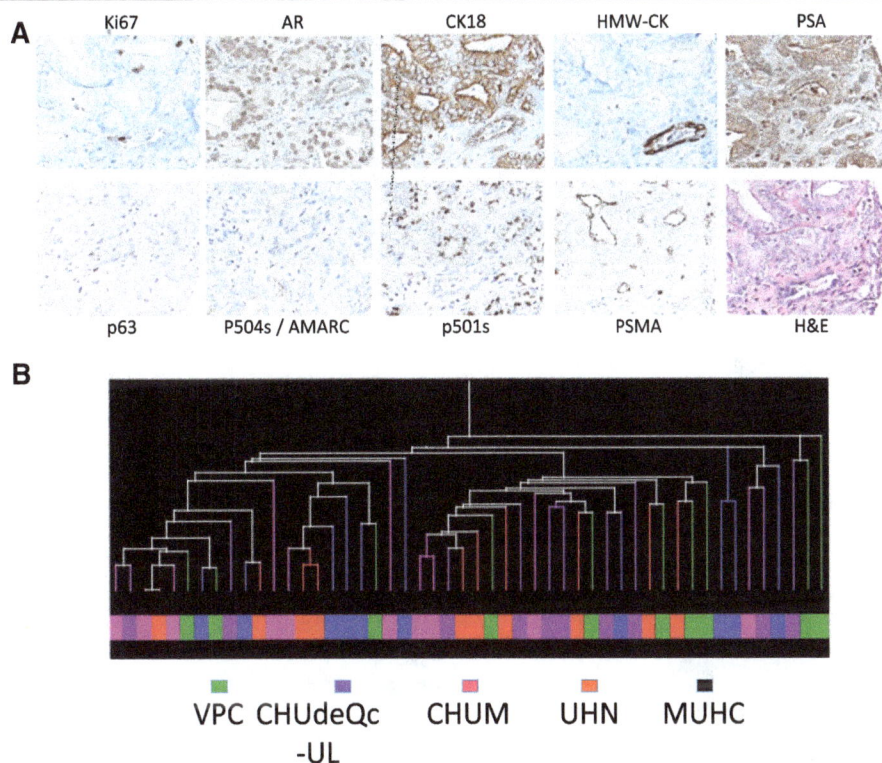

Fig. 2 Immunohistochemistry and hierarchal clustering analysis of biobanked specimens arrayed in the QC-TMA, representing 50 radical prostatectomy cases from five different centres (total of 150 cores). **a** IHC evaluation with nine protein tissue markers. **b** Hierarchal clustering based on IHC detection of the nine different markers in samples of different center origin, corresponding to the colour legend below

Design and strategy of a biomarker validation process

Under the pipeline scheme (Fig. 1, right column), a study committee comprised of pathologists, clinicians and researchers selects promising markers for access to TMA resources and clinical data according to specific criteria (Table 1). This is followed by sequential evaluation through the TMA series starting with the OPT-TMA, which confirms reproducibility and reliability of staining conditions and reagents on different tissues. Upon successful completion of this step, the Test-TMA ($n = 250$), which evaluates the biomarker strength within a small subset representing the RP cohort, is released to the investigator. Finally, after evaluation of the performance of the biomarker, the large Validation-TMA, which contains the remaining cases of the entire RP cohort ($n = 1262$) is released. Both the OPT-TMA and Test-TMA represent checkpoints that determine whether biomarkers can advance along the pipeline. In the end, raw data and images are compiled and transferred to the coordinating center (CHUM) for repository and central pathology review, and secured for future nomogram development. This nomogram, once validated, could be used in a clinical setting to discriminate patients that would need a more aggressive treatment compared to those with a favorable prognosis.

Test and validation TMA evaluation

Each center selected 300 RP cases to build the Test and Validation TMAs. A central pathologist reviewed each TMA block to ensure the high quality of the resource (Table 2). Core assessments for sufficient material and accurate tissue representation (cancer or adjacent benign) determined which patient samples required additional cores. At least 2 cores of tumor tissues were arrayed from a total of 1429 patients (95%) whereas 1047 patients (69%) had 3 cores or more (Table 3). For the benign adjacent tissue, at least 1 core was obtained for 1496 patients (99%) and 2 cores for 1212 patients (80%) (Table 3).

Clinical data management

A central ATiM database was created and customized for the CPCBN repository in which clinical data were entered and yearly updated using a standardized process. The database was subjected to quality control measures to assess the degree of entry error or missing information across all centers (Fig. 1, left panel). An audit was performed on entries for 10% of patients contributed by each site. Based on this exercise, 6 out of 6309 data entries resulted in an error rate of 0.09%, which was taken

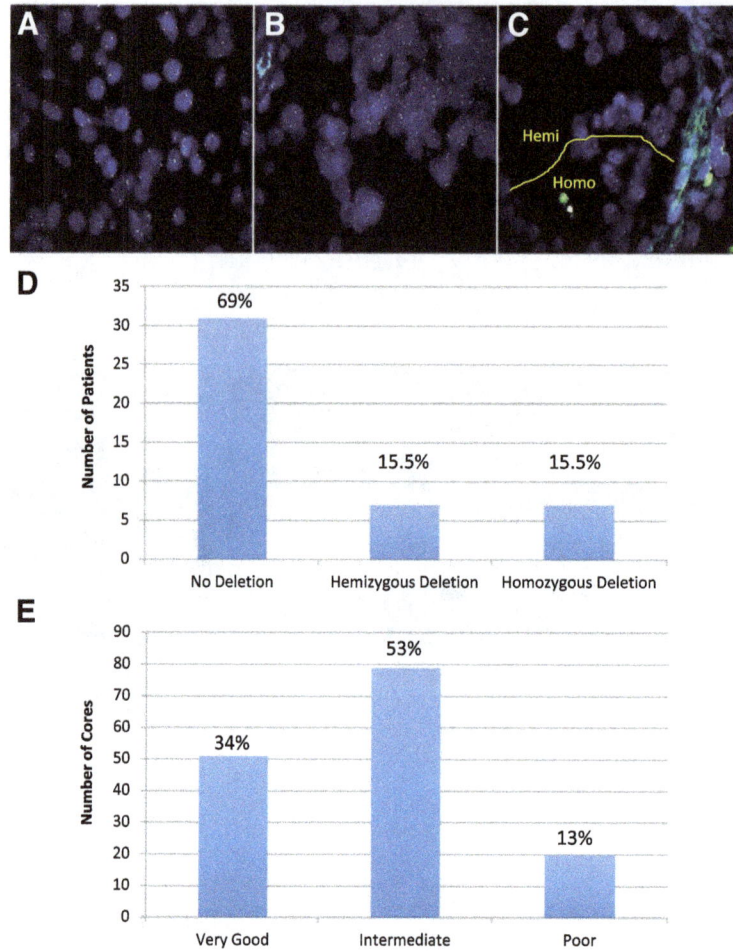

Fig. 3 Fluorescence in-situ hybridization of the QC-TMA, with DNA probes detecting *PTEN* (orange), *WAPAL* (green), *FAS* (aqua), and *CEP* 10 (red). **a** Cells representing no *PTEN* deletion. **b** Cells showing homozygous *PTEN* deletion with relative hemizygous loss of *WAPAL* and *FAS* signal. **c** Cells in the same gland showing homozygous (Homo) and hemizygous (Hemi) *PTEN* deletions. **d** *PTEN* deletion status among the 50 patients in the QC-TMA. **e** Overall quality assessment of 150 cores for FISH analysis. Intermediate quality was assigned to 53% of cores that had a detectable *PTEN* deletion status but also had high background to signal ratios or had areas that were over-digested. Very good quality was observed for 34% of cores that produced strong signal over low background and even digestion throughout (Additional file 2)

Table 1 Biomarker selection criteria and considerations

Interest of the biomarker based on extensive preliminary data

Relevance to CPCBN objectives and clinical impact for prostate cancer

Cohort size used to determine biomarker status

Assay performed on paraffin-embedded tissue or TMA

Staining quality and requirements that include the following:
 • Reliable staining against controls and background levels using an automated stainer
 • Antibody specificity validated by western blot or IHC/immunofluorescence with appropriate controls
 • Preferences towards monoclonal antibody use
 • Preferences towards digital image analysis

Specific role in prostate cancer prognosis and supporting statistical data (BCR, development of metastasis, *p* value)

Sufficient resources for biomarker analysis (proposed laboratory, supportive infrastructure, funding, and partners)

Table 2 Central pathology review of all tissue cores contributing to the Test- and Validation-TMA series

	Sites				
	CHUM	CHUdeQ-UL	MUHC	UHN	VPC
EXPECTED BENIGN CORES	623	545	627	773	691
Reviewed as Benign	597	436	485	673	511
Reviewed as Cancer	0	19	67	25	88
Reviewed as Uninformative[a]	26	90	75	75	92
EXPECTED TUMOR CORES	954	1269	953	1042	1135
Reviewed as Cancer	845	944	707	825	825
Reviewed as Benign	52	133	109	109	192
Reviewed as Uninformative[a]	57	192	137	108	118

[a]Prostatic intraepithelial neoplasia, intraductal carcinoma, atypical small acinar proliferation, < 5% tumor cells, stroma only, muscle or inflammation

Table 3 Number and nature of cores included in the Test- and Validation-TMA series after central pathology review

Sites	Number of Patients	Number of Tumor Cores per Patient					Number of Benign Adjacent Cores per Patient				
		0	1	2	3	> 4	0	1	2	3	> 4
CHUM	304	2	6	55	236	5	1	16	241	37	9
CHUdeQ-UL	301	1	9	65	98	128	4	130	104	36	27
MUHC	304	6	26	93	167	12	5	50	208	37	4
UHN	303	9	10	111	119	54	1	37	177	28	60
VPC	300	5	9	58	165	63	5	51	162	49	33
Total	1512	23	60	382	785	262	16	284	892	187	133

into account for standardization of data and future database updates (data not shown).

Demographic of the CPCBN cohort

The median patient follow-up of patients was approximately 9.8 years, and a sufficient number of patients presented with endpoint elements such as BCR (34%), development of bone metastasis (4.3%) and death from PC (2.6%) to perform statistical analyses. Details on the clinico-pathological data of cohorts of patients whose prostate tissues were included in the Test-TMA as well as the Validation-TMA are presented in Table 4. In order to determine if the CPCBN cohort was representative of a general PC cohort, Cox regression analyses and Kaplan-Meier curves coupled with log-rank tests were performed using clinical parameters known to be associated with patient prognosis. As expected, PSA serum levels prior to surgery, pathological TNM, Gleason grade and margin status showed an association with BCR in both Test and Validation cohorts (Table 5 and Fig. 4). All clinical parameters except for margin status were also associated with the development of bone metastasis (Table 5 and Additional file 3: A-H) and death (Table 5 and Additional file 3: I-L).

Discussion

The mandate of the CPCBN is to identify the best set of molecular markers that will complement current parameters for clinical decision-making in PC. The underlying incentive behind this pursuit is to minimize adverse health complications that result from overtreatment of clinically-indolent PC. Current diagnostics are unable to resolve the range of heterogeneity and individualized risk of patients. Although active surveillance is now an option, still too many newly diagnosed patients with early-stage tumors are aggressively treated to safeguard them against the potential fraction of tumors that progress or cause lethal disease. Despite several reports of proposed biomarkers with prognostic impact, most have been reported in the context of small cohorts, same-institution studies, or lack follow-up patient data, introducing a level of bias that limits their validation for

Table 4 Clinico-pathological features of prostate cancer patients treated by radical prostatectomy

TMA series		Test		Validation	
Number of patients		250		1262	
Mean age at diagnosis		61		61	
Median follow-up (months)		113		120	
		N	%	N	%
Gleason score at RP	≤3 + 3	64	25.6	392	31.1
	3 + 4	104	41.6	499	39.5
	4 + 3	42	16.8	188	14.9
	≥4 + 4	36	14.4	175	13.9
	NA	4	1.6	8	0.6
pTNM	2	171	68.4	788	62.4
	3	77	30.8	453	35.9
	4	2	0.8	21	1.7
Margin status	Negative	156	62.4	837	66.3
	Positive	91	36.4	418	33.1
	NA	3	1.2	7	0.6
Biochemical relapse	No	173	69.2	828	65.6
	Yes	77	30.8	434	34.4
Type of biochemical relapse	Rising PSA	54	21.6	264	20.9
	Failed RP	16	6.4	85	6.7
	Treatment	7	2.8	85	6.7
Bone metastasis	No	239	95.6	1208	95.7
	Yes	11	4.4	54	4.3
Castrate resistant	No	237	94.8	1201	95.2
	Yes	13	5.2	61	4.8
Mortality	PC specific	4	1.6	36	2.9
	Other cause(s)	17	6.8	119	9.4
	Overall	21	8.4	155	12.3

TMA tissue microarray, *RP* radical prostatectomy, *pTNM* pathological staging, *NA* not available, *Rising PSA* serum level of prostate-specific antigen (PSA) of 0.2 ng/mL and rising, *Failed RP* PSA level after surgery > 0.2 ng/mL, *PC* prostate cancer

Table 5 Cox regression analyses of clinico-pathological parameters on the Test- and Validation-TMA cohorts

Endpoint	Clinical parameter	Test-TMA cohort				Validation-TMA cohort			
		P	Exp(B)	95.0% CI		P	Exp(B)	95.0% CI	
				Lower	Upper			Lower	Upper
BCR	Serum PSA level	< 0.001	1.064	1.042	1.086	< 0.001	1.031	1.026	1.036
	Gleason score at RP (6, 3 + 4, 4 + 3, > 8)	< 0.001	2.035	1.631	2.54	< 0.001	1.946	1.778	2.13
	pTNM	< 0.001	4.673	3.133	6.97	< 0.001	2.599	2.202	3.067
	Margin status	< 0.001	2.392	1.517	3.77	< 0.001	2.362	1.955	2.852
Bone metastasis	Serum PSA level	0.051	1.047	1	1.096	0.047	1.018	1	1.036
	Gleason score at RP (6, 3 + 4, 4 + 3, > 8)	0.001	3.159	1.6	6.237	< 0.001	3.333	2.476	4.487
	pTNM	< 0.001	8.396	3.043	23.162	< 0.001	3.882	2.422	6.22
	Margin status	0.125	2.624	0.765	9.008	0.988	0.996	0.569	1.743
PC specific death	Serum PSA level	–	–	–	–	0.046	1.02	1	1.039
	Gleason score at RP (6, 3 + 4, 4 + 3, > 8)	0.001	3.159	1.6	6.237	< 0.001	3.333	2.476	4.487
	pTNM	–	–	–	–	< 0.001	3.263	1.843	5.78
	Margin status	–	–	–	–	0.117	1.689	0.877	0.3252

TMA tissue microarray, *95% CI* 95% confidence interval, *BCR* biochemical recurrence, *PSA* prostate-specific antigen, *RP* radical prostatectomy, *pTNM* pathological staging, *PC* prostate cancer. Bold indicate significance

broad clinical use [3, 5, 11, 12]. The CPCBN addresses the outstanding need for validating existing biomarkers with a TMA-based platform to validate tissue markers. With large cohorts of adequate power, standardized protocols, and extensive clinical information centralized into one database, the CPCBN validation platform provides a resource to refine a panel of markers that can be readily integrated into clinical practice.

The first phase of this initiative involved the construction of the QC-TMA, which demonstrated the quality and feasibility of a multi-center TMA resource. The results of this exercise provided a logistical assurance in building large-scale cohorts from five participating biobanks, without site-specific bias. More noteworthy was the overall informative quality of cores that were evaluated by IHC and FISH

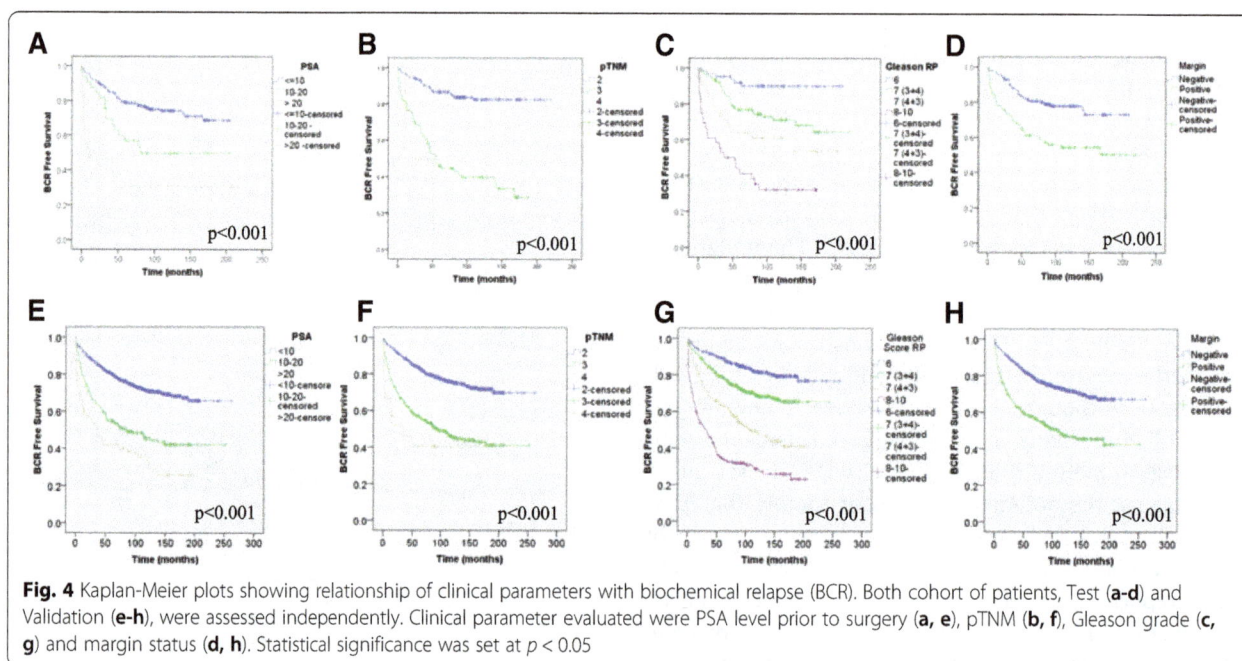

Fig. 4 Kaplan-Meier plots showing relationship of clinical parameters with biochemical relapse (BCR). Both cohort of patients, Test (**a-d**) and Validation (**e-h**), were assessed independently. Clinical parameter evaluated were PSA level prior to surgery (**a, e**), pTNM (**b, f**), Gleason grade (**c, g**) and margin status (**d, h**). Statistical significance was set at p < 0.05

techniques already used in clinical pathology practice and diagnostic labs. With H&E staining and reference markers of tissue integrity and malignancy, we were able to assess that 94% of samples provided at least two informative cores of high quality. FISH results also demonstrated a distribution of *PTEN* deletions among tumor cores that were aligned with previous reports in the literature [13]. With a homogeneous patient cohort, we were able to accumulate a large sample size ($n = 1512$) based on power calculations that would bestow statistical significance on biomarker performance. Division of the RP cohort into a Test-TMA ($n = 250$) and Validation-TMA ($n = 1262$) enhances the selection process and power of the platform, centered upon a rigorous checkpoint scheme in which biomarker status is assessed at several stages with a "Go or No-Go" decision tree. With the addition of an OPT-TMA to ensure the efficacy of conditions and staining protocols with prospective candidates, the sequence of testing from OPT-TMA to Test-TMA to Validation-TMA guards against wasting efforts with weak biomarkers, and preserving the Validation-TMA for the most robust candidates.

CTRNet policies and SOPs, patient information is updated each year on the ATiM database. In addition updates regarding the progress status of biomarkers and associated TMAs that are assigned to each project are also entered into the database. The centralized database can also coordinate several projects for meta-analysis and help to develop nomograms that will combine current parameters with biomarker analyses and integrate age, co-morbidity, clinico-pathological staging to ultimately define an accurate profile indicating individual risk for each PC patients. The application of emerging nomograms including biomarkers could be useful in the decision-making process with correlative evidence-based science to guide patient care.

Conclusions

In conclusion, the CPCBN RP TMA has been constructed, controlled for quality and is available, in a step-wise manner, for researchers who intend to validate prognostic biomarkers in prostate cancer (for more information see http://www.tfri.ca/en/research/translational-research/cpcbn/cpcbn_access.aspx). As the first completed TMA series of the CPCBN-TMA platform, this RP cohort will serve as a prototype model that will facilitate the assembly of future retrospective and prospective cohorts for biomarker validation. Altogether the CPCBN-TMA platform will serve as an invaluable resource for the entire PC research community, accelerating breakthroughs in PC research, and supporting the establishment of nomograms to predict progression.

Abbreviations
ASAP: Atypical small acinar proliferation; ATiM: Advanced Tissue Management; BCR: Biochemical relapse; CHUdeQ-UL: Centre hospitalier universitaire de Québec-Université Laval CHUdeQ-UL; CHUM: Centre hospitalier de l'Université de Montréal; CPCBN: Canadian prostate cancer biomarker network; CTRNet: Canadian Tumor Repository Network; FFPE: Formalin-fixed paraffin-embedded; FISH: Fluorescence in situ hybridization; GS: Gleason score; H&E: Hematoxylin and eosin; IDC: Intraductal carcinoma; IHC: Immunohistochemistry; IRB: Institutional Review Board; MUHC: McGill University Health Centre; OPT-TMA: Optimization TMA; PC: Prostate cancer; PIN: Prostatic intraepithelial neoplasia; PSA: Prostate-specific antigen; QC-TMA: Quality control TMA; RP: Radical prostatectomy; SOPs: Standard operating procedures; TMA: Tissue microarray; UHN: University Health Network; VPC: Vancouver Prostate Centre

Acknowledgements
Authors are grateful to patients who generously agreed to participate in this research by providing specimens and data to the CPCBN affiliated repositories (for a full list and for biomarker proposal form see http://www.tfri.ca/en/research/translational-research/cpcbn/cpcbn). We are also grateful to Véronique Barrès (CRCHUM), Nathalie Delvoye (CRCHUM), Jennifer Good (Kingston University), Dr. Eleonora Scarlata (MUHC-RI), Dr. Lucie Hamel (MUHC-RI), Hélène Hovington (CHUdeQ-UL), Céline Veilleux (CHUdeQ-UL), Alireza Moeen (VPC), and Karen Chadwick (UHN) for their technical support. We thank the molecular pathology core facility of the CRCHUM for performing the sections, IHC and slide scanning. We thank Jacqueline Chung for editing this manuscript. The CPCBN was funded by the Terry Fox Research Institute and the Canadian Partnership against cancer. This networks are managed and supervised by the CRCHUM. The authors declare that they have no competing interests.

Funding
This research was part of a pan-Canadian initiative named the Canadian Prostate Biomarker Network and funded by the Terry Fox Research Institute (TFRI) and the Canadian Partnership Against Cancer (CPAC). The funding body did not had any role in the design of the study and collection, analysis, and interpretation of data and in writing the manuscript in this section.

Authors' contributions
Participation in the conception and initial design: VO, AA, AB, RGB, SC, LF, NEF, MG, PK, LK, LL, JBL, TvdK, ML, DT, AMMM, FS, Participation in the acquisition: VO, AA, AB, FB, SC, LF, LL, NEF, MG, TvdK, JAS, ML, DT, AMMM, FS. Participation in the analysis and interpretation: VO, AA, AB, FB, RGB, SC, DD, LF, LL, NEF, MG, PK, LK, JBL, TvdK, JAS, ML, DT, AMMM, F. Participation in the drafting and/or revision of the manuscript: VO, AA, AB, FB, RGB, SC, DD, LF, NEF, MG, PK, LK, LL, JBL, TvdK, JAS, ML, DT, AMMM, FS. All authors have read and approved the manuscript.

Competing interests
The authors declare that they have no competing interests.

Author details
[1]Institut du cancer de Montréal and Centre de recherche du Centre hospitalier de l'Université de Montréal, 900, St-Denis St, room R10-464, Montréal, Québec H2X 0A9, Canada. [2]Research Institute of McGill University Health Center and Department of Surgery (Urology), McGill University, Montréal, Québec, Canada. [3]CHU de Québec-Université Laval and Department of Surgery, Université Laval, Québec City, Québec, Canada. [4]Department of Pathology, McGill University Health Centre, Montréal, Québec, Canada. [5]Department of Medical Biophysics and Department of Radiation Oncology, University of Toronto, Toronto, ON, Canada. [6]University Health Network, Toronto, ON, Canada. [7]University of Manitoba and Manitoba Prostate Centre, Winnipeg, MB, Canada. [8]Vancouver Prostate Centre,

Vancouver, BC, Canada. [9]Division of Urology, Department of Surgery of
University Health Network, University of Toronto, Toronto, ON, Canada.
[10]Department of Urologic Sciences, Vancouver, BC, Canada. [11]Cancer
Prognostics and Health Outcomes Unit, Centre hospitalier de l'Université de
Montréal, Montréal, Québec, Canada. [12]Department of Surgery, Université de
Montréal, Montréal, Québec, Canada. [13]Sunnybrook Health Sciences Centre,
Toronto, ON, Canada. [14]Department of Pathology and Molecular Medicine,
Queen's University, Kingston, ON, Canada. [15]Department of Pathology and
Cellular Biology, Université de Montréal, Montréal, Québec, Canada.
[16]Department of Medicine, Université de Montréal, Montréal, Québec,
Canada. [17]Department of Genetics and Pathology, Ribeirão Preto Medical
School, University of São Paulo, Ribeirão Preto, Brazil.

References

1. Frank SB, Miranti CK. Disruption of prostate epithelial differentiation
    pathways and prostate cancer development. Front Oncol. 2013;3:273.
2. Auprich M, Bjartell A, Chun FK, de la Taille A, Freedland SJ, Haese A, et al.
    Contemporary role of prostate cancer antigen 3 in the management of
    prostate cancer. Eur Urol. 2011;60(5):1045–54.
3. Huber F, Montani M, Sulser T, Jaggi R, Wild P, Moch H, et al. Comprehensive
    validation of published immunohistochemical prognostic biomarkers of
    prostate cancer -what has gone wrong? A blueprint for the way forward in
    biomarker studies. Br J Cancer. 2015;112(1):140–8.
4. Mohler JL, Kantoff PW, Armstrong AJ, Bahnson RR, Cohen M, D'Amico
    AV, et al. Prostate cancer, version 2.2014. J Natl Compr Canc Netw.
    2014;12(5):686–718.
5. Prensner JR, Rubin MA, Wei JT, Chinnaiyan AM. Beyond PSA: the next
    generation of prostate cancer biomarkers. Sci Transl Med. 2012;4(127):
    127rv3.
6. Fraser M, Berlin A, Ouellet V, Saad F, Bristow RG. Prostate Cancer genomics
    as a driver of personalized medicine-Chapter 14. In: Dellaire G, Berman JN,
    Arceci RJ, editors. Cancer genomics: Academic Press; 2014.
7. Boutros PC, Fraser M, Harding NJ, de Borja R, Trudel D, Lalonde E, et al.
    Spatial genomic heterogeneity within localized, multifocal prostate cancer.
    Nat Genet. 2015;47(7):736–45.
8. Kristiansen G. Diagnostic and prognostic molecular biomarkers for prostate
    cancer. Histopathology. 2012;60(1):125–41.
9. Yoshimoto M, Ludkovski O, Good J, Pereira C, Gooding RJ, McGowan-Jordan
    J, et al. Use of multicolor fluorescence in situ hybridization to detect
    deletions in clinical tissue sections. Lab Invest. 2018;98(6):839.
10. Leyh-Bannurah SR, Trudel D, Latour M, Zaffuto E, Grosset AA, Tam C, et al. A
    multi-institutional validation of Gleason score derived from tissue microarray
    cores. Pathol Oncol Res. 2018.
11. Hawley S, Fazli L, McKenney JK, Simko J, Troyer D, Nicolas M, et al. A model
    for the design and construction of a resource for the validation of
    prognostic prostate cancer biomarkers: the canary prostate Cancer tissue
    microarray. Adv Anat Pathol. 2013;20(1):39–44.
12. Narayan VM, Konety BR, Warlick C. Novel biomarkers for prostate
    cancer: an evidence-based review for use in clinical practice. Int J Urol.
    2017;24(5):352–60.
13. Troyer DA, Jamaspishvili T, Wei W, Feng Z, Good J, Hawley S, et al. A
    multicenter study shows PTEN deletion is strongly associated with seminal
    vesicle involvement and extracapsular extension in localized prostate
    cancer. Prostate. 2015;75(11):1206–15.

22

Site-dependent differences in the composite fibers of male pelvic plexus branches: an immunohistochemical analysis of donated elderly cadavers

Kuniyasu Muraoka[1,5*], Shuichi Morizane[1], Keisuke Hieda[2], Masashi Honda[1], Takehiro Sejima[1], Gen Murakami[3], Shin-ichi Abe[4] and Atsushi Takenaka[1]

Abstract

Background: Although the pelvic autonomic plexus branches are considered to be a mixture of sympathetic and parasympathetic nerves, little is known regarding the composite fibers of the pelvic plexus branches. This study aimed to investigate the immunohistochemical features of sympathetic and parasympathetic nerves in the pelvic autonomic plexus branches.

Methods: Using 10 donated elderly male cadavers, the detailed topohistology of nerve fibers at and around the bladder, seminal vesicle, prostate, and rectum was examined. Neuronal nitric oxide synthase (nNOS) and vasoactive intestinal polypeptide (VIP) were used as parasympathetic nerve markers; tyrosine hydroxylase (TH) was used as a sympathetic nerve marker. The myenteric plexus of the colon was utilized as a positive control.

Results: Most nerve fibers in the bladder, seminal vesicle, prostate, and rectum were both nNOS- and TH-positive. Thus, pelvic plexus branches were classified into two types: 1) triple-positive mixed nerves (nNOS+, VIP+, TH+, thick myelinated fibers + or -) and 2) double-positive mixed nerves (nNOS+, VIP-, TH+, thick myelinated fibers + or -). Notably, triple-positive nerves were localized within the posterosuperior part of the plexus (near the rectum) and travelled anteroinferiorly toward the posterolateral corner of the prostate. The posteriorly and inferiorly located nerves were predominantly composed of parasympathetic, rather than sympathetic, fibers. In contrast, nerve fibers within and along the bladder and seminal vesicle contained either no or few VIP-positive nerves. These superiorly located nerves were characterized by clear sympathetic nerve dominance.

Conclusions: The nerves of the pelvic plexus branches were clearly classified into nerves around the bladder and seminal vesicle (VIP-negative) and nerves around the prostate (VIP-positive). Although nNOS- and VIP-positive nerve fibers are candidate cavernous nerves, cavernous nerve identity cannot be definitively concluded for these nerves in the periprostatic region.

Keywords: Pelvic autonomic nerve plexus, Fiber composition, Neuronal nitric oxide synthase, Vasoactive intestinal polypeptide, Tyrosine hydroxylase

* Correspondence: knys1970108@outlook.jp
[1]Department of Urology, Tottori University Faculty of Medicine, Yonago, Japan
[5]Division of Urology, Department of Surgery, Tottori University Faculty of Medicine, 36-1 Nishi-cho, Yonago 683-8504, Japan
Full list of author information is available at the end of the article

Background

Autonomic innervation of the pelvic viscera is formed by sympathetic fibers from the inferior hypogastric plexus and parasympathetic fibers from the pelvic splanchnic nerves [1, 2]. The genital organs and lower urinary tract are controlled by the autonomic nervous system, as well as the somatic nerves. Because functional disruptions, such as urinary incontinence and sexual dysfunction, represent important determinants of quality of life, detailed anatomical studies of the pelvic neuro-anatomy are essential to preserve continence, erection, and bladder function after pelvic surgery [3, 4].

Immunohistochemistry is widely applied in pelvic nerve research. However, as evaluation of the peripro-static nerve distribution is typically performed using sur-gically acquired specimens [5–7], the staining of a large area, including adjacent organs, is generally not possible. Therefore, to investigate the anatomy of the pelvic plexus, use of the entire pelvic block of cadavers is ideal. Nitric oxide synthase (nNOS) and vasoactive intestinal polypeptide (VIP) are used as parasympathetic nerve markers, whereas tyrosine hydroxylase (TH) is used as a marker of sympathetic nerves [8]. Recent reports have demonstrated that, in the human pelvic floor, a portion of the pelvic plexus branches contained VIP-, nNOS-, and TH-positive nerve fibers [9–11].

The aim of this study was to investigate the topohistol-ogy of three types of pelvic nerve fibers (nNOS-, VIP-, and TH-positive fibers) by comparison of the peripro-static nerve configuration and distribution with that of adjacent regions.

Methods

This study examined 10 donated male cadavers with a mean age of 73 years (range, 64–82 years). The cause of death was either ischemic heart failure or intracranial bleeding; none of the cadavers had undergone abdom-inal or pelvic surgery, as confirmed by review of patient medical histories, as well as by macroscopic observation of the abdominopelvic cavity. The 10 cadavers were do-nated to Tokyo Dental College for research and educa-tion on human anatomy in accordance with their consent, and their use in research was approved by the Ethics Committee of Tottori University Faculty of Medi-cine. The study was performed in accordance with the provisions of the Declaration of Helsinki 1995, as revised in Edinburgh in 2000.

The donated cadavers had been fixed by arterial perfu-sion of 10% v/v formalin solution, then stored in 50% v/v ethanol solution for >3 months. From each of the ca-davers, a large tissue block, including the bladder, seminal vesicle, urethra, prostate, and rectum, as well as any con-nective tissue around these viscera, was prepared. After bi-section along the midsagittal line, each of the hemiblocks

was cut into 15-mm thick sections; then, routine proce-dures for paraffin-embedded histology were performed. From each of the macroslices, large horizontal or sagittal sections (70 × 50 mm) were prepared at 2–3-mm inter-vals, then stained with hematoxylin and eosin (H&E). After reviewing the large sections to identify target re-gions, sections (50 × 20 mm) for immunohistochemistry were cut, in close proximity to the former plane. Ultim-ately, we obtained 2–5 large sections and 8–20 standard-sized sections from a single paraffin block con-taining a 15-mm-thick slice.

Most sections were stained with H&E, whereas others were stained via immunohistochemistry and elastic-tissue Masson staining (a variation of Masson-Goldner staining). Primary antibodies for nerve immunohistochemistry were used based on the methods of Hinata et al. [12]; these com-prised mouse monoclonal anti-human S100 protein (1:200 dilution, Dako Z0311; Dako, Glostrup, Denmark), rabbit polyclonal anti-human nNOS (1:200 dilution; Cell Signaling Technology, Beverly, MA, USA), mouse monoclonal anti-human VIP (1:100 dilution, Santa Cruz sc25347; Santa Cruz, CA, USA), and rabbit polyclonal anti-human TH (1:500 dilution, Millipore-Chemicon ab152; Temecula, CA, USA). When possible, the four immunohistochemical stains were applied on adjacent sections; occasionally, non-adjacent sections were sometimes used because of failed immunostaining. As a positive control for immuno-histochemistry, the myenteric plexus of the descending colon was acquired from the 10 specimens; the colic my-enteric nerves invariably exhibit a dense distribution of nNOS-/VIP-coreactive nerve fibers, even in centenarians [13]. The secondary antibody was labeled with horseradish peroxidase (HRP), and antigen-antibody reactions were de-tected via the HRP-catalyzed reaction with diaminobenzi-dine. The immunohistochemistry-labeled samples were counterstained with hematoxylin. Negative controls com-prised samples without primary antibody.

Results

The tissue blocks that were prepared for horizontal sec-tions contained the posterior part of the bladder, nearly the entire seminal vesicle, the superoposterior part of the prostate, the anterior wall of the rectum, and parts of the levator ani muscle. The horizontal sections were suitable for a better understanding of the topographical anatomy in and around the bladder and seminal vesicle. However, the periprostatic neurovascular bundle could not easily be included in a block because of the large mass of the prostate. Thus, to easily identify the peripro-static nerves, sagittal sections were necessary. A complete set of observations of most branches of the pelvic plexus was performed in two specimens (all hori-zontal sections), whereas in the other eight specimens (combination of horizontal and sagittal sections), either the superior or inferior group of nerves was examined. Figures 1, 2, 3, 4 and 5 were prepared from a combination of observations from two specimens.

In all 10 cadavers, the colic myenteric plexus expressed all three markers (nNOS, VIP, and TH; Fig. 1), although TH expression was typically weak and found in very few fibers. For descriptive purposes, the pelvic plexus branches to the urogenital organs were divided into four areas: 1) the middle and superior area between the seminal vesicle and rectum (Fig. 1b); 2) the anterosuperior area between the bladder and seminal vesicle (Fig. 1c); 3) the posterosuperior area between the rectum and levator ani muscle (Fig. 1d); and, 4) the posteroinferior area at and along the posterolateral corner of the prostate (Fig. 5b). The third group of nerves traveled anteroinferiorly toward the posterolateral corner of the

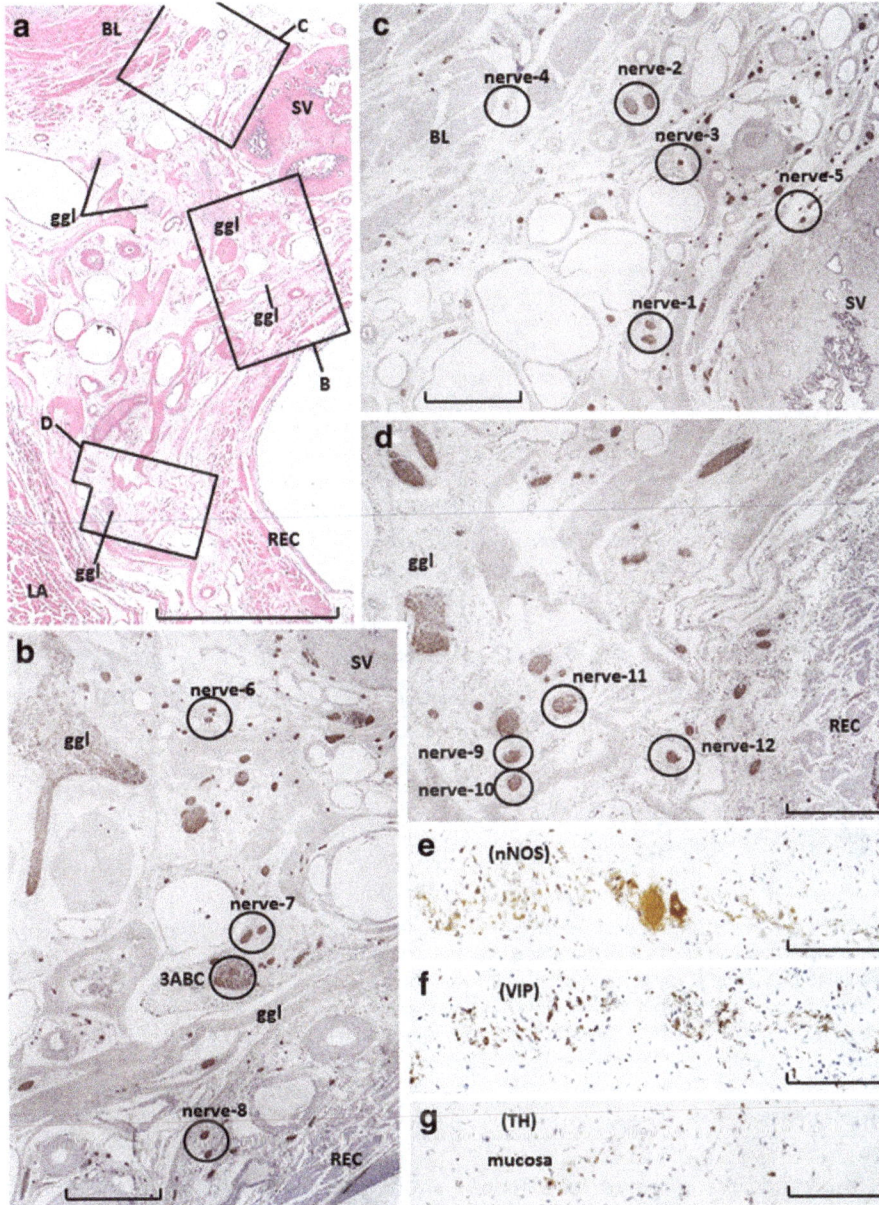

Fig. 1 Topohistology of nerves for immunohistochemistry. Near-horizontal sections of specimens from a 76-year-old man. Panel a (hematoxylin and eosin staining; scale bar, 10 mm) displays topographical anatomy, including the bladder (BL), seminal vesicle (SV), rectum (REC), and levator ani muscle (LA). There are five ganglion cell clusters (ggl) in the panel. Panel b (an area between the seminal vesicle and rectum), panel c (an area between the bladder and seminal vesicle), and panel d (an area between the rectum and levator ani muscle), corresponding to squares b, c, or d within panel a, exhibit immunohistochemistry of S100-labeled nerves that are shown in Figs. 2, 3, 4 and 5. Scale bars in panels b–d are 1 mm. Panels e, f, and g (nearby sections; scale bars, 0.1 mm) depict the colic myenteric plexus in the same specimen as the positive control: the plexus strongly expresses nNOS and VIP, whereas TH-positive cells are scarce

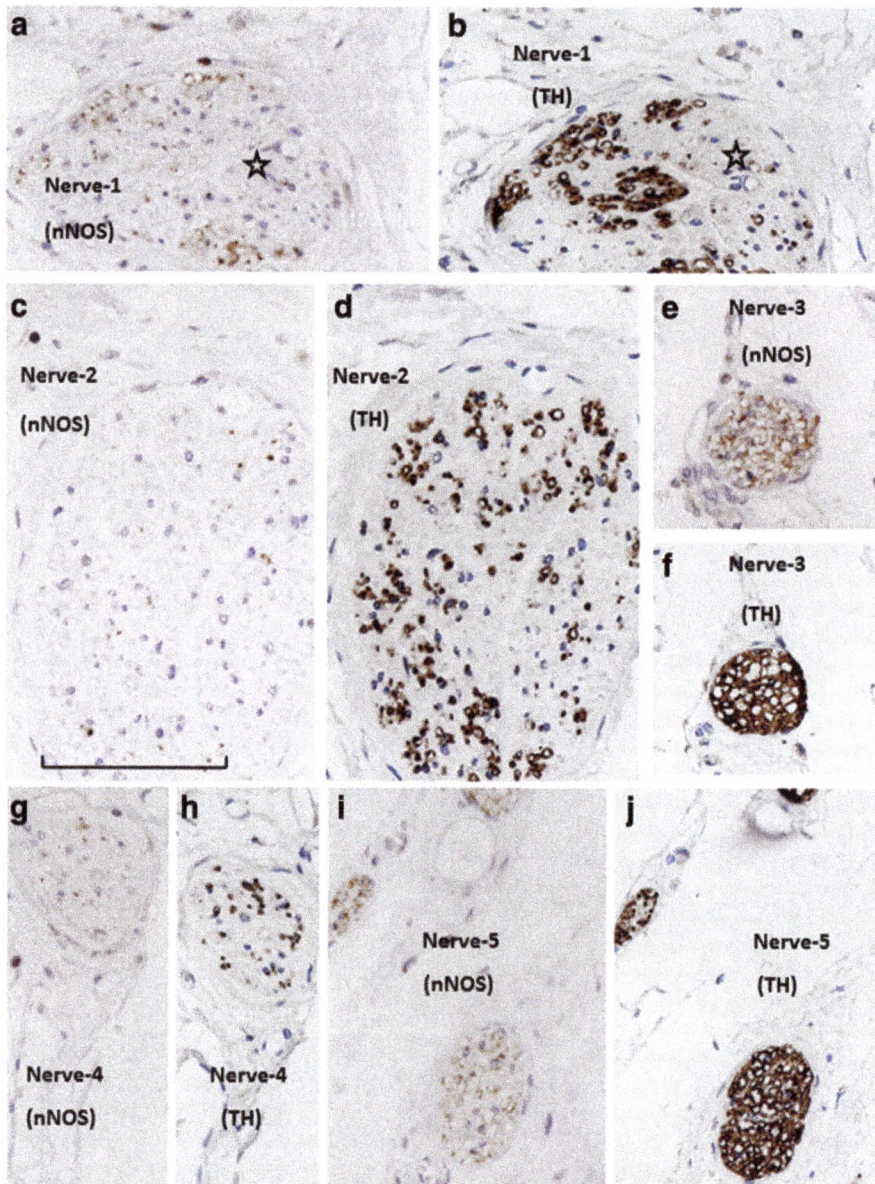

Fig. 2 Immunohistochemistry of nerves in an area between the bladder and seminal vesicle (anterosuperior group of the pelvic plexus branches). Topographical nerve anatomy is shown in Fig. 1c. Panels **a**, **c**, **e**, **g**, and **i** exhibit nNOS immunostaining, while panels **b**, **d**, **f,** and **i** display TH immunostaining. Panels **a** and **b** (or **i** and **j**) are adjacent sections, whereas panels **c** and **d** (or **e** and **f**, **g** and **h**) are proximal sections. These nerves did not contain fibers that were reactive for VIP (not shown). In all of these nerves, nNOS- and TH-positive fibers appear to be intermingled, without clear localization. However, in panels **a** and **b**, triple-negative areas (putative myelinated sensory fiber-dominant areas; stars) are visible. Panels **g** and **h** display nerves in the bladder detrusor, while panels **i** and **j** show nerves attaching to the seminal vesicle. Nerves along the seminal vesicle are characterized by an abundance of TH-positive fibers. In contrast, bladder detrusor nerves contain an abundance of triple-negative fibers (putative sensory fibers). All panels were prepared at the same magnification (scale bar in panel **f**, 0.1 mm)

prostate, such that the third area appeared to be connected to the fourth area. All four areas of nerves exhibited ganglion cell clusters, but the second and third areas (3–10 clusters per horizontal section) contained greater numbers than the others (1–5 clusters per horizontal section). Numbers of cut nerve profiles per mm^2 in each horizontal section ranged from 15 to 25 in the first area, 22 to 38 in the second area, 8 to 13 in the

third area, and 5 to 18 in the fourth area. Therefore, nerve density was consistently highest in the first (anterosuperior) area of nerves, located between the bladder and seminal vesicle.

More than 70% of nerves in the anterosuperior area were thin (< 0.05-mm diameter), and the density was higher along the seminal vesicle than the bladder (Fig. 1c). In these nerves, TH-positive sympathetic fibers

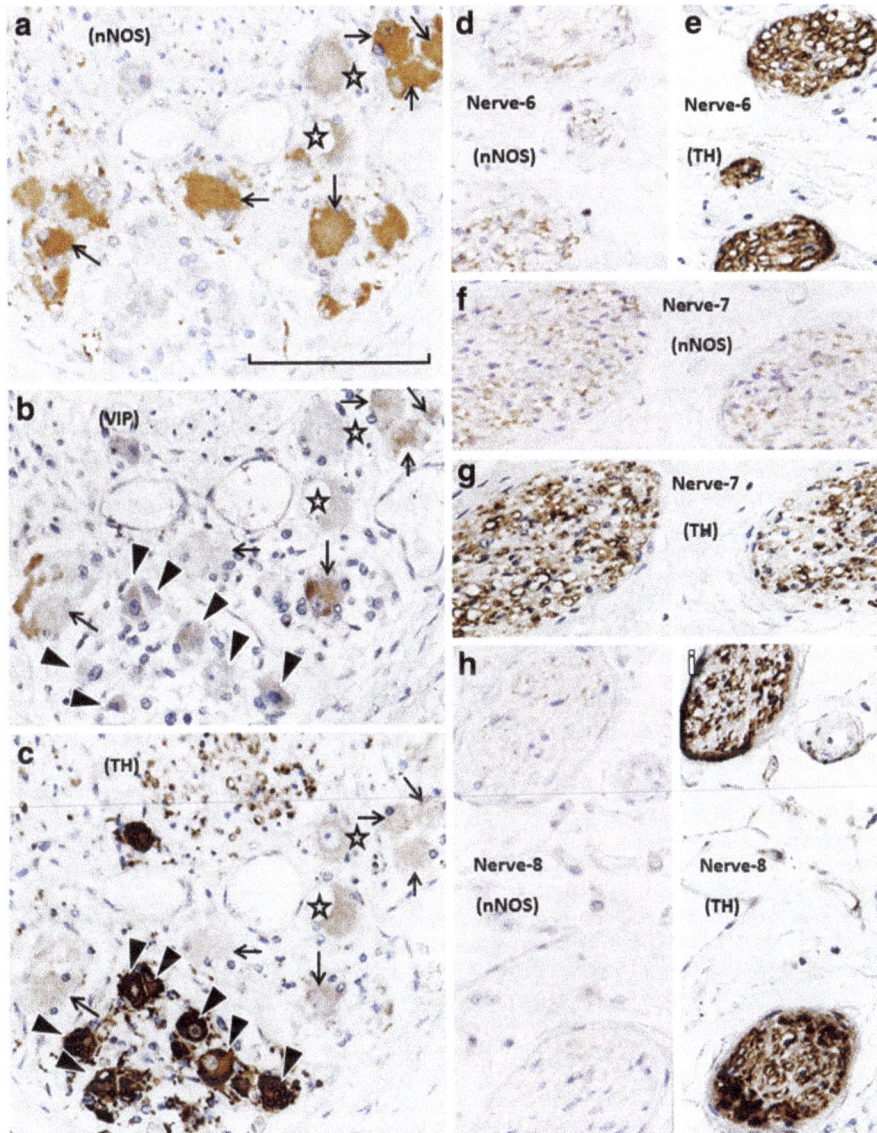

Fig. 3 Immunohistochemistry of nerves in an area between the rectum and seminal vesicle (middle and superior group of the pelvic plexus branches). Topographical nerve anatomy is shown in Fig. 1b. Panels **a**, **d**, **f**, and **h** display nNOS immunostaining, while panels **c**, **e**, **g**, and **i** exhibit TH immunostaining. Only panel **b** displays VIP immunostaining: the other nerves in this figure did not contain VIP-positive fibers (not shown). Panels **a–c** (or **f** and **g**; **h** and **i**) are adjacent sections, whereas panels **d** and **e** are proximal sections. Arrows, arrowheads, and stars in panels **a–c** indicate ganglion cells corresponding to each panel: two ganglion cells (stars) appear to be negative for all three markers. All VIP-positive cells (panel **b**) appear to express nNOS (panel **a**). All TH-positive cells (panel **c**) do not express either nNOS or VIP. In all of these nerves, nNOS- and TH-positive fibers appear to be intermingled and do not exhibit a clear localization. All panels were prepared at the same magnification (scale bar in panel **a**, 0.1 mm)

were much more abundant than parasympathetic fibers, especially in the thinner nerves (Fig. 2). The proportion of TH-positive fibers in the nerve along the seminal vesicle was much higher than the corresponding proportion along the bladder. Sympathetic nerve dominance was also observed in the first (middle and superior) area between the seminal vesicle and rectum (Fig. 3). In contrast to the first and second areas, nerves in the third (posterosuperior) and fourth (posteroinferior) areas contained VIP-positive fibers, although the number per section was consistently lower than for nNOS-positive nerves (Figs. 4 and 5). Furthermore, in these posterior areas, the number of nNOS-positive fibers was often equal to or greater than the number of TH-positive fibers. In addition, with respect to intra-organ nerves, both nNOS-positive fibers and TH-positive fibers were present; these were adjacent to and alongside the glands and mucosa of the prostate, seminal vesicle, and bladder.

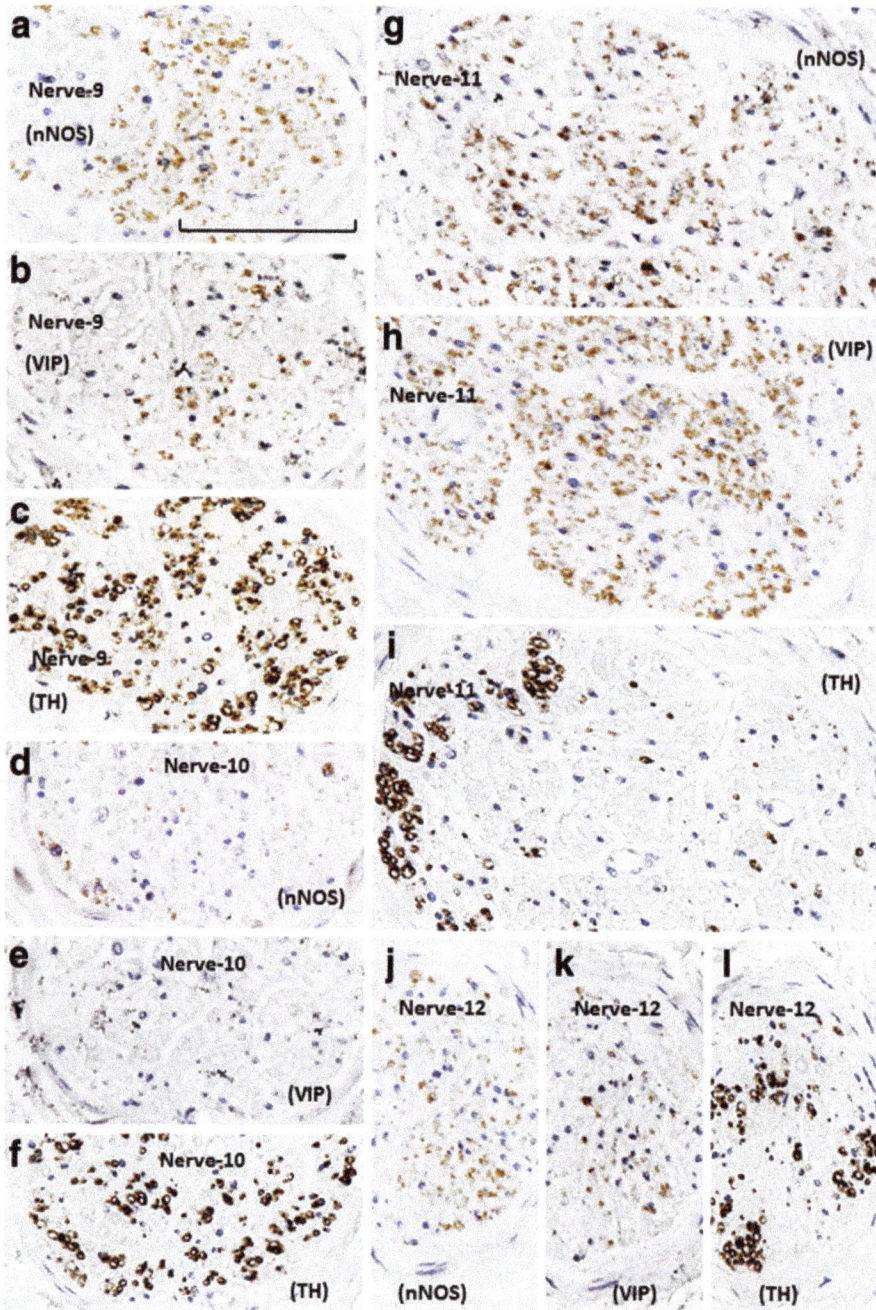

Fig. 4 Immunohistochemistry of nerves in an area between the rectum and levator ani muscle (posterosuperior group of the pelvic plexus branches). This area is characterized by the existence of VIP-positive nerves. The topographical relationship of the four nerves is shown in Fig. 1d. Panels **a**, **d**, **g**, and **j** display nNOS immunostaining; panels **b**, **e**, **h**, and **k** exhibit VIP immunostaining; panels **c**, **f**, **i**, and **l** exhibit TH immunostaining. One of the four nerves (panel **e**) does not express VIP. In a single nerve, panel **d** does not correspond to the site shown in panels **e** and **f**, as nNOS- (or TH-) positive nerves are restricted to the upper (or lower) side of the panel. VIP-positive fibers appear to be intermingled with nNOS-positive fibers. In panel **i**, TH-positive fibers are restricted to the left-hand side of the nerve. All panels were prepared at the same magnification (scale bar in panel **a**, 0.1 mm)

Similarly, the smooth muscles of the prostate and seminal vesicle contained a very high proportion of TH-positive fibers, as well as multiple nNOS-positive fibers. However, immunoreactive nerves were not found in the bladder detrusor smooth muscles. Other areas of nerves were characterized according to sympathetic nerve dominance. Of note, in all four areas, the intrapelvic nerves consistently contained both nNOS-positive and TH-positive fibers. In contrast, the pelvic nerve branches, such as those surrounding the levator ani

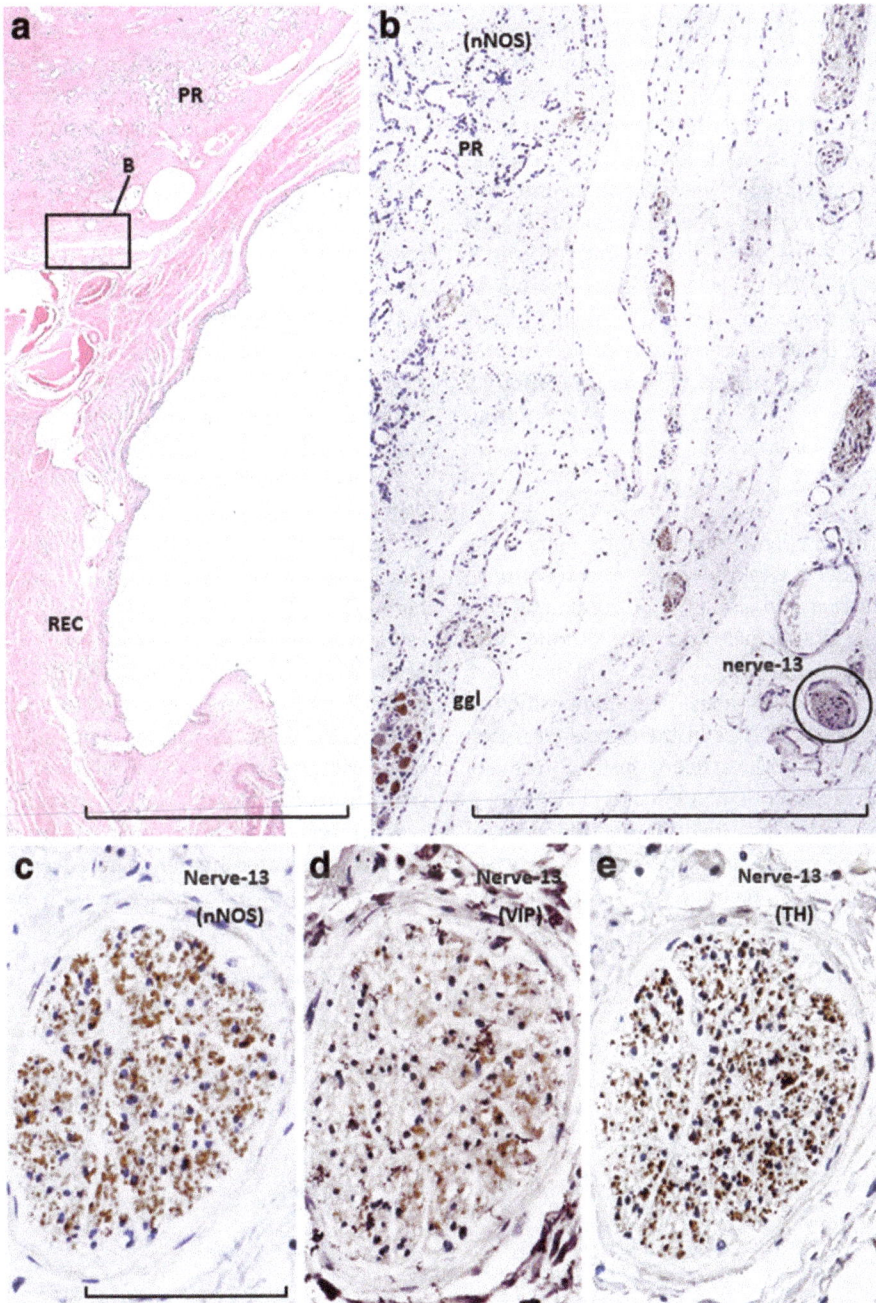

Fig. 5 Immunohistochemistry of nerves at and along the posterolateral corner of the prostate (posteroinferior group of the pelvic plexus branches). Near-sagittal sections of specimens from a 77-year-old man. Panel **a** (HE staining; scale bar, 10 mm) displays the topographical anatomy of nerves within the prostate (PR) and rectum (REC). After rotation, a square in panel **a** is shown in panel **b**. Panel **b** displays nNOS immunostaining in a part of the periprostatic nerves: at this lower magnification (scale bar, 1 mm), strong expression of nNOS can be identified. Panels **c**, **d**, and **e** (adjacent sections), corresponding to a nerve indicated by a circle in panel **b**, show nNOS, VIP, and TH immunostaining, respectively (scale bar in panel **c**, 0.1 mm). The periprostatic nerve contains abundant nNOS- and TH-positive fibers, but VIP-positive fibers are rare

muscle, did not contain either nNOS- or VIP-positive fibers (data not shown). Ganglion cells, albeit rare, contained triple-negative fibers (Figs. 2a, b; 3a, b, c).

In a ganglion cell cluster (Figs. 3a, b, c; 5b), nNOS-positive ganglion cells were consistently highest in number, followed by TH-positive cells. Some nNOS-positive cells also appeared to express VIP when observed in serial sections. The maximum diameter of cell bodies ranged from 15 to 25 μm, irrespective of their sympathetic or parasympathetic function. TH-positive cells were found either intermingled with, or in clusters separated from, nNOS-positive cells (Fig. 3c).

Sympathetic nerve fibers were most frequently observed in the superiorly located branches of the pelvic plexus near the bladder and seminal vesicle; in contrast, parasympathetic fibers, a portion of which expressed VIP, were dominant in the inferiorly or posteriorly located nerves near the prostate. Based on these observations, the pelvic plexus branches were classified into two types: 1) triple-positive mixed nerves (nNOS+, VIP+, TH +, thick myelinated fibers + or -); and, 2) double-positive mixed nerves (nNOS+, VIP-, TH+, thick myelinated fibers + or -). Figure 6 depicts representative pelvic plexus branches, including both triple-positive mixed nerves and double-positive mixed nerves. The composition of nerve fibers shown in Figs. 1, 2, 3, 4 and 5 is summarized in Table 1.

Discussion

This study focused on the pelvic plexus branches, from the lateral site of the bladder, seminal vesicle, and rectum, to the posteroinferior site at and along the posterolateral corner of the prostate, in elderly male cadavers. Although limited regions of the peripheral pelvic plexus were examined, several patterns were identified in the fiber composition of the pelvic plexus branches. Nerves in the examined region consistently included TH-positive fibers; further, many of the plexus branches were both nNOS- and TH-positive. Notably, the anterosuperior area (between the bladder and seminal vesicle) and the middle and superior area (between the seminal vesicle and rectum) did not contain VIP-positive nerve fibers. On the contrary, the posterosuperior area (between the rectum and levator ani muscle) and the posteroinferior area (at and along the posterolateral corner of the prostate) contained VIP-positive nerve fibers. The hypogastric and pelvic splanchnic nerves both contain nNOS-, VIP-, and TH-positive nerves [14, 15]. Kraima et al. [15] reported that VIP-positive fibers were not present in tissues isolated from the lumbar sympathetic chain; thus, areas that do not include VIP-positive nerves may be supplied by the lumbar sympathetic chain. In addition, a non-parasympathetic pattern [−, −, +] was not evident in the plexus branches, but was observed both inside and outside of the levator ani muscle; these nerves appeared to be pudendal nerve branches. Few triple-negative fibers were observed; these are candidate pure sensory nerves [10].

TH is the rate-limiting enzyme in the synthetic pathway of norepinephrine, a neurotransmitter that is found in peripheral sympathetic nerves and their related ganglia; thus, TH is often used as a marker of sympathetic nerves [10, 14–17]. Both nNOS and VIP have been used as parasympathetic nerve markers of the pelvic plexus branches [8–11]; nNOS is found in peripheral parasympathetic nerves and catalyzes the formation of nitric oxide [18], whereas, VIP is generally considered to be the primary transmitter released from cholinergic smooth muscle vasodilator and secretomotor fibers [19].

With regard to lower urinary function, the bladder neck is innervated by dense noradrenergic nerves, which have been shown to cause smooth muscle contraction

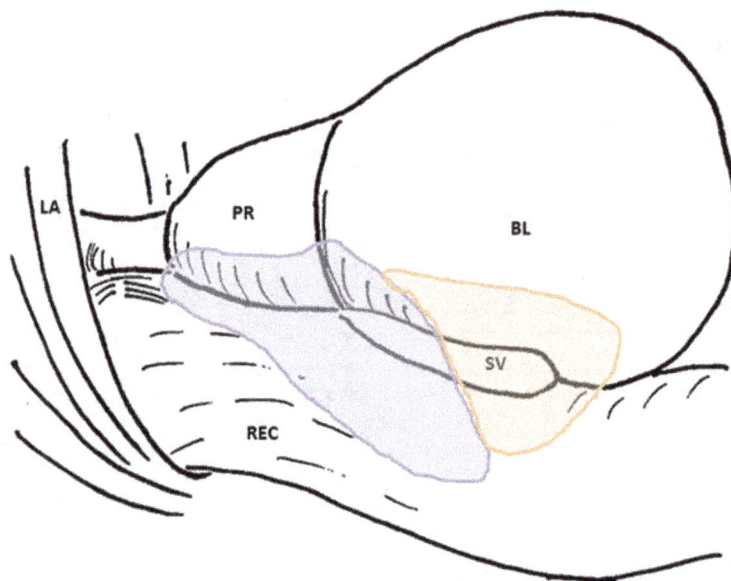

Fig. 6 Schema of pelvic plexus branches. The dominance of VIP-positive nerve fibers varied by site; nerves of the pelvic plexus branches were clearly classified into two types. The purple and orange areas indicate triple-positive mixed nerves (nNOS+, VIP+, TH+) and double-positive mixed nerves (nNOS+, VIP-, TH+), respectively. VIP-positive nerve fibers are distributed to the posterosuperior area between the rectum and levator ani, as well as to the posteroinferior area at and along the posterolateral corner of the prostate. BL, bladder; PR, prostate; SV, seminal vesicle; LA, levator ani muscle; REC, rectum

Table 1 Summary of composite nerve fibers of the pelvic plexus branches

	nNOS	VIP	TH
The anterosuperior group between the bladder and seminal vesicle			
nerve-1	++	–	++
nerve-2	+	–	++
nerve-3	+++	–	+++
nerve-4	+	–	+
nerve-5	+++	–	+++
The middle and superior group between the seminal vesicle and rectum			
nerve-6	+++	–	+++
nerve-7	+++	–	+++
nerve-8	+++	–	+++
The posterosuperior group between the rectum and levator ani			
nerve-9	++	+	+++
nerve-10	+	–	++
nerve-11	+++	++	+
nerve-12	++	+	+
The postero-inferior group at and along the posterolateral corner of the prostate			
nerve-13	+++	+	+++
Nerves to BL	+	–	+
Nerves to SV	+	–	+++
Nerves to PR and CTs	+++	+ or ±	+

+, > 10 positive nerve fibers were seen in the nerve; ++, positive nerves occupied 30–70% of a cross-sectional area of the nerve; +++, positive fibers occupied nearly all parts of the nerve with a high density
BL bladder, *CTs* cavernous tissues, *PR* prostate, *SV* seminal vesicle

and subsequent closure of the bladder neck during the storage of urine [20]. During micturition, inhibition of the sympathetic pathway may lead to opening of the bladder neck and prostatic urethra [21]. Additionally, high NOS activity was found in the urethra, whereas intermediate activity was found in the bladder neck, and comparatively low activity was found in the detrusor muscle. VIP-containing nerves form a dense subepithelial plexus and project to the detrusor muscle bundles of the bladder [22]. VIP plays an important role in bladder neck opening by promoting relaxation of the smooth muscle [20]. With regard to sexual function, TH- and VIP-positive nerve fibers are very abundant in the human prostate [23, 24] and are considered to play a role in the expulsion of the contents of the prostate gland during seminal emission, as well as during ejaculation, which is largely under adrenergic control [21]. Sympathetic innervation mediates corporeal vasoconstriction and corporeal smooth muscle contraction; further, it causes penile detumescence after orgasm, and (in the absence of sexual arousal) maintains the penis in the flaccid state [25]. The perivascular and trabecular nerve fibers within the corpus cavernosum exhibit positive

immunostaining for both nNOS and VIP [16, 26]. Nitric oxide is released by parasympathetic fibers and is a potent vasodilator associated with the physiology of the male erection. Nitric oxide and VIP participate in the erectile process via activation of the nitric oxide/cGMP and adenylyl cyclase/cAMP pathways, respectively [23, 24].

The present study demonstrated that nNOS-positive fibers are present in the pelvic plexus branches, as well as in the prostate, seminal vesicle, and bladder; further, the number of cut nerves per mm^2 decreases with proximity to the periphery. Ganzer et al. reported that nerve planimetry, using a polyclonal antibody against the neural protein S100, revealed that 75% of nerves from the seminal vesicles do not reach the striated urethral sphincter level along the prostate [27]. Thus, the nerves around the prostatic apex may be the remaining nerves of the pelvic plexus, after distribution to the prostate, seminal vesicle, and bladder. Although nNOS immunoreactivity has been used to identify cavernous nerves, previous data, suggesting that nNOS-positive periprostatic nerves are cavernous nerves, may have been overstated.

VIP immunoreactivity is also found in the human penis, where the largest concentrations of VIP are present in the cavernosum body [28]. The present study demonstrated that approximately 10% of nerve fibers progressing toward the prostate and cavernous tissues were VIP-positive. Hinata et al. reported that there were few VIP-positive fibers adjacent to, and posterior to, the rhabdosphincter area [11]. Ehmke et al. reported that > 50% of perivascular nerve fibers and > 90% of trabecular nerve fibers within the corpus cavernosum stained positive for both nNOS and VIP. Furthermore, NOS/VIP immunoreactivity was reduced (diabetes) or absent (lesion of the cavernous nerve) in penile tissue taken from patients with neurogenic impotence [26]. Although nNOS- and VIP-positive nerve fibers from the prostatic apex toward the periphery are regarded as candidate cavernous nerves, there may be considerable interindividual variation in nNOS and VIP immunoreactivity, corresponding to erectile function.

Many excellent studies have been published regarding the macro- and microscopic anatomy of the pelvic autonomic nerve plexus and its branches. Takenaka et al. reported that the main route of the cavernous nerve branches from a location near the root of the pelvic splanchnic nerves, then joins in a spray-shaped distribution to the central area of the neurovascular bundle, travelling along the distal side of the pelvic plexus [2]. The distal pelvic plexus, including the cavernous nerves, passes through the rectourethral muscle [29, 30]. Clinically, even after non-nerve sparing prostatectomy, erectile function may be maintained [31, 32], which implies that the cavernous nerves along the posterior side of the prostate and urethra are preserved, in some cases, after resecting the so-called neurovascular bundle. Furthermore, differences in the postoperative recovery of erectile function depend on the quantity of damaged cavernous nerves. Therefore, athermal dissection and reduced traction may lead to the preservation of function, even when non-nerve-sparing procedures are used.

There are several limitations to the present study. Because of the lack of immunohistochemical analysis of the hypogastric and pelvic splanchnic nerves, it was not possible to propose a complete scheme from a preganglionic fiber, via a ganglion cell and postganglionic fibers, to the target organs. Additionally, nNOS immunohistochemistry is difficult to successfully perform in cadaveric specimens that have undergone long periods of preservation [9]. Because the quality of nNOS immunohistochemistry varies among individuals, we did not perform a quantitative evaluation, which might have included a determination of the percentages of each nerve type.

Conclusions

Because the dominance of VIP-positive nerve fibers varied by site, nerves of the pelvic plexus branches were clearly categorized as those nerves around the bladder and seminal vesicle (VIP-negative) and those nerves around the prostate (VIP-positive). Furthermore, the results confirmed that nNOS expression is a general characteristic of the pelvic plexus branches, rather than a specific characteristic of the cavernous nerve. Although nNOS- and VIP-positive nerve fibers are candidate cavernous nerves, the periprostatic nNOS-positive fibers may not be cavernous nerves, even when they are observed alongside VIP-positive fibers.

Abbreviations
H&E: hematoxylin and eosin; HRP: horseradish peroxidase; nNOS: nitric oxide synthase; TH: tyrosine hydroxylase; VIP: vasoactive intestinal polypeptide

Acknowledgments
We are grateful to the individuals who donated their bodies to Tokyo Dental College for research and education in human anatomy without any economic benefit. We also thank their families for agreeing to the donation, as well as for their patience in waiting for return of the bodies after completion of the study.

Authors' contributions
Conception and design: KM, SM, GM, SA, and AT. Acquisition of data: KM, SM, KH, and MH. Analysis and interpretation of data: KM, SM, and TS. Drafting of the manuscript: KM, GM, and AT. Critical review of the manuscript for important intellectual content: KM and AT. Statistical analysis: KM and AT. Administrative, technical, or material support: GM and SA. All authors read and approved the final manuscript.

Competing interests
The authors declare that they have no competing interests.

Author details
[1]Department of Urology, Tottori University Faculty of Medicine, Yonago, Japan. [2]Department of Urology, Hiroshima University Faculty of Medicine, Hiroshima, Japan. [3]Division of Internal Medicine, Iwamizawa Kojin-kai Hospital, Iwamizawa, Japan. [4]Department of Anatomy, Tokyo Dental College, Tokyo, Japan. [5]Division of Urology, Department of Surgery, Tottori University Faculty of Medicine, 36-1 Nishi-cho, Yonago 683-8504, Japan.

References
1. Mauroy B, Demondion X, Drizenko A, Goullet E, Bonnal JL, Biserte J, Abbou C. The inferior hypogastric plexus (pelvic plexus): its importance in neural preservation techniques. Surg Radiol Anat. 2003;25(1):6–15.
2. Takenaka A, Murakami G, Soga H, Han SH, Arai Y, Fujisawa M. Anatomical analysis of the neurovascular bundle supplying penile cavernous tissue to ensure a reliable nerve graft after radical prostatectomy. J Urol. 2004;172(3):1032–5.
3. Sanda MG, Dunn RL, Michalski J, Sandler HM, Northouse L, Hembroff L, Lin X, Greenfield TK, Litwin MS, Saigal CS, et al. Quality of life and satisfaction with outcome among prostate-cancer survivors. N Engl J Med. 2008;358(12):1250–61.
4. Beveridge TS, Johnson M, Power A, Power NE, Allman BL. Anatomy of the nerves and ganglia of the aortic plexus in males. J Anat. 2015;226(1):93–103.
5. Kiyoshima K, Yokomizo A, Yoshida T, Tomita K, Yonemasu H, Nakamura M, Oda Y, Naito S, Hasegawa Y. Anatomical features of periprostatic tissue and its surroundings: a histological analysis of 79 radical retropubic prostatectomy specimens. Jpn J Clin Oncol. 2004;34(8):463–8.
6. Lee SB, Hong SK, Choe G, Lee SE. Periprostatic distribution of nerves in specimens from non-nerve-sparing radical retropubic prostatectomy. Urology. 2008;72(4):878–81.
7. Hisasue S, Hashimoto K, Kobayashi K, Takeuchi M, Kyoda Y, Sato S, Masumori N, Tsukamoto T. Baseline erectile function alters the cavernous nerve quantity and distribution around the prostate. J Urol. 2010;184(5):2062–7.
8. Butler-Manuel SA, Buttery LD, A'Hern RP, Polak JM, Barton DP. Pelvic nerve plexus trauma at radical and simple hysterectomy: a quantitative study of nerve types in the uterine supporting ligaments. J Soc Gynecol Investig. 2002;9(1):47–56.
9. Hieda K, Cho KH, Arakawa T, Fujimiya M, Murakami G, Matsubara A. Nerves in the intersphincteric space of the human anal canal with special reference to their continuation to the enteric nerve plexus of the rectum. Clin Anat. 2013;26(7):843–54.
10. Hinata N, Hieda K, Sasaki H, Murakami G, Abe S, Matsubara A, Miyake H, Fujisawa M. Topohistology of sympathetic and parasympathetic nerve fibers in branches of the pelvic plexus: an immunohistochemical study using donated elderly cadavers. Anat Cell Biol. 2014;47(1):55–65.
11. Hinata N, Murakami G, Miyake H, Abe S, Fujisawa M. Histological study of the cavernous nerve mesh outside the periprostatic region: anatomical basis for erectile function after nonnerve sparing radical prostatectomy. J Urol. 2015;193(3):1052–9.
12. Hinata N, Hieda K, Sasaki H, Kurokawa T, Miyake H, Fujisawa M, Murakami G, Fujimiya M. Nerves and fasciae in and around the paracolpium or paravaginal tissue: an immunohistochemical study using elderly donated cadavers. Anat Cell Biol. 2014;47(1):44–54.
13. Bernard CE, Gibbons SJ, Gomez-Pinilla PJ, Lurken MS, Schmalz PF, Roeder JL, Linden D, Cima RR, Dozois EJ, Larson DW, et al. Effect of age on the enteric nervous system of the human colon. Neurogastroenterol Motil. 2009;21(7):746–e746.
14. Jang HS, Cho KH, Hieda K, Kim JH, Murakami G, Abe S, Matsubara A. Composite nerve fibers in the hypogastric and pelvic splanchnic nerves: an immunohistochemical study using elderly cadavers. Anat Cell Biol. 2015;48(2):114–23.
15. Kraima AC, van Schaik J, Susan S, van de Velde CJ, Hamming JF, Lakke EA, DeRuiter MC. New insights in the neuroanatomy of the human adult superior hypogastric plexus and hypogastric nerves. Auton Neurosci. 2015;189:60–7.
16. Tamura M, Kagawa S, Kimura K, Kawanishi Y, Tsuruo Y, Ishimura K. Coexistence of nitric oxide synthase, tyrosine hydroxylase and vasoactive intestinal polypeptide in human penile tissue–a triple histochemical and immunohistochemical study. J Urol. 1995;153(2):530–4.
17. Takenaka A, Kawada M, Murakami G, Hisasue S, Tsukamoto T, Fujisawa M. Interindividual variation in distribution of extramural ganglion cells in the male pelvis: a semi-quantitative and immunohistochemical study concerning nerve-sparing pelvic surgery. Eur Urol. 2005;48(1):46–52. discussion 52

18. Stanarius A, Uckert S, Machtens SA, Stief CG, Wolf G, Jonas U. Immunocytochemical distribution of nitric oxide synthase in the human corpus cavernosum: an electron microscopical study using the tyramide signal amplification technique. Urol Res. 2001;29(3):168–72.
19. Lundberg JM. Evidence for coexistence of vasoactive intestinal polypeptide (VIP) and acetylcholine in neurons of cat exocrine glands. Morphological, biochemical and functional studies. Acta Physiol Scand Suppl. 1981;496:1–57.
20. Gosling JA, Dixon JS, Jen PY. The distribution of noradrenergic nerves in the human lower urinary tract. A review. Eur Urol. 1999;36(Suppl 1):23–30.
21. Iwata T, Ukimura O, Inaba M, Kojima M, Kumamoto K, Ozawa H, Kawata M, Miki T. Immunohistochemical studies on the distribution of nerve fibers in the human prostate with special reference to the anterior fibromuscular stroma. Prostate. 2001;48(4):242–7.
22. Smet PJ, Moore KH, Jonavicius J. Distribution and colocalization of calcitonin gene-related peptide, tachykinins, and vasoactive intestinal peptide in normal and idiopathic unstable human urinary bladder. Lab Investig. 1997;77(1):37–49.
23. Gonzalez-Cadavid NF, Ignarro LJ, Rajfer J. Nitric oxide and the cyclic GMP system in the penis. Mol Urol. 1999;3(2):51–9.
24. Andersson KE. Mechanisms of penile erection and basis for pharmacological treatment of erectile dysfunction. Pharmacol Rev. 2011;63(4):811–59.
25. Kandeel FR, Koussa VK, Swerdloff RS. Male sexual function and its disorders: physiology, pathophysiology, clinical investigation, and treatment. Endocr Rev. 2001;22(3):342–88.
26. Ehmke H, Junemann KP, Mayer B, Kummer W. Nitric oxide synthase and vasoactive intestinal polypeptide colocalization in neurons innervating the human penile circulation. Int J Impot Res. 1995;7(3):147–56.
27. Ganzer R, Stolzenburg JU, Neuhaus J, Weber F, Fuchshofer R, Burger M, Bründl J. Anatomical study of pelvic nerves in relation to seminal vesicles, prostate and urethral sphincter: Immunohistochemical staining, computerized Planimetry and 3-dimensional reconstruction. J Urol. 2015; 193(4):1205–12. https://doi.org/10.1016/j.juro.2014.10.001. Epub 2014 Oct 6.
28. Polak JM, Bloom SR. Localisation and measurement of VIP in the genitourinary system of man and animals. Peptides. 1984;5(2):225–30.
29. Takenaka A, Murakami G, Matsubara A, Han SH, Fujisawa M. Variation in course of cavernous nerve with special reference to details of topographic relationships near prostatic apex: histologic study using male cadavers. Urology. 2005;65(1):136–42.
30. Takenaka A, Leung RA, Fujisawa M, Tewari AK. Anatomy of autonomic nerve component in the male pelvis: the new concept from a perspective for robotic nerve sparing radical prostatectomy. World J Urol. 2006;24(2):136–43.
31. Tewari AK, Srivastava A, Huang MW, Robinson BD, Shevchuk MM, Durand M, Sooriakumaran P, Grover S, Yadav R, Mishra N, et al. Anatomical grades of nerve sparing: a risk-stratified approach to neural-hammock sparing during robot-assisted radical prostatectomy (RARP). BJU Int. 2011;108(6 Pt 2):984–92.
32. Moskovic DJ, Alphs H, Nelson CJ, Rabbani F, Eastham J, Touijer K, Guillonneau B, Scardino PT, Mulhall JP. Subjective characterization of nerve sparing predicts recovery of erectile function after radical prostatectomy: defining the utility of a nerve sparing grading system. J Sex Med. 2011;8(1): 255–60.

23

Is there still a place for retroperitoneal lymph node dissection in clinical stage 1 nonseminomatous testicular germ-cell tumours? A retrospective clinical study

K.-P. Dieckmann[1,2,5*†] (iD), P. Anheuser[1†], M. Kulejewski[1], R. Gehrckens[3] and B. Feyerabend[4]

Abstract

Background: Primary retroperitoneal lymph node dissection (RPLND) ultimately lost its role as the standard management of clinical stage (CS) 1 nonseminomatous (NS) testicular germ cell tumours (GCTs) in Europe when the European Germ Cell Cancer Consensus Group released their recommendations in 2008. Current guide-lines recommend surgery only for selected patients but reasons for selection remain rather ill-defined. We evaluated the practice patterns of the management of CS1 patients and looked specifically to the role of RPLND among other standard treatment options.

Methods: We retrospectively evaluated the treatment modalities of 75 consecutive patients treated for CS1 NS at one centre during 2008–2017. The patients undergoing RPLND were selected for a closer review. Particular reasons for surgery, clinical features of patients, and therapeutic outcome were analyzed using descriptive statistical methods.

Results: Twelve patients (16%) underwent nerve-sparing RPLND, nine surveillance, 54 had various regimens of adjuvant chemotherapy. Particular reasons for surgery involved illnesses precluding chemotherapy ($n = 2$), patients' choice ($n = 4$), and teratomatous histology of the primary associated with equivocal radiologic findings ($n = 6$). Five patients had lymph node metastases, two received additional chemotherapy. Antegrade ejaculation was preserved in all cases. One patient had a grade 2 complication that was managed conservatively. All RPLND-patients remained disease-free.

Conclusions: Primary RPLND is a useful option in distinct CS1 patients, notably those with concurrent health problems precluding chemotherapy, and those with high proportions of teratoma in the primary associated with equivocal radiological findings. Informed patient's preference represents another acceptable reason for the procedure. RPLND properly suits the needs of well-selected patients with CS1 nonseminoma and deserves consideration upon clinical decision-making.

Keywords: Testicular germ cell tumour, Nonseminomatous tumour, Lymph node dissection , Teratoma

* Correspondence: DieckmannKP@t-online.de
†K.-P. Dieckmann and P. Anheuser contributed equally to this work.
[1]Albertinen-Krankenhaus Hamburg, Klinik für Urologie, Hamburg, Germany
[2]Asklepios Klinik Altona, Urologische Abteilung, Hodentumorzentrum Hamburg, Hamburg, Germany
Full list of author information is available at the end of the article

Background

Patients with clinical stage (CS) 1 nonseminomatous (NS) testicular germ cell tumors (GCTs) can be successfully managed with quite different treatment methods [1]. Retroperitoneal lymph node dissection (RPLND) used to be the standard of care for a fifty years period from the end of world war II [2, 3] to the late nineties of the last century [4, 5]. In European countries, it was then gradually replaced by surveillance strategies with chemotherapy to be applied at the time of progression [6–9]. Primary prophylactic chemotherapy with two cycles of the cisplatin-etoposide-bleomycin (PEB) regimen came into use as another alternative around the turn of the century [10]. Currently, a risk-adapted strategy using vascular invasion (VI) of the primary tumour as a risk indictor [11] is the most preferred option with surveillance in the absence of the risk factor and prophylactic chemotherapy with one cycle of PEB if vascular invasion is detected in the primary [12]. In 2008, the European Germ Cell Cancer Consensus Group (EGCCCG) released guide-lines that virtually abandoned RPLND as the standard of management of CS1 NS in European countries [13]. Since that time patients underwent stratifying with regard to the presence of risk factors for progression. If vascular invasion of the primary was present, adjuvant chemotherapy became the standard way of care while surveillance and RPLND were considered merely as options for rare and specific cases. In patients without risk factor, surveillance was considered the standard way of treatment assigning RPLND only a role for exceptional circumstances. In the most recent guide-line of the European Association of Urology (EAU), surveillance is considered one standard option for all patients with nonseminoma CS1 while risk-adapted strategy is regarded another equally effective standard option [14]. RPLND is justified only in the few cases when "conditions are against surveillance and chemotherapy". Unfortunately, no further definitions were given to clarify those "conditions" and thus, decision-making was left to care-givers and patients. Currently, the degree of utilization of RPLND in European countries is largely unknown [15, 16]. The aim of the present study is to evaluate the patterns of care applied to NS CS1 patients in a testicular cancer unit in Northern Germany and to specifically look to the utilization of RPLND.

Patients, methods

From 1993 through 2017, a total of 722 patients with testicular GCT were treated at Albertinen-Krankenhaus, Hamburg. We elected the cohort treated from 2008 to 2017 ($n = 378$) for review because the EGCCCG guide-lines with the changing role of RPLND came into use in 2008 [13]. Histologies and stage distribution of that cohort are shown in Fig. 1. All patients were managed in line with contemporary guide-lines. Histological work-up of orchiectomy specimens was accomplished according to pathological guide-lines [13]. Clinical staging involved tumor marker measurement prior to orchiectomy and re-evaluation five days postoperatively, also abdominal and chest computed tomography scan with application of intravenous and oral contrast material [17]. A total of 75 cases with NS CS1 were identified in the patient cohort. We retrospectively evaluated the treatment strategies applied in these patients and selected the patients who had undergone RPLND for a closer review. The latter cases were tabulated regarding age, percentage of teratoma and vascular invasion in the primary tumour, numbers of lymph nodes surgically removed and numbers of metastatic nodes, and the particular individual reasons for surgery. The surgical approach consisted of open unilateral nerve-sparing lymph node dissection (Fig. 2) in the Indiana technique [18, 19] and was performed by a single surgeon in all cases (KPD). Frozen section examination was not employed. All patients received a postoperative abdominal drain that was usually

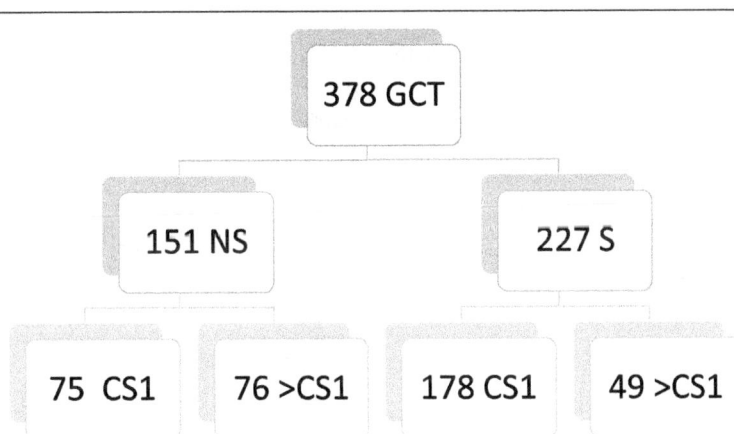

Fig. 1 Histology and clinical stages in 378 patients with testicular germ cell tumours treated in a single institution, 2008–2017 (numbers of patients). GCT germ cell tumours; S seminoma; NS nonseminoma; CS clinical stage

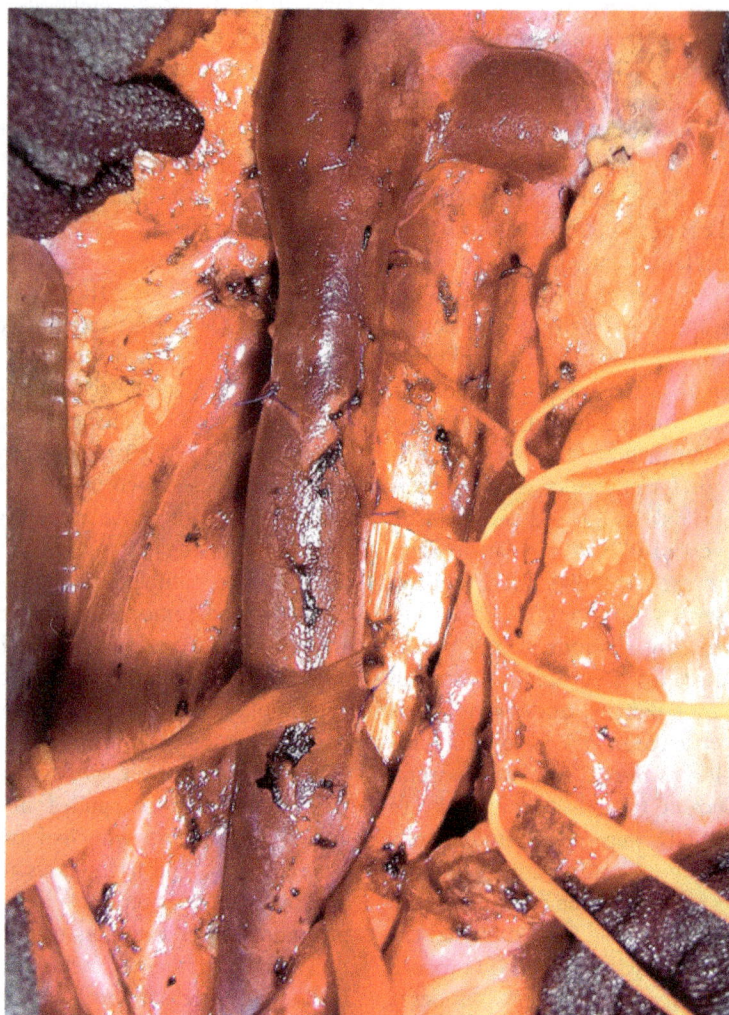

Fig. 2 Intraoperative site during right sided nerve sparing retroperitoneal lymph node dissection of pt #12 showing two lumbar postganglionic sympathetic nerve fibres between inferior vena cava and aorta. IVC inferior vena cava

removed after 3 to 4 days postoperatively. The rationale for this procedure was to monitor lymphatic fluid drainage and to early detect chylous lymphatic leakage. Statistical analysis involved descriptive statistical methods with calculation of proportions and medians with interquartile ranges (IQRs). The study obtained institutional ethical approval (U3/2015 AKH).

Results

The treatment strategies applied in the CS1 patients are listed in Table 1. Twelve patients (16%) had received RPLND, clinical details of whom are listed in Table 2. The median ages of surgical patients and those managed with other modalities are 29 years (IQR 25–38, range 18–53 years) and 32 years (IQR 27–40 yrs., range 18–74 years), respectively, and are obviously not dissimilar in view of the widely overlapping interquartile ranges. Regarding histology, all except one patients had primary

tumours with components of teratoma, thereof six with proportions of more than 50% teratoma. Among the NS patients managed without RPLND only 35% had components of teratoma in the primary. Vascular invasion was present in 5 of the 12 cases. With regard to tumour markers, alpha fetoprotein was increased prior to orchiectomy in three cases and beta chorionic gonadotropin in one. All patients were marker-negative at the time of

Table 1 Treatment modalities applied after orchiectomy in 75 patients with nonseminomatous testicular germ cell tumours clinical stage 1

	(Number)	(Percent)
Adjuvant chemotherapy [a]	54	72.0
Surveillance	9	12.0
RPLND	12	16.0

[a]Chemotherapy consisted of two courses of PEB in 35 patients and of one course in 18; one had other chemotherapy

Table 2 Synopsis of patients undergoing primary RPLND

Patient (#)	Primary tumour: % teratoma	Primary tumour: Vascular inavasion	Individual reason for RPLND	Surgical result: nodes involved/nodes excised (n/n)	Additional treatment	Outcome
1	75%	no	Teratoma plus equivocal radiological finding	5/15	2xPEB	NED 8 yr
2	20%	no	Patient's choice	1/27	F/U	NED 7 yr
3	40%	no	Lupus erythematodes, chronic glomerulonephritis	0/42	F/U	NED 7 yr
4	60%	yes	Teratoma plus equivocal radiological finding	0/27	F/U	NED 6 yr
5	20%	yes	chronic kidney disease due to congenital polycystic disease	0/22	F/U	NED 5 yr
6	40%	yes	Equivocal radiological findings	0/30	F/U	NED 4 yr
7	50%	no	Patient's choice	0/26	F/U	NED 4 yr
8	10%	yes	Equivocal radiological findings	1/33	F/U, NHL 1 year later	AWSM 1 yr
9	95%	no	Teratoma plus equivocal radiological finding	0/24	F/U	NED 3 yr
10	60%	no	Patient's choice	0/39	F/U	NED 3 yr
11	90%	no	Teratoma plus equivocal radiological finding	1/29	F/U	NED 2 yr
12	0	yes	Patient's choice	1/10	2x PE	NED 1 yr.

PEB chemotherapy with cisplatin, etoposide, bleomycin; *F/U* follow-up, *NHL* Non Hodgkin lymphoma, *NED* no evidence of disease, *AWSM* alive with second malignancy, *yr* years

decision-making for additional treatment. The particular reasons for electing RPLND instead of chemotherapy or surveillance were unsuitability of chemotherapy due to chronic illnesses in 2 cases (Fig. 3), patient's choice in 4 cases, and equivocal radiological findings in the presence of teratomatous primary tumour in the remaining six cases (Fig. 4). A median number of 27 (range 10–42) lymph nodes were excised upon surgery. Lymph node metastases were identified in 5 cases (Fig. 5) none of whom had extranodal extension and all were excised completely. Two of the five pN1 patients received adjuvant chemotherapy. The reasons for additional treatment were an apparently high risk of recurrence in the patient with 5 nodes involved (21 yrs., #1, Table 2), and the individual wish for highest probability of disease-free survival in the other one (29 yrs., #12, Table 2).

No major surgical complications were noted in any of the patients and in all of whom antegrade ejaculation was preserved. One grade 2 complication according to the Clavien/Dindo classification involved chylous lymph secretion after restarting of oral nutrition that was amply detectable in the fluid collected via the abdominal drainage tube. This patient required intravenous nutrition for three days until cessation of chylous leakage. All patients remained disease-free with respect to GCT, however, one patient developed malignant Non-Hodgkin lymphoma one year after treatment for GCT and is currently undergoing chemotherapy for that second malignancy.

Of the patients managed with surveillance, two relapsed and were salvaged with chemotherapy. No relapse was recorded in those undergoing adjuvant chemotherapy. However, one patient succumbed to treatment-related vascular complications involving mesenterial infarction with bowel gangrene resulting from cisplatin-based chemotherapy.

Discussion

Retroperitoneal lymph node dissection is clearly no more the standard way of management of CS1 nonseminoma in European countries [20]. But, as shown in the present series, a well selected sub-cohort of patients might well benefit from it. RPLND is particularly useful in cases where chemotherapy is precluded by concurrent health problems. This constellation was given in two of our patients, one of whom had chronic kidney disease due to congenital polycystic disease (Fig. 3) and the other suffered from lupus erythematosus auto-immune disease. The surgical approach employed in these cases not only obviated the need for upfront chemotherapy but in light of high relapse rates upon surveillance it also minimized the need of chemotherapy during follow-up.

Four patients of our series refused chemotherapy for personal reasons and opted for surgery. All of these decisions were made by the patients after full information about advantages and disadvantages of the available treatment modalities representing the expression of

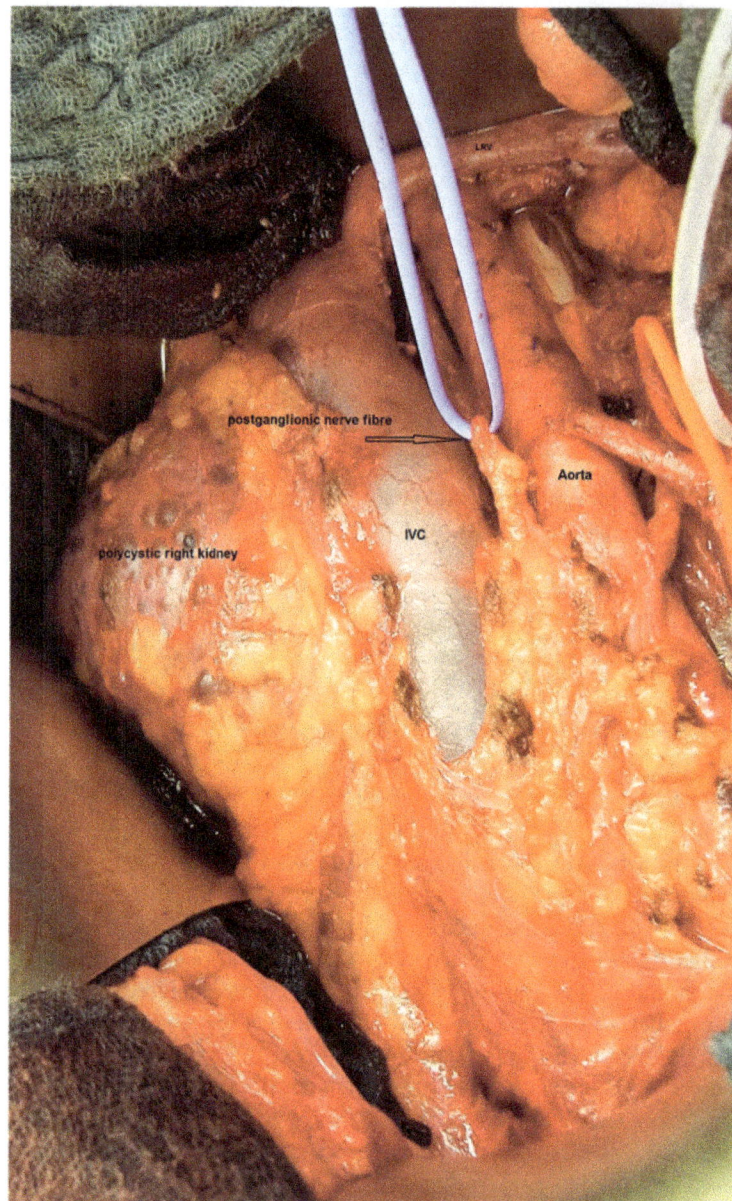

Fig. 3 Intraoperative site during RPLND of a patient #5 with polycystic kidney disease. IVC inferior vena cava; LRV left renal vein

patient autonomy as recently advocated by a joint statement of leading European GCT experts [21]. According to that report, a personalized approach to management decisions should be favoured because the over-all cure rates are excellent regardless of the treatment modality employed [14, 22]. Further, patient autonomy is to be strictly respected by care givers, and professionals are not supposed to influence their patients′ decisions. A full definition of patient autonomy is given on the MedicineNet website (www.medicinenet.com).

In six patients the decision for RPLND was based on equivocal radiological findings in the presence of teratomatous elements in the primary tumour. Retroperitoneal

lymph node metastases are radiologically defined by nodes sized > 10 mm in diameter and located in the primary landing zone of the testicular tumour [13, 23, 24]. However, as shown in large series of patients undergoing primary RPLND, around 20–25% of patients may harbor metastatic seeds in lymph nodes despite negative radiological findings [25, 26]. Clearly, a lot of clinical uncertainty exists in cases with lymph nodes sized around 1 cm particularly in those with negative markers. Adjuvant chemotherapy may overcome this problem because 1 or 2 cycles of cisplatin-based chemotherapy will usually sterilize micrometastatic spread [10, 27]. But of note, the subgroup of teratoma does not respond to chemotherapy

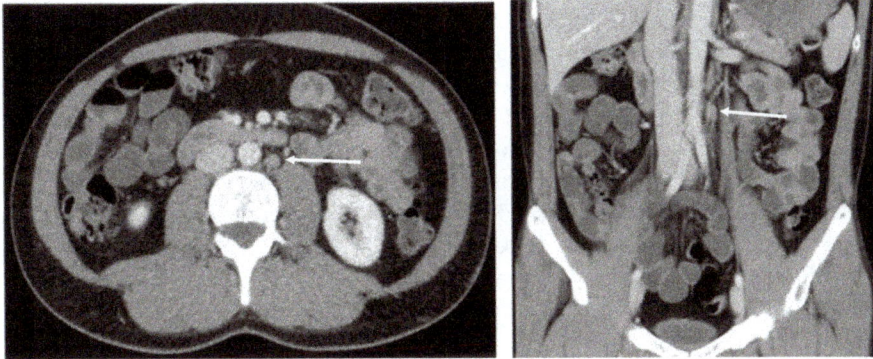

Fig. 4 (left) abdominal computed tomography (pt #9) showing lymph node of equivocal size (arrow) in the para-aortal template (axial scan). (right) same patient, CT showing suspicious para-aortal lymph node in coronal scan. Histologically, no metastasis was found in this lymph node

[28]. In patients having a high proportion of teratoma in the primary tumour, such chemotherapy-resistent elements must also be expected in the secondaries [29–31]. This constellation must be particularly considered when equivocally enlarged para-aortal lymph nodes are found upon abdominal imaging. Accordingly, in three of our six patients with these features, metastases were detected in the RPLND specimens. In two of whom, only one microscopic focus was found and surgery was considered sufficient for cure (Fig. 5).

When RPLND lost its role as the standard way of management of CS1 nonseminoma, the reasoning was mainly based on two arguments, the perioperative risk of this major surgical procedure being the leading one [12, 32]. Perioperative morbidity is clearly undisputable, but it is constantly decreasing ever since the employment of nerve-sparing surgical techniques. Furthermore, reduced complication rates result from rising experience of surgeons based on the increasing acceptance of guide-line recommendations to refer GCT patients requiring specific treatment modalities to recognized centres of excellence [33–36]. A further reduction of perioperative morbidity might be achieved with the upcoming implementation of laparoscopic or robotic-assisted surgical techniques [37].

The other argument against RPLND was the expectation of an over-all increased treatment burden in surgical patients relating to additional measures required in those with metastases found upon surgery (i.e. pathological stage [pS] 2a,b) [12, 32]. By comparison, primary adjuvant chemotherapy usually does not necessitate second treatment measures. However, dual treatment (i.e. RPLND plus adjuvant chemotherapy) is actually required

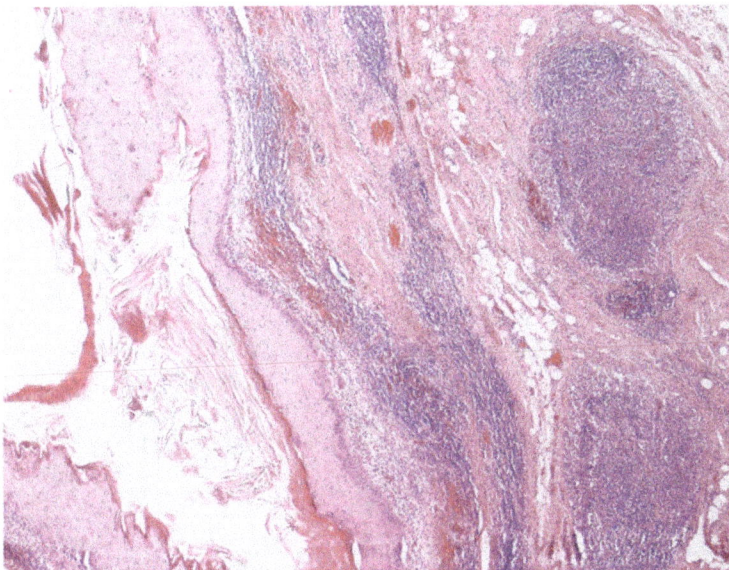

Fig. 5 Histologic section of lymph node specimen from RPLND (pt #11). Metastasis consisting of pure teratoma with cystic elements lined by squamous cell epithelium (left side of figure). Intact lymph node tissue on the right side. Hematoxylin eosin stain, original × 100

only by a minority of patients. Roughly, one third of CS1 patients undergoing primary RPLND will have pS2a,b [26]. But as shown in the classic reports on primary RPLND, about one half of the patients with surgically proven lymph node metastases do not progress and are thus virtually cured with the procedure [5, 33]. Accordingly, this way of management was successfully applied in two of our cases. Cisplatin-based chemotherapy does effectively eradicate microscopic foci of GCT. One course of PEB is sufficient to control CS1 disease [27].Two courses of PE (without bleomycin) have been shown to be safe in the adjuvant setting of pS2a cases [38] which was confirmed in one of our patients. In conclusion, only a small proportion of about 10–15% of the patients undergoing RPLND will need adjuvant chemotherapy as a second treatment modality, and notably, that treatment can be safely shaped to reduced doses with reduced toxicity. The over-all burden of additional therapy of the surgical patients is probably not as extensive as initially believed.

When weighting the arguments for and against the treatment modalities available for CS1 nonseminoma (i.e. chemotherapy, surveillance, RPLND) it should be noted that we are facing increasing knowledge about hazardous late effects of chemotherapy, particularly in light of the long-term exposure to circulating platinum owing to an estimated half-life of as long as 3.7 years [39]. The risk of second malignancies is significantly increased after cisplatin-based chemotherapy depending on cumulative dosages [40]. An excess of haematological malignancies has repeatedly been reported but also increased rates of renal carcinomas, thyroid cancer and soft tissue neoplasms [41–43]. In addition, multiple organ late toxicities have been reported notably a 1.9–3.1 fold risk of cardiovascular diseases including myocardial infarctions and cerebral strokes [44, 45], but also decreased pulmonary function [46] as well as other significant late sequelae of chemotherapy in a variety of organs [47, 48]. Although all of these late toxicities have been documented so far only in cases receiving full course chemotherapy it is not irrational to assume that late toxicities of lesser extent might occur in patients receiving the abbreviated prophylactic regimens. Particularly in view of the young ages of the nonseminoma patients potential late toxicities of systemic therapy must not be ignored.

Limitations of our analysis mainly involve the low number of patients. Also, selection bias cannot be ruled out because of the single-centre setting and the retrospective design of the study.

Conclusions

In Europe, primary RPLND is clearly not the standard way of managing nonseminoma CS1 patients. However, as documented herein it can be a valuable option in well-selected patients, particularly those with concurrent chronic diseases. Also, patients with equivocal radiological findings upon abdominal imaging in the presence of teratoma in the primary might benefit from surgery. Finally, a few patients may prefer RPLND after full information about the treatment modalities mirroring the increasing awareness and acceptance of patient autonomy.

Abbreviations
CI: Confidence intervals; CS: Clinical stage; GCT: Germ cell tumour; IQR: Interquartile range; NS : Nonseminoma; PEB: Chemotherapy with cisplatin, etoposide, bleomycin; pS: Pathological stage; RPLND: Retroperitoneal lymph node dissection

Acknowledgements
The authors are grateful to Prof. Thomas Löning for reviewing pathohistological slides of many of the surgical specimens. Dr. Raphael Ikogho and Mrs. Evelyn Stolle provided help compiling the clinical data.

Funding
This study did not receive any funding.

Authors' contributions
KPD conceived and designed the study, drafted the manuscript. PA co-conceived the study, participated in its design, performed data acquisition, and helped to draft the manuscript. MK participated in designing the study, performed data acquisition, performed most of the clinical management of patients. RG provided substantial help in data acquisition, did all of the imaging studies of the patients reported, participated in designing the study. BF performed histopathological examinations, participated in designing the study, gave substantial input to drafting the manuscript. All authors read and approved the final manuscript.

Competing interests
The authors declare that they have no competing interests.

Author details
[1]Albertinen-Krankenhaus Hamburg, Klinik für Urologie, Hamburg, Germany. [2]Asklepios Klinik Altona, Urologische Abteilung, Hodentumorzentrum Hamburg, Hamburg, Germany. [3]Albertinen-Krankenhaus Hamburg, Klinik für Diagnostische Radiologie, Hamburg, Germany. [4]MVZ Hanse Histologikum, Hamburg, Germany. [5]Asklepios Klinik Altona, Hodentumorzentrum Hamburg, Paul Ehrlich Strasse 1, 22763 Hamburg, Germany.

References
1. Chovanec M, Hanna N, Cary KC, Einhorn L, Albany C. Management of stage I testicular germ cell tumours. Nat Rev Urol. 2016;13(11):663–73.
2. Lewis LC. Testis tumors: report on 250 cases. J Urol. 1948;59:763–72.
3. Staubitz WJ, Magoss IV, Oberkircher OJ, Lent MH, Mitchell FD, Murphy WT. Management of testicular tumors. J Am Med Assoc. 1958;166(7):751–8.
4. Weissbach L, Boedefeld EA, Horstmann Dubral B. Surgical treatment of stage-I non-seminomatous germ cell testis tumor. Final results of a prospective multicenter trial 1982-1987. Testicular tumor study group. Eur Urol. 1990;17(2):97–106.
5. Donohue JP. Evolution of retroperitoneal lymphadenectomy (RPLND) in the management of non-seminomatous testicular cancer (NSGCT). Urol Oncol. 2003;21:129–32.
6. Peckham MJ, Barrett A, Husband JE, Hendry WF. Orchidectomy alone in testicular stage I non-seminomatous germ-cell tumours. Lancet. 1982; 2(8300):678–80.

7. Sturgeon JF, Moore MJ, Kakiashvili DM, Duran I, Anson-Cartwright LC, Berthold DR, Warde PR, Gospodarowicz MK, Alison RE, Liu J, et al. Non-risk-adapted surveillance in clinical stage I Nonseminomatous germ cell tumors: the Princess Margaret Hospital's experience. Eur Urol. 2011;59:556–62.

8. Daugaard G, Gundgaard MG, Mortensen MS, Agerbæk M, Holm NV, Rørth M, von der Maase H, Christensen IJ, Lauritsen J. Surveillance for stage I nonseminoma testicular Cancer: outcomes and long-term follow-up in a population-based cohort. J Clin Oncol. 2014;32(34):3817–23.

9. Yap SA, Yuh LM, Evans CP, Dall'Era MA, Wagenaar RM, Cress R, Lara PNJ. Evolving patterns of care in the management of stage I non-seminomatous germ cell tumors: data from the California Cancer registry. World J Urol. 2017;35(2):277–83.

10. Cullen M, James N. Adjuvant therapy for stage I testicular cancer. Cancer Treat Rev. 1996;22(4):253–64.

11. Pont J, Albrecht W, Postner G, Sellner F, Angel K, Höltl W. Adjuvant chemotherapy for high-risk clinical stage I nonseminomatous testicular germ cell cancer: long-term results of a prospective trial. J Clin Oncol. 1996;14(2):441–8.

12. Beyer J, Albers P, Altena R, Aparicio J, Bokemeyer C, Busch J, Cathomas R, Cavallin-Stahl E, Clarke NW, Claßen J, et al. Maintaining success, reducing treatment burden, focusing on survivorship: highlights from the third European consensus conference on diagnosis and treatment of germ-cell cancer. Ann Oncol. 2013;24(4):878–88.

13. Krege S, Beyer J, Souchon R, Albers P, Albrecht W, Algaba F, Bamberg M, Bodrogi I, Bokemeyer C, Cavallin-Ståhl E, et al. European consensus conference on diagnosis and treatment of germ cell Cancer: a report of the second meeting of the European germ cell Cancer consensus group (EGCCCG): part I. Eur Urol. 2008;53:478–96.

14. Albers P, Albrecht W, Algaba F, Bokemeyer C, Cohn-Cedermark G, Fizazi K, Horwich A, Laguna MP, Nicolai N, Oldenburg J. Guidelines on testicular Cancer: 2015 update. Eur Urol. 2015;68:1054–68.

15. Sun M, Abdollah F, Budäus L, Liberman D, Tian Z, Morgan M, Johal R, Schmitges J, Shariat SF, Montorsi F, et al. Trends of retroperitoneal lymphadenectomy use in patients with nonseminomatous germ cell tumor of the testis: a population-based study. Ann Surg Oncol. 2011; 18(10):2997–3004.

16. Clemons J, Zahnd WE, Nutt M, Sadowski D, Dynda D, Alanee S. Impact of urologist density and county rurality on the practice of retroperitoneal lymph node dissection and Cancer-specific death in patients with Nonseminomatous germ cell tumors. J Adolesc Young Adult Oncol. 2017; 6(1):83–90.

17. Sohaib SA, Koh DM, Husband JE. The role of imaging in the diagnosis, staging, and management of testicular cancer. AJR Am J Roentgenol. 2008; 191(2):387–95.

18. Donohue JP, Foster RS, Rowland RG, Bihrle R, Jones J, Geier G. Nerve-sparing retroperitoneal lymphadenectomy with preservation of ejaculation. J Urol. 1990;144(2 Pt 1):287–91.

19. Dieckmann KP, Gross AJ, Huland H. A test for the identification of relevant sympathetic nerve fibers during nerve-sparing retroperitoneal lymphadenectomy. J Urol. 1992;148:1450–2.

20. Hugen CM, Hu B, Jeldres C, Burton C, Nichols CR, Porter CR, Daneshmand S. Utilization of retroperitoneal lymph node dissection for testicular cancer in the United States: Results from the National Cancer Database (1998–2011). Urol Oncol. 2016;34:487.e487–11.

21. Oldenburg J, Aparicio J, Beyer J, Cohn-Cedermark G, Cullen M, Gilligan T, De Giorgi U, De Santis M, de Wit R, Fosså SD, et al. Personalizing, not patronizing: the case for patient autonomy by unbiased presentation of management options in stage I testicular cancer. Ann Oncol. 2015;26:833–8.

22. Isharwal S, Risk MC. Management of clinical stage I nonseminomatous germ cell tumors. Expert Rev Anticancer Ther. 2014;14:1–12.

23. Koh DM, Hughes M, Husband JE. Cross sectional imaging of nodal metastases in the abdomen and pelvis. Abdom Imaging. 2006;31(6):632–43.

24. Heidenreich A, Albers P, Classen J, Graefen M, Gschwend J, Kotzerke J, Krege S, Lehmann J, Rohde D, Schmidberger H, et al. Imaging studies in metastatic urogenital cancer patients undergoing systemic therapy: recommendations of a multidisciplinary consensus meeting of the Association of Urological Oncology of the German Cancer society. Urol Int. 2010;85(1):1–10.

25. Bussar-Maatz R, Weissbach L. Retroperitoneal lymph node staging of testicular tumours. TNM Study Group. Br J Urol. 1993;72(2):234–40.

26. Spermon JR, Roeleveld TA, van der Poel HG, Hulsbergen-van de Kaa CA, Ten Bokkel Huinink WW, van de Vijver M, Witjes JA, Horenblas S. Comparison of

surveillance and retroperitoneal lymph node dissection in stage I nonseminomatous germ cell tumors. Urology. 2002;59:923–9.

27. Tandstad T, Ståhl O, Håkansson U, Dahl O, Haugnes HS, Klepp OH, Langberg CW, Laurell A, Oldenburg J, Solberg A, et al. One course of adjuvant BEP in clinical stage I nonseminoma mature and expanded results from the SWENOTECA group. Ann Oncol. 2014;25(11):2167–72.

28. Rabbani F, Gleave ME, Coppin CM, Murray N, Sullivan LD. Teratoma in primary testis tumor reduces complete response rates in the retroperitoneum after primary chemotherapy. The case for primary retroperitoneal lymph node dissection of stage IIb germ cell tumors with teratomatous elements. Cancer. 1996;78(3):480–6.

29. Beck SD, Foster RS, Bihrle R, Ulbright T, Koch MO, Wahle GR, Einhorn LH, Donohue JP. Teratoma in the orchiectomy specimen and volume of metastasis are predictors of retroperitoneal teratoma in post-chemotherapy nonseminomatous testis cancer. J Urol. 2002;168(4 Pt 1):1402–4.

30. Heidenreich A, Moul JW, McLeod DG, Mostofi FK, Engelmann UH. The role of retroperitoneal lymphadenectomy in mature teratoma of the testis. J Urol. 1997;157(1):160–3.

31. Sheinfeld J, Motzer RJ, Rabbani F, McKiernan J, Bajorin D, Bosl GJ. Incidence and clinical outcome of patients with teratoma in the retroperitoneum following primary retroperitoneal lymph node dissection for clinical stages I and IIA nonseminomatous germ cell tumors. J Urol. 2003;170:1159–62.

32. Hotte SJ, Mayhew LA, Jewett M, Chin J, Winquist E. Genitourinary Cancer disease site Group of the Cancer Care Ontario Program in evidence-based care: management of stage I non-seminomatous testicular cancer: a systematic review and meta-analysis. Clin Oncol (R Coll Radiol). 2010;22:17–26.

33. Heidenreich A, Paffenholz P, Haidl F, Pfister D. When is surgical resection of metastases in testicular germ cell tumors indicated and is there a scientific basis? [Article in German]. Urologe A. 2017;56(5):627–36.

34. Tandstad T, Kollmannsberger CK, Roth BJ, Jeldres C, Gillessen S, Fizazi K, Daneshmand S, Lowrance WT, Hanna NH, Albany C, et al. Practice makes perfect: the rest of the story in testicular Cancer as a model curable neoplasm. J Clin Oncol. 2017;35(31):3525–8.

35. Albany C, Adra N, Snavely AC, Cary C, Masterson TA, Foster RS, Kesler K, Ulbright TM, Cheng L, Chovanec M, et al. Multidisciplinary clinic approach improves overall survival outcomes of patients with metastatic germ cell tumors. Ann Oncol. 2018;29(2):341–6.

36. Woldu SL, Matulay JT, Clinton TN, Singla N, Krabbe LM, Hutchinson RC, Sagalowsky A, Lotan Y, Margulis V, Bagrodia A. Impact of hospital case volume on testicular cancer outcomes and practice patterns. Urol Oncol. 2018;36(1):14.e17–5.

37. Kunit T, Janetschek G. Minimally invasive retroperitoneal lymphadenectomy: current status. Urol Clin North Am. 2015;42(3):321–9.

38. Motzer RJ, Sheinfeld J, Mazumdar M, Bajorin DF, Bosl GJ, Herr H, Lyn P, Vlamis V. Etoposide and cisplatin adjuvant therapy for patients with pathologic stage II germ cell tumors. J Clin Oncol. 1995;13(11):2700–4.

39. Boer H, Proost JH, Nuver J, Bunskoek S, Gietema JQ, Geubels BM, Altena R, Zwart N, Oosting SF, Vonk JM, et al. Long-term exposure to circulating platinum is associated with late effects of treatment in testicular Cancer survivors. Ann Oncol. 2015;26(11):2305–10.

40. Kier MG, Hansen MK, Lauritsen J, Mortensen MS, Bandak M, Agerbaek M, Holm NV, Dalton SO, Andersen KK, Johansen C, et al. Second malignant neoplasms and cause of death in patients with germ cell cancer: a Danish Nationwide cohort study. JAMA Oncol. 2016;2(12):1624–1.

41. Fung C, Sesso HD, Williams AM, Kerns SL, Monahan P, Abu Zaid M, Feldman DR, Hamilton RJ, Vaughn DJ, Beard CJ, et al. Multi-institutional assessment of adverse health outcomes among north American testicular Cancer survivors after modern cisplatin-based chemotherapy. J Clin Oncol. 2017;35(11):1211–22.

42. Maroto P, Anguera G, Martin C. Long-term toxicity of the treatment for germ cell-cancer. A review. Crit Rev Oncol Hematol. 2018;121:62–7.

43. Haugnes HS, Bosl GJ, Boer H, Gietema JA, Brydøy M, Oldenburg J, Dahl AA, Bremnes RM, Fosså SD. Long-term and late effects of germ cell testicular Cancer treatment and implications for follow-up. J Clin Oncol. 2012;30(30): 3752–63.

44. Huddart RA, Norman A, Shahidi M, Horwich A, Coward D, Nicholls J, Dearnaley DP. Cardiovascular disease as a long-term complication of treatment for testicular cancer. J Clin Oncol. 2003;21:1513–23.

45. Meinardi MT, Gietema JA, van der Graaf WT, van Veldhuisen DJ, Runne MA, Sluiter WJ, de Vries EG, Willemse PB, Mulder NH, van den Berg MP, et al. Cardiovascular morbidity in long-term survivors of metastatic testicular cancer. J Clin Oncol. 2000;18:1725–32.

24

Increased expression of immediate early response gene 3 protein promotes aggressive progression and predicts poor prognosis in human bladder cancer

Jianheng Ye[1,2†], Yanqiong Zhang[2,3†], Zhiduan Cai[4], Minyao Jiang[1], Bowei Li[1], Guo Chen[1], Yanru Zeng[1], Yuxiang Liang[1], Shulin Wu[2], Zongwei Wang[2], Huichan He[1,6*], Weide Zhong[1,5*] and Chin-Lee Wu[2*]

Abstract

Background: Immediate early response gene 3 (IER3) is a stress-inducible gene, which exerts diverse effects in regulating cell apoptosis and cell cycle. Growing evidence shows that IER3 functions either as an oncogene or a tumor suppressor in various human cancers with a cancer type-dependent manner. However, the involvement of IER3 in human bladder cancer (BCa) has not been elucidated. In the current study, we aimed to investigate the expression pattern and the clinical significance of IER3 in BCa.

Methods: We performed immunohistochemistry analysis to examine the subcellular localization and the expression levels of IER3 protein in 88 BCa specimens obtained from Department of Pathology in Massachusetts General Hospital. The associations of IER3 protein expression with various clinicopathological features and patients' overall survival were statistically evaluated.

Results: IER3 protein was mainly expressed in the cytoplasm in bladder cancer cell. Of 88 BCa tissue specimens, 39 (44.3%) showed high expression of IER3 protein and 49 (55.7%) showed low expression. High IER3 protein expression was significantly associated with high pathologic nodal stage ($p = 0.018$). Kaplan-Meier analysis revealed that the overall survival of BCa patients with overexpression of IER3 protein was shorter than that with low expression ($p < 0.01$). Multivariate analysis by Cox regression further identified IER3 as an independent prognostic factor of BCa patients ($p = 0.010$).

Conclusions: Our findings suggest for the first time that the increased expression of IER3 protein may promote the aggressive progression of BCa. Importantly, IER3 may be a potential prognostic marker for BCa patients.

Keywords: Immediate early response gene 3, Bladder cancer, Clinicopathological feature, Prognosis

* Correspondence: xiaohejian@21cn.com; zhongwd2009@live.cn; cwu2@mgh.harvard.edu
†Jianheng Ye and Yanqiong Zhang contributed equally to this work.
[1]Department of Urology, Guangdong Key Laboratory of Clinical Molecular Medicine and Diagnostics, Guangzhou First People's Hospital, Guangzhou Medical University, Guangzhou 510180, China
[2]Departments of Urology and Pathology, Massachusetts General Hospital and Harvard Medical School, Boston, MA 02114, USA
Full list of author information is available at the end of the article

Background

Bladder cancer (BCa) was the fourth most common cancer in men and the twelfth most common cancer in women in United States in 2016 [1]. Although there have been great advances in bladder carcinogenesis, the mortality rate of BCa is still high, due to its complex etiology and insufficient therapeutic strategies. A multivariate analysis showed that an increasing death rate of BCa was associated with multiple environmental exposures, such as smoking, air pollution, well water, urban residence and mining employment [2]. Most of BCa occur as non-muscle-invasive cancer, but there are still approximately 25% of them have muscle-invasive or metastatic disease, which leads to a poor outcome [3]. Therefore, it is of great clinical significance to discover novel and efficient molecular markers to develop more accurate diagnosis and prognosis methods for BCa patients.

Immediate early response gene 3 (IER3), also known as IEX-1, Dif-2, gly96 or p22/PRG-1, is a stress-inducible gene, which is rapidly regulated by multiple factors, including transcription factors, inflammatory cytokines, viral infection, chemical carcinogens, growth factors and hormones [4]. Under a wide range of stress, IER3 activation exerts diverse effects in regulating cell apoptosis and cell cycle with its distinct domains [5]. Accumulating studies have reported that IER3 may be associated with various signaling pathways, such as Nuclear factor kappa B (NF-κB) pathway and Mitogen-activated protein kinase (MAPK) /Extracellular regulated protein kinases (ERK) pathway, and may functions either as an oncogene or a tumor suppressor [6–8].

IER3 expression has been observed in a wide range of human epithelial tissues [9]. Growing evidence also shows that the aberrant expression of IER3 may be associated with prognosis in patients with multiple cancers [4]. However, the involvement of IER3 in BCa has not been elucidated. In this present study, we aimed to examine the expression pattern of IER3 protein in BCa tissues, and to evaluate its clinical significance in this malignancy.

Methods

Patients and tissues

This study used the same cohorts of BCa patients and tissue samples with our previous study [10]. All eighty-eight BCa tissue samples obtained from eighty-eight BCa patients who underwent cystectomy were collected from Massachusetts General Hospital between 2002 and 2010. The BCa patients' detail clinical information was shown in Table 1. All cases were re-reviewed by CLW and JHY (two authors) according to the newest version of World Health Organization classification of tumor of the bladder [11].

Table 1 Associations between IER3 protein expression and various clinicopathological characteristics of 88 BCa patients underwent cystectomy between 2002 and 2010

	IER3 (low)	IER3 (high)	P
Number of patients, no. %	49(55.7)	39(44.3)	
Gender, no.%			0.799
Female	12(24.5)	8(20.5)	
Male	37(75.5)	31(79.5)	
Age at Surgery, median(IQR)	70(62–75)	72(62–80)	0.462
pT, no. %			0.493
< =pT2	16(32.7)	10(25.6)	
> =pT3	33(67.3)	29(74.4)	
pN, no. % (n = 79)			**0.018**
pN(−)	33(76.7)	18(50.0)	
pN(+)	10(23.3)	18(50.0)	
LVI, no. %			0.284
LVI(−)	31(63.3)	20(51.3)	
LVI(+)	18(36.7)	19(48.7)	
PNI, no. %			0.808
PNI(−)	37(75.5)	28(71.8)	
PNI(+)	12(24.5)	11(28.2)	
STSM, no. %			0.781
margin(−)	40(81.6)	33(84.6)	
margin(+)	9(18.4)	6(15.4)	
Metastasis, no. %			1.000
Mets(−)	29(59.2)	23(59.0)	
Mets(+)	20(40.8)	16(41.0)	

Bold values indicate that they are less than 0.05

Immunohistochemistry and Immunoreactive score

Following the immunohistochemistry (IHC) protocol we described in our previous study [10], IER3 protein expression level was assessed by IHC using a polyclonal goat anti-IER3 antibody (Santa-Cruz biotechnology, CA). Detail information of IHC protocol was provided in Additional file 1. After performing IHC, the IER3 protein expression level in each tissue section was evaluated according to the immunostaining intensity and percentage. Immunoreactive score (IRS) was obtained by multiplying intensity and percentage of immunostaining. The intensity of immunostaining graded from 0 to 3: 0 (negative), 1 (weak), 2 (moderate), and 3 (strong); the percentage of staining cells were classified as 0–4: 0 (negative), 1 (<=10%), 2 (11–50%), 3 (51–80%), and 4 (> 80%). The final IRS (ranged from 0 to 12) was determined: 0–3 as low IER3 protein expression, and 4–12 as high IER3 protein expression [12]. The IRS of IER3 immunostaining of each tissue section was scored by two investigators (CLW and JHY) independently in a blind manner without any knowledge of the patient clinical characteristics.

The IRSs evaluated by two investigators respectively were compared. In order to reach a consensus, different IRSs of the same tissue section were reevaluated through a re-examination of the intensity of IER3 immunostaining by both investigators.

Statistics

All statistical analyses in this study were performed using Stata14 software (College Station, TX, USA).The associations between expression level of IER3 protein and BCa patients' clinicopathological data were analyzed by two statistical methods (Pearson's Chi-squared test or Fisher's exact test). Kaplan-Meier method was using to estimate the BCa patients' overall survival. Then, log-rank test was used for assessing differences. Cox proportional hazard regression models were used to perform univariate and multivariate survival analyses. Hazard ratios (HR) and the corresponding 95% confidence intervals (CI) were used to express the relative risks of dying. Two-sided with $p < 0.05$ was considered as statistically significant.

Results

Protein expression of IER3 in BCa

IER3 protein's expression in 88 BCa patients' tissue samples was identified by IHC. As shown in Fig. 1, IER3 protein was mainly localized in the cytoplasm of BCa cells. All specimens were divided into 2 groups: high IER3 protein expression group, containing 39 (44.3%) BCa patients; low IER3 protein expression group, containing 49 (55.7%) BCa patients. Statistical analysis showed that BCa patients with high expression of IER3 protein more frequently had high pathologic nodal stage (pN) ($p = 0.018$, Table 1). However, no significant associations were observed between IER3 protein expression level and other clinicopathological features, including patients' age, pathological stage (pT), gender, perineural

invasion (PNI), lymphvascular invasion (LVI), soft tissue surgical margins (STSM) and distant metastasis.

High IER3 protein expression was an independent indicator of poor prognosis in BCa patients

After analyzed by Kaplan-Meier method, the curves showed that BCa patients in high IER3 protein expression group had worse overall survival compared with those in low IER3 protein expression group ($p = 0.002$,Fig. 2). Additionally, the univariate analysis demonstrated that old patients' age ($p = 0.029$), high pT ($p = 0.006$), high pN ($p < 0.001$), positive LVI ($p = 0.006$), positive STSM ($p = 0.002$), positive distant metastasis ($p = 0.001$) and high expression of IER3 protein ($p = 0.003$) were all associated with poor survival of BCa patients significantly (Table 2). The multivariate survival comparison indicated that patients' age ($p = 0.012$), pN ($p = 0.007$) and IER3 protein expression ($p = 0.010$) can act as the independent prognostic indicators of BCa (Table 2).

Discussion

IER3 was initially identified as a radiation-inducible protein in squamous carcinomas [13]. It has been demonstrated to response to quite distinct stress or cellular stimuli immediately. Among these stimulating factors, NF-κB, p53, SP1 and AP1 are well-known to be involved into tumor development [6]. Increasing evidence show that IER3 may play complex roles in cell apoptosis in different manners [4–6]. In a mitochondria-dependent environment, IER3 up-regulated can reduce the production of intracellular reactive oxygen species by facilitating the degradation of the inhibitor of F1 catalytic sector, which can prevent apoptosis at its initial phase [14]. On the other hand, IER3 was identified to mediate the NF-κB signaling pathway by interacting with RelA/p65 subunit. This modification can contribute to inducing the expression of

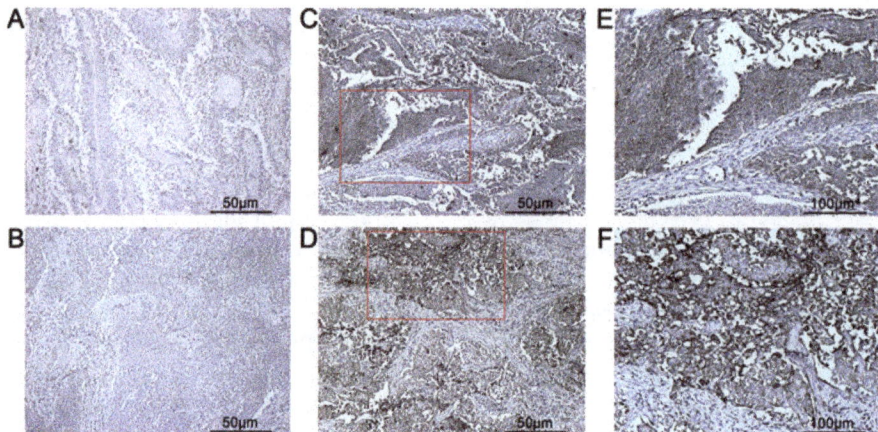

Fig. 1 Representative images of IER3 immunostaining in BCa tissue specimens. Negative (**a** and **b**) and positive (**c** and **d**) expression of IER3 protein are shown (Magnification: 100X). Magnified images (**e** and **f**) of two immunostaining regions marked by red boxes in **c** and **d** (Magnification: 200X)

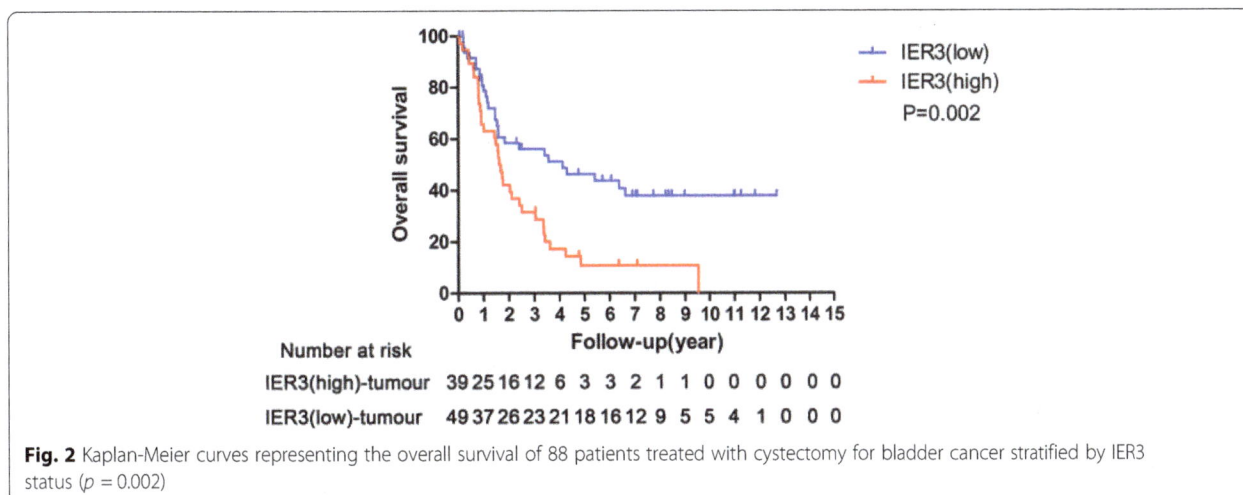

Fig. 2 Kaplan-Meier curves representing the overall survival of 88 patients treated with cystectomy for bladder cancer stratified by IER3 status (p = 0.002)

anti-apoptotic NF-κB target genes and then supporting cell apoptosis [15]. Besides the impact of IER3 on NF-κB signaling pathway, some studies indicated the IER3 might act as a regulator of ERK1/2 pathway. A phenomenon found by Letourneux et al. [16] showed that ERK activation led to IER3 phosphorylation. Simultaneously, the p-IER3 can enhance ERK phosphorylation by preventing its dephosphorylation factor B56-containing PP2A. The roles of IER3 sustaining ERK1/2 phosphorylation and promoting the tumor development were found in pancreatic cancer [17], lung adenocarcinoma [18] and Hodgkin lymphoma [19]. Moreover, IER3 were found to play

crucial roles in regulating tumor growth. Han et al. [20] analyzed the clinical significance of IER3 expression in 77 ovarian carcinoma patients by using immunohistochemistry, and found a decreased expression of IER3 in ovarian carcinoma tissues compared to cystadenoma and borderline tumors tissues. They also indicated that the decreased expression of IER3 was associated with a short survival time of patients with this cancer. They subsequently showed a positive correlation between IER3 expression and anti-apoptotic activity of ovarian cancer cell. In breast cancer, estrogen was reported to effectively up-regulated the expression of IER3 [21]. Furthermore, Yang et al. [22]

Table 2 Prognostic value of IER3 protein expression for the overall survival by Cox proportional hazards model

	Univariable			Multivariable		
	Hazard Ratio	95% CI	*P*	Hazard Ratio Ratio	95% CI	*p*
Gender						
Male vs. Female	1.14	0.62–2.10	0.681			
Age	1.03	1.00–1.05	**0.029**	1.04	1.01–1.07	**0.012**
pT						
>=pT3 vs. <=pT2	2.39	1.29–4.42	**0.006**	1.54	0.71–3.32	0.272
pN						
pN(+) vs. pN(−)	3.41	1.95–5.99	**< 0.001**	2.35	1.26–4.38	**0.007**
LVI						
LVI(+) vs. LVI(−)	2.03	1.22–3.37	**0.006**	0.99	0.52–1.89	0.987
PNI						
PNI(+) vs. PNI(−)	1.03	0.56–1.87	0.935			
STSM						
STSM(+) vs. STSM(−)	2.62	1.41–4.88	**0.002**	2.02	0.96–4.27	0.065
Metastasis						
Mets(+) vs. Mets(−)	2.35	1.41–3.97	**0.001**	1.81	0.98–3.33	0.058
IER3 IHC						
IER3(high) vs. IER3(low)	2.16	1.29–3.13	**0.003**	2.21	1.21–4.04	**0.010**

Bold values indicate that they are less than 0.05

showed IER3 was overexpressed in invasive breast cancer tissues compared with preinvasive cancer tissues. In vitro experimental system, IER3 was found to reduce the apoptotic activity of T47D and MCF-7 cells. Akilov et al. [23] revealed that IER3 up-regulation in Sézary cells might result in decreased expression levels of reactive oxygen species; as a downstream target of TNF-α-induced pathway, IER3 could protect Sézary cells from TNF-α-induced apoptosis. Sasada et al. [24] found that IER3 protein showed high expression in 41 patients and low expression in 37 patients with pancreatic cancer; statistically, patients with IER3 overexpression had a significantly better survival than those with low expression. In colon cancer, Nambiar et al. [25] built two different mouse models with hyperplasic or dysplastic preneoplastic aberrant crypt foci (ACF). The gene expression analysis based on ACF lesions showed that IER3 expression was increased in low risk ACF mice compared to high risk ACF mice; further immunohistochemistry analysis showed the positive staining of IER3 in adjacent normal-appearing colonic while the negative staining in the tumor crypts from the same patients. These findings suggest that the aberrant expression of IER3 may be implicated into carcinogenesis, progression and patients' outcome of various human cancers.

In present study, we determined that IER3 protein was overexpressed in the cytoplasm of cancer cells in BCa tissues specimens and that high IER3 protein expression was distinctly associated with high pathologic nodal stage. Notably, high IER3 protein expression also predicted poor overall survival in BCa patients.

Conclusions

Our findings suggest for the first time that the increased expression of IER3 protein may promote the aggressive progression of BCa. Importantly, IER3 may be a potential prognostic marker for BCa patients. Further investigations on molecular mechanisms underlying IER3 involvement in BCa are required.

Abbreviations

ACF: Aberrant crypt foci; AP-1: Activator protein 1; BCa: Bladder cancer; CI: Confidence intervals; ERK: Extracellular regulated protein kinases; HR: Hazard ratios; IER3: Immediate early response gene 3; IHC: Immunohistochemistry; IQR: Interquartile Range; IRS: Immunoreactive score; LVI: Lymphvascular invasion; MAPK: Mitogen-activated protein kinase; Mets: Metastasis; NF-κB: Nuclear factor kappa B; P: p-value; pN: Pathologic nodal stage; PNI: Perineural invasion; pT: Pathological stage; SP1: Specificity protein 1; STSM: Soft tissue surgical margins; TNFα: Tumor necrosis factor alpha

Funding
This work was supported by grants from National Key Basic Research Program of China (2015CB553706), National Natural Science Foundation of China (81571427, 81470983, 81641102), Science and Technology Project of Guangdong Province (2016A020215018, 2013B021800055), Guangzhou Municipal Science and Technology Project (2014 J4100072), Projects of Guangzhou Key Laboratory of Clinical Molecular Medicine and Diagnostics & NIH/NCI P01 CA120964. These foundations did not interfere in the design of the study and collection, analysis, and interpretation of data and in writing the manuscript.

Authors' contributions
WDZ, CLW, HCH: participated in study design and coordination, analysis and interpretation of data, material support for obtained funding, and supervised study. JHY and YQZ: performed most of the experiments, drafted and revised the manuscript. SLW and ZWW: performed statistical analysis. ZDC, MYJ, BWL, GC, YRZ and YXL: carried out the experiments and samples collection. All authors have read and approved the final version of the manuscript.

Competing interests
The authors declare that they have no competing interests.

Author details
[1]Department of Urology, Guangdong Key Laboratory of Clinical Molecular Medicine and Diagnostics, Guangzhou First People's Hospital, Guangzhou Medical University, Guangzhou 510180, China. [2]Departments of Urology and Pathology, Massachusetts General Hospital and Harvard Medical School, Boston, MA 02114, USA. [3]Institute of Chinese Materia Medica, China Academy of Chinese Medical Sciences, Beijing 100700, China. [4]Southern Medical University, Guangzhou 510515, China. [5]Department of Urology, Guangzhou First People's Hospital, Guangzhou Medical University, Guangzhou 510180, China. [6]Urology Key Laboratory of Guangdong Province, The First Affiliated Hospital of Guangzhou Medical University, Guangzhou Medical University, Guangzhou 510230, China.

References
1. Siegel RL, Miller KD, Jemal A. Cancer statistics, 2016. CA Cancer J Clin. 2016; 66(1):7–30.
2. Smith ND, Prasad SM, Patel AR, Weiner AB, Pariser JJ, Razmaria A, Maene C, Schuble T, Pierce B, Steinberg GD. Bladder Cancer mortality in the United States: a geographic and temporal analysis of socioeconomic and environmental factors. J Urol. 2016;195(2):290–6.
3. Kamat AM, Hahn NM, Efstathiou JA, Lerner SP, Malmström PU, Choi W, Guo CC, Lotan Y, Kassouf W. Bladder cancer. Lancet. 2016;388(10061):2796–810.
4. Wu MX, Ustyugova IV, Han L, Akilov OE. Immediate early response gene X-1, a potential prognostic biomarker in cancers. Expert Opin Ther Targets. 2013; 17(5):593–606.
5. Shen L, Guo J, Santos-Berrios C, Wu MX. Distinct domains for anti- and pro-apoptotic activities of IER3. J Biol Chem. 2006;281(22):15304–11.
6. Arlt A, Schäfer H. Role of the immediate early response 3 (IER3) gene in cellular stress response, inflammation and tumorigenesis. Eur J Cell Biol. 2011;90(6–7):545–52.
7. Wu MX, Ao Z, Prasad KV, Wu R, Schlossman SF. IEX-1L, an apoptosis inhibitor involved in NF-kappaB-mediated cell survival. Science. 1998; 281(5379):998–1001.
8. de Laval B, Pawlikowska P, Barbieri D, Besnard-Guerin C, Cico A, Kumar R, Gaudry M, Baud V, Porteu F. Thrombopoietin promotes NHEJ DNA repair in hematopoietic stem cells through specific activation of Erk and NF-κB pathways and their target, IEX-1. Blood. 2014;123(4):509–19.
9. Feldmann KA, Pittelkow MR, Roche PC, Kumar R, Grande JP. Expression of an immediate early gene, IER3, in human tissues. Histochem Cell Biol. 2001; 115(6):489–97.
10. Wu S, Ye J, Wang Z, Lin SX, Lu M, Liang Y, Zhu X, Olumi AF, Zhong WD, Wu CL. Expression of aromatase in tumor related stroma is associated with human bladder cancer progression. Cancer Biol Ther. 2018;19(3):175–80.
11. Humphrey PA, Moch H, Cubilla AL, Ulbright TM, Reuter VE. The 2016 WHO classification of Tumours of the urinary system and male genital organs-part B: prostate and bladder Tumours. Eur Urol. 2016;70(1):106–19.

12. Specht E, Kaemmerer D, Sänger J, Wirtz RM, Schulz S, Lupp A. Comparison of immunoreactive score, HER2/neu score and H score for the immunohistochemical evaluation of somatostatin receptors in bronchopulmonary neuroendocrine neoplasms. Histopathology. 2015; 67(3):368–77.

13. Kondratyev AD, Chung KN, Jung MO. Identification and characterization of a radiation-inducible glycosylated human early-response gene. Cancer Res. 1996;56(7):1498–502.

14. Shen L, Zhi L, Hu W, Wu MX. IEX-1 targets mitochondrial F1Fo-ATPase inhibitor for degradation. Cell Death Differ. 2009;16(4):603–12.

15. Arlt A, Rosenstiel P, Kruse ML, Grohmann F, Minkenberg J, Perkins ND, Fölsch UR, Schreiber S, Schäfer H. IEX-1 directly interferes with RelA/p65 dependent transactivation and regulation of apoptosis. Biochim Biophys Acta. 2008;1783(5):941–52.

16. Letourneux C, Rocher G, Porteu F. B56-containing PP2A dephosphorylate ERK and their activity is controlled by the early gene IEX-1 and ERK. EMBO J. 2006;25(4):727–38.

17. Garcia MN, Grasso D, Lopez-Millan MB, Hamidi T, Loncle C, Tomasini R, Lomberk G, Porteu F, Urrutia R, Iovanna JL. IER3 supports KRAS^{G12D} dependent pancreatic cancer development by sustainingERK1/2 phosphorylation. J Clin Invest. 2014;124(11):4709–22.

18. Ito T, Ozaki S, Chanasong R, Mizutani Y, Oyama T, Sakurai H, Matsumoto I, Takemura H, Kawahara E. Activation of ERK/IER3/PP2A-B56γ-positive feedback loop in lung adenocarcinoma by allelic deletion of B56γ gene. Oncol Rep. 2016;35(5):2635–42.

19. Locatelli SL, Careddu G, Stirparo GG, Castagna L, Santoro A, Carlo-Stella C. Dual PI3K/ERK inhibition induces necroptotic cell death of Hodgkin lymphoma cells through IER3 downregulation. Sci Rep. 2016;6:35745.

20. Han L, Geng L, Liu X, Shi H, He W, Wu MX. Clinical significance of IEX-1 expression in ovarian carcinoma. Ultrastruct Pathol. 2011;35(6):260–6.

21. Rasmussen LM, Frederiksen KS, Din N, Galsgaard E, Christensen L, Berchtold MW, Panina S. Prolactin and oestrogen synergistically regulate gene expression and proliferation of breast cancer cells. Endocr Relat Cancer. 2010;17(3):809–22.

22. Yang C, Trent S, Ionescu-Tiba V, Lan L, Shioda T, Sgroi D, Schmidt EV. Identification of cyclin D1- and estrogen- regulated genes contributing to breast carcinogenesis and progression. Cancer Res. 2006;66(24):11649–58.

23. Akilov OE, Wu MX, Ustyugova IV, Falo LD Jr, Geskin LJ. Resistance of Sézary cells to TNF-α-induced apoptosis is mediated in part by a loss of TNFR1 and a high level of the IER3 expression. Exp Dermatol. 2012;21(4):287–92.

24. Sasada T, Azuma K, Hirai T, Hashida H, Kanai M, Yanagawa T, Takabayashi A. Prognostic significance of the immediate early response gene X-1 (IER3) expression in pancreatic cancer. Ann Surg Oncol. 2008;15(2):609–17.

25. Nambiar PR, Nakanishi M, Gupta R, Cheung E, Firouzi A, Ma XJ, Flynn C, Dong M, Guda K, Levine J, Raja R, Achenie L, Rosenberg DW. Genetic signatures of high- and low-risk aberrant crypt foci in a mouse model of sporadic colon cancer. Cancer Res. 2004;64(18):6394–401.

Epidermal growth factor expression as a predictor of chemotherapeutic resistance in muscle-invasive bladder cancer

Ahmed M. Mansour[1,2], Mona Abdelrahim[1], Mahmoud Laymon[1], Mamdouh Elsherbeeny[1], Mohammed Sultan[1], Ahmed Shokeir[1], Ahmed Mosbah[1], Hassan Abol-Enein[1], Amira Awadalla[1], Eunho Cho[3], Vikram Sairam[3], Taeeun D. Park[4], Muhammad Shahid[5] and Jayoung Kim[3,5*]

Abstract

Background: Epidermal growth factor receptor (EGFR) overexpression is believed to be associated with bladder cancer (BC) progression and poor clinical outcomes. In vivo studies have linked EGFR subcellular trafficking and chemo-resistance to cisplatin-based chemotherapies. This has not been studied in the clinical adjuvant setting. We aimed to investigate the prognostic significance of EGFR expression in patients receiving cisplatin-based adjuvant chemotherapy following radical cystectomy for advanced BC.

Methods: The database from the Urology and Nephrology Center at Mansoura University was reviewed. BC patients who were treated with radical cystectomy and adjuvant chemotherapy for adverse pathological features or node positive disease were identified. Patients who underwent palliative cystectomy, had histological diagnoses other than pure urothelial carcinoma, or received adjuvant radiotherapy were excluded from the study. Immunohistochemical staining for EGFR expression was performed on archived bladder specimens. The following in vitro functional analyses were performed to study the relationship of EGFR expression and chemoresponse.

Results: The study included 58 patients, among which the mean age was 57 years old. Majority of patients had node positive disease ($n = 53$, 91%). Mean follow up was 26.61 months. EGFR was overexpressed in 25 cystectomy specimens (43%). Kaplan-Meier analysis revealed that EGFR over-expression significantly correlated with disease recurrence ($p = 0.021$). Cox proportional hazard modeling identified EGFR overexpression as an independent predictor for disease recurrence ($p = 0.04$). Furthermore, in vitro experiments demonstrated that inhibition of EGFR may sensitize cellular responses to cisplatin.

Conclusions: Our findings suggest that EGFR overexpression is associated with disease recurrence following adjuvant chemotherapy for advanced BC. This may aid in patient prognostication and selection prior to chemotherapeutic treatment for BC.

Keywords: EGFR, Bladder cancer, Survival, Adjuvant chemotherapy

---

* Correspondence: Jayoung.kim@csmc.edu
[3]University of California Los Angeles, Los Angeles, CA, USA
[5]Departments of Surgery and Biomedical Sciences, Samuel Oschin Comprehensive Cancer Institute, Cedars Sinai Medical Center, 8700 Beverly Blvd, Los Angeles, CA 90048, USA
Full list of author information is available at the end of the article

Background

Bladder cancer (BC) is the second most common genito-urinary malignancy and the fourth most common cancer in the United States (U.S.). Over an estimated $4 billion/year is spent on BC treatment annually in the U.S., making BC one of the most expensive cancer treatments to date [1–3]. Currently, BC is also the most common cancer in Egyptian males, representing about 30% of all cancer types [4]. Thus, BC is a major burden on the health services and economic resources at an international level [5]. Despite the drastic decrease in the prevalence of schistosomiasis in Egypt due to nationwide anti-bilharzial campaigns, there has been an increase in incidences of bladder urothelial carcinoma. This could possibly be due to smoking and carcinogenic chemical exposure [6, 7].

The gold standard therapy for patients with muscle-invasive bladder cancer (MIBC) is radical cystectomy with regional lymphadenectomy. Despite local aggressive therapy, nearly half of patients eventually develop metastasized tumors and, ultimately, die from the disease [8]. In an attempt to improve survival, integration of systemic chemotherapy with surgical management has been suggested to control micrometastasis [9]. However, around 40% of patients receiving neoadjuvant chemotherapy are termed "non-responders", with a complete pathological down-staging rate of only 14–38% [10, 11]. MIBC patients who do not respond to adjuvant chemotherapy generally have a poor prognosis [12]. The incidence of BC recurrence following chemotherapy remains high with a modest survival advantage of 5–15%. Thus, there is an important and urgent need to identify prognostic marker(s) that will identify patients who are at risk and to better understand the functional contribution of potential predictive markers in aggressive BC.

Prior research has shown that epidermal growth factor receptor (EGFR) overexpression has been associated with BC progression and poor clinical outcomes [13, 14]. In vivo studies have linked EGFR subcellular trafficking and chemo-resistance in many tumor types [15, 16]. However, this has not yet been studied in the clinical adjuvant setting.

In this study, we aimed to investigate the prognostic significance of EGFR expression in patients receiving adjuvant chemotherapy. Our study was conducted on an Egyptian cohort. Our findings suggest that EGFR protein expression may be indicative of aggressive BC and these expression patterns possibly involve direct action on signaling pathways in BC cells.

Methods

Patients and tissue samples

All of the enrolled patients had been treated with similar or identical regimens with at least four cycles of cisplatin-based chemotherapy. Patients previously treated with radical cystectomy and had completed adjuvant chemotherapy for adverse pathological features or node positive diseases were selected. Exclusion criteria were applied to patients who underwent palliative cystectomy, those with histological diagnosis other than pure transitional cell carcinoma, and patients who received adjuvant radiotherapy. Bladder tumors were staged according to the 2002 TNM classification. Disease progression was defined as newly diagnosed distant metastases with a $\geq 20\%$ increment increase in tumor mass following radical cystectomy. Surgical tumor tissues were macro-dissected, typically within 15 min of surgical resection. Each BC specimen was confirmed as representative by analysis of adjacent tissue in fresh frozen sections from radical cystectomy specimens.

Reagents

Cisplatin was purchased from Sigma. Antibodies against EGFR and β-actin were obtained from Cell Signaling Technology (for Western blot analysis), Abcam (for IHC analysis) and Santa Cruz Biotechnology. The ECL detection kit was from BioRad and New England Nuclear. All other biochemical reagents were purchased from Sigma or BD Biosciences.

Immunohistochemical staining

Immunohistochemical (IHC) analysis for EGFR expression was performed on archived bladder specimens. The relationship of EGFR expression and clinical outcomes was assessed. In vitro studies were performed to determine whether EGFR expression was associated with resistance to chemotherapeutic reagents. Paraffin blocks from 58 BC cases were used for immunohistochemical analysis. Tissue sections were cut and placed on Superfrost Plus microscope slides. Using the Benchmark XT automated immunohistochemistry stainer (Ventana Medical Systems, Inc., Tucson, AZ, USA), slides were stained following typical procedure. Detection was done using the Ventana Ultraview DAB Kit (Ventana Medical Systems).

Sections were deparaffinized using EZ Prep solution. CC1 standard (pH 8.4 buffer contained Tris/Borate/EDTA) was used for antigen retrieval. DAB inhibitor (3% H_2O_2, Endogenous peroxidase) was blocked for 4 min at 37 °C temperature. Sections were incubated with an anti-EGFR (Cat # ab32077, Abcam Inc., San Diego, CA, dilution 1/100) primary antibody for 40 min at 37 °C, and then incubated with a secondary antibody of Universal HRP Multimer for 8 min at 37 °C. Slides were then incubated with DAB + H_2O_2 substrate for 8 min, followed by hematoxylin and bluing reagent counterstain at 37 °C. Reaction buffer (pH 7.6 Tris buffer) was used as the washing solution. Staining intensity and proportion of positively-stained cells were evaluated. Staining intensity

Table 1 Baseline characteristics of the patients in this study

Variables		Incidence (SD or %)
Age mean (SD)		57 (6.6)
No. gender (%)	Male	53 (91.4)
	Female	5 (8.6)
No. clinical T stage (%)	T2	7 (12.1)
	T3	30 (51.7)
	T4a	18 (31.1)
	T4b	3 (5.2)
No. pathologic T stage (%)	TIS	1 (1.7)
	T1	1 (1.7)
	T2a	7 (12.1)
	T2b	7 (12.1)
	T3a	22 (37.9)
	T3b	15 (25.9)
	T4a	5 (8.6)
No. pathologic N status (%)	N0	5 (8.6)
	N1	14 (24.1)
	N2	37 (63.8)
	N3	2 (3.4)
No. lymphovascular invasion (%)	Yes	45 (77)
	No	13 (23)
No. strong EGFR expression (%)	Yes	10 (17.2)
	No	48 (82.8)

was classified as follows: none (score 0), weak (score 1), moderate (score 2) and strong (score 3). Each specimen was examined and scored separately by two pathologists, and discrepancies were discussed until agreements were reached.

Cell culture and transfection

TCCSUP or T24 human BC cells were purchased from American Type Culture Collection (ATCC, Manassas, VA) and maintained in DMEM or RPMI1640 (Invitrogen, Carlsbad, CA) with 10% FBS and 1% Penicillin/Streptomycin at 37 °C under 5% CO_2. The day before transfection, TCCSUP or T24 cells were trypsinized and counted. Cells were plated in 6-well plate with approximately 6.25×10^5 cells per well in 2 ml of complete growth medium. When cell density reached 80–90% confluence, TCCSUP or T24 BC cells were transiently transfected with 25-50 nM of small interfering RNAs (siRNAs) targeting EGFR (SignalSilence® EGF Receptor siRNA, Cell Signaling #6482) using Lipofactamine 2000. For transfection controls, empty (Ctrl) or non-target siRNAs (siCtrl) were used.

Cell viability assay

Experiments were performed in 6-well plates after cell density reached to about 90% (2×10^3/well). TCCSUP or T24 cells were transfected with various constructs or siRNAs and cisplatin simultaneously for 48 h (siRNA added 2 h before cisplatin). Cells were then incubated with cisplatin containing serum-free medium (RPMI1640

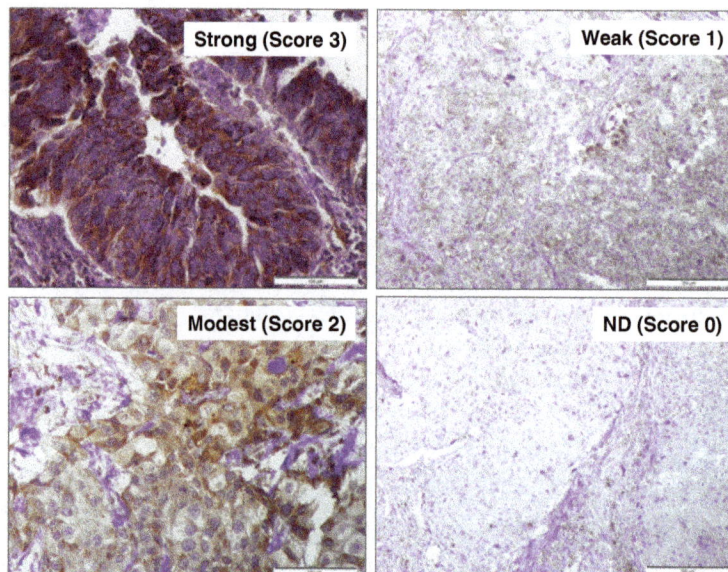

Fig. 1 Representative figures showing IHC slides with different scores. Immunohistochemical staining for EGFR in BC tissue samples. Four representative fields are shown after IHC staining with anti-EGFR (1:1000 dilution). Negative (Score 0), weak (Score 1), intermediate (Score 2), and strong (Score 3). EGFR expression was observed in the cytoplasm, membrane, and/or nucleus in our BC specimens. The intensity of EGFR staining was often heterogeneous within the same cancer tissue.

Epidermal growth factor expression as a predictor of chemotherapeutic resistance in muscle-invasive...

207

Table 2 Cox proportional hazard model of overall survival predictors

Covariate	Univariate		Multivariate	
	HR (95% CI)	P value	HR (95% CI)	P value
Age	1.41 (1.02–2.45)	0.029	1.34 (0.94–1.77)	0.056
Sex (M vs F)	1.88 (1.06–3.34)	0.048	1.48 (0.26–1.80)	0.479
EGFR expression (strong vs negative/weak/moderate)	1.55 (1.30.-2.33)	0.002	1.38 (1.201–2.744)	0.004
Chemotherapy Regimen (MVAC vs GemCis)	1.72 (0.84–3.75)	0.159		
pT stage (T2 or less vs greater than T2)	2.88 (1.92–3.99)	0.003	3.28 (1.54–4.62)	< 0.001
pN stage (N0 vs greater than N0)	2.31 (1.88–2.93)	< 0.001	1.81 (1.23–2.74)	< 0.001

or DMEM) for the indicated time. Cell viability was determined using MTS reagents, as instructed by the company's protocol (Promega Corporation, Madison, WI).

Statistical analysis

Univariate analysis with the Pearson chi-square was performed to analyze associations between strong EGFR expression and pT stage, pN stage, (N0 and greater than N0) and lymphovascular invasion. A Kaplan-Meier estimator curve with the log rank test and a Cox proportional hazard model were used to test whether observed

response to chemotherapy predicted disease specific survival.

Results

Baseline characteristics

The study included 58 patients. The mean age of the 57 patients who received adjuvant therapy was 57 ± 6.6 years, and the mean follow-up period was 26.61 months. A majority of patients had node positive disease ($n = 53$, 91%). Forty-five patients (77%) had lymphovascular invasion. Other baseline characteristics of the patients are presented in Table 1.

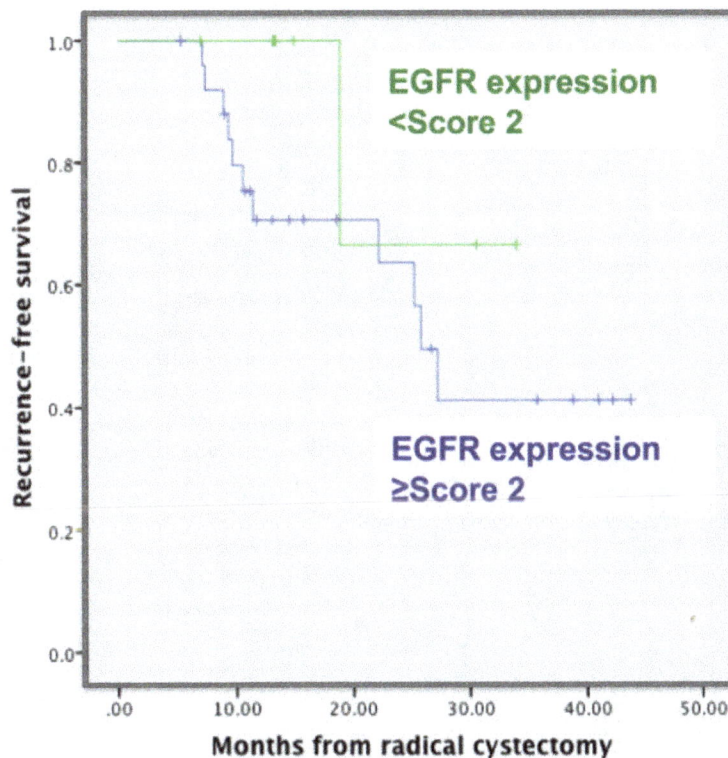

Fig. 2 Cancer-specific survival in BC patients stratified by EGFR staining

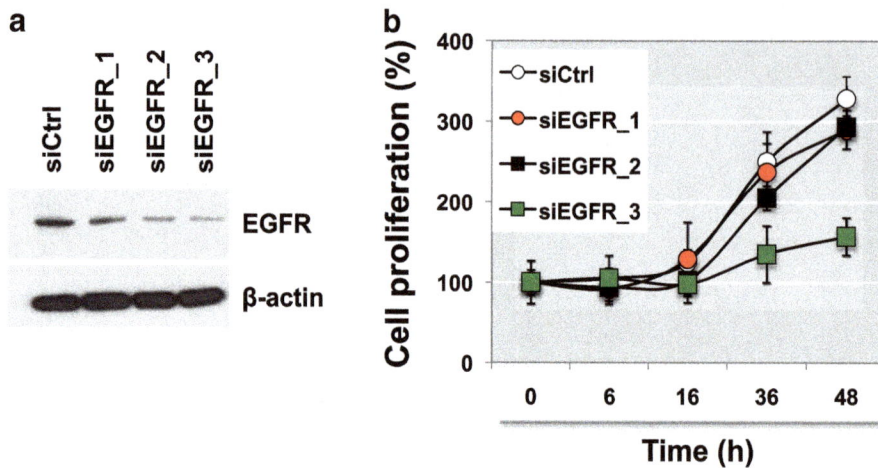

Fig. 3 EGFR expression is associated with drug sensitivity to cisplatin treatment. **a, b** TCCSUP cells were transiently transfected with varying doses of siRNA against EGFR. Knockdown of EGFR with control and EGFR-targeted siRNAs shows that proliferation in TCCSUP BC cells decreases in a dose-dependent manner (siEGFR_1, siEGFR_2, siEGFR_3). Cell proliferation assay was performed at the indicated time points (0, 6, 16, 36, or 48 h after transient transfection with siRNAs) using MTT assay at the varying time points. *$p < 0.05$ (Student's t-test)

EGFR expression is negatively correlated with survival

To measure EGFR expression in our cohort, IHC analysis was performed. IHC images were scored from 0 (negative staining) to 3 (highest staining intensity). Representative images are shown in Fig. 1. Cox proportional hazard modeling identified EGFR overexpression as an independent predictor for disease recurrence (OR, 1.38 (1.201–2.744), $p = 0.004$) in the Egyptian cohort (Table 2). Kaplan-Meier analysis revealed that EGFR overexpression (score ≥ 2)

significantly correlated with disease recurrence ($p = 0.021$) (Fig. 2).

EGFR silencing alters cell proliferation, viability and response to cisplatin-induced apoptosis

We further performed loss-of-function studies on TCCSUP human BC cells to assess the biological role of EGFR. EGFR was knocked-down using iRNAs and this was subsequently confirmed via western blot analysis (Fig. 3a). Silencing of EGFR did not induce a

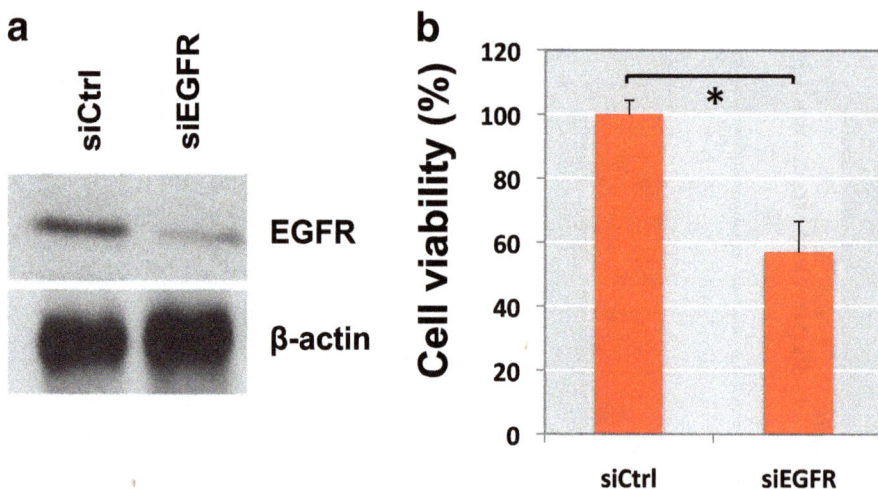

Fig. 4 Knockdown of EGFR suppresses recovery from cisplatin treatment. **a** EGFR silenced TCCSUP cells (siEFGR) or control TCCSUP cells (siCtrl) were challenged with cisplatin treatment. TCCSUP cells were incubated with cisplatin (10 μM) and siRNAs for 48 h and then re-treated with cisplatin alone for an additional 6 h. After, the cisplatin was removed from the culture media and cells were incubated in normal growth medium for 24 h. **b** Cell viability was measured using MTT assay. Cell viability levels of three wells of transfected cells were determined. The graph was plotted as %, compared to control, no cisplatin treatment in siCtrl group (± SD). *$P < 0.05$ (Student's t-test). All experiments were done in at least triplicates

morphological switch. However, in vitro functional analysis demonstrated that EGFR expression levels can alter cell proliferation rates in TCCSUP BC cells. A dose dependent transfection of EGFR siRNAs (siEGFR_1, _2, or _3) revealed that EGFR deficiency evoked an approximately 50% decrease in cell proliferation (Fig. 3b). This data implicates that EGFR loss as an important mechanism through which BC cells keep proliferating.

We next assessed whether loss of EGFR expression can result in cell viability responses in relation to the effects of cisplatin and whether inhibition of EGFR can enhance the sensitivity of BC cells to cisplatin. We found that EGFR expression is associated with resistance to cisplatin-induced cytotoxicity. EGFR knockdown delayed cell recovery from 10 μM cisplatin treatment (Fig. 4).

Viability of control cells (siCtrl) in serum-free medium was compared with or without a challenge by 10 μM cisplatin. Cell viability assay revealed that silencing of EGFR sensitized TCCSUP BC cells to cisplatin treatment. Knockdown of EGFR was validated by western blot analysis (Fig. 4a). Cells transfected with EGFR siRNAs showed around 50% viability after cisplatin treatment compared to control TCCSUP cells (siEGFR). Removal of cisplatin from the culture medium of control cells resulted in 100% recovery of cell viabilitya (siCtrl) (Fig. 4b).

We next sought to determine whether gene silencing of EGFR might also increase drug sensitivity to cisplatin. TCCSUP BC cells were transfected with EGFR siRNAs or control siRNAs for 48 h. Immunoblotting confirmed that EGFR expression was significantly reduced in siEGFR-transfected cells (Fig. 5a). Interestingly, loss of EGFR made TCCSUP cells more sensitive to cisplatin-induced cell apoptosis, leading to reduced cell viability. TCCSUP cells were ~2x more sensitive to 5 or 10 μM cisplatin treatments (Fig. 5b). These results were further validated in T24 BC cells (Fig. 5c-d). These

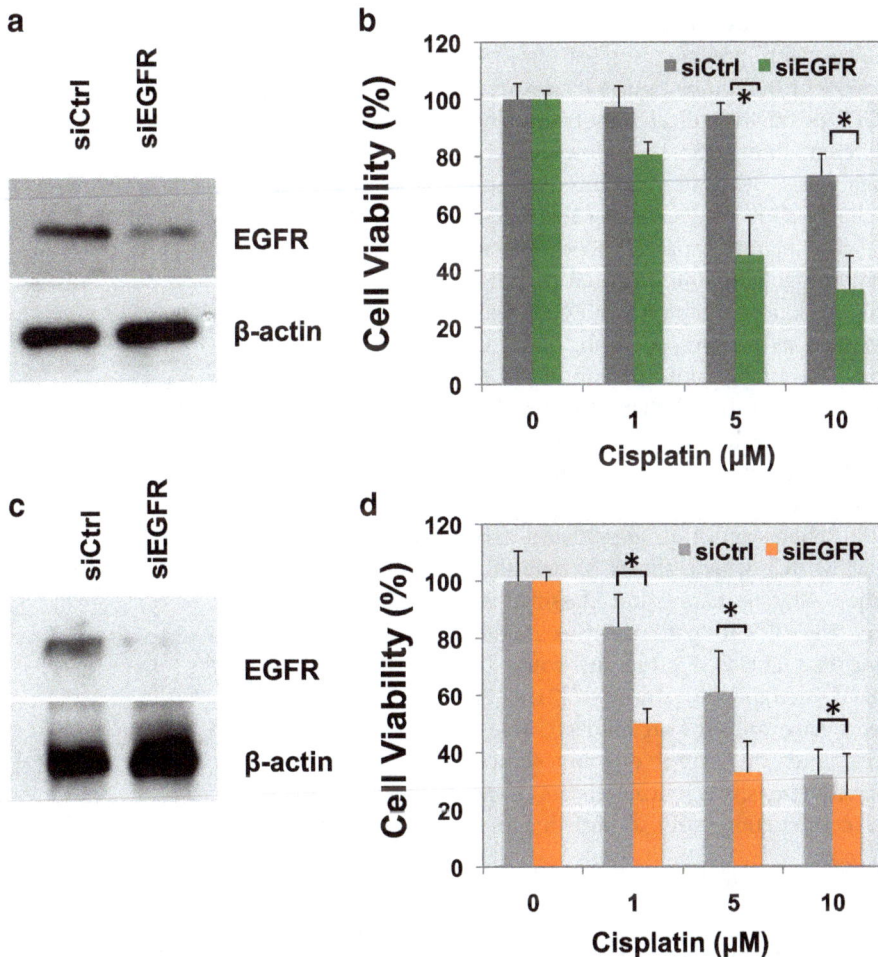

Fig. 5 Gene silencing of EGFR enhances drug sensitivity to cisplatin treatment. (a and b, TCCSUP; c and d; T24) Transiently transfected TCCSUP (a) or T24 (c) cells with siRNA of EGFR were treated with cisplatin (0, 1, 5 and 10 μM). Cisplatin was added together with siNRA for 48 h and then re-treated with cisplatin. Cell viability was measured by MTS assay after 2 days. Overexpression of siEGFR, but not a control siRNA, in TCCSUP (c) or T24 (d) cells reduced cell proliferation (Student's t-test, *p < 0.05)

findings suggest that EGFR knockdown not only suppresses the recovery of BC cells from cisplatin-reduced cell viability but also enhances the sensitivity of BC cells to cisplatin's cytotoxicity.

Discussion

Systemic chemotherapy is currently being used as the first line of treatment in advanced stages of BC. However, it is still unclear which group of patients will benefit and which patients will be more sensitive to cisplatin-based therapy. Our findings suggest that EGFR overexpression is associated with disease recurrence following adjuvant chemotherapy for advanced BC [17, 18]. Determining EGFR expression status may help predict prognoses and assist in deciding which patients would best benefit from adjuvant chemotherapy. Our findings also suggest that patients with higher EGFR expression may have a worse prognosis than those with little to no EGFR expression. An evaluation of intratumoral molecular marker(s) could be used to identify BC patients more likely to respond to cisplatin-based chemotherapy.

These findings align with previous studies showing that approximately 50% of BC tumor tissues overexpress EGFR and that EGFR positivity indicates more invasive cells and poor differentiation [13, 14]. However, the mechanisms through which BC tumors acquire cisplatin resistance are still elusive. Our results suggest that EGFR silencing may enhance cisplatin's capability to shrink tumors. This observation highlights the potential of EGFR targeting strategies (e.g., kinase inhibitors or EGFR neutralizing antibodies such as gefitini, erlotinib, trastuzumab, cetuximab, matuzumutab, panitumumab et al.) to improve the effects of cisplatin-based chemotherapy. Recent reports have demonstrated that a subgroup of muscle-invasive bladder carcinomas with a basal-like phenotype are sensitive to EGFR kinase blockers, such as erlotinib [19, 20]. Rebouissou et al. identified a subgroup of aggressive MIBC, which shows a basal-like phenotype using their 40-gene expression classifier. In this BC subgroup, the EGFR pathway was highly activated, suggesting that anti-EGFR therapy could be used as a powerful therapeutic strategy [21, 22]. EGFR-targeted agents have only shown modest success due to acquired resistance in current ongoing clinical trials. Therefore, comprehensive clinical studies using EGFR-targeting in combination with other therapies would be more attractive.

Conclusions

Many questions regarding EGFR silencing strategies remain unanswered. For example, what signaling cascades are modulated by high EGFR expression? How can these be regulated pharmacologically? Will BC cells obtain resistance to cisplatin? Can cells become resistant to EGFR

silencing? In this study, our experimental results present EGFR as a marker of recurrence in Egyptian BC patients. Further studies are needed to better understand the regulatory mechanisms of EGFR overexpression and its downstream signaling pathways in BC, particularly in the context of squamous cell carcinoma (SCC) and transitional cell carcinoma (TCC). Our findings also suggest that elucidating some of these facets of EGFR and BC drug resistance might improve pharmacologic intervention.

Abbreviations
BC: Bladder cancer; EGFR: Epidermal growth factor receptor; MIBC: Muscle-invasive bladder cancer; siCtrl: Control cells; siRNAs: Small interfering RNAs

Acknowledgements
None

Funding
The authors acknowledge support from National Institutes of Health grants (1U01DK103260, 1R01DK100974, U24 DK097154, NIH NCATS UCLA CTSI UL1TR000124), Department of Defense grants (W81XWH-15-1-0415), Centers for Disease Controls and Prevention (1U01DP006079), IMAGINE NO IC Research Grant, the Steven Spielberg Discovery Fund in Prostate Cancer Research Career Development Award, and the U.S.-Egypt Science and Technology Joint Fund (to J.K.). J.K. is former recipient of Interstitial Cystitis Association Pilot Grant, a Fishbein Family IC Research Grant, New York Academy of Medicine, and Boston Children's Hospital Faculty Development. The funders had no role in the experimental design, data collection, analysis, preparation of the manuscript, or decision to publish. In addition, this article is derived from the Subject Data funded in whole or part by National Academies of Sciences, Engineering, and Medicine (NAS) and The United States Agency for International Development (USAID). Any opinions, findings, conclusions, or recommendations expressed in this article are those of the authors alone, and do not necessarily reflect the views of USAID or NAS.

Authors' contributions
JK and AMM conceived of the study, designed experiments, evaluated data and wrote the paper. AMM, ML, EC, VS, TP, MS, AM, MA, AA, and ME performed experiments. MS, AS, and AM provided expertise and supervised data interpretation. JK, AMM, and HA-E have contributed conceptually and intellectually and to the writing of the manuscript. All authors have read and approved the final manuscript.

Competing interests
The authors declare that they have no competing interests.

Author details
[1]Urology and Nephrology Center, Mansoura University, Mansoura, Egypt. [2]University of Texas Health Science Center, San Antonio, USA. [3]University of California Los Angeles, Los Angeles, CA, USA. [4]University of California, Berkerly, CA, USA. [5]Departments of Surgery and Biomedical Sciences, Samuel Oschin Comprehensive Cancer Institute, Cedars Sinai Medical Center, 8700 Beverly Blvd, Los Angeles, CA 90048, USA.

References

1. Antoni S, Ferlay J, Soerjomataram I, Znaor A, Jemal A, Bray F. Bladder Cancer incidence and mortality: a global overview and recent trends. Eur Urol. 2017;71(1):96–108.
2. Kamat AM, Hahn NM, Efstathiou JA, Lerner SP, Malmstrom PU, Choi W, Guo CC, Lotan Y, Kassouf W. Bladder cancer. Lancet. 2016;388(10061):2796–810.
3. Kaplan AL, Litwin MS, Chamie K. The future of bladder cancer care in the USA. Nature reviews Urology. 2014;11(1):59–62.
4. Mahdavifar N, Ghoncheh M, Pakzad R, Momenimovahed Z, Salehiniya H. Epidemiology, incidence and mortality of bladder cancer and their relationship with the development index in the world. Asian Pac J Cancer Prev. 2016;17(1):381–6.
5. Ibrahim AS, Khaled HM, Mikhail NN, Baraka H, Kamel H. Cancer incidence in Egypt: results of the national population-based cancer registry program. J Cancer Epidemiol. 2014;2014:437971.
6. Zaghloul MS, Nouh A, Moneer M, El-Baradie M, Nazmy M, Younis A. Time-trend in epidemiological and pathological features of schistosoma-associated bladder cancer. J Egyp Natl Cancer Inst. 2008;20(2):168–74.
7. Mostafa MH, Sheweita SA, O'Connor PJ. Relationship between schistosomiasis and bladder cancer. Clin Microbiol Rev. 1999;12(1):97–111.
8. Ghoneim MA, Abdel-Latif M, el-Mekresh M, Abol-Enein H, Mosbah A, Ashamallah A, el-Baz MA. Radical cystectomy for carcinoma of the bladder: 2,720 consecutive cases 5 years later. J Urol. 2008;180(1):121–7.
9. Grossman HB, Natale RB, Tangen CM, Speights VO, Vogelzang NJ, Trump DL, deVere White RW, Sarosdy MF, Wood DP Jr, Raghavan D, et al. Neoadjuvant chemotherapy plus cystectomy compared with cystectomy alone for locally advanced bladder cancer. N Engl J Med. 2003;349(9):859–66.
10. Mansour AM, Soloway MS, Eldefrawy A, Singal R, Joshi S, Manoharan M. Prognostic significance of cystoscopy findings following neoadjuvant chemotherapy for muscle-invasive bladder cancer. Can J Urol. 2015;22(2):7690–7.
11. Rosenblatt R, Sherif A, Rintala E, Wahlqvist R, Ullen A, Nilsson S, Malmstrom PU, Nordic Urothelial Cancer G. Pathologic downstaging is a surrogate marker for efficacy and increased survival following neoadjuvant chemotherapy and radical cystectomy for muscle-invasive urothelial bladder cancer. Eur Urol. 2012;61(6):1229–38.
12. Black PC, Dinney CP. Growth factors and receptors as prognostic markers in urothelial carcinoma. Curr Urol Rep. 2008;9(1):55–61.
13. Abbosh PH, McConkey DJ, Plimack ER. Targeting signaling transduction pathways in bladder Cancer. Curr Oncol Rep. 2015;17(12):58.
14. van Kessel KE, Zuiverloon TC, Alberts AR, Boormans JL, Zwarthoff EC. Targeted therapies in bladder cancer: an overview of in vivo research. Nature Rev Urol. 2015;12(12):681–94.
15. Lee HH, Wang YN, Hung MC. Non-canonical signaling mode of the epidermal growth factor receptor family. Am J Cancer Res. 2015;5(10):2944–58.
16. Tan X, Lambert PF, Rapraeger AC, Anderson RA. Stress-induced EGFR trafficking: mechanisms, functions, and therapeutic implications. Trends Cell Biol. 2016;26(5):352–66.
17. Kim WT, Kim J, Yan C, Jeong P, Choi SY, Lee OJ, Chae YB, Yun SJ, Lee SC, Kim WJ. S100A9 and EGFR gene signatures predict disease progression in muscle invasive bladder cancer patients after chemotherapy. Ann Oncol. 2014;25(5):974–9.
18. Symanowski JT, Kim ES. Gene expression and prognosis in bladder cancer--real progress? Editorial on 'S100A9 and EGFR gene signatures predict disease progression in muscle invasive bladder cancer patients after chemotherapy. Ann Oncol. 2014;25(5):919–20.
19. Choi W, Czerniak B, Ochoa A, Su X, Siefker-Radtke A, Dinney C, McConkey DJ. Intrinsic basal and luminal subtypes of muscle-invasive bladder cancer. Nature Rev Urol. 2014;11(7):400–10.
20. Shah JB, McConkey DJ, Dinney CP. New strategies in muscle-invasive bladder cancer: on the road to personalized medicine. Clin Cancer Res. 2011;17(9):2608–12.
21. Bladder cancers respond to EGFR inhibitors. Cancer discovery. 2014, 4(9):980–981.
22. Rebouissou S, Bernard-Pierrot I, de Reynies A, Lepage ML, Krucker C, Chapeaublanc E, Herault A, Kamoun A, Caillault A, Letouze E, et al. EGFR as a potential therapeutic target for a subset of muscle-invasive bladder cancers presenting a basal-like phenotype. Sci Transl Med. 2014;6(244):244ra291.

26

Patient centred care for the medical treatment of lower urinary tract symptoms in patients with benign prostatic obstruction: a key point to improve patients' care

Cosimo De Nunzio[1*], Fabrizio Presicce[1], Riccardo Lombardo[1], Alberto Trucchi[1], Mariangela Bellangino[1], Andrea Tubaro[1] and Egidio Moja[2,3]

Abstract

Background: Even though evidence based medicine, guidelines and algorithms still represent the pillars of the management of chronic diseases (i.e: hypertension, diabetes mellitus), a patient centred approach has been recently proposed as a successful strategy, in particular to improve drug adherence. Aim of the present review is to evaluate the unmet needs in LUTS/BPH management and the possible impact of a patient centered approach in this setting.

Methods: A National Center for Biotechnology Information (NCBI) PubMed search for relevant articles published from January 2000 until December 2016 was performed by combining the following MESH terms: patients centred medicine, patient centered care, person centered care, patient centered outcomes, value based care, shared decision making, male, Lower Urinary Tract Symptoms, Benign Prostatic Hyperplasia, treatment. We followed the Preferred Reporting Items for Systematic Review and Meta-Analysis (PRISMA). All studies reporting on patient centred approach, shared decision making and evidence-based medicine were included in the review. All original article, reviews, letters, congress abstracts, and editorials comments were included in the review. Studies reporting single case reports, experimental studies on animal models and studies not in English were not included in the review.

Results: Overall 751 abstracts were reviewed, out of them 87 full texts were analysed resulting in 36 papers included. The evidence summarised in this systematic review confirmed how a patient centred visit may improve patient's adherence to medication. Although a patient centred model has been rarely used in urology, management of Low Urinary Tract Symptoms (LUTS) and Benign Prostatic Obstruction (BPO) may represent the perfect ground to experiment and improve this approach. Notwithstanding all the innovations in LUTS/BPO medical treatment, the real life picture is far from ideal.

Conclusions: Recent evidence shows a dramatical low drug adherence and satisfaction to medical treatment in LUTS/BPH patients. A patient centred approach may improve drug adherence and some unmet needs in this area, potentially reducing complications and costs. However further well designed studies are needed to confirm this data.

Keywords: Prostate, BPO, LUTS, Centred care, Treatment

* Correspondence: cosimodenunzio@virgilio.it
[1]Department of Urology, Ospedale Sant'Andrea, "Sapienza" University of Rome, Rome, Italy
Full list of author information is available at the end of the article

Background

In the last decades Evidence Based Medicine (EBM) has been the cornerstone of the clinical practice [1, 2]. Physicians' personal experience and expertise are often limited by several knowledge biases and gaps, thus EBM intends to ameliorate the decision-making process by collecting and summarising evidence from well-designed and well-conducted clinical trials, developing and updating international, widely-accepted guidelines [1, 2]. Following this approach, a safer, more reliable, and more cost-effective clinical practice may be achieved.

Conversely, critics were concerned that the emphasis on EBM could undervalue the tacit knowledge that physicians may accumulate with clinical experience [1–3]. In addition they questioned whether results from designed research could apply strictly about real patients, who often differ significantly from those included in clinical trials [1–3]. Lastly EBM frequently ignores patients' preferences and values, theoretically reducing their adherence to the proposed treatment [1–3].

Therefore, recently the patient centred approach has emerged as an important new paradigm in the clinical management of patients in many specialties including urology [1–3]. Impressive evidence supports positive associations between physician communication behaviours and positive patient outcomes, such as patient recall, patient understanding, and patient adherence to therapy [2]. Nonetheless, incorporating patient values, preferences and circumstances is probably the most difficult and important step in the management of urological diseases and frequently it does not receive the appropriate interest. As recently suggested by Hoffmann "Without shared decision making, EBM could turn into evidence tyranny" [4]. Lower urinary tract symptoms (LUTS) are a common complaint in adult men with a great impact on quality of life [5]. Medical treatment of LUTS due to Benign Prostatic Obstruction (BPO) represents the standard treatment aiming to improve symptoms, patient's quality of life and reduce disease progression [6]. Despite EBM, algorithms and guidelines are the highway to guide LUTS/BPO treatment, outlooks are sometime far from reality and we know from daily practice that different medical needs remain unmet in this area. Therefore, the medical management of LUTS/BPO seems to be a fertile ground to experiment a patient centred approach. Probably LUTS/BPO patients may benefit from a shared decision method, aiming at discussing harms and benefits of different treatment options, taking into account personal expectations and personal feelings generated by the illness. LUTS/BPH management is based on evidence-based medicine although a patient centred approach could be proposed and integrated. Previous experiences in chronic diseases as diabetes and BPCO have confirmed that an integrated

approach including evidenced based and patient centred medicine have a significant impact on patients care without contraindications.

Aim of the present review is to evaluate the unmet needs in LUTS/BPH management and the possible impact of a patient centered approach in this setting.

Methods

A National Center for Biotechnology Information (NCBI) PubMed search for relevant articles published from January 2000 until December 2016 was performed by combining the following MESH terms: patients centred medicine, patient centered care, person centered care, patient centered outcomes, value based care, shared decision making, male, Lower Urinary Tract Symptoms, Benign Prostatic Hyperplasia, treatment, drug adherence and measurements of adherence. We followed the Preferred Reporting Items for Systematic Review and Meta-Analysis (PRISMA). Only articles published in the English language and with an available full text were selected. In addition, sources in the reference sections of the identified publications were added to the list. Furthermore, all the abstracts presented at the annual congresses of the European Association of Urology (EAU) and American Urology Association (AUA), were evaluated and selected if relevant. All studies reporting on patient centred approach, shared decision making and evidence-based medicine were included in the review. All original article, reviews, letters, congress abstracts, and editorial comments were included in the review. Studies reporting single case reports, experimental studies on animal models, congress abstracts and studies not in English were not included in the review. The initial search resulted in 818 citations (Fig. 1). After initial title screening and manual reduplication, 749 references remained for abstract review. Four authors (CDN, FP, RL and EM) selected the initial studies based on selection criteria by abstract screening. These studies were categorised in three categories: excluded, included and possibly relevant. Included and possibly relevant studies were rescreened by three authors (CDN, FP and EM) to confirm eligibility. Overall 715 studies were excluded (not relevant to the topic or not original research). All authors then participated in full-text evaluation for the remaining 36 citations identified by abstract review or by manual search of references list (Fig. 1). Full texts were analysed by four reviewers (CDN, FP, RL, EM) and two subheadings were identified to summarize the results: LUTS/BPO medical treatment: unmet needs and Patient centered medicine in LUTS/BPO management (Table 1).'

Results

Overall 36 articles were selected for the quantitative synthesis and divided in two topics: LUTS/BPO medical treatment: unmet needs and Patient centered medicine in LUTS/BPO management.

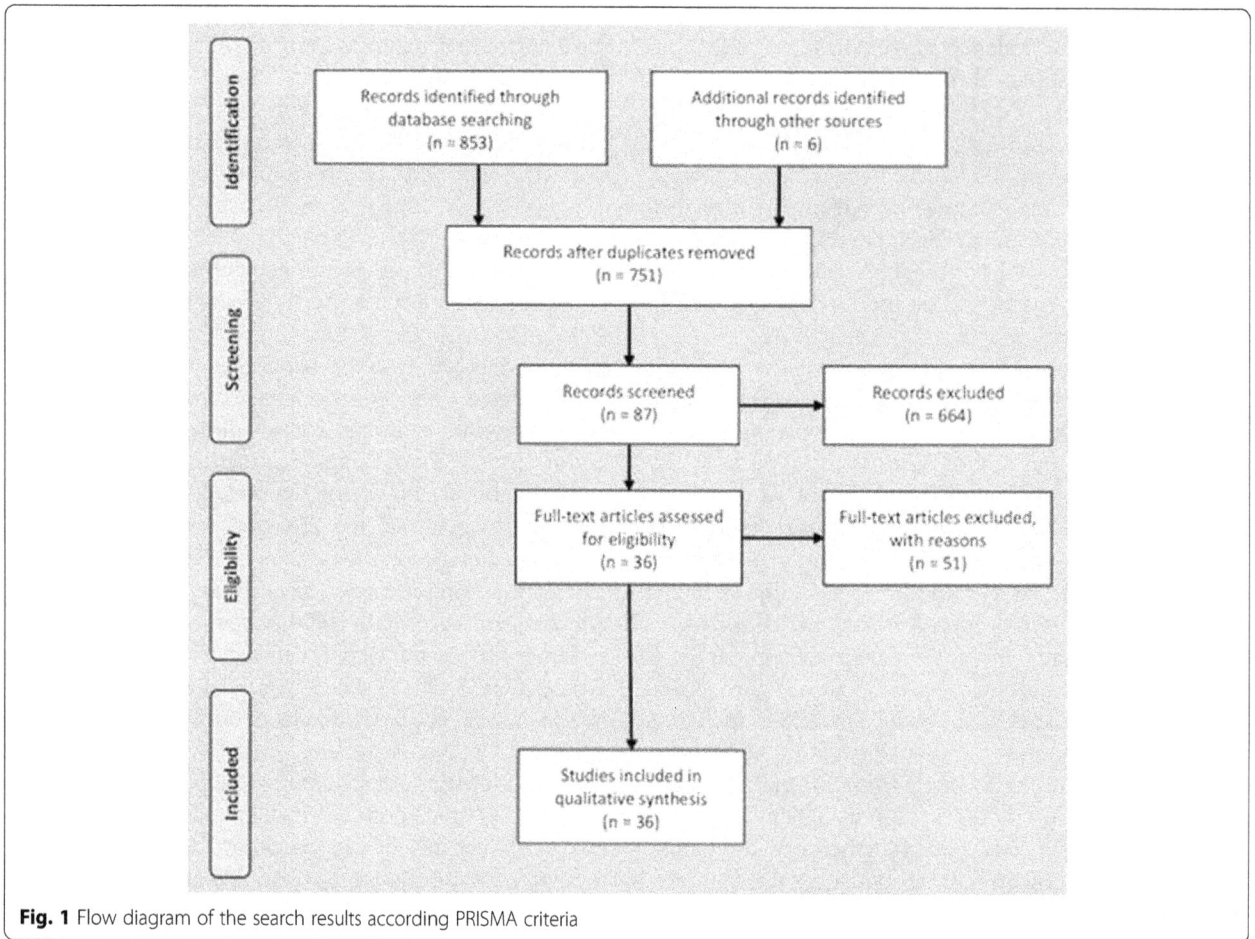

Fig. 1 Flow diagram of the search results according PRISMA criteria

LUTS/BPO medical treatment: unmet needs

LUTS can be divided into storage, voiding and post-micturition symptoms [6]. LUTS are highly prevalent, cause bother and impact on QoL. LUTS are strongly associated with ageing processes; therefore associated costs and burden are likely to increase with future demographic changes. Most elderly men suffer at least of one LUTS. LUTS evolve dynamically: for some patients LUTS persist and progress over long time periods, and for others they remit [6]. Six pharmacological classes [alpha blockers (ABs), 5-alpha reductase inhibitors (5ARIs), phytotherapeutics, antimuscarinics (AMs), beta-3 agonists and phosphodiesterase type 5 inhibitors] are available alone or in combination for the treatment of male LUTS [7]. However, notwithstanding all these different therapeutic options, medical treatment of LUTS/BPO is far from the ideal situation and different unmet needs remain in this area [8, 9].

Despite most of the European countries adopt the same guidelines for the management of patients with LUTS/BPO, different prescription strategies exist between European countries [10]. The overall prescription index is three times more important in southern

countries than in northern countries [10]. In addition, when three classes of medications are compared, alpha-blockers are continuously widely used, 5-ARI prescriptions are variable (highest in Poland and Italy), and the prescription of plants is strictly country dependent (significantly higher in France and Hungary) [10].

Fourcarde et al., in a cross-sectional observational study, described the profile and management of patients receiving medical therapy for BPH in primary care-centres in France [11]. Half of the BPO patients medically treated report unsatisfactory outcomes and only 60% of patients received a stable treatment without modifications over a year time [11, 12]. Moreover, only 17.3% of the patients start with combination treatment and curiously the most prescribed combination therapy was alpha blockers + plant extract (49.7%), non-considered as a recommended combination treatment in the current guidelines, highlighting that only a small number of physicians adhere to guidelines and algorithms [11, 12].

LUTS/BPO patients are managed by urologists and general practitioners (GPs) and some differences in drug prescription can be commonly observed. The BPH

Table 1 Characteristics of the studies retrieved

Study and year	Design	Main findings
ACCF 2012 [40]	Guidelines	Patient centered approach should be implemented in the management of the cardiological patient.
Agarwal 2014 [25]	Observational	Patient perception of urinary incontinence may differe from clinicians perception.
Balint 1969 [33]	Lecture	A shift of emphasis in the research from expecting the doctor to be a sort of detective inspector to a study of the varieties of response open to the doctor; or to put it in other words to the variety of ways the doctor can be used. This may be one of the changes which will lead to understand the possibilities and techniques of 'patient-centred medicine' and thus to undo the split in the doctor.
Bertaccini 2001 [29]	Observational	Quality of life is a major determinant in LUTS/BPH patients evaluated by the ICS-Qol questionnaire.
Cindolo 2014 [20]	Observational	Adherence to pharmacological therapy for BPH is low and could affect clinical outcomes. Our findings suggest the need for new strategies to increase patient adherence to prescribed treatment and more appropriate prescribing by physicians.
Cindolo 2015 [21]	Retrospective	Adherence to pharmacological therapy of BPH-associated LUTS is low and varies depending on drugs class. Patients under CT have a higher likelihood of discontinuing treatment for a number of reasons that should be better investigated. The study suggests that new strategies aiming to increase patient's adherence to the prescribed treatment are necessary in order to prevent BPH progression.
Cornu 2010 [8]	Review	Major variations were seen among European countries concerning the prescriptions related to BPH, although the prevalence of the disease and the guidelines are similar. Analysis of actual prescription levels would complement evidence-based medicine as critical material for public health analysis, recommendations, and health insurance policies.
Coyne 2009 [31]	Observational	In this large population study of three countries, LUTS are highly prevalent among men and women aged > 40 years. In general, LUTS experienced 'often' or more are bothersome to most people.
Chung 2013 [27]	Prospective	LUTS are important risk factors in predicting the presence of clinically relevant depressive symptoms. In elderly men, increased awareness and possible screening are needed to detect the increased risk of clinically relevant depressive symptoms.
De Nunzio 2016 [7]	Review	The possibility of tailoring BPH treatment according to different patient characteristics and expectations, using two or more drugs, seems a promising path in the field of LUTS/BPH management; however, physicians should consider the risk of increasing costs without proven long-term efficacy with most of these combination treatments.
Epstein 2005 [24]	Rieview	PCC is regarded by the public, health care organizations, funding agencies and licensure bodies as a component of high-quality care. Defining outcomes of patient centeredness is essential to measure the clinical impact of a PCC approach.
Foo 2010 [9]	Review	The final decision for management of LUTS/BPH patient can then be tailored and individualized to achieve cost-effectiveness
Emberton 2007 [23]	Observational	This study highlights discrepancies between views and beliefs of patients and physicians regarding BPH and current practice in Europe.
Emberton 2010 [24]	Review	Improved physician–patient communication will help determine the best treatment option for patients with BPH and may ensure greater compliance and treatment success.
Foo 2017 [10]	Review	Treatment of prostatic adenoma can be individualized and tailored. Final decision-making would be personalized to the patient's age, comorbidity and preferences (values). This would be in line with the recent emphasis on patient-centered care in evidence-balanced medicine, treating the patient not just the disease.
Fourcade 2008 [11]	Observational	There were geographical discrepancies that could be attributed to either different cultural habits or merely organisational differences, e.g. the presence of office urologists in Germany or diverse modes of access to phytotherapy (prescription vs 'over the counter') in the various countries.
Fourcade 2012 [12]	Observational	Around half of BPH patients medically treated report unsatisfactory outcomes, suggesting consequential unmet medical needs in general practice. A patient centered approach may improve outcomes.
Garraway 1993 [28]	Observational	Further investigation of these possible influences on non-consultation is required before any programme of health education can be considered which would encourage a higher proportion of men with bothersome urinary symptoms to come forward for attention at an earlier stage in the natural history of benign prostatic hyperplasia.

Table 1 Characteristics of the studies retrieved *(Continued)*

Study and year	Design	Main findings
Greenhald 2014 [35]	Essay	Evidence based medicine has not resolved the problem sit set out to address (especially evidence biases and the hidden hand of vested interests),which have become subtler and harder to detect. Despite lip service to shared decision making, patients can be left confused and even tyrannised when their clinical management is inappropriately driven by algorithmic protocols,top-down directives and population targets.
Hong 2005 [5]	Review	Patient perceptions are receiving greater emphasis as part of clinical decision-making. Selecting an inappropriate treatment, or not including the patient's preference, may lead to a cascade of therapies and unmet expectations, and increase the economic and human burden of the disease.
Hollingsworth 2009 [13]	Retrospective	On average, urologists had a higher intensity practice style for benign prostatic hyperplasia than primary care physicians. Further studies are needed to determine how these practice style differences relate to patient clinical outcomes.
Lamiani 2008 [37]	Prospective	Results suggest that the concept and practice of patient-centred care is variable and may be influenced by culture. The study methodology improved participants' self-awareness of cultural values, and has potential as a cost-effective, experiential educational approach
Little 2001 [1]	Observational	Components of patients'perceptions can be measured reliably and predict different outcomes.If doctors don't provide a positive,patient centred approach patients will be less satisfied,less enabled,and may have greater symptom burden and higher rates of referral.
Makoul 2001 [17]	Review	The group identified seven essential sets of communication tasks: (1) build the doctor-patient relationship; (2) open the discussion; (3) gather information; (4) understand the patient's perspective; (5) share information; (6) reach agreement on problems and plans; and (7) provide closure. These broadly supported elements provide a useful framework for communication-oriented curricula and standards
Miner 2009 [15]	Review	General Practitioners and Urologist manage LUTS/BPH patients differently and not always according to the guidelines. Increasing communication between patients, GPs and Urologist may improve management of LUTS/BPH patients.
Mozes 1999 [26]	Observational	The relative weight of the impact of a symptom or disease on QoL domains is changed by the presence of other competingfactors, such as co-morbidities or sociodemographic attributes. Social context and quality of life is essential for a correct management of LUTS/BPH patients
Murray 2001 [3]	RCT	An interactive multimedia decision aid in the NHS would be popular with patients, reduce decisional conflict, and let patients play a more active part in decision making without increasing anxiety. The use of web based technology would reduce the cost of the intervention.
Piercy 1999 [46]	Observational	A shared decision making program is beneficial for the patient and should be implemented in clinical practice specially for LUTS/BPH patients. Patients were enthusiastic and physician-patient relationship could be enhanced.
Ridder 2015 [30]	Observational	The prevalence of LUTS, especially nocturia and urgency, is high and a significant number of men indicated to be seriously bothered. Increasing awareness of male LUTS, and storage symptoms in particular, is warranted to discuss management options that could increase quality of life.
Sells 2000 [32]	Prospective	The study confirmed the presence of significant morbidity in the partners of patients with BPE. The degree of partnermorbidity was related to the severity of the patients' symptoms. Including the social entourage when managing LUTS/BPH patient may improve its management.
Stewart 2001 [34]	Editorial	Patients "may not prefer a patient centred approach" and hence its universal adoption would be "unwise." Patient centred clinical practice is a holistic concept in which components interact and unite in a unique way in each patient doctor encounter.
Wei 2011 [14]	Observational	Significant differences in practice patterns were observed between primary care physicians and urologists in the evaluation of and management for lower urinary tract symptoms/benign prostatic hyperplasia. These data establish valuable benchmarks and identify possible interventions that may improve the standard of care.
Wagg 2012 [19]	Observational	Need for a better understanding of non-persistent patients treated with antimuscarinics and for the development of initiatives to improve the quality of drug therapy management. Further studies are required to investigate the reasons underlying this trend, such as lack of effi cacy, poor tolerability or inconvenient dosing, why patients are lost to follow-up, whether symptoms resolve at some point during the prescribed treatment, and whether lack of patient understanding about the need for long-term management is a factor.

Table 1 Characteristics of the studies retrieved *(Continued)*

Study and year	Design	Main findings
Weston 2001 [22]	Comment	When you and your patient disagreeabout management, be sure to listen carefully to thepatient's ideas and paraphrase them so that the patient knows that you understand his or her point of view. Then, express your concerns and engage in a discussion that seeks to find common ground.
WHO 2003 [16]	Review	Methods and interventions to improve drug adeherence.

Registry and Patient Survey is a longitudinal, observational, disease registry cohort of patients enrolled from January 2004 to February 2005 in the United States [13]. It includes 402 urologist and primary care physician practices throughout the United States. Several differences in prescription patterns may be seen between urologist and GPs. GPs tend to prescribe more likely ABs (77,4% vs 58,4%) than 5ARIs (14% vs 6,3%), AB plus 5ARI combination therapy (22,7% vs 13,8%) or anticholinergic therapy (4,8% vs 2,5%) [26]. Nonetheless, the abovementioned results are confirmed by other experiences in European and Asian cohorts [14, 15]. Therefore this evidence emphasizes the low observance of international guidelines from Urologists and GPs, and prompts a better collaboration between GPs and Urologists.

Another important concern in the LUTS/BPO management is represented by the poor drug adherence. Adherence to medication is best defined by the extent to which patients take medications as prescribed by their health care providers [16]. Persistence is defined as the mean number of days that a patient remained on therapy. The non-adherence and the lack of persistence to a certain medication have been recognized as a public health problem [16]. The current guidelines offer multiple and different chronic drug regimens for the treatment of BPO/LUTS [17, 18]. However very little is known on the patient adherence to the LUTS/BPO medications. Wagg et al. investigated patterns of persistence with oral AMs drugs across different age groups in UK [19]. The mean persistence rate ranged between 77 and 157 days depending on AM type and age (older patients presented better persistence rates) [19]. The same issue has recently been addressed by Cindolo et al. in their study including 1,5 million patients under LUTS/BPO medications [20]. The number of patients who received prescriptions for at least 6 months was 97,407, decreasing to 61,298 (63%) at 10 months and 28,273 (29%) at 12 months (26%). The proportion of patients who continued the drugs up to 10 months was 70, 59, and 34% respectively for AB, 5ARI, and combination therapy, respectively [20]. These results confirmed by similar experiences [21] showed as medical treatment of LUTS/BPO is far from the ideal treatment and that several factors could influence the long-term efficacy in relation to the poor drug adherence and persistence observed in real life studies.

Several factors as race, insurance coverage, information technology, type of medication and prescription burden can influence drug adherence in LUTS/BPO patients, however recent evidence support that drug adherence is mostly influenced by patient's perception of discomfort and inconvenience and patient's expectations [19, 21].

Therefore, the clinicians should not limit their attention to the correct diagnosis and treatment of the disease (LUTS/BPO); they are required to provide a comprehensive assessment of the patient's illness experience. Nevertheless a thorough exploration of the illness experience requires insight, tools, and practice. One helpful acronym, that could summarize the issues to be considered in a patient centered approach, is FIFE: Feelings, Ideas, Function, and Expectations [22].

Feelings: what emotions have your experiences given rise to?

The occurrence of lower urinary tract symptoms unsurprisingly generates in the minds of patients several feelings, especially fears, related to this illness condition. According data from Emberton and coworkers survey, the main concerns first experienced by symptomatic patients seeking healthcare consultation were the fear of cancer, disruption to sleep, discomfort and embarrassment [23, 24]. In particular almost one-third of patients (32%) mentioned a fear of cancer, as the reason for seeking medical assistance, and those with more severe symptoms, were more likely to harbour this underlying concern. Other common complaints triggered by LUTS onset are: frustration with symptoms (18%), impact of symptoms on work life (10% of patients), impact of symptoms on social activities (9%), affection of the relationships with people (5%) [23, 24]. Furthermore Agarwal and coworkers reported that urgency, nocturia and urinary incontinence are the most bothersome symptoms in the their study population [25]. Interestingly, 10 weeks delay occurs usually from symptoms' onset to medical advice [23]. The main motivations that induce patients to defer consultation are the hope that the symptoms would go away or the belief that symptoms were an expected component of ageing [23].

Ideas: what do you think is causing this?

Despite more than half of patients (56%) affirmed that they felt 'fairly' or 'very' well-informed about health issues related to prostate problems, the prevalent Idea

(32%) about what causes their symptoms was once again a cancer [23, 24]. When the disease is recognised as benign condition, patients' concerns usually shift to a fear of subsequent disease progression. In particular 57% of subjects were significantly worried about the possibility of acute urinary retention (AUR), and 67% about surgery, while 68% believed that the insertion of a catheter would have a worse impact on their quality of life (QoL) than surgery [23, 24].

Function: how has this affected your work? Relationships? Hobbies? Self-care?

We should not underestimate the impact of LUTS on the quality of life since LUTS affect patients' Functions as do several chronic diseases such as epilepsy, asthma [5]. Using the SF-36 and EuroQoL questionnaires Hong and coworkers reported that increasing symptom severity was significantly associated with worsening physical role, social functioning, vitality, mental health and perception of general health [5]. Furthermore, in all domains except physical functioning, patients with BPO had a worse QoL than patients with epilepsy or chronic pulmonary disease [5]. Sameway, Mozes et al. [37] showed a remarkable negative impact of LUTS on the mental health domain of QoL, which was greater than other disease states such as pulmonary disease. Consistently, in an Asian cohort of patients Chung et al. reported that the presence of moderate-to-severe LUTS at baseline were significantly associated with a three times increased risk for being depressed at two-year follow-up (OR = 2.97; CI: 1.70–5.20) [27]. In addition, in a Scottish community-based survey, half of men with LUTS/BPO experienced limitations with at least one living activity (e.g. the ability to sleep, participate in outdoor sports or to travel), while this degree of interference was reached by only 3% of subjects in the same age group without LUTS/BPO [28]. In accordance with these findings, in a cohort of Italian patients with bothersome LUTS (IPSS more than 7), Bertaccini et al. found that 95% of subjects would not be completely happy to spend the rest of their life with their actual condition and that LUTS/BPO presence influences their life from 'a little' to 'a lot' in 79% of patients [29]. All these surveys on the quality of life are agreed that storage symptoms are the most bothersome ones. In fact in all these studies QoL are more positively associated with storage symptoms (frequency, urgency or nocturia) than voiding symptoms (weak stream, hesitancy, etc.) or objective parameters (urinary flow, prostate volume, etc.) [26–28]. These conclusions were recently further confirmed in a large cohort of 5890 Belgium men aged ≥ 40 years (mean age: 61.2 years) [30]. Nocturia (69.2%) and urgency (58.3%) were the most prevalent and bothersome symptoms. Both prevalence and bother of all LUTS increased with age.

Additionally, 28.9% of men reported to be a little bothered by their LUTS condition in everyday life, while 11.9% were bothered a lot/very much (2.5% in age group 40–49 years increasing to 29.2% in those > 80 years) [30].

Expectations: what are you hoping to leave here with?

When clinicians plan a possible BPO/LUTS treatment, they should bear in mind the patients' Expectations. In the PROBE survey Emberton and co-workers reported that more than half of all patients had discussed the topic of prostate-related surgery or AUR with their healthcare provider, and most of them reported that they were 'fairly' or 'very' concerned about developing these complications [23, 24]. Further analysis from the PROBE survey and the Kaplan survey study has provided a better understanding of preferences and satisfaction with BPH (Benign Prostatic Hyperplasia) treatments, suggesting that patient and physician expectations may not always coincide [23, 31]. In the PROBE study, patients considered that the ideal treatment option is a drug providing a 50% reduction in the risk of surgery and symptom relief even if after 6 months, while the worst treatment is drug providing relief from symptoms within 2 weeks but no reduction in the risk of surgery in the long term [23]. The Kaplan survey confirmed how most of BPH patients are interested about long-term effect of treatment and their beliefs are completely different when compared with physicians. Most of them supposed that patients were more interested about immediate symptom relief than with long-term effects [31].

Finally another important element to consider during the shared decision-making is the "whole person" and the social context. In the attempt to give relief to urinary problems, we should also consider the other personal areas that might be involved and affected by this decision. Medical LUTS/BPH medications have a moderate impact on sexual life and in particular incidence of sexual AEs with combination therapy may be as high as 30% [21, 22]. Nevertheless clinicians often underrate the patients' concerns about their sexual life. Fourcarde et al. described the profile and management of patients receiving medical therapy for BPH in primary care in four European countries [24, 25]. Even in return for complete suppression of urinary problems, most patients (> 50%) declared they would not agree to continue the treatment if they had to experience sexual adverse events [12].

If the patients agree, family members and in particular the partners should always be involved in the decision-making, as they are the main actors in the social context that surrounds the patients.

In fact, partners play a specific role in patient's life as well as in in LUTS/BPH treatment. Sells and co-workers evaluated 90 partners using a dedicated questionnaire to assess partners' morbidity associated with BPH/LUTS management [32]. Almost all partners experienced some morbidity as a consequence of the patients' condition, with the most common issues being sleep disturbance, fear of cancer and surgery and limitations in social life including sexual life [32].

In conclusion, during this process, the clinician should not focus exclusively on the disease, but he should consider the whole person and the social context that surrounds him. In particular, in the case of LUTS/BPH, the clinician should evaluate carefully the sexual functions of the patient, involving as much as possible the partner in the decision-making.

Patient centered medicine in LUTS/BPO management

The term "patient-centred" has been first used in a paper by Enid Balint in 1969 to indicate that the 'whole person' has to be considered in the clinical consultations [33]. Medical world showed a delayed reaction to this term and concept but in the last 20 years, there was progressively widespread acceptance that a 'patient-centred' approach may be beneficial [1, 2], although, as Stewart wrote: "Patient-centredness... may be most commonly understood for what it is not – technology-centred, doctor-centred, hospital-centred, disease-centred" [34]. Probably the rapid diffusion of a patient-centred model in several fields of medicine in the last decade has been linked to the crisis of the "Evidence-Based Medicine" model. As highlighted even by some members of the Centre for Evidence-Based Medicine of University of Oxford, evidence based medicine has not resolved all the problems it set out to address, which have become subtler and harder to detect [35]. In fact, patients often report that many of their informational and emotional needs remain unmet during encounters with their physicians and all this results in low levels of patient recall, a poor understanding of treatment recommendations, and a reduced adherence to those recommendations [35]. Therefore as suggested by the members of the Centre for EBM of University of Oxford, an exceeding of the standard EBM is needed, the research agenda should become broader and more interdisciplinary, embracing the experience of illness, the psychology of evidence interpretation, the negotiation and sharing of evidence by clinicians and patients [35]. Following these suggestions some authors have begun to explore the advantages of a patient centred approach in some chronic diseases, as hypertension, diabetes and arthritis [1, 2]. These studies showed that patients usually preferred patient centred care, and those who received it report enhanced health outcomes [1, 2]. In particular patient-centred encounters resulted in: better patient satisfaction, greater patient adherence to plans made, higher physician satisfaction, and fewer malpractice complaints [36].

Even if a patient-centred care has been interpreted and enacted differently among the different studies [37], it is possible to recognize two different dimensions of the concept. The first dimension means that in a patient-centred consultation the physician has to explore both the patients' disease and four dimensions of the illness experience including: their feelings about being ill, their ideas about what is wrong with them, the impact of the problem on their daily functioning, and their expectations of what should be done [38]; the second dimension means that a patient-centred consultation has to encourage a more sharing, participative, and equal approach with the patient [38, 39]. The two dimensions are not mutually exclusive and affect the consultation and its outcomes. Therefore, the term "patient-centred" includes the patient perspective, and the psychosocial context along with shared understanding, power, and responsibility [40, 41]. In a recent consensus statement developed by representatives from medical education and professional organizations, seven essential communication tasks were identified: 1) build the doctor–patient relationship; 2) open the discussion; 3) gather information; 4) understand the patient's perspective; 5) share information; 6) reach agreement on problems and plans; and 7) provide closure [17]. These tasks should be adopted in medical education, providing a template for the assessment of the various elements of patient-centred approach. Moreover the awareness of suboptimal health literacy and the importance of cultural competence in communication are imperative for effective patient communication and have been identified as key contributors to patient safety by the Joint Commission [18]. To reach significant enhancements of all these physicians' communication skills, an effort by National Health Institutions is awaited, likely requiring changes in instruction at both the undergraduate and graduate levels of training [40]. Furthermore the challenge of assessing communication skills should not be underestimated [42]. This assessment should use well-established instruments for measurement of physicians' communication skills in patient encounters [42].

In conclusion the patient-centred model has come a long way since the pioneering work of Enid Balint was published [33]. The scope of communication skills, important for successful clinical encounters, has been broadened and better defined. Moreover it has been successfully demonstrated that a patient-centred approach is positively associated with better health outcomes for patients in some fields of medicine [1, 2]. However, the potential of this method have not yet been explored in full, whereas in many areas of medicine, such as urology, the experiences with this approach although promising are still very rare. Further studies with this model are waited to confirm the positive outcomes of these preliminary findings.

A patient centered approach seems an innovative option to overcome the current limitations in the pharmacological treatment of LUTS/BPO patients, improving outcomes and drug adherence. As suggested in the last paragraph of the EAU guidelines on non-neurogenic LUTS, a patient centred care should be preferred and treatment should follow patients' preferences and expectations in terms of efficacy, morbidity, speed of onset and disease progression [43]. Similarly the first paragraph of the NICE guidelines about the treatment of LUTS highlights a better communication between physicians and patients is mandatory, possibly using different communication skills and instruments in relation to patients' education and needs [44]. Unfortunately, despite all these considerations, in the field of urology the use of this approach is still very limited. In particular, a total of seven survey studies, widely mentioned in the previous paragraph, have assessed LUTS/BPO treatment preference [11, 12]. Of these, two studies evaluated preferences in patients [11, 12], three studies examined preferences in physicians [13–15] and two studies investigated preferences in both patients and physicians [23, 24]. However, to our knowledge only two studies specifically addressed the impact of a shared-decision making approach for LUTS/BPO treatment outcomes [45, 46]. A preliminary RCT was performed in UK in the early 2000s to evaluate whether a decision aid on benign prostatic enlargement influenced patient decision-making, health outcomes, and resource use [45]. This study involved 33 GPs and 99 BPO patients, the decision aid consisted in interactive multimedia programme with booklet and printed summary [45]. Information included probabilities of the risks and benefits of each treatment, estimated on the basis of information on age, severity of symptoms, and general health entered by the patient at the beginning of the session. The final outcomes were promising, in fact the decision aid was highly acceptable to both the patients and their GPs; the decisional conflict was reduced in the intervention group and patients who accessed to the decision aid reported a more active part in the decision making process and were less anxious than control patients [45]. The study failed to reduce the rate of BPH surgical procedure, however the small sample size and the short follow up (9 months) may explain this inconclusive resul [45]. In the second study, including 678 patients with symptomatic BPH from eight Canadian centers, Piercy et al. examined the impact of a shared decision-making program (SDP) on perceived knowledge and treatment preference [46]. The SDP required by this study protocol, was rudimentary, consisting simply in viewing an educational programme designed to inform LUTS/BPO patients about their condition and treatment options [46]. SDP showed only a minor impact in changing the preferences of those subjects who had expressed an initial preference (89.7 and 89.4% of patients preferring surgical and non-surgical

therapy respectively, maintaining their preferences after viewing the programme), although it helped almost half of those initially undecided in forming a preference, reducing the percentage of doubtful patients to 14.8% [46].

Figure 2 shows a possible suggestion of a patient centred approach in LUTS/BPH patients. Evidence based medicine includes etiology, diagnosis, current medications and guidelines/algorithms which should be integrated with patient illness, social context and partner. All the actors of a clinical consultation (GPs, urologist and patients) should participate together and actively communicate to achieve an integrated evidence based/patient centered approach. The disease and the patient are to be treated as a whole.

Discussion

The present review analyses the possible impact of a patient centred approach in LUTS/BPH patients. The available literature on patient centred medicine has successfully demonstrated that this approach is positively associated with better health outcomes for patients in some fields of medicine. Medical treatment of LUTS/BPO is far from ideal, several factors could influence the long-term efficacy in relation to the poor drug adherence and persistence observed in real life studies. When managing LUTS/BPO patients, diagnostic and treatment algorithms should consider feelings, ideas, functions and expectations of the patient to tailor the management. Few studies evaluated the impact of a shared-decision making approach in the management of LUTS/BPO patients. Preliminary findings appear to be encouraging, even if definitive conclusions cannot be drawn from the scarcity of the available data. So far, our analysis should be considered as a preliminary summary of the role of a patient centred approach in managing patients with LUTS/BPO.

We strongly believe that LUTS/BPO is a particularly fertile ground for the implementation of a patient-centred approach. First, the plethora of guidelines and evidence-based therapies constitute a solid foundation from which evidence can be extracted and shared with patients [6, 7, 44]. Furthermore, several validated risk models of outcomes exist and can be used to advise patients of their likely outcomes, based on the results of previously treated patients [6, 7, 44]. Finally, there are many treatments for which no differences in outcomes are well defined; consequently the treatment plan may depend on patients' feelings and expectations being then the appropriate driving force in decision-making.

Further studies on this topic are needed to confirm this hypothesis, however the experiences, derived from other specialties ahead of ours in this field [40, 47–49], suggest that in the next future the art of medicine probably will move more and more from a "one fit all" model to a "tailored" model, specifically for each patient's

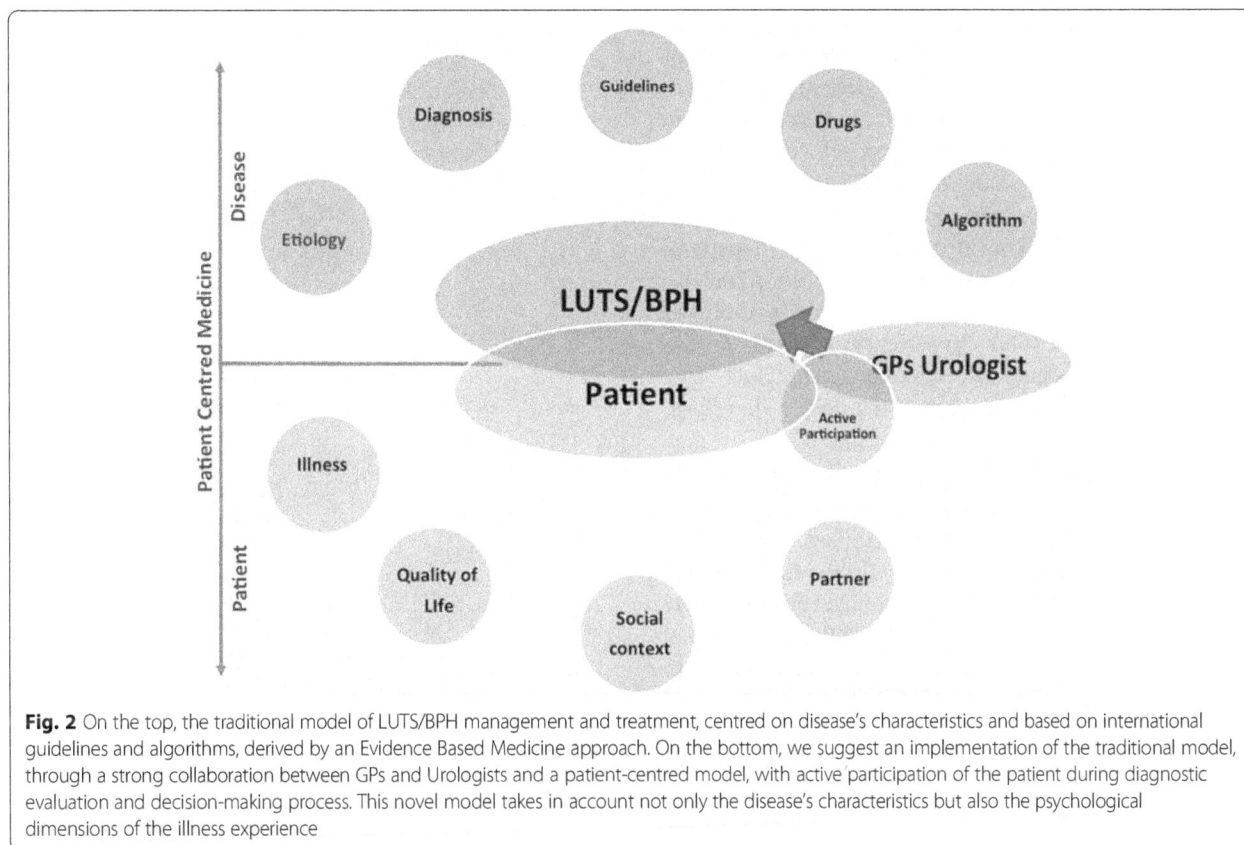

Fig. 2 On the top, the traditional model of LUTS/BPH management and treatment, centred on disease's characteristics and based on international guidelines and algorithms, derived by an Evidence Based Medicine approach. On the bottom, we suggest an implementation of the traditional model, through a strong collaboration between GPs and Urologists and a patient-centred model, with active participation of the patient during diagnostic evaluation and decision-making process. This novel model takes in account not only the disease's characteristics but also the psychological dimensions of the illness experience

needs. We support that in the near future Urologist and GP will enter a patient's centered path for the management of LUTS/BPO where patient's expectations, illness, ideas, social and familiar context were integrated with the disease and its relative possible treatment. The adoption of a patient centered model should improve patient's care, the key is on focusing our attention rather than on the disease, on the patient who have the disease.

Additional studies should evaluate if a patient centered model, in a BPH/LUTS patient, can improve drug adherence, reduce the risk of doctor shopping and the number of legal controversies as already observed in other chronic diseases.

The management of the disease is then driven by the evidence based medicine however Feelings, Ideas, Function, Expectations, Social Context and partner take part into the decision making process where participation of each component of the central core represents the key for the successful treatment of the patient (Fig. 2). The next step will be how to translate effectively this theoretical model in a clinical scenario. The possible types of intervention could range between educational meetings, distribution of educational materials, audit and feedback, barriers assessment, and educational outreach visits and they could be divided in three categories of implementation intervention: 1) interventions targeting patients, 2)

interventions targeting healthcare professionals, and 3) interventions targeting both. Anyway, regardless of the selected practical interventions to increase the SDP, the assessments of their efficacy should be addressed in terms of both patients' satisfaction and clinical outcomes.

We have to acknowledge some limitations in our study. The few of studies retrieved on patient centred medicine in Urology do not allow definitive conclusion. Moreover, studies available on the subject have no common outcomes and therefore a quantitative analysis is limited. As well the studies available on patient centred medicine in other medical areas have different definitions of patient centred approach and analyse different aspects of the topic [40]. Probably, common outcomes are needed to better understand the real impact of a patient centred approach in the every day clinical practice. In particular, drug adherence in LUTS/BPH patients could serve as a proxy to evaluate the impact of a patient centred model. Notwithstanding all these limitations a patient centred approach may help clinicians in the management of LUTS/BPH patients and standing to the available evidence no real complications seem to emerge from this approach.

Conclusion

LUTS/BPO medical treatment is a successful story in the field of Urology and it is based on excellent evidence and several International guidelines. However recent evidence shows a dramatically low drug adherence and satisfaction coming from LUTS/BPO patients on medical treatment. Urologists and general practitioners should be aware that a patient centred approach could improve drug adherence and some unmet needs in this area, potentially reducing complications and costs. Medical treatment should be considered in relation to patients' illness, preference and expectations. The adoption of a patient-centered model in other chronic pathologies, such as diabetes and hypertension, have further improved drug adherence, patients' compliance to a chronic treatment and have reduced a doctor shopping.

Similarly LUTS/BPH management may represent the perfect ground to experiment and improve this approach, considering the richness of the agenda's components in these patients, the low drug-adherence rate reported in the literature, and the choice between several therapies of similar efficacy but with different effects on the patient's QoL (with the importance to strongly involve every single patients in the treatment decision). However, the benefits of this approach, albeit reasonably deducible, are difficult to demonstrate in accordance with the criteria of the evidence base medicine and the adoption of a shared decision making is still very limited in the field of urology. The selection criteria in the medical treatment of LUTS remain primarily, as emerged from the aforementioned surveys, the personal preferences of the clinicians and the habit of prescribing a certain class of medication and this may explain the geographical spread above reported.

We proposed and support a patient centered model to improve drug adherence and some unmet needs in this area, potentially reducing complications and costs. Further studies in this area are awaited to support this hypothesis.

Abbreviations
5ARIs: 5-alpha reductase inhibitors; ABs: Alpha blockers; AMs: Antimuscarinics; AUA: American Urology Association; AUR: Acute urinary retention; BPH: Benign Prostatic Hyperplasia; BPO: Benign Prostatic Obstruction; EAU: European Association of Urology; EBM: Evidence Based Medicine; LUTS: Low Urinary Tract Symptoms; PRISMA: Preferred Reporting Items for Systematic Review and Meta-Analysis; SDP: Shared decision-making program

Authors' contributions
CDN made substantial contribution to conception, design, interpretation and analysis of data, has been involved in drafting the manuscript and revising it critically for important intellectual content. FP made substantial contributions to analysis and interpretation of data; has been involved in drafting the manuscript and revising it critically for important intellectual content. RL, AT, MB made substantial contributions to acquisition of data; have been involved in drafting the manuscript. AT and EM made substantial contributions to analysis and interpretation of data; have been involved in revising the manuscript critically for important intellectual content. All the authors read and approved the final version of the manuscript.

Competing interests
The authors declare that they have no competing interests.

Author details
[1]Department of Urology, Ospedale Sant'Andrea, "Sapienza" University of Rome, Rome, Italy. [2]Unit of Clinical Psychology, Department of Health Sciences, University of Milan, San Paolo Hospital, Milan, Italy. [3]CURA Centre, University of Milan, Milan, Italy.

References
1. Little P, Everitt H, Williamson I, Warner G, Moore M, Gould C, et al. Observational study of effect of patient centredness and positive approach on outcomes of general practice consultations. BMJ. 2001;323:908–11.
2. Légaré F, Stacey D, Turcotte S, Cossi M-J, Kryworuchko J, Graham ID, et al. In: Légaré F, editor. Cochrane Database Syst. Rev Interventions for improving the adoption of shared decision making by healthcare professionals. Chichester: Wiley; 2014. p. CD006732.
3. Murray E, Davis H, Tai SS, Coulter A, Gray A, Haines A. Randomised controlled trial of an interactive multimedia decision aid on hormone replacement therapy in primary care. BMJ. 2001;323:490–3.
4. Hoffmann TC, Montori VM, Del Mar C. The connection between evidence-based medicine and shared decision making. JAMA. 2014;312:1295.
5. Hong SJ, Rayford W, Valiquette L, Emberton M. The importance of patient perception in the clinical assessment of benign prostatic hyperplasia and its management. BJU Int. 2005;95:15–9.
6. Gravas S, Cornu JN, Drake MJ, Gacci M, Gratzke C, Herrmann TRW, Madersbacher S, Mamoulakis C, Tikkinen KAO. Management of Non-Neurogenic Male Lower Urinary Tract Symptoms (LUTS), incl. Benign Prostatic Obstruction (BPO) EAU Guidelines on. [cited 2018 Apr 26]; Available from: https://uroweb.org/wp-content/uploads/EAU-Guidelines-on-the-Management-of-Non-neurogenic-Male-LUTS-2018-large-text.pdf.
7. De Nunzio C, Presicce F, Tubaro A. Combination therapies for improved management of lower urinary tract symptoms/benign prostatic hyperplasia. Drugs Today. 2016;52:501.
8. Cornu J-N, Cussenot O, Haab F, Lukacs B. A widespread population study of actual medical Management of Lower Urinary Tract Symptoms Related to benign prostatic hyperplasia across Europe and beyond official clinical guidelines. Eur Urol. 2010;58:450–6.
9. Foo KT. Decision making in the management of benign prostatic enlargement and the role of transabdominal ultrasound. Int J Urol [Internet]. 2010;17:974–9. Available from: http://doi.wiley.com/10.1111/j.1442-2042.2010.02668.x. [cited 2018 Jun 7].
10. Foo KT. From evidence-based medicine to evidence-balanced medicine for individualized and personalized care: as applied to benign prostatic hyperplasia/male lower urinary tract symptoms. Int J Urol [Internet]. 2017;24:94–5. Available from: http://www.ncbi.nlm.nih.gov/pubmed/28191718. [cited 2018 Jun 7].
11. Fourcade R-O, Théret N, Taïeb C. Profile and management of patients treated for the first time for lower urinary tract symptoms/benign prostatic hyperplasia in four European countries. BJU Int Blackwell Publishing Ltd. 2008;101:1111–8.
12. Fourcade R-O, Lacoin F, Rouprêt M, Slama A, Le Fur C, Michel E, et al. Outcomes and general health-related quality of life among patients medically treated in general daily practice for lower urinary tract symptoms due to benign prostatic hyperplasia. World J Urol. 2012;30:419–26.
13. Hollingsworth JM, Hollenbeck BK, Daignault S, Kim SP, Wei JT. Differences in initial benign prostatic hyperplasia management between primary care physicians and urologists. J Urol. 2009;182:2410–4.
14. Wei JT, Miner MM, Steers WD, Rosen RC, Seftel AD, Pasta DJ, et al. Benign prostatic hyperplasia evaluation and management by urologists and primary care physicians: practice patterns from the observational BPH registry. J Urol. 2011;186:971–6.
15. Miner MM. Primary care physician versus urologist: how does their medical management of LUTS associated with BPH differ? Curr Urol Rep. 2009;10:254–60.
16. Evidence for action. http://www.who.int/chp/knowledge/publications/adherence_full_report.pdf.
17. Makoul G. Essential elements of communication in medical encounters: the Kalamazoo consensus statement. Acad Med. 2001;76:390–3.

18. Wilson-Stronks A, Galvez E. Hospitals, Language, and Culture: A Snapshot of the Nation Exploring Cultural and Linguistic Services in the Nation's Hospitals A Report of Findings. Oakbrook Terrace: Joint Commission; 2007.
19. Wagg A, Compion G, Fahey A, Siddiqui E. Persistence with prescribed antimuscarinic therapy for overactive bladder: a UK experience. BJU Int. 2012;110:1767–74.
20. Cindolo L, Pirozzi L, Fanizza C, Romero M, Tubaro A, Autorino R, et al. Drug adherence and clinical outcomes for patients under pharmacological therapy for lower urinary tract symptoms related to benign prostatic hyperplasia: population-based cohort study. Eur Urol. 2015;68:418–25.
21. Cindolo L, Pirozzi L, Sountoulides P, Fanizza C, Romero M, Castellan P, et al. Patient's adherence on pharmacological therapy for benign prostatic hyperplasia (BPH)-associated lower urinary tract symptoms (LUTS) is different: is combination therapy better than monotherapy? BMC Urol. 2015;15:96.
22. Weston WW. Informed and shared decision-making: the crux of patient-centered care. CMAJ. 2001;165:438–9.
23. Emberton M, Marberger M, de la Rosette J. Understanding patient and physician perceptions of benign prostatic hyperplasia in Europe: the prostate research on behaviour and education (PROBE) survey. Int J Clin Pract Wiley-Blackwell; 2008;62:18–26.
24. Emberton M. Medical treatment of benign prostatic hyperplasia: physician and patient preferences and satisfaction. Int J Clin Pract. 2010;64:1425–35.
25. Agarwal A, Eryuzlu LN, Cartwright R, Thorlund K, Tammela TLJ, Guyatt GH, et al. What is the most bothersome lower urinary tract symptom? Individual- and population-level perspectives for both men and women. Eur Urol. 2014;65:1211–7.
26. Mozes B, Maor Y, Shmueli A. The competing effects of disease states on quality of life of the elderly: the case of urinary symptoms in men. Qual Life Res. 1999;8:93–9.
27. Chung RY, Leung JCS, Chan DCC, Woo J, Wong CKM, Wong SYS. Lower urinary tract symptoms (LUTS) as a risk factor for depressive symptoms in elderly men: results from a large prospective study in southern Chinese men. Tu Y-K, editor. PLoS One. 2013;8:e76017.
28. Garraway WM, Russell EB, Lee RJ, Collins GN, McKelvie GB, Hehir M, et al. Impact of previously unrecognized benign prostatic hyperplasia on the daily activities of middle-aged and elderly men. Br J Gen Pract. 1993;43:318–21.
29. Bertaccini A, Vassallo F, Martino F, Luzzi L, Rocca Rossetti S, Di Silverio F, et al. Symptoms, bothersomeness and quality of life in patients with LUTS suggestive of BPH. Eur Urol. 2001;40(Suppl 1):13–8.
30. De Ridder D, Roumeguère T, Kaufman L. Urgency and other lower urinary tract symptoms in men aged ≥ 40 years: a Belgian epidemiological survey using the ICIQ-MLUTS questionnaire. Int J Clin Pract. 2015;69:358–65.
31. Coyne KS, Sexton CC, Thompson CL, Milsom I, Irwin D, Kopp ZS, et al. The prevalence of lower urinary tract symptoms (LUTS) in the USA, the UK and Sweden: results from the epidemiology of LUTS (EpiLUTS) study. BJU Int. 2009;104:352–60.
32. Sells H, Donovan J, Ewings P, MacDonagh RP. The development and validation of a quality-of-life measure to assess partner morbidity in benign prostatic enlargement. BJU Int. 2000;85:440–5.
33. Balint E. The possibilities of patient-centered medicine. J R Coll Gen Pract. 1969;17:269–76.
34. Stewart M. Towards a global definition of patient centred care. BMJ. 2001;322:444–5.
35. Greenhalgh T, Howick J, Maskrey N. Evidence based medicine renaissance group. Evidence based medicine: a movement in crisis? BMJ. 2014;348:g3725.
36. Kurtz SM, Silverman J, Draper J. Teaching and learning communication skills in medicine. Manchester: Radcliffe Medical; 2005.
37. Lamiani G, Meyer EC, Rider EA, Browning DM, Vegni E, Mauri E, et al. Assumptions and blind spots in patient-centredness: action research between American and Italian health care professionals. Med Educ. 2008;42:712–20.
38. Schofield T. Patient-centered medicine: transforming the clinical method. BMJ. 1995;311:1580.
39. PS B, BE L. Doctors talking to patients. A study of the verbal behaviour of general practitioners consulting in their surgeries. London: London England Her Majestys stationery Office; 1976.
40. Norine Walsh M, Bove AA, Cross RR, Ferdinand KC, Forman DE, Freeman AM, et al. ACCF 2012 health policy statement on patient-centered Care in Cardiovascular Medicine. J Am Coll Cardiol. 2012;59:2125–43.
41. Epstein RM, Franks P, Fiscella K, Shields CG, Meldrum SC, Kravitz RL, et al. Measuring patient-centered communication in patient–physician consultations: theoretical and practical issues. Soc Sci Med. 2005;61:1516–28.
42. King A, Hoppe RB. "Best practice" for patient-centered communication: a narrative review. J Grad Med Educ. 2013;5:385–93.
43. Gratzke C, Bachmann A, Descazeaud A, Drake MJ, Madersbacher S, Mamoulakis C, et al. EAU guidelines on the assessment of non-neurogenic male lower urinary tract symptoms including benign prostatic obstruction. Eur Urol. 2015;67:1099–109.
44. Lower urinary tract symptoms in men: management | Guidance and guidelines | NICE. NICE. https://www.nice.org.uk/guidance.
45. Murray E, Davis H, Tai SS, Coulter A, Gray A, Haines A. Randomised controlled trial of an interactive multimedia decision aid on benign prostatic hypertrophy in primary care. BMJ. 2001;323:493–6.
46. Piercy GB, Deber R, Trachtenberg J, Ramsey EW, Norman RW, Goldenberg SL, et al. Impact of a shared decision-making program on patients with benign prostatic hyperplasia. Urol. 1999;53:913–20.
47. Treatment of Non-neurogenic Male LUTS | Uroweb. https://uroweb.org/guideline/treatment-of-non-neurogenic-male-luts/.
48. Benign Prostatic Hyperplasia: American Urological Association. http://www.auanet.org/benign-prostatic-hyperplasia-(2010-reviewed-and-validity-confirmed-2014).
49. Kinmonth AL, Woodcock A, Griffin S, Spiegal N, Campbell MJ. Randomised controlled trial of patient centred care of diabetes in general practice: impact on current wellbeing and future disease risk. The diabetes care from diagnosis research team. BMJ. 1998;317:1202–8.

27

Longitudinal recovery patterns of penile length and the underexplored benefit of long-term phosphodiesterase-5 inhibitor use after radical prostatectomy

Young Suk Kwon[1,2†], Nicholas Farber[2†], Ji Woong Yu[3], Kevin Rhee[1], Christopher Han[2], Patrick Ney[4], Jeong Hee Hong[5], Paul Lee[1], Nikhil Gupta[2], Wun-Jae Kim[6] and Isaac Yi Kim[1,2*]

Abstract

Background: Penile length (PL) shortening is an underreported phenomenon following radical prostatectomy (RP) and risk factors are not fully explored. We aimed to describe longitudinal patterns of PL recovery and evaluate factors predicting complete return to baseline PL.

Methods: PL measurement was performed during a preoperative and postoperative follow-up visits at 7 days and 3, 6, 9, and 12 months. Patients who completely recovered (CR: $N = 397$) their preoperative stretched PL measured during at least one of their follow-up visits were compared to those with incomplete recovery (IR: $N = 131$). Recovery patterns were analyzed for both groups and were also compared in regards to demographics, nerve-sparing techniques, prostate size, cardiovascular risk profiles, and phosphodiesterase-5 inhibitor (PDE5i) uses. Logistic regression analyses were performed using age and other relevant clinicopathologic variables to predict PL recovery.

Results: 60.2% of the total study population regained their preoperative PL at 12 months. Average percent (length) differences from baseline were -1.70% (-0.25 cm) and -16.42% (-2.35 cm) in the CR and the IR groups, respectively ($p < 0.001$). Multivariate logistic regression demonstrated that younger age (OR 0.962; 95%CI 0.931–0.994; $p = 0.019$), high preoperative erectile function (EF) (OR 1.028; 95%CI 1.001–1.056; $p = 0.046$), and consistent PDE5i use (OR 1.998; 95%CI 1.166–3.425; $p = 0.012$) were independent predictors of CR. At 12-month follow up, PL difference for consistent PDE5iusers was statistically different from those who did not use PDE5i consistently (-3.25%vs. -6.64%; $P = 0.001$).

Conclusion: Age, preoperative EF, and consistent use of PDE5i were associated with complete recovery of baseline PL after RP. The therapeutic effect of PDE5i was most pronounced at 12-month visit, suggesting an added benefit with long-term use.

Keywords: Penile length, PDE5 inhibitor, Radical prostatectomy, RP

* Correspondence: kimiy@cinj.rutgers.edu
†Equal contributors
[1]Section of Urologic Oncology, Rutgers Cancer Institute of New Jersey, 195 Little Albany Street, New Brunswick, NJ 08903, USA
[2]Division of Urology, Rutgers Robert Wood Johnson Medical School, New Brunswick, NJ, USA
Full list of author information is available at the end of the article

Background

Urinary incontinence and erectile dysfunction (ED) are well-described postoperative complications associated with radical prostatectomy (RP). However, additional side effects of sexual nature have also been reported in the literature, such as orgasm-associated incontinence, altered orgasmic function, orgasm-associated pain, and penile length (PL) shortening [1].

In particular, PL shortening (PS) is a common occurrence and is experienced in 15–68% of patients after RP, with losses often greater than 1 cm in stretched penile length (SPL) [1, 2]. PS has been associated with compromised quality of life and self-esteem [3]. There are multiple mechanisms proposed for post-RP PS, including anatomic changes related to urethral shortening, neural damage and attendant ED, sympathetic overactivity associated with chronic contractions of the cavernous smooth muscle, and arterial insufficiency leading to hypoxia-induced smooth muscle apoptosis with subsequent fibrous tissue deposition [4]. However, the precise mechanism of PS remains unclear.

Additional evidence is necessary to resolve conflicting perspectives on the reversibility and natural history of post-RP PS. While some have argued that patients are unlikely to regain original PL and that permanent PS is inevitable at long-term follow-up [5, 6], others report that PL eventually returns to preoperative baseline at 9–48 months [7, 8]. The differences in recovery rate may be attributed to the heterogeneous study populations with varying demographic and clinical characteristics, and intraoperative techniques.

Several factors are suggested to be associated with better PL recovery including the presence of preoperative erectile function (EF) and a nerve-sparing (NS) RP [8, 9]. In addition, the use of phosphodiesterase-5 inhibitors (PDE5i) has been demonstrated to promote PL recovery, as PDE5i use has consistently shown to aid smooth muscle preservation after cavernosal nerve injury in animal models and in a randomized clinical trial [10–12]. However, whether anatomic alteration involving shortening of the urethra and pre-existing cardiovascular comorbidity contribute to PL recovery has not been adequately explored. Therefore, the aim of our study was to describe longitudinal patterns of PL recovery and evaluate potential factors predictive of complete PL recovery. We hypothesize that PDE5i use leads to long-term PL recovery compared to non-use.

Methods

Study cohort

Following Institutional Review Board (IRB) approval, a total of 602 patients who underwent robotic RP for localized prostate cancer (PCa) between May 2010 and December 2014 were queried after excluding subjects with Peyronie's disease, previous penile surgery, or any other preexisting penile abnormalities. No individuals in our study cohort received vacuum, penile stretcher, or intracavernous injection therapies within the 12-month follow up period. Also, there were no cases of de-novo Peyronie's diseases.

Demographic parameters [age, race, height, weight, cardiovascular (CV) risk factors, prostate-specific antigen (PSA), sexual health inventory for men (SHIM), history of transurethral resection of the prostate (TURP), and history of neo/adjuvant therapy], perioperative parameters [operative room (OR) time, estimated blood loss (EBL)], and postoperative parameters (pathologic stage, prostate weight, length, volume) were reviewed for each patient. Prostate volume was determined by measuring the overall size of the excised specimen in three dimensions, (i.e. apex-to-base, right-to-left, and anterior-to-posterior). Prostate length was measured in the vertical dimension from apex-to-base.

Penile length

PL was measured in both flaccid and stretched states to the nearest 0.5 cm [13]. SPL was measured from pubic bone to coronal sulcus with the phallus maximally extended manually. SPL was utilized for all study analyses as a proxy for erected PL. All measurements of PL were performed by a single surgeon during a pre-operative visit before RP (defined as baseline PL), and then at post-operative visits at 7 days, and 3, 6, 9, and 12 months after RP. Although no repeat measurements were performed, each evaluation was performed blindly to prior measurements. The assessment took place in an exam room kept at a temperature $\geq 22\ °C$.

Comparisons were made between patients who had completely recovered (CR) their preoperative SPL within 1 year (CR: $N = 397$) and those who had incompletely recovered (IR: $N = 131$). Complete recovery was considered for men who achieved 100% of their preoperative PL in at least one of the five postoperative measurements without any specific follow-up requirement. Patients who did not achieve a full PL recovery were placed in IR group if they met a minimum of two separate follow-up visits, one of which included a 6 month-visit or later. Patients who failed to meet the follow-up requirement were excluded from the analysis ($N = 74$).

Nerve sparing technique and pelvic lymph node dissection

The initial decision to preserve neurovascular bundle was made by thorough review of preoperative characteristics. However, the final decision to perform NS procedure was ultimately determined by intraoperative findings. In order to ensure that patients have optimal functional outcomes, efforts are made to perform NS techniques in the majority of patients, except for those with extensive high-volume disease. At our institution, two types of nerve sparing (NS) techniques are used: traditional interfacial approach (IF) and athermal intra-fascial robotic (AIR) technique [14]. Hence, NS type was categorized as none, IF, or AIR. Additionally, patients were dichotomized by pelvic lymph node dissection (PLND) status.

Cardiovascular risk factor

The presence of CV risk factors was determined based on past medical and surgical history along with the list of home medications queried from electronic medical records. Advanced CV risk was determined by the presence of coronary heart disease (CHD) or CHD-risk equivalents [15]. Men with a history significant for angina, myocardial infarction and/or surgical history of cardiac stent or coronary artery bypass graft were considered to have CHD-equivalent disease. Those with abdominal aortic aneurysm, peripheral vascular disease, and carotid artery disease were considered to have CHD-equivalents. Lastly, patients with regular use of clopidogrel were considered to have advanced CV risks as clopidogrel has been demonstrated to be a reliable surrogate marker for CV damage [16].

Phosphodiesterase-5 inhibitor (PDE5i)

Post-operatively, patients were routinely recommended to take a daily PDE5i (Sildenafil, vardenafil, or tadalafil). Patients were placed on all three types of PDE5Is within the one-year period in the following sequential order: sildenafil 50 mg (Day 9–3 months), tadalafil 20 mg (4–6 months), sildenafil 100 mg (7–9 months), and vardenafil 20 mg (10–12 months). Using a three-point scale, PDE5i use was quantified as one of the following based on medication history as reported by patients: 1) almost always/always, 2) inconsistently, or 3) almost never/never.

Erectile function rehabilitation

Patients who desired to engage in sexual intercourse were placed on our institutional erectile function rehabilitation protocol. The rehabilitation protocol utilized was a 12-month regimen that consisted of 2 parts: sexual stimulation and oral medication (Additional file 1: Table S1).

Statistical analysis

PL recovery, in absolute length (cm) and percent (%) reduction from baseline, was compared at each postoperative visit using unpaired t-tests. Demographical and clinical variables were compared using chi-square (χ^2) tests for categorical variables, and t-tests for continuous variables. Cohrane-Mantel-Haenszel chi-square test (χ^2_{CMH}) as well as Cochran-Armitage Trend Test were employed to measure the linear trend between PL

recovery (CR vs. IR) and key demographic characteristics: age (< 50 vs. 50–60 vs. ≥ 60) and SHIM groups (1–7: low vs. 8–16: medium vs. ≥ 17: high).

Univariate and multivariate logistic regression analyses were performed using age and other variables to predict PL recovery. Logistic regression analysis was conducted with the inclusion of an interaction term to account for possible interaction between PDE5i use and preoperative SHIM. Longitudinal recovery patterns were analyzed according to PDE5i use and median age. All analyses were performed using SAS version 9.3 (SAS, Carry, NC). A two-sided $p < 0.05$ was considered significant.

Results

In the analysis of the PL recovery at various times, about half of the total study population regained their preoperative PL at 9 months in both flaccid and stretched lengths: 44.6% vs. 48.3%, respectively. Of those examined at 12 months, 59.4% and 60.2% of patients fully recovered in terms of flaccid and stretched measurements, respectively (Table 1). The percent reductions of PL in postoperative visits were significantly different between the CR and the IR group (all $p < 0.002$) (Fig. 1). Among those in the CR group, the mean initial PL reduction at 7-day follow-up was 14.13% (1.9 cm) and the final reduction at 12-month visit was 1.7% (0.25 cm) of the preoperative PL. The mean initial percent reduction in the IR group was 23.8% (3.38 cm), whereas the final reduction was 16.4% (2.36 cm) of the preoperative PL (Fig. 1a). The CR group showed steady recovery throughout the follow-up measurements, reaching less than 1 cm PL reduction (0.51 cm) by 9 months. The IR group showed a slower recovery, with mean reductions at 6, 9, and 12 months measured at – 2.51 cm, – 2.44 cm, and – 2.36 cm, respectively (Fig. 1b).

When comparing the 373 patients in the CR group with the 131 patients in the IR group, the CR group was younger (59.3 years vs. 62.0 years; $p < 0.001$) and had shorter preoperative penile measurements (8.38 cm vs. 8.93 cm; $p < 0.0001$). The CR group also had lower preoperative PSA (5.11 ng/ml vs. 5.50 ng/ml; $p = 0.029$) and had lower pathologic staging (≤T2: 78.9% vs. 68.5%;

Table 1 Penile length recovery at various follow-up intervals

	Flaccid penile length		Stretched penile length	
	Analyzed, N	Recovered, N (%)	Analyzed, N	Recovered, N (%)
7 days	507	159 (31.4)	507	120 (23.7)
3 months	496	157 (31.7)	495	152 (30.7)
6 months	463	184 (39.7)	459	187 (40.7)
9 months	404	180 (44.6)	404	195 (48.3)
12 months	352	209 (59.4)	352	212 (60.2)

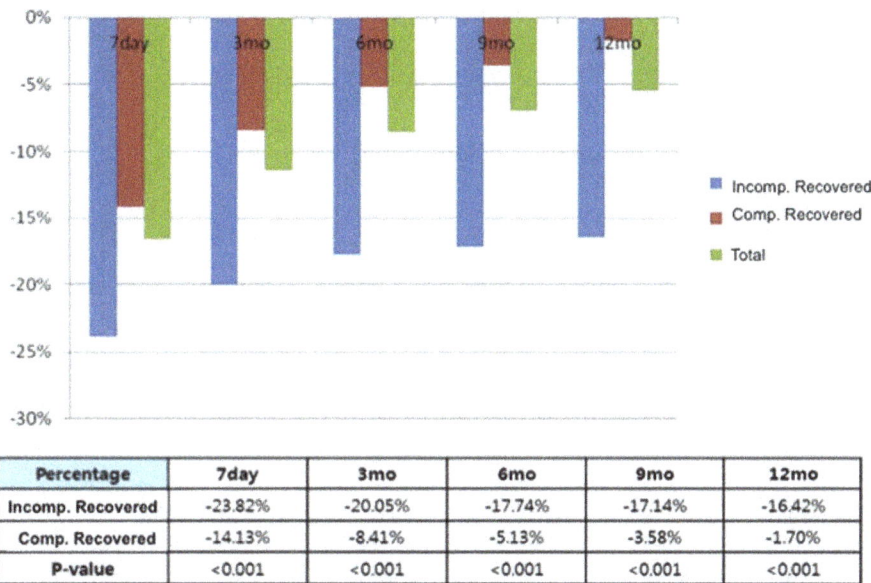

Percentage	7day	3mo	6mo	9mo	12mo
Incomp. Recovered	-23.82%	-20.05%	-17.74%	-17.14%	-16.42%
Comp. Recovered	-14.13%	-8.41%	-5.13%	-3.58%	-1.70%
P-value	<0.001	<0.001	<0.001	<0.001	<0.001

Fig. 1 Comparing penile length recovery pattern between the completely recovered group and the incompletely recovered group, (**a**) Percent difference (preoperative-postoperative), % and (**b**) Length difference (preoperative-postoperative), cm

$p = 0.017$) (Additional file 2: Table S2). In terms of CV risk factors, the CR group had fewer patients with hypertension (40.3% vs. 50.8%; $p = 0.047$) and CAD (6.9% vs. 13.7%; $p = 0.026$).

While it appeared that a greater proportion of intraoperative NS was in the CR group versus the IR group (97.5% vs. 93.9%; $p = 0.075$), the anatomical parameters of the prostate including the weight ($p = 0.56$), volume ($p = 0.93$), and length ($p = 0.46$) were not associated with a full PL recovery. Regarding therapeutic management, a greater proportion of CR patients used PDE5i consistently when compared to the IR patients (31.7% vs. 16.0%; $p = 0.002$) (Additional file 2: Table S2).

The linear trends of PL recovery [CR within 3 months ('Fast' CR) vs. CR within 12 months ('Slow' CR) vs. IR] with respect to age (< 50 vs. 50–60 vs. > 60) and SHIM groups (1–7: low vs. 8–16: medium vs. > 17: high) were statistically significant ($\chi^2_{CMH} = 9.0447$ and 12.83; $p = 0.003$ and 0.003, respectively). A decreasing trend of PL recovery with respect to age (< 50 vs. 50–60 vs. > 60) and increasing trend of recovery with respect to SHIM groups (1–7: low vs. 8–16: medium vs. > 17: high) were statistically significant (Cochran-Armitage Trend Test Z = − 3.74 and 3.85; $p = 0.0002$ and 0.0001, respectively).

Upon univariate logistic analysis, younger age (OR 0.944; 95%CI 0.916–0.973; $p < 0.0001$), higher preoperative SHIM (OR 1.049; 95%CI 1.023–1.075; $p < 0.0001$), and consistent use of PDE5i (OR 2.435; 95%CI 1.459–4.065; $p = 0.001$) were predictive of complete PL recovery. NS in either approach (AIR or IF), as opposed to a wide resection, showed a marginal association with complete PL recovery (OR 2.511; 95%CI 0.969–6.502; $P = 0.058$). In multivariate logistic

analysis, however, only younger age (OR 0.962; 95%CI 0.931–0.994; $p = 0.019$), high preoperative SHIM (OR 1.028; 95%CI 1.001–1.056; $p = 0.046$), and consistent use of PDE5i (OR 1.998; 95%CI 1.166–3.425; $p = 0.012$) remained as the significant predictors of complete PL recovery when adjusting for NS status and other pertinent clinical parameters (Table 2). Evaluation of the effect of PDE5i use on PL stratified by the three SHIM categories revealed that the effect of PDE5i is significant at median SHIM level between 8 and 17 (OR 11.497; 95% CI 1.475–89.608; $p = 0.020$), but not at low SHIM level between 1 and 8 (OR 1.56; 95% CI 0.387–6.253; $p = 0.53$) or at high SHIM level between 17 and 25 (OR 1.47; 95% CI 0.777–2.773; $p = 0.24$) (Data not shown).

When stratified by PDE5i use, patients with consistent PDE5i use had improved recovery patterns at the 12-month visit compared to those who did not take PDE5i consistently (− 3.25% vs. -6.64%; $p < 0.001$) (Fig. 2). Alternatively, the study population was divided based on whether patients had attained median study age (≥ 60 vs. < 60). These two age groups showed comparable recovery patterns (Data not shown).

Discussion

Despite concerns that post-RP PS may be irreversible [5, 6], our results demonstrate that 59.4% and 60.2% of patients returned to their baseline stretched and flaccid PL, respectively, suggesting that PS is not a permanent consequence. Additionally, our study demonstrated that younger age, high preoperative erectile function, and consistent PDE5i use were independent predictors of complete PL recovery. It appears that these therapeutic effects of PDE5i were only

Table 2 Univariate and multivariate model predictive of complete penile length recovery

Variable	Univariate		Multivariate	
	Odds ratio (95% CI)	P value	Odds ratio (95%CI)	P value
Age	0.944 (0.916–0.973)	< 0.0001	0.962 (0.931–0.994)	0.019
PSA	0.977 (0.947–1.007)	0.13		
SHIM	1.049 (1.023–1.075)	< 0.0001	1.028 (1.001–1.056)	0.046
PDEi5				
None or Not consistent	Ref.		Ref.	
Always	2.435 (1.459–4.065)	0.001	1.998 (1.166–3.425)	0.012
NSS				
None	Ref.		Ref.	
AIR or Interfascial	2.511 (0.969–6.502)	0.058	1.676 (0.602–4.665)	0.32

Abbreviations: *PSA* Prostate-specific antigen, *SHIM* Sexual health index of male, *PDEi5* Phosphodiesterase inhibitor-5, *NSS* Nerve-sparing surgery, *AIR* Athermal intrafacial robotic technique

appreciated for long-term users, and in individuals with medium preoperative SHIM scores. Neither prostate anatomy nor metabolic risk factors were significant predictors of complete PL recovery.

Older patients were less likely to reach complete PL recovery when controlled for other variables. This finding agrees with the results of a recent report that analyzed postoperative EF and continence, confirming the correlation between senility and delayed recovery from surgical trauma [17]. Among other variables associated with complete recovery was a high baseline preoperative EF, which has also been previously identified as a protective factor in PL recovery [8, 9]. Similarly, our multivariate logistic regression model revealed that high preoperative SHIM, a marker for intact erectile function, was an independent predictor of complete PL recovery.

NS techniques have frequently been reported as an independent predictor of reduced PL loss [5]. One study demonstrated that patients undergoing NS RP had no changes in penile measurements at 6-months postoperative visit when compared to preoperative baseline [9]. Our univariate logistic regression showed that both types of NS RP approach were marginally predictive of complete PL recovery (OR 2.511; 95%CI 0.969–6.502; $p = 0.058$). The lack of association at the multivariate level could be related to the distribution of our study cohort where 96. 6% of men were operated on using a NS technique - either IF or AIR. No difference was appreciated in PL recovery between these two types of NS techniques ($p = 0.24$) although AIR was found to be a superior NS technique when compared to IF in terms of preserving sexual function in our earlier report [14].

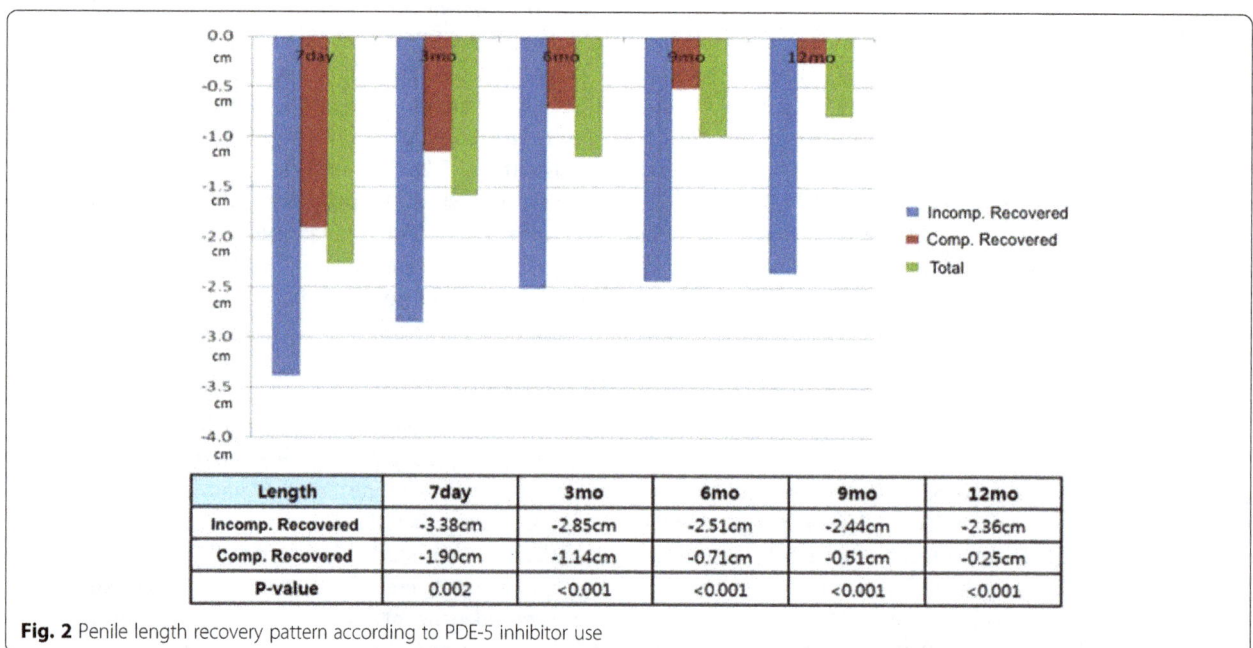

Length	7day	3mo	6mo	9mo	12mo
Incomp. Recovered	-3.38cm	-2.85cm	-2.51cm	-2.44cm	-2.36cm
Comp. Recovered	-1.90cm	-1.14cm	-0.71cm	-0.51cm	-0.25cm
P-value	0.002	<0.001	<0.001	<0.001	<0.001

Fig. 2 Penile length recovery pattern according to PDE-5 inhibitor use

Prostate anatomic factors have been implicated in the pathophysiology of PL shortening because a part of prostatic urethra will be resected during surgery [13]. However, recent studies demonstrated that prostate size and weight were not correlated with PS, suggesting that the length of prostatic urethra is fixed at the urogenital diaphragm [2, 5]. However, no study has investigated the effects of post-surgical anatomic alteration using more than two parameters. The incorporation of comprehensive anatomic parameters in our study has shown that prostate length (4.4 cm vs. 4.3 cm; $p = 0.93$), volume (63.7 ml vs. 64.1 ml; $p = 0.46$), and weight (49.1 g vs. 50.7 g; $p = 0.40$) were not significantly different between the CR and the IR groups, demonstrating that prostate size itself does not affect PL recovery.

We also investigated the effects of metabolic derangement and CV risk factors on PL recovery. In our findings, the CR group had a smaller proportion of men affected by hypertension and CAD when compared to the IR group (40.3% vs. 50.8%; $p = 0.047$ and 6.9% vs. 13.7%; $p = 0.026$, respectively), but the associations with CV factors did not remain significant in logistic regression analyses, suggesting that they might be an age-related phenomenon. Similarly, the proportion of diabetic patients who reached a complete recovery were similar in both the CR and the IR groups (13.0% vs. 12.1%; $p = 0.877$).

The literature suggests that patients can improve PL recovery by consistently taking PDE5i. Recently, Brock et al. reported on 423 patients who were randomized to receive 1) 5-mg tadalafil once daily (OaD), 2) 20-mg tadalafil on-demand ("pro renata", PRN), or 3) placebo [12]. The authors found that at the end of 9 months, PS was significantly less for patients treated with tadalafil OaD than those treated with placebo, with a least-squares mean difference in stretched PL change from preoperative PL of 4.1 mm (95% CI, 0.4–7.8; $P = 0.032$). No significant difference in PL change was observed between tadalafil PRN and placebo.

Our results are in line with previous studies and support the routine use of PDE5i after RP. Our multivariate logistic analysis demonstrated that consistent use of PDE5i was predictive of PL recovery (OR 1.998; 95%CI 1.166–3.425; $p = 0.012$). Moreover, when the study population was analyzed according to PDE5i use, the difference in penile recovery was only significant at 12-month postoperative visit (Fig. 2).

Our study is unique in that it not only attempted to describe longitudinal patterns of PL recovery between the CR and the IR groups, but also analyzed comprehensive factors associated with complete recovery within a one-year follow-up. Our study has confirmed many previous findings, and also has tested claims that were largely speculative. Importantly, our study further supports the long-term efficacy of consistent PDE5i use for PL recovery. This benefit of PDE5i in this patient population was first proved in the recent clinical trial that demonstrated that tadalafil has therapeutic potential beyond its conventional indication. To add to this, our study has found that the PL protective effect is not just unique to patients using tadalafil, but also to patients using sildenafil and vardenafil, thereby better representing the current clinical practice where different types of PDE5i are utilized in a heterogeneous patient population. For example, our study population is not limited to patients with Gleason 6 disease and PSA < 10 ng/mL, two of the inclusion criteria listed for the clinical trial. To our knowledge, our study is also the first to describe the temporal patterns of PDE5i efficacy and identify SHIM scores that would benefit from PDE5i use for PL recovery, defining a target population for intervention. The results of our study are also important to patients, as PL shortening has been consistently associated with a decreased quality of life, including reduced self-esteem, interference with close relationships, and ultimately treatment regret [18, 19]. The potential of PDE5is to potentially improve PL recovery, and consequently quality of life, is a concept that many patients may wish to embrace.

Nonetheless, our study is limited by several weaknesses. First, limited by its retrospective design with inherent selection bias, our study necessitates a randomized clinical trial for a higher level of evidence and confirmation of our results. Second, it is possible that the frequency of sexual intercourse and patient/partner satisfaction are correlated with the rate of PL recovery, but this information was unattainable in our study. Third, a longer follow-up beyond 1 year would be more useful to understand patterns of PL recovery in patients who demonstrated slower PL recovery. Fourth, measurement errors were inevitable. Although inter-observer bias was eliminated as a single surgeon evaluated patients throughout the study period, intra-observer variability may not have been well-controlled for as repeat measurements were not made for each visit. Fifth, the design of our penile habitation protocol also makes a direct comparison of the three PDE5I agents not possible because our PDE5i assignment regimen entails that a patient would take all three types in an assigned, sequential order. But it also provided an opportunity for patients to explore because it is reported that up to 40% patients are kept from best drug of choice if they only try one type of PDE5Is [20]. Sixth, patients who received adjuvant or salvage radiation therapies were not excluded from the study, but the relationship between penile length recovery and radiation therapy was not statistically significant in our study cohort (Additional file 2:

Table S2). The cost of PDE5is is a potential financial limitation and may be prohibitive to some patients, though a generic version of sildenafil is now currently available. Lastly, our penile measurement did not include penile girth, and the standardized approximation of erect PL from SPL could be a source of systemic bias. However, it is not feasible to perform direct measurement of erect PL, and SPL is considered an accepted alternative [13].

Conclusion

Our study demonstrated that more than half of post RP patients regain their preoperative PL by one-year follow up. There is evidence that a long-term use of PDE5i may aide PL recovery, particularly in individuals with medium SHIM scores. In agreement with current literature, age and preoperative erectile function were also associated with complete recovery of baseline PL.

Abbreviations

χ^2: Chi-square; AIR: Athermal intrafascial robotic; CAD: Coronary artery disease; CHD: Coronary heart disease; CI: Confidence interval; CR: Complete recovery; CV: Cardiovascular; EBL: Estimated blood loss; ED: Erectile dysfunction; EF: Erectile function; IF: Interfascial approach; IR: Incomplete recovery; NS: Nerve-sparing; OR: Operative room (OR); PCa: Prostate cancer; PDE5i: Phosphodiesterase-5 inhibitor; PL: Penile length; PLND: Pelvic lymph node dissection; PRN: Pro re nata; PS: Penile length shortening; PSA: Prostate-specific antigen; RP: Radical prostatectomy; SHIM: Sexual health inventory for men; SPL: Stretched penile length; TURP: Transurethral resection of the prostate

Authors' contributions

YSK and NF reviewed the pertinent literature, analyzed the results, and drafted and edited the manuscript. IYK was responsible for the entire project. He designed the study concept, guided the study design, conducted data acquisition, and revised the manuscript critically for important intellectual content. JWY, KR, CH, PN, JHH, PL, NG, and WJK collected data, analyzed data, and revised the manuscript. All authors read and approved the final manuscript.

Competing interests

None of the contributing authors have any competing interest, including specific financial interests and relationships and affiliation relevant to the subject matter or materials discussed in the manuscript.

Author details

[1]Section of Urologic Oncology, Rutgers Cancer Institute of New Jersey, 195 Little Albany Street, New Brunswick, NJ 08903, USA. [2]Division of Urology, Rutgers Robert Wood Johnson Medical School, New Brunswick, NJ, USA. [3]Samsung Medical Center, Sungkyunkwan University School of Medicine, Seoul, Korea. [4]Department of Biostatistics, Rutgers School of Public Health, Piscataway, NJ, USA. [5]Department of Urology, Dankook University College of Medicine, Chungnam, Korea. [6]Department of Urology, Chungbuk National University College of Medicine, Cheongju, Korea.

References

1. Frey AU, Sonksen J, Fode M. Neglected side effects after radical prostatectomy: a systematic review. J Sex Med. 2014;11(2):374–85.
2. Savoie M, Kim SS, Soloway MS. A prospective study measuring penile length in men treated with radical prostatectomy for prostate cancer. J Urol. 2003;169(4):1462–4.
3. Carlsson S, Nilsson AE, Johansson E, Nyberg T, Akre O, Steineck G. Self-perceived penile shortening after radical prostatectomy. Int J Impot Res. 2012;24(5):179–84.
4. Mulhall J. Can penile size be preserved after radical prostatectomy? Eur Urol. 2007;52(3):626–8. discussion 8-9
5. Gontero P, Galzerano M, Bartoletti R, Magnani C, Tizzani A, Frea B, et al. New insights into the pathogenesis of penile shortening after radical prostatectomy and the role of postoperative sexual function. J Urol. 2007;178(2):602–7.
6. Fraiman MC, Lepor H, McCullough AR. Changes in penile Morphometrics in men with erectile dysfunction after nerve-sparing radical Retropubic prostatectomy. Mol Urol. 1999;3(2):109–15.
7. Engel JD, Sutherland DE, Williams SB, Wagner KR. Changes in penile length after robot-assisted laparoscopic radical prostatectomy. J. Endourol. 2011;25(1):65–9.
8. Vasconcelos JS, Figueiredo RT, Nascimento FL, Damiao R, da Silva EA. The natural history of penile length after radical prostatectomy: a long-term prospective study. Urology. 2012;80(6):1293–6.
9. Briganti A, Fabbri F, Salonia A, Gallina A, Chun FK, Deho F, et al. Preserved postoperative penile size correlates well with maintained erectile function after bilateral nerve-sparing radical retropubic prostatectomy. Eur Urol. 2007;52(3):702–7.
10. Mulhall JP, Muller A, Donohue JF, Mullerad M, Kobylarz K, Paduch DA, et al. The functional and structural consequences of cavernous nerve injury are ameliorated by sildenafil citrate. J Sex Med. 2008;5(5):1126–36.
11. Ferrini MG, Davila HH, Kovanecz I, Sanchez SP, Gonzalez-Cadavid NF, Rajfer J. Vardenafil prevents fibrosis and loss of corporal smooth muscle that occurs after bilateral cavernosal nerve resection in the rat. Urology. 2006;68(2):429–35.
12. Brock G, Montorsi F, Costa P, Shah N, Martinez-Jabaloyas JM, Hammerer P, et al. Effect of Tadalafil once daily on penile length loss and morning erections in patients after bilateral nerve-sparing radical prostatectomy: results from a randomized controlled trial. Urology. 2015;85(5):1090–6.
13. Munding MD, Wessells HB, Dalkin BL. Pilot study of changes in stretched penile length 3 months after radical retropubic prostatectomy. Urology. 2001;58(4):567–9.
14. Potdevin L, Ercolani M, Jeong J, Kim IY. Functional and oncologic outcomes comparing interfascial and intrafascial nerve sparing in robot-assisted laparoscopic radical prostatectomies. J. Endourol. 2009;23(9):1479–84.
15. Third Report of the National Cholesterol Education Program (NCEP) Expert panel on detection, evaluation, and treatment of high blood cholesterol in adults (adult treatment panel III) final report. Circulation 2002;106(25):3143–421.
16. Wisman PP, Roest M, Asselbergs FW, de Groot PG, Moll FL, van der Graaf Y, et al. Platelet-reactivity tests identify patients at risk of secondary cardiovascular events: a systematic review and meta-analysis. J Thromb Haemost. 2014;12(5):736–47.
17. Hatzichristodoulou G, Wagenpfeil S, Wagenpfeil G, Maurer T, Horn T, Herkommer K, et al. Extended versus limited pelvic lymph node dissection during bilateral nerve-sparing radical prostatectomy and its effect on continence and erectile function recovery: long-term results and trifecta rates of a comparative analysis. World J Urol. 2016;34(6): 811–20.
18. Parekh A, Chen MH, Hoffman KE, Choueiri TK, Hu JC, Bennett CL, et al. Reduced penile size and treatment regret in men with recurrent prostate cancer after surgery, radiotherapy plus androgen deprivation, or radiotherapy alone. Urology. 2013 Jan;81(1):130–4.
19. Carlsson S, Nilsson AE, Johansson E, Nyberg T, Akre O, Steineck G. Self-perceived penile shortening after radical prostatectomy. Int J Impot Res. 2012 Sep;24(5):179–84.
20. Stroberg P, Hedelin H, Ljunggren C. Prescribing all phosphodiesterase 5 inhibitors to a patient with erectile dysfunction–a realistic and feasible option in everyday clinical practice–outcomes of a simple treatment regime. Eur Urol. 2006;49(5):900–7. discussion 7

28

The application of a novel integrated rigid and flexible Nephroscope in percutaneous nephrolithotomy for renal staghorn stones

Huan Yang[1], Jianxing Li[2], Gang Long[3] and Shaogang Wang[1*] (iD)

Abstract

Background: Renal staghorn stones are challenging for urologists to ensure maximum stone clearance and minimal morbidity. Percutaneous nephrolithotomy (PCNL) has become the gold standard treatment for renal staghorn stones. To assess the safety and efficacy of a novel integrated rigid and flexible percutaneous nephroscope(Rigi-flex nephroscope) in PCNL for renal staghorn stones.We present our initial experience with this new technique.

Methods: From March to July 2016, a prospective analysis of 3 patients with staghorn stones treated with Rigi-flex nephroscope in PCNLunder totally ultrasound guidance by paravertebral block (PVB) anesthesia was done. PCNL was performed with the rigid section of a 13-Fr Rigi-flex nephroscope firstly and the stones were disintegrated into fragments by holmium laser.Then the stones were removed by active flushout, followed by a search for residual stones in other inaccessible calyces with the flexible section. Finally, the residual stones were disintegrated into small fractions by holmium laser in situ or repositioned with a set of disposable retrieval baskets to pelvic or other accessible areas. The whole procedure was accomplished via only one nephrostomy tract. The operating time, stone-free rates (SFR), postoperative hemoglobin drop, complications, length of hospitalization, were recorded.

Results: The operation time were 89, 62 and 45 min, respectively, the postoperative hemoglobin drop was 1, 0.8 and 0. 9 mg/dl, respectively.The postoperative Kidney-Ureter-Bladder (KUB) radiograph of the three patients showed no residual fragment >3 mm. No patients needed blood transfusion and suffered significant complications. The length of hospitalization was 9, 6 and 4 days, respectively. No patient needed multiple tracts PCNL or staged auxiliary measures one month after the operation.

Conclusions: The application of Rigi-flex nephroscope in PCNL under ultrasound guidance for staghorn stones has its unique advantages as monotherapy with increasing procedural stone free rate (SFR) via single nephrostomy tract, hence there is less morbidity as it does not require additional tracts dilation and staged auxiliary procedures combination. However, SFR should also be evaluated at a longer follow-up, particularly for staghorn stone, further large-scale multicenter prospective clinical trial are needed to verify its feasibility.

Keywords: Integrated rigid and flexible Nephroscope, Percutaneous nephrolithotomy, Ultrasound guidance, Renal staghorn stones, Single nephrostomy tract

* Correspondence: sgwangtjm@163.com
[1]Dartment of Urology, Tongji Hospital,Tongji Medical School, Huazhong University of Science and Technology, Wuhan 430030, China
Full list of author information is available at the end of the article

Background

Percutaneous nephrolithotomy (PCNL) has become the gold standard treatment for large renal stones and currently is recommended for staghorn stones, as it has stone-free rate three times higher than extracorporeal shock wave lithotripsy (ESWL), along with lower morbidity, shorter length of hospital stayand operating time as well as faster return to work than open stone extraction surgery [1–3].Retrograde intrarenal surgery (RIRS) is becoming popular, due to the advances in flexible ureteroscope and holmium laser lithotripsy. It allows retrograde access to the entire intrarenal collecting system in treating renal stones. However, RIRS has high rates of fiber breakage and lower efficiency for larger stones [4].

Most of staghorn stones were approached with PCNL primarily in accordance with existing techniques, but the large stone burden volume and scattered distribution in various parts of the pelvocalyceal system are challenging for most urologists to ensure maximum stone clearance and minimal morbidity.As a rigid endoscope, conventional nephroscope or semi-rigid ureteroscope can not access the renal calyces situated at an acute angle with the calyx of entry, which may increase needs of multiple tracts PCNL or staged auxiliary measures(PCNL or ESWL or RIRS et al.). Creation of multiple tracts to maneuver into various parts of the pelvocalyceal system, for staghorn stones or migrated stone fragments, increases potential risks of access-related morbidity of the procedure [5]. Staged auxiliary measures often accompanied by more medical expenses, with more instruments and procedures [6]. So the preoperative decision of therapeutic schedule should be made to accurately balance cost-efficacy and safety .

It is necessary to explore a new concept and definition of PCNL.So we proposed that PCNL is redefined beyond a surgical technique as a new requirement for the operation procedure:P-Patient oriented, C-Cost efficient, N-New features, L-Less invasive. The new concept of "PCNL" indicates that: the therapeutic schedule including the selection of surgical technique and instruments shall be individualized based on cost-efficacy and safety. The operation shall be completed by novel less-invasive and high-efficacy instruments. Surgeon's expertise, experience and skills, as well as the new instruments are of upmost impotantance in the new "PCNL" for precise treatment of complex nephrolithiasis.

Based on the new concept of "PCNL", we proposed "integrated rigid and flexible Percutaneous Nephrolithotomy(Rigi-flex PCNL)" via a novel integrated rigid and flexible nephroscope (Rigi-flex nephroscope) (Youcare, Wuhan, China) for accessing all calyces of the pelvocalyceal system through only one nephrostomy tract, with the objective of assessing the feasibility and safety of this new technique, especially in increasing procedural SFR.

The seamless switching of Rigi-flex nephroscope between rigid mode and flexible mode is straightforward. Technical parameters and pictures of Rigi-flex nephroscope are shown in Table 1 and Fig. 1.

No reference to a similar study or use of a similar instrument could be found during a thorough literature search. To the best of our knowledge, this is the first clinical study using this endoscope anywhere in the world.

Methods

Our study was a small-scale clinical observational trial, which used the Rigi-flex nephroscope to evaluate the efficacy and safety of PCNL for patients with staghorn stones. The study was approved by the ethics committees of our hospital. All patients gave written informed consent for the Rigi-flex PCNL and the use of their information in our research, according to the Helsinki II declaration.

From March to July 2016, three patients (two female and one male) with staghorn stones were admitted in our department. Eligible patients were 18 years of age or older with staghorn stones that required PCNL.The demographic characteristics are reported in Table 2. The age of patients was 47, 65 and 53 years, respectively. Two patients had staghorn stones in the right kidney, and one patient had staghorn stones in the left kidney. The maximum diameters of the stones were 4 cm, 3.5 cm and 4.2 cm, respectively.

In addition to routine preoperative examination, urine culture and sensitivity was also tested. Preoperative Kidney-ureter-bladder (KUB) radiograph and abdominal non-contrast computed tomography (NCCT) were used to proved staghorn stones and delineate kidney (renal parenchyma, and the distribution in pelvocalyceal system) and adjacent viscera.All patients with urinary tract infection were treated with culture specific antibiotic therapy until repeat urine culture was negative. All other patients with negative urine culture received empiric antibiotic therapy for three days before operation.

After total paravertebral block (PVB) anesthesia was accomplished.An externalized ureteric stent was placed into ureter retrogradely with cystoscope in lithotomy position for retrograde saline injection if intraoperative artificial hydronephrosis is needed, and a 18-Fr Foley catheter was remained in the bladder.Then, the patients were repositioned to prone position with a pillow under the abdomen for establishment of percutaneous nephrostomy tract under totally ultrasound guidance with 3.5-MHz convex abdominal ultrasound probe (BK flex Focus 500, Denmark). The percutaneous renal puncture was finished by an 18G access needle with echogenic tip (Urovision, Germany). First, the surgeons observed the kidney (renal outline and parenchyma, the stone size and distribution in pelvocalyceal system) and adjacent viscera in lower

Table 1 Technical Parameters of Rigi-flex nephroscope

Working length (mm)		
Rigid section	220	
Flexible section	56.5	
Outer diameter (F)		
Rigid section	13	
Flexible section	10.5	
Max deflection angle		
Unloaded	290	
Loaded with 200um Holmium Laser Fiber	270	
Loaded with COOK HWS-035150 Loach Guidewire	210	
Working Channel ID1 (F)	3	
Working Channel ID2 (F)	6	
Unloaded bending times	720	
Minimum bending radius (mm)	10	
Imaging	CMOS	
Using style	One-time use	
Water discharge rate (ml/min)	Lower pressure (13.3 kpa)	Higher pressure (26 kpa)
Unloaded working channel	300	400
4.5 F Ultrasonic Probe	120	140
1 F Holmium Laser Fiber	200	300
1.5 F Holmium Laser Fiber	180	220
2 F Holmium Laser Fiber	170	200
COOK HWS-035150 Loach Guidewire	150	188

paravertebral region by ultrasound, and then selected an optimum percutaneous puncture spot (The preset spot in skin was pressed by the index finger with low frequency impact from the caudal position behind ultrasound probe, and the shock wave direction of pressed impact wave from the preset spot to the target calyx in ultrasonic imaging plane as the simulative ultrasound-guided needle access was observed and adjusted) usually through the posterior middle calyx, which led straight to maximum stone burden, and kept the adjacent viscera out of the preset needle access. Two-steps precise puncture method was performed for good visualization of entire needle from preset spot into target cylax:First, the echogenic tip of the access needle was moved from skin into the perinephric fat tissue where the direction of the needle can be adjusted accompanying respiratory movement.Second, the echogenic tip of needle was inserted into target cylax fornix quickly.

If percutaneous renal puncture was accomplished successfully with the flow-out of clear and transparent urine from needle, a hydrophilic 0.035-inch J-tip coaxial guidewire was placed into the collecting system through

access needle (ultrasound can detect the J-tip in collecting system). After 1 cm skin surrounding the access needle was incised, tract dilatation was serially performed by 10 to 22-Fr fascia dilators (Cook, USA) through the guidewire and a 22-Fr working access sheath was kept in the collecting system.A 13-Fr Rigi-flex nephroscope was advanced into pelvocalyceal system in its rigid section through working access sheath along the longitudinal axial direction of nephrostomy access. The stones were disintegrated into fragments by holmium laser fiber (PowerSuite 100w, lumenis, USA). A 500-μm laser fiber was used for rigid mode with power setting 3.0/20 Hz.The stones were actively flushed out with transportion of stone fragments by continuous irrigation backflow through access sheath alongside the nephroscope or by filling of collecting system with high pressure and quickly removing the nephroscope resulting in immediate inversion of irrigation water-flow with spillage-like removal of stones via the access sheath [7, 8].All visible accessible stones were broken into fraction and flushed out, then the working access sheath and Rigi-flex nephroscope were pulled back to the renal calyx neck when the rigid section couldn't access the peripheral calyces situated at an acute angle with the calyx of entry.The flexible section of Rigi-flex nephroscope stretched out and deflected for residual stones and migrated stone fragments, then the stones was broken into fraction with laser in situ or repositioned with a set of disposable retrieval baskets to pelvic or other easily accessible area. A 200-μm laser fiber was used for flexible mode with power setting 1.2 J/20 Hz.The interior pictures of Rigi-flex nephroscope in operation were captured and shown in Fig. 2.

The operations were terminated when no residual fragments could be detected with the help of Rigi-flex nephroscope and ultrasound screening.A double J-tip ureteric stent (Bard, USA) was inserted into ureter antegradly and a 20-Fr nephrostomy tube was placed in each patient.All patients were initially evaluated with KUB in postoperative 1st day.Nephrostomy tubes were removed in postoperative 2nd day.The patients were reevaluated with KUB about one month post-operation and double J-tip ureteric stents were removed. NCCT was performed when the stone status were suboptimally evaluated with KUB.Residual fragment <3 mm were defined as clinically insignificant residual fragments (CIRF). Larger stones >3 mm were defined as residual stones. Patients who were complete stone free or had only CIRF were considered to have a successful surgery.Stone free rate (SFR), postoperative hemoglobin drop and length of hospitalization was recorded. All complications occurring within one month post-operation were recorded according to the modified Clavien Classification system..

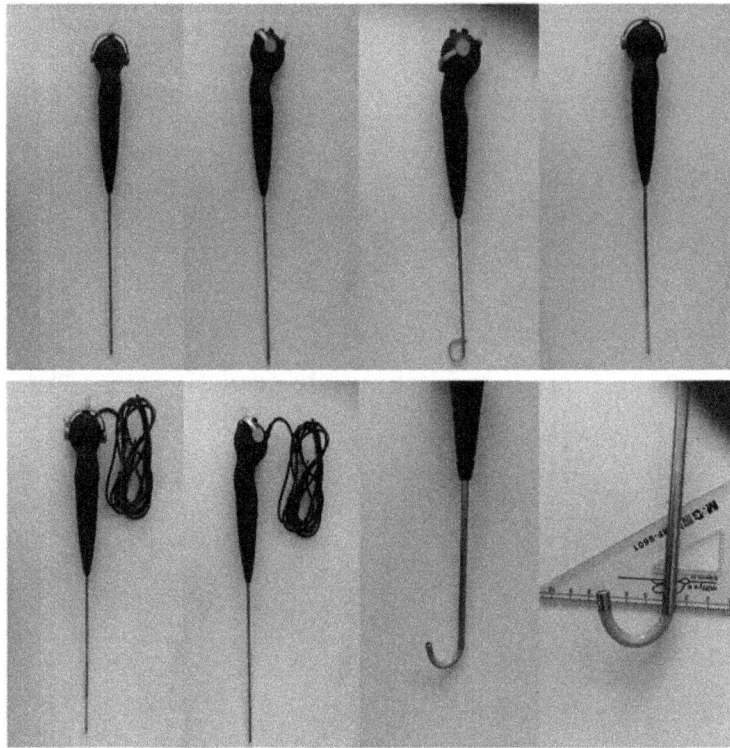

Fig. 1 External view of Rigi-flex nephroscope

Results

Theperioperative data and postoperative complications were reported in Table 2 too. No patients complained of pain during operation. Early ambulation could be achieved in 1 h after the operations. The postoperative KUB radiographs of all three patients showed no residual fragment >3 mm.Pre and post-operative radiology for the 3 patients were shown in Fig. 3.2 patients had postoperative fever, which were treated with diclofenac sodium and penicillium carbon alkene respectively. No patients needed blood transfusion and no patients suffered severe complications.The operation time was 89, 62 and 45 min, respectively. The postoperative hemoglobin drop was 1, 0.8 and 0.9 mg/dl, respectively. The lengths of hospitalization were 9, 6 and 4 days, respectively.No patient needed multiple tracts PCNL or staged auxiliary measures (PCNL or ESWL or RIRS) one month after the operation.

Discussion

The first description of percutaneous renal stone extraction was reported by Fernstrom and Johansson in 1976 [9].Wickham and Kollett officially reported and named the Percutaneous Nephrolithotomy (PCNL) in 1981 [10].

The indications for PCNL include stone factors (stone size, stone composition, and stone location), patient factors (habitus and renal anomalies), and failure of other treatment modalities (ESWL and flexible ureteroscopy). The accepted indications for PCNL are stones larger than 20 mm^2, staghorn and partial staghorn calculi. American Urological Association (AUA) recommends that all newly diagnosed staghorn stones should be actively treated, because untreated staghorn stones have a tendency to destroy the kidney and cause life-threatening urosepsis [2]. It is crucial to completely remove all staghorn calculi, because residual stones can form nuclei for stone recurrence (85% recurrence rate) that may lead to infection [11].

As compared to ESWL as well as RIRS, althrough PCNL with the highest SFR after one-stage single treatment in case of large or multiple renal stones [12, 13].However, It is challenging for the urologist to perform PCNL on staghorn stones and ensure complete stone clearance and minimise morbidity, which may increase the need for multiple tracts PCNL and incidence of staged procedures (Including PCNL, RIRS, ESWL). Conventional PCNL procedure uses a rigid nephroscope or semi-rigid ureteroscope as the level and the neck of access calyx as the pivot, at various angles inside pelvocalyceal system to search for and clear all visible stones in a singe nephrostomy tract. This could cause some certain kidney damage, and even accidental calyx neck avulsion if nephroscope was forced to see the calyx of which the axis form an acute angle with the nephrostomy access for higher stone clearance rate. In

Table 2 The demographics, perioperative data, and complications of patient

Num	Age(years)	Gender	Store Side	Maximum diameter of stone(cm)	Operation time(min)	Operation time with rigid section (min)	Operation with flexible section (min)	Hospitalization Stay (day)	Postoperative haemoglobin drop rate	Stone free rates(%)	Postoperative recovery time(h)	Complications
1	47	Female	Right	4	89	27	62	9	1	100%	1	fever
2	65	Male	Right	3.5	62	23	39	6	0.8	100%	1	haematuria
3	53	Female	Left	4.2	45	15	30	4	0.9	100%	1	fever

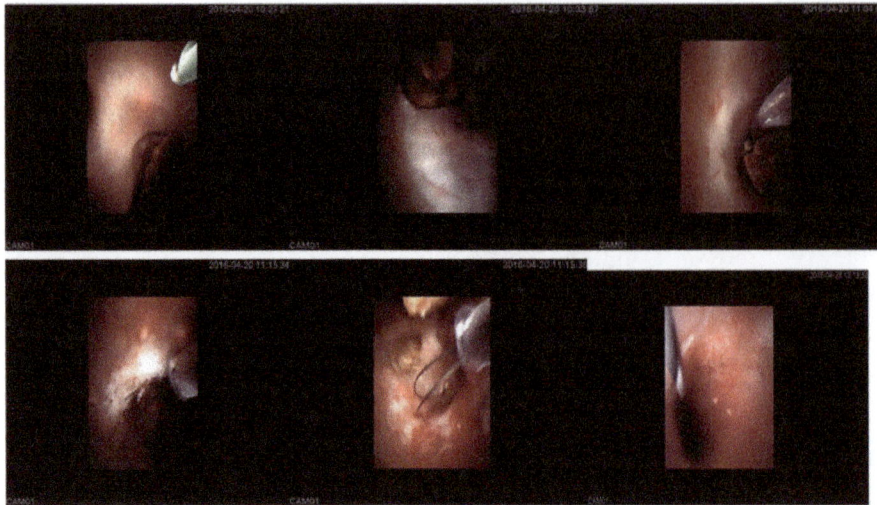

Fig. 2 Endoscopic view from Rigi-flex nephroscope demonstrating the digital image quality in operation

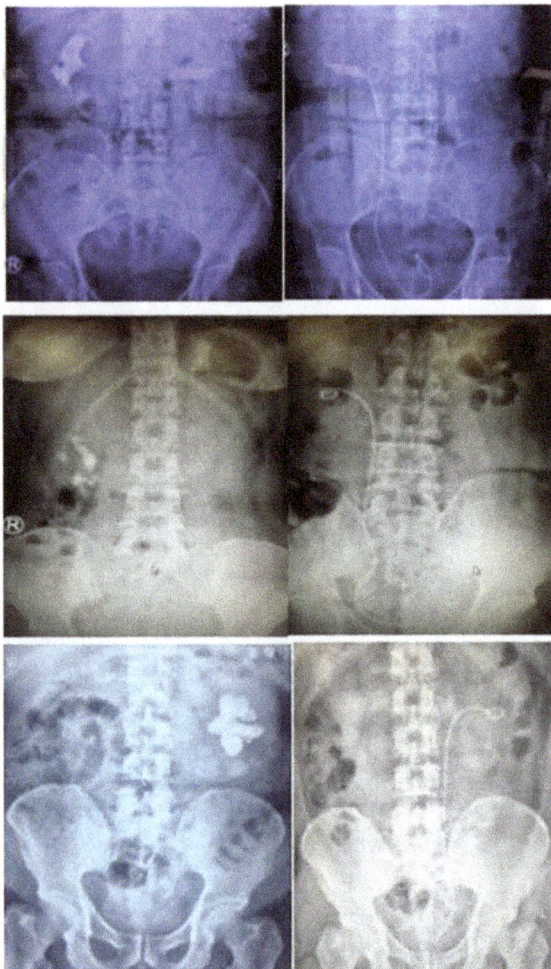

Fig. 3 Pre and post-operative radiology for the 3 patients

severe cases, massive haemorrhage might occur, which blurs the operative vision and hence the procedure needs to be terminated. In such cases, emergency embolization is required, which further increases the medical expense. So to achieve higher complete stone clearance rate for treating multiple stones or staghorn stones, multiple tracts or staged procedure needs to be adopted.

Of the 1466 patients with staghorn stones undergoing PCNL in the CROES database, the SFRs was only 56.9% [14]. SFRs for staghorn stones were even lower in the UK registry [15]. Increasing staghorn volume and complexity may predict the need for multiple tracts and staged procedures for successful stone clearance [16]. Although multiple-tract access did not lead to a more severe reduction in renal function than singe-tract access [17], but multiple-tract access may lead to higher complication rate [18]. Akman et al.demonstrated that >60% of patients with residual stones after PCNL required a second intervention [19]. So PCNL needs continuous improvements for better cost efficacy and less complications.

To the best of our knowledge, this is the first clinical study to use this novel type device-integrated rigid and flexible percutaneous nephroscope in PCNL under totally ultrasound guidance by total PVB anesthesia.As compared with traditional PCNL, Rigi-flex PCNL has its unique advantages:Rigi-flex percutaneous nephroscope can find almost all stones in various calyces with single nephrostomy tract through intraoperative seamless switching of Rigi-flex nephroscope between rigid mode and flexible mode. Medical expenses and access-related morbidity were reduced as it does not require multiple tracts and staged procedures with less instruments. In our initial experience, three patients with staghorn stones underwent Rigi-flex PCNL and were almost completely stone free. The postoperative complications were fewer and minor. The length of hospitalization was slightly longer than before due to treatment of postoperative fever with urosepsis and hematuria. It is a promising tool that has the potential to reduce the morbidity of PCNL in cases of multiple or staghorn stones and improve stone clearance rates.

However, there were certain limitations in our study:- This is the initial experience of a new technique from a single center.Since the number of patients included in this study was small, the results were not statistically significant.The SFR should be evaluated in a longer follow-up, particularly for staghorn stones.Further large-scale multicenter prospective clinical trials are needed to verify the cost efficacy and safety of the device.

Conclusion

The application of Rigi-flex nephroscope in PCNL under ultrasound guidance for staghorn stones has its unique advantages as monotherapy with increasing procedural stone free rate (SFR) via single nephrostomy tract, hence there is less morbidity as it does not require additional tracts dilation and staged auxiliary procedures combination. Given the limited case number, further large-scale multicenter prospective clinical trials are still required.

Abbreviation

AUA: American Urological Association; CIRF: Clinically insignificant residual fragments; ESWL: Extracorporeal shock wave lithotripsy; KUB: Kidney-Ureter-Bladder; NCCT: Non-contrast computed tomography; PCNL: Percutaneous nephrolithotomy; PVB: Paravertebral block; Rigi-flex nephroscope: Integrated rigid and flexible percutaneous nephroscope; Rigi-flex PCNL: Integrated rigid and flexible Percutaneous Nephrolithotomy; RIRS: Retrograde intrarenal surgery; SFR: Stone free rate

Acknowledgements
None.

Funding
National Natural Science Foundation (81500534);The institution of higher learning doctoral discipline specific program of scientific research fund for new teachers supported by National Ministry of Education (20130142120072).

Authors' contributions
SGW conceived and designed this study. HY and JXL performed the surgeries and collected clinical data.GL provided and introduced the applied devices. HY and SGW drafted the manuscript. All the authors read and approved the final manuscript.

Competing interests
The authors declare that they have no competing interests.

Author details
[1]Dartment of Urology, Tongji Hospital,Tongji Medical School, Huazhong University of Science and Technology, Wuhan 430030, China. [2]Department of Urology, Beijing Tsinghua changgung Hospital, Beijing, China. [3]YouCare Technology Co., Ltd, Wuhan, China.

References

1. Al-Kohlany KM, Shokeir AA, Mosbah A, et al. Treatment of complete staghorn stones: a prospective randomized comparison of open surgery versus percutaneous nephrolithotomy. J Urol. 2005;173(2):469–73.
2. Türk C, Petrik A, Sarica K, et al. EAU guidelines on interventional treatment for Urolithiasis. Eur Urol. 2016;69(3):475–82.
3. Assimos D, Krambeck A, Miller NL, et al. Surgical Management of Stones: American urological association/Endourological society guideline PART II. J Urol. 2016;196(4):1161–9.
4. Bryniarski P, Paradysz A, Zyczkowski M. Et al.a randomized controlled study to analyze the safety and efficacy of percutaneous nephrolithotripsy and retrograde intrarenal surgery in the management of renal stones more than 2 cm in diameter. J Endourol. 2012;26(1):52–7.
5. Ahmed R, El-Nahas IE, Shokeir AA, et al. Percutaneous nephrolithotomy for treating staghorn stones: 10 years of experience of a tertiary-care centre. Arab J Urol. 2012;10(3):324–9.
6. Ghani KR, Andonian S. Bultitude M, et alPercutaneous Nephrolithotomy: update, trends, and future directions. Eur Urol. 2016;70(2):382–96.
7. Rassweiler J, Rassweiler MC, Klein J. New technology in ureteroscopy and percutaneous nephrolithotomy. Curr Opin Urol. 2016;26(1):95–106.
8. Zeng G, Wan S, Zhao Z, et al. Super-mini percutaneous nephrolithotomy (SMP):a new concept in technique and instrumentation. BJU Int. 2016;117(4):655–61.
9. Fernström I, Johansson B. Percutaneous pyelolithotomy. A new extraction technique. Scand J Urol Nephrol. 1976;10:257–9.
10. Wickham JE, Kellett MJ. Percutaneous Nephrolithotomy. Br J Urol. 1981;53(4):297–9.
11. Meng M.: Struvite and staghorn calculi. Http://emedicine.medscape.com/article/439127-overview#a7. Accessed: Aug 22, 2016.
12. Wiesenthal JD, Ghiculete D, D'A Honey RJ, et al. A comparison of treatment modalities for renal calculi between 100 and 300 mm2: are shockwave lithotripsy, ureteroscopy, and percutaneous nephrolithotomy equivalent? J Endourol. 2011;25:481–5.
13. De S, Autorino R, Kim FJ, et al. Percutaneous nephrolithotomy versus retrograde intrarenal surgery: a systematic review and meta-analysis. Eur Urol. 2015;67:125–37.
14. Desai M, De Lisa A, Turna B, et al. The clinical research office of the endourological society percutaneous nephrolithotomy global study: staghorn versus nonstaghorn stones. J Endourol. 2011;25:1263–8.
15. Armitage JN, Irving SO, Burgess NA. British Association of Urological Surgeons Section of Endourology. Percutaneous nephrolithotomy in the United Kingdom: results of a prospective data registry. Eur Urol. 2012;61:1188–93.
16. Mishra S, Sabnis RB, Desai M. Staghorn morphometry: a new tool for clinical classification and prediction model for percutaneous nephrolithotomy monotherapy. J Endourol. 2012;26:6–14.
17. El-Nahas AR, Eraky I, Shokeir AA, et al. Long-term results of percutaneous nephrolithotomy for treatment of staghorn stones. BJU Int. 2011;108:750–4.
18. El-Nahas AR, Shokeir AA, El-Assmy AM, et al. Post-percutaneous nephrolithotomy extensive hemorrhage: a study of risk factors. J Urol. 2007; 177:576–9.
19. Akman T, Binbay M, Kezer C, et al. Factors affecting kidney function and stone recurrence rate after percutaneous nephrolithotomy for staghorn calculi: outcomes of a long-term followup. J Urol. 2012;187:1656–61

29

Changes in the outcome of prostate biopsies after preventive task force recommendation against prostate-specific antigen screening

Ahmed S. Zakaria[1] (iD), Alice Dragomir[1], Fadi Brimo[2], Wassim Kassouf[1], Simon Tanguay[1] and Armen Aprikian[1*]

Abstract

Background: The benefits of PSA-based screening for prostate cancer (PCa) are controversial. The Canadian and American Task Forces on Preventive Health Care (CTFPHC & USPSTF) have released recommendations against the use of routine PSA-based screening for any men. We thought to assess the impact of these recommendations on the outcomes and trends of prostate needle biopsies.

Methods: A complete chart review was conducted for all men who received prostate needle biopsies at McGill University Health Center between 2010 and 2016. Of those, we included 1425 patients diagnosed with PCa for analysis. We Compared 2 groups of patients (pre and post recommendations' release date) using Welch's t-tests and Chi-square test. A multivariate logistic regression model was used to analyze variables predicting worse pathological outcomes.

Results: When the release date of the USPSTF draft (October 2011) was used as a cut-off, we found an average annual decrease of 10.6% in the total number of biopsies. The median (IQR) baseline PSA levels were higher in post-recommendations group ($n = 977$) when compared to pre-recommendations group ($n = 448$) [8 ng/ml (5.7–12.9) versus 6.4 ng/ml (4.9–10.1), respectively. $P = 0.0007$]. Also, post-recommendations group's patients had higher Gleason score (G7: 35.4% versus 28.4% and G8-G10: 31.2% versus 18.1%, respectively. $P < 0.0001$). Moreover, they had higher intermediate and high-risk PCa classification (36.4% versus 32.8% and 35.5% versus 22.1%, respectively. $P < 0.0001$). The recommendations release date was an independent variable associated with higher Gleason score in prostate biopsies (OR: 2.006, 95%CI: 1.477–2.725). Using the CTFPHC recommendations release date (October 2014) as a cut-off in further analysis, revealed similar results.

Conclusions: Our results revealed a reduction in the number of prostate needle biopsies performed over time after the recommendations of the preventive task forces. Furthermore, it showed a significant relative increase in the higher risk PCa diagnosis. The oncological outcomes associated with this trend need to be examined in further studies.

Keywords: Prostate-specific antigen, Prostate cancer screening, Task force recommendations, Prostate biopsies

* Correspondence: armen.aprikian@muhc.mcgill.ca
[1]Department of Surgery, Division of Urology, McGill University, McGill
University Health Centre, 1001 Boulevard Decarie, Montreal, Quebec H4A 3J1,
Canada
Full list of author information is available at the end of the article

Background

Prostate cancer (PCa) is the most frequently diagnosed cancer in men, with an estimated 202,490 new cases diagnosed in North America in 2016 [1, 2]. In Canada, it is expected that 1 in 8 males will develop PCa in their lifetime and last year it accounted for 10% of cancer-related death in Canadian men [2].

Owing to the high incidence rate and the potential for cure with early detection, screening for PCa using the prostate specific antigen (PSA) blood test, is a common practice. Since its emergence in 1986 [3] and its approval by the Food and Drug Administration in 1994 [4], along with the digital rectal exam (DRE), PSA has been shown to be a valuable oncological marker. Epidemiologically this approach was associated with a dramatic increase in PCa detection rates and substantial decline in PCa mortality rates that have fallen by over 50% [5].

However during the last decade, results from major randomized trials, showed mixed evidence regarding the utility of PSA screening, with questionable survival benefit and significant harms associated with PCa diagnosis and overtreatment [6–8]. Following these results, the US Preventive Services Task Force (USPSTF) issued a first recommendation in 2008 advising against routine screening in men older than 75 years [9]. Few years later in October 2011 they issued the highly publicized draft recommendation against PSA screening of all ages, that was finalized as (Grade D recommendation) in May 2012 [10]. Recently, in October 2014 the Canadian Task Force on Preventive Health Care (CTFPHC) issued a similar recommendation against PCa screening with PSA.

The USPSTF and CTFPHC recommendations may have changed screening practice and referral patterns among primary care physicians [11–14]. In the current study, we aimed to characterize the trends of prostate needle biopsies as well as to assess for changes in the pathological outcomes before and after these recommendations, in a tertiary-care academic hospital.

Methods

Data source and study population

The study cohort was built retrospectively through complete chart review, during the period between January 2010 and December 2016, to analyze data of all patients who underwent prostate biopsies at McGill University Health Center. Patients' information was collected in a database with an institutional review board-approved protocol for the collection of data. Our cohort's patients were referred to our tertiary-hospital by primary care providers and were offered trans-rectal ultrasound (TRUS)--guided prostate biopsy to rule out PCa due to abnormal laboratory or clinical findings. Data collected included: demographics, laboratory, clinical, and pathological data in relation to the first recorded prostate needle biopsy.

From our whole cohort, the exclusion criteria of this study were: 1) patients who were previously diagnosed with PCa; 2) repeated biopsies of active surveillance patients; 3) absent baseline PSA test result; and 4) non-standard needle biopsies (non-TRUS-guided prostate biopsy and biopsies with less than 10 cores).

Biochemical, clinical and pathological evaluation

The baseline serum PSA level was defined as the last PSA measured before the diagnostic biopsy and up to 3 months before biopsy. PSA was categorized based on D'Amico risk score criteria as patients with a PSA of 10.00 ng/ml or less (sub-categorized into: 4.00 ng/ml or less and 4.01 to 10.00 ng/ml), 10.01 to 20.00 ng/ml and greater than 20.00 ng/ml. Patient's PSA density (PSAD) was calculated by dividing baseline PSA to prostate volume measured by TRUS at time of diagnostic biopsy. Clinical staging was determined from the TRUS findings at the time of diagnostic biopsy or by digital rectal exam (DRE) at the time of first encounter with the urologist. Individual D'Amico risk classification score was calculated for each patient using previously published criteria [15].

Prostate needle biopsies were performed during the study period by six attending urologists and radiologists, with the number of cores taken per biopsy varying according to the time period of the biopsy (range, 10–20 cores). All prostate biopsies specimens were reviewed by a team of four attending pathologists led by dedicated genitourinary pathologist (F.B.). The biopsy findings analyzed in this study included: the Gleason score (primary and secondary predominant patterns), the total number of cores, the number of positive cores, and the maximum percentage of cancer on each core. The modifications of the Gleason grading system, implemented by the International Society of Urological Pathology over the previous years, were taken in account during reporting.

Statistical analysis

Descriptive statistics [percentages for categorical variables and mean (standard deviation = SD or range) and medians (inter quartile range = IQR) for continuous variables], respectively, were used to summarize the characteristics of the study population. Age, age categories, baseline PSA, PSA categories, baseline prostate volume, PSA density, Gleason score on biopsy, clinical stage and D'Amico risk classification were compared between patients who underwent prostate needle biopsies before recommendation date (USPSTF draft on 7 October 2011 and CTFPHC recommendations on 27 October 2014) with those who underwent prostate needle biopsies after the recommendation release date. Comparison between groups was performed using Chi-square and Welch's t-tests. Multivariate logistic regression models were used to assess the association between the time period of prostate biopsy (pre- versus post-recommendation date) and worse pathological outcomes while adjusting for potential confounding factors and other covariables. Analyses were performed using the Statistical Analysis System Software (Version 9 SAS Institute, Cary, North Carolina). All tests were two-sided with a significance threshold of 5%.

Results

Our study flowchart is shown in Fig. 1. From our main cohort of all patients (4362 patients) who underwent prostate biopsies between January 2010 and December 2016, 1823 (41.7%) patients were diagnosed with PCa and finally 1425 (32.6%) patients were included for analysis after applying the study's exclusion criteria (excluded 298 (9.1%) patients).

During the study time period, there was a trend of decline in the total number of prostate needle biopsies performed over years as shown in Fig. 2, with an average annual decrease of 10.6% after the recommendations, this trend was consistent for biopsies pathologically diagnosed as PCa and biopsies that showed no evidence of cancer. Also, our results revealed that relative PCa detection rate did not change significantly over study period ($p = 0.24$), specially before and after the (USPSTF & CTFPHC) recommendations, but what actually has changed was the percentage of pathologically high grade cancer diagnosed, namely G8–10, that increased by at least 11% in the years immediately after the release of the 2011 USPSTF draft recommendations.

The baseline clinical, biochemical and pathological characteristics of the study population were noted in Table 1. Basically, at the time of diagnosis, the cohort mean (SD) age was 68.6 (8.72) years, The baseline PSA was ≤10 ng/mL in 948 (66.5%) patients, 566 (39.7%) patients had a Gleason score of ≤6 and 477 (33.4%)

patients were classified as having low risk PCa according to D'Amico risk classification criteria.

The absolute numbers of different pathological grades diagnosed in biopsies during the study time period are shown in Table 2, where there was an increase in the number of G8–10 cases after the USPSTF recommendation, associated with decline in low grade cancer, especially G6 cases during the same time period.

Based on USPSTF draft recommendation as a cut-off, Table 3 is comparing characteristics of 448 patients in the pre-recommendation group with 977 patients in the post-recommendation group. Generally, patients in the post-recommendation group were relatively younger, and had significantly higher median baseline PSA of 8 ng/ml compared to a median baseline PSA of 6.4 ng/ml in the pre-recommendation group ($p = 0.0007$). Moreover, 37.4% of the post-recommendation group had a PSA more than 10 ng/ml at diagnosis in comparison to 25.2% in the pre-recommendation group ($p < .0001$). With respect to the clinical and pathological criteria, patients in the post-recommendation group were more likely to have higher clinical stage, where 171 (17.5%) patients had T2c-3a compared to 40 (9%) patients with the same stage in the pre-recommendation group, as well as higher Gleason score at diagnostic biopsies, where 305 (31.2%) patients in the post-recommendation group had Gleason grades 8–10 in comparison to 81 (18.1%) patients in the pre-recommendation group ($p < .0001$). Post recommendation patients were more likely to be classified into the D'Amico high risk PCa category (35.5% versus 22.1%, $p < .0001$).

Applying the Canadian Task force recommendation date and dividing the cohort similarly into two groups, before and after the recommendation date yielded similar results as shown on Table 4.

Results from the multivariate logistic analyses for the variables predicting worse pathological outcomes in the prostate needle biopsies, showed that the US task force recommendation release date was an independent variable associated with higher Gleason score (G8–10) in biopsies, with patients who had their biopsies performed after the recommendation release date having double the odds of being diagnosed with Gleason score 8–10 (OR: 2.006, 95%CI: 1.477–2.725) as illustrated in Table 5.

Discussion

Over the past few decades, the introduction of the serum PSA test has been associated with a greater than 50% significant reduction in PCa mortality rates in many areas around the world [5]. It is believed that this downward mortality path is attributed mainly to the PSA-based screening programs and improved treatment strategies. However, despite this decline in PCa specific mortality

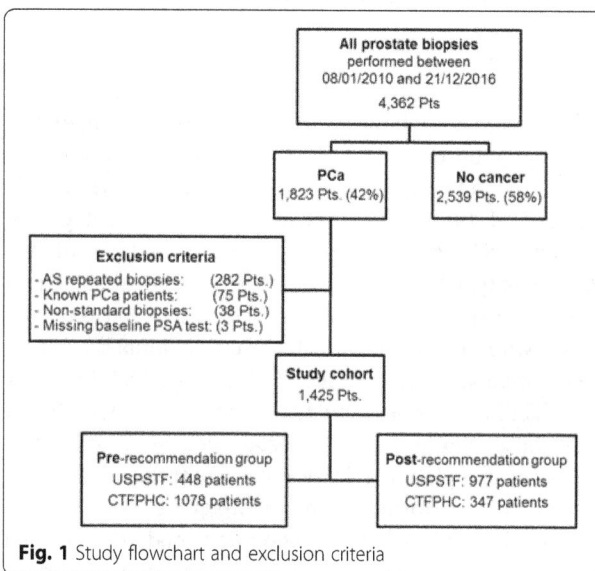

Fig. 1 Study flowchart and exclusion criteria

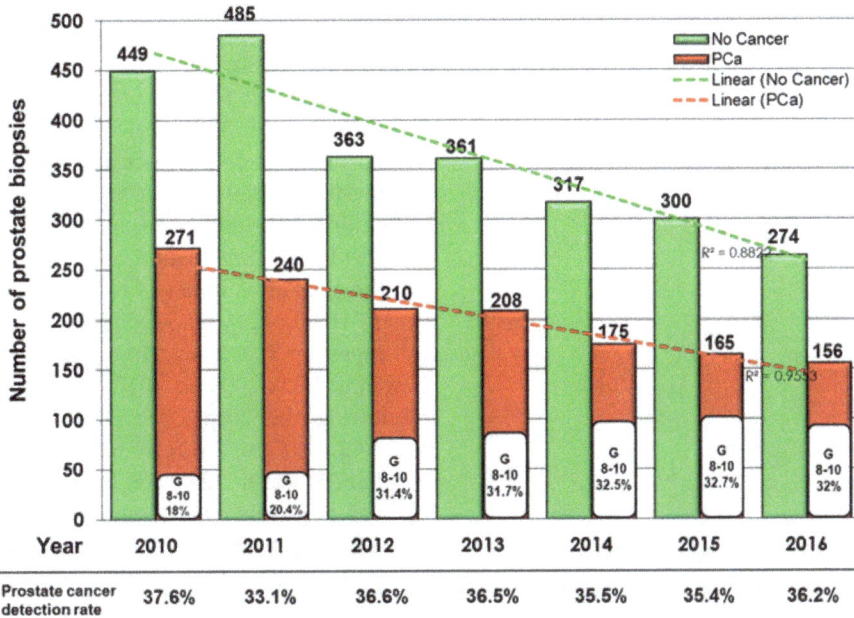

Fig. 2 Rate of prostate needle biopsies performed over study period (2010–2016), with absolute numbers of cases negative for PCa (represented by green columns) and absolute numbers of cases positive for PCa (represented by red columns), percentage of cases diagnosed with Gleason grades G8–10 were calculated to the year positive cases (represented by white columns)

rates since the early 1990s, controversy about the harms and benefits of PSA based screening still exist [16].

The harms of PSA screening are well known including overdiagnosis and overtreatment. The USPSTF and CTFPHC recommendations against PSA screening were based mainly on three significant randomized controlled trials, namely, the Prostate, Lung, Colon and Ovarian (PLCO) screening trial, the European Randomized Study of Screening for Prostate Cancer (ERSPC) and the Goteborg trial [6, 7, 17].

The task forces have a significant effect on the practice patterns of primary and specialty healthcare professionals, as seen with primary care providers with whom the decision to offer screening usually lies [18].

Following the draft guidelines in October 2011 and the official recommendations against PSA screening in May 2012 in US and October 2014 in Canada, multiple studies demonstrated a significant decrease in PSA screening. Shoag et al. [11] used the US National Ambulatory Medical Care Survey (NAMCS) data and recently reported a relative 64% decrease in DRE and a 39% decrease in PSA testing after the recommendations. The decrease was significant among men 55 to 69 years old, where the number of visits in which DRE and PSA testing were performed decreased 65% and 39%, respectively ($p < 0.001$).

Drazer et al. [12] reported a significant decline in PSA-based screening after the recommendations, using the US National Health Interview Survey (NHIS) data, with the largest decline among men aged 50–59 years, where relative screening rates decreased by 25% from 2010 to 2013. Similarly, Jemal et al. [13] showed a decrease in the PSA screening rates by 18% between 2010 and 2013 and as in the previous reports, the highest decline was seen among men aged 50–74 years.

On the other hand, Hutchinson et al. [19] did not identify a significant change in the use of PSA-based screening as measured by the total annual number of resultant PSA examinations in their single-center analysis. However, they reported that patients were referred at progressively higher average PSA levels. Also, Rahbar et al. [20] in their recent update of their already published data (14) extended the previous data analysis with additional years to determine if the downward trend continued past the immediate response to the recommendation, and they showed that from 2013 to 2015 there was a non-significant decrease in PSA screening (only 0.4%). According to them, the absence of a change between these years might highlight the contrasting recommendations by different guideline panels regarding the use of this test.

In our study we present the finding of a significant decline in prostate biopsy volume following the USPSTF and CTFPHC recommendations, where we found an average annual decrease of 10.6%. Our results matched a recent report from a community-based urology practice, where Gaylis et al. [21] examined a total of 3915 prostate biopsies performed during 4 years, with 1581 (40.4%) of these prostate biopsies performed in men referred for newly elevated PSA. They found a 22.8% reduction in biopsies performed in newly referred men. Also in Canada, Bhindi et al. [22] conducted a time series analysis during

Table 1 Baseline clinical, biochemical and pathological features of the cohort

Parameters	Value
Clinical:	
Cohort total number of patients:	1425
Age at diagnosis, years, mean (SD):	68.6 (8.72)
Age categories, n (%)	
- < 50 years	8 (0.6%)
- 50–74 years	861 (60.4%)
- ≥75 years	556 (39%)
Baseline prostate volume (ml³), median [IQR]:	36.4 [27–49.8]
Clinical stage: n (%)	
- T1-2a	859 (60.3%)
- T2b	355 (24.9%)
- T2c-3a	211 (14.8%)
Biochemical:	
Baseline PSA (ng/ml), median [IQR]	7.55 [5.4–12]
PSA categories, ng/ml, n (%)	
- ≤ 4:	113 (7.9%)
- 4.1–10:	835 (58.6%)
- 10.1–20:	293 (20.6%)
- > 20	184 (12.9%)
PSA density (ng/ml/ml³), median [IQR]	0.21 [0.13–0.36]
Pathological:	
Gleason score, n (%)	
- Gleason ≤6:	566 (39.7%)
- Gleason 7:	473 (33.2%)
- Gleason 8:	194 (13.6%)
- Gleason 9:	168 (11.8%)
- Gleason 10:	24 (1.7%)
D'Amico risk classification, n (%)	
- Low:	477 (33.4%)
- Intermediate:	503 (35.3%)
- High	445 (31.2%)

SD Standard Deviation, *IQR* Inter Quartile Range, *n (%)*: Number of patients (Percentage)

Table 2 Absolute numbers of Gleason grades diagnosed during the study time period

Grade	Year						
	2010	2011	2012	2013	2014	2015	2016
G8–10	49	49	66	66	57	54	50
G7	77	71	55	75	68	75	59
G6	145	120	89	67	50	36	47
Total	271	240	210	208	175	165	156

2008 to 2013 of prostate biopsies performed at University Health Network in Toronto, and reported a decline in the median number of biopsies performed per month from 58.0 (IQR 54.5–63.0) before the USPSTF recommendations to 35.5 (IQR 27.0–41.0) afterward ($p = 0.003$). Likewise, Banerji et al. [23] assessed the number of needle biopsies done at an academic institution in the US during the 30-month period before and after the USPSTF recommendation and reported a 31% decrease in the absolute number of biopsies. Furthermore, Gershman et al. [24], showed that prostate biopsy rates dropped by 33% from 64.1 to 42.8 per 100,000 person/months from 2005 to 2014, with the greatest decrease following the 2012 USPSTF recommendation (– 13.8; 95% CI, – 21.0 to – 6.7; $p < 0.001$).

Halpern et al. [25] conducted a US national study across academic and community practice settings and health plans to evaluate variations in prostate biopsy volumes from 2009 through 2015, they demonstrated geographic variation in prostate biopsy volumes and an overall decrease in prostate biopsies after USPSTF recommendation, the median biopsy volume per urologist significantly decreased from 29 to 21 (IQR 12–34; $p < 0.001$), and the total number of annual biopsies decreased by 12.7%. After adjustment for practice and physician characteristics, they reported an overall decrease of 28.7% in biopsy volume following 2012. The greatest decrease in biopsy volume was observed in men with abnormal PSA, whereas biopsy volume in men under surveillance for confirmed PCa significantly increased by 28.8%.

Conversely, Misra-Hebert et al. [26] in their study conducted over 160,211 men aged ≥40 years with at least one visit to a primary care clinic during the years 2007–2014, reported higher rates of first prostate biopsy in men who were screened with a PSA test, especially for men with an increased risk of PCa (African Americans and men with positive family history). However, when they used all men aged ≥40 years with a primary care clinic visit each year as the denominator, overall yearly rates of prostate biopsy were similar between 2007 and 2014 and for men ≥70 years, biopsy rates decreased in 2014 in comparison to 2007.

In our study, PSA assessments over time revealed that for men presenting for prostate biopsy, the median PSA values showed a rising trend after recommendations. This trend was significant for both USPSTF and CTFPHC recommendations ($p = 0.0007$ and 0.037, respectively). In addition the percentage of men presenting with PSA value > 10 ng/ml was significantly higher in the post recommendation era ($p < .0001$ and 0.011, respectively). These findings are consistent with previous two studies [21, 23], where one reported that post-USPSTF patients had a higher median PSA ($p < 0.001$), and was significantly more

Table 3 Comparison between groups (according to USPSTF recommendation)

Characteristics	Pre-recommendation 448 Pts. (31.5%)	Post-recommendation 977 Pts. (68.5%)	P-value
Age, median [IQR]	74 [68–80]	71 [65–77]	
Age at diagnosis, mean [range]	68.2 [41–96]	68.8 [40–93]	0.258
Age categories, n (%)			<.0001
- < 50 years	1 (0.2%)	7 (0.7%)	
- 50–74 years	234 (52.2%)	627 (64.2%)	
- ≥75 years	213 (47.6%)	343 (35.1%)	
PSA (ng/ml), median [IQR]	6.4 [4.9–10.1]	8 [5.7–12.9]	0.0007
PSA categories, n (%)			<.0001
- ≤4	48 (10.7%)	65 (6.6%)	
- 4.01–10	287 (64.1%)	548 (56.1%)	
- 10.01–20	76 (16.9%)	217 (22.2%)	
- > 20	37 (8.3%)	147 (15.1%)	
Prostate volume (ml3), median [IQR]	34.9 [26–46.2]	37.2 [27.1–51]	0.126
PSA density (ng/ml/ml3), median [IQR]	0.19 [0.13–0.33]	0.22 [0.14–0.39]	0.132
Gleason score			<.0001
- Gleason 6	240 (53.5%)	326 (33.4%)	
- Gleason 7	127 (28.4%)	346 (35.4%)	
- Gleason 8–10	81 (18.1%)	305 (31.2%)	
Clinical stage			<. 0001
- T1-2a	301 (67.1%)	558 (57.1%)	
- T2b	107 (23.9%)	248 (25.4%)	
- T2c-3a	40 (9%)	171 (17.5%)	
D'Amico risk classification			<. 0001
Low	202 (45.1%)	275 (28.1%)	
Intermediate	147 (32.8%)	356 (36.4%)	
High	99 (22.1%)	346 (35.5%)	

likely to have a PSA between 6.1 and 10 ng/ml ($P = 0.019$) or 10.1 and 20 ng/ml ($p = 0.002$) than the pre-USPSTF patients. The second study reported that the proportion of men presenting with PSA > 10 ng/ml increased from 28.1 to 36.8% ($p = 0.009$).

Among our cohort, we found no significant changes in the relative PCa detection rate (33.1% to 37.6%) over the study period. However, we noted worse pathological outcomes in terms of slight higher absolute numbers and rates of Gleason grades [8–10] and higher risk classification PCa cases diagnosed in the years after the recommendations. Similarly, Hu et al. [27] Using the most recent Surveillance, Epidemiology, and End Results (SEER) release, identified 1,107,111 men 40 years or older diagnosed with PCa from 2004 to 2013 and reported increase in the percentage presenting with intermediate and high-grade PCa, from 46.3 to 56.4% ($p < .01$), in men younger than 75 years, and increase in the proportion of men presenting with distant metastases from 2.7 to 4.0% ($p < .01$). Bhindi

et al. [22] in their study also reported no significant differences in relative cancer detection rates in the year after versus the year before USPSTF recommendations, but In contrast with our results, they found significant decrease ($p < 0.001$) in the absolute rates of cancer detection after the USPSTF recommendation statement, where the median number of Gleason 7–10 PCa detected per month decreased from 17.5 (IQR 14.5–21.5) to 10.0 (IQR 9.0–12.0), however, their report was limited to only one year after the recommendation.

Although our results showed higher rates of high-risk PCa after the recommendation, the actual absolute number was a little higher, which may be explained by the pattern of less aggressive screening during the years after the recommendations, which led to decreased absolute numbers and rates of low grade PCa detected during screening.

Barocas et al. [28] investigated the incident diagnoses of PCa after the USPSTF draft recommendation, based on US national cancer database, they reported 28% decrease

Table 4 Comparison between groups (according to CTFPHC recommendation)

Characteristics	Pre-recommendation 1078 Pts. (75.6%)	Post-recommendation 347 Pts. (24.3%)	P-value
Age, median [IQR]	73 [67–79]	69 [64–76]	
Age at diagnosis, mean [range]	68.4 [40–96]	69.1 [47–91]	0.274
Age categories, n (%)			<.0001
- < 50 years	4 (0.4%)	4 (1.1%)	
- 50–74 years	615 (57%)	246 (70.8%)	
- ≥75 years	459 (42.6%)	97 (27.9%)	
PSA (ng/ml), median [IQR]	7.1 [5.2–11.5]	8.8 [6.4–13.4]	0.037
PSA categories, n (%)			0.011
- ≤4	90 (8.4%)	23 (6.6%)	
- 4.01–10	652 (60.4%)	183 (52.7%)	
- 10.01–20	204 (18.9%)	89 (25.7%)	
- > 20	132 (12.2%)	52 (15%)	
Prostate volume (ml3), median [IQR]	34.8 [26.4–47.1]	40.3 [29.6–56.9]	<.0001
PSA density (ng/ml/ml3), median [IQR]	0.21 [0.14–0.336	0.22 [0.12–0.38]	0.756
Gleason score			<.0001
- Gleason 6	473 (43.9%)	93 (26.8%)	
- Gleason 7	327 (30.3%)	146 (42.1%)	
- Gleason 8–10	278 (25.8%)	108 (31.1%)	
Clinical stage			0.035
- T1-2a	669 (62.1%)	190 (54.7%)	
- 2b	252 (23.4%)	103 (29.7%)	
- 2c-3a	157 (14.5%)	54 (15.6%)	
D'Amico risk classification			<.0001
- Low	399 (37%)	78 (22.4%)	
- Intermediate	356 (33%)	147 (42.4%)	
- High	323 (30%)	122 (34.8%)	

Table 5 multivariate analyses of factors predicting higher Gleason score on biopsies

Variable	Odds ratio estimates		
	Point estimate	95% Confidence interval	P-Value
Post USPSTF recommendation	2.006	1.477–2.725	<.0001
Post CTFPHC recommendation	1.359	0.980–1.868	0.058
Age at diagnosis	1.047	1.032–1.063	<.0001
Baseline PSA	1.074	1.032–1.063	<.0001
Baseline prostate volume	0.990	0.983–0.997	0.006
Baseline PSA density	1.181	0.596–2.343	0.633
Number of cores per biopsy	1.035	0.953–1.124	0.409
TRUS operator (Urologist versus Radiologist)	1.326	0.989–1.778	0.060
Pathology reviewer (F.B. versus others)	1.013	0.793–1.294	0.916

in the incidence, they noted that the monthly PCa diagnoses decreased by 1363 cases (12.2%, $p < 0.01$) in the month after the USPSTF draft and continued to decrease by 164 cases per month relative to baseline (-1.8%, $p < 0.01$). Jemal et al. [13] reported more specific decreases in the early-stage PCa incidence following the 2012 USPSTF recommendations. The largest decrease occurred between 2011 and 2012, from 498.3 to 416.2 per 100,000 men aged 50 years and older. In addition they recently updated their results [29] and reported a continuing decline in incidence rates for early-stage PCa in men aged over 50 years, the decrease rate was lower in 2012–2013 than that from 2011 to 2012 (6% versus 19%).

Of note, recently the US task force initiated a new update process of the 2012 recommendation on PCa screening and in April 2017 they issued a new draft recommendation, that was published as final recommendation as of May 2018 [30], proposing the following modification based on additional evidence published since the 2012 recommendation: - For men aged 55–69: The decision about whether to be screened for PCa should be an individual one. The USPSTF recommends that clinicians inform men ages 55 to 69 years about the potential benefits and harms of PSA–based screening for PCa. (Grade C).

Our study has some limitations including its retrospective nature, single center experience (related to local network of primary care physician), and being an observational study that cannot confirm causality. Despite these limitations, the strengths of our study include being the first study to assess and report on prostate biopsy outcomes after both (the US and Canadian) recommendations, the fair number of patients included and the longer follow up time after the recommendations. We believe that our study results with the results of others could be informative to the health policy makers.

Conclusions

In conclusion, our results revealed a reduction in the total number of prostate needle biopsies performed over time after the recommendations of the American and Canadian preventive task forces against PSA-based screening for prostate cancer. Furthermore, it showed a slight increase in absolute high-risk PCa diagnoses and a significant relative increase in higher risk PCa diagnosis. The oncological outcomes associated with this trend need to be examined in further studies.

Abbreviations

CTFPHC: Canadian Task Force on Preventive Health Care; DRE: Digital rectal exam; IQR: Inter Quartile Range; PCa: Prostate Cancer; PSA: Prostate Specific Antigen; PSAD: Prostate Specific Antigen Density; SD: Standard Deviation; TRUS: Trans-Rectal Ultrasound; USPSTF: US Preventive Services Task Force

Funding

This study was supported by Urology division of McGill University and no external funds were obtained to support this study.

Authors' contributions

AsZ: Project development, Data collection, Data analysis, Manuscript writing. AD: Project development, Data analysis, Manuscript writing. FB: Project development, Data collection, Manuscript writing. WK: Project development, Manuscript writing. ST: Project development, Manuscript writing. AA: Project development, Data analysis, Manuscript writing. All authors read and approved the final manuscript.

Competing interests

The authors declare that they have no competing interests.

Author details

¹Department of Surgery, Division of Urology, McGill University, McGill University Health Centre, 1001 Boulevard Decarie, Montreal, Quebec H4A 3J1, Canada. ²Department of Pathology, McGill University, Montreal, Quebec, Canada.

References

1. Siegel RL, Miller KD, Jemal A. Cancer statistics, 2016. CA Cancer J Clin. 2016; 66(1):7–30.
2. Canadian Cancer Society's Advisory. Committee on Cancer Statistics. Canadian Cancer Statistics 2016. Toronto, : Canadian Cancer society 2016. October 2016.
3. Stamey TA, Yang N, Hay AR, McNeal JE, Freiha FS, Redwine E. Prostate-specific antigen as a serum marker for adenocarcinoma of the prostate. N Engl J Med. 1987;317(15):909–16.
4. Stanford JL, Stephenson RA, Coyle LM, Cerhan J, Correa R, Eley J, et al. SEER program, National Cancer Institute. NIH pub. 1973–1995;1999(99–4543)
5. Etzioni R, Gulati R, Tsodikov A, Wever EM, Penson DF, Heijnsdijk EA, et al. The prostate cancer conundrum revisited. Cancer. 2012;118(23):5955–63.
6. Andriole GL, Crawford ED, Grubb RL III, Buys SS, Chia D, Church TR, et al. Mortality results from a randomized prostate-cancer screening trial. N Engl J Med. 2009;360(13):1310–9.
7. Schröder FH, Hugosson J, Roobol MJ, Tammela TL, Ciatto S, Nelen V, et al. Screening and prostate-cancer mortality in a randomized European study. N Engl J Med. 2009;360(13):1320–8.
8. Andriole GL, Crawford ED, Grubb RL III, Buys SS, Chia D, Church TR, et al. Prostate cancer screening in the randomized prostate, lung, colorectal, and ovarian Cancer screening trial: mortality results after 13 years of follow-up. J Natl Cancer Inst. 2012;104(2):125–32.
9. Force UPST. Screening for prostate cancer: US preventive services task force recommendation statement. Ann Intern Med. 2008;149(3):185.
10. Moyer VA. Screening for prostate cancer: US preventive services task force recommendation statement. Ann Intern Med. 2012;157(2):120–34.
11. Shoag J, Halpern JA, Lee DJ, Mittal S, Ballman KV, Barbieri CE, et al. Decline in prostate Cancer screening by primary care physicians: an analysis of trends in the use of digital rectal examination and prostate specific antigen testing. J Urol. 2016;196(4):1047–52.
12. Drazer MW, Huo D, Eggener SE. National Prostate Cancer Screening Rates after the 2012 US preventive services task force recommendation discouraging prostate-specific antigen-based screening. J Clin Oncol Off J Am Soc Clin Oncol. 2015;33(22):2416–23.
13. Jemal A, Fedewa SA, Ma J, Siegel R, Lin CC, Brawley O, et al. Prostate Cancer incidence and PSA testing patterns in relation to USPSTF screening recommendations. JAMA. 2015;314(19):2054–61.
14. Sammon JD, Abdollah F, Choueiri TK, Kantoff PW, Nguyen PL, Menon M, et al. Prostate-specific antigen screening after 2012 US preventive services task force recommendations. JAMA. 2015;314(19):2077–9.
15. D'amico AV, Whittington R, Malkowicz SB, Schultz D, Blank K, Broderick GA, et al. Biochemical outcome after radical prostatectomy, external beam radiation therapy, or interstitial radiation therapy for clinically localized prostate cancer. JAMA. 1998;280(11):969–74.
16. Brawley OW. Trends in prostate cancer in the United States. J Natl Cancer Inst Monogr. 2012;2012(45):152–6.
17. Hugosson J, Carlsson S, Aus G, Bergdahl S, Khatami A, Lodding P, et al. Mortality results from the Göteborg randomised population-based prostate-cancer screening trial. The lancet oncology. 2010;11(8):725–32.

18. Tasian GE, Cooperberg MR, Cowan JE, Keyashian K, Greene KL, Daniels NA, et al., editors. Prostate specific antigen screening for prostate cancer: knowledge of, attitudes towards, and utilization among primary care physicians. Urologic Oncology: Seminars and Original Investigations; 2012: Elsevier.

19. Hutchinson R, Akhtar A, Haridas J, Bhat D, Roehrborn C, Lotan Y. Testing and referral patterns in the years surrounding the US preventive services task force recommendation against prostate-specific antigen screening. Cancer. 2016;122(24):3785–93.

20. Rahbar H, Karabon P, Menon M, Trinh Q-D, Abdollah F. Trends in Prostate-Specific Antigen Screening Since the Implementation of the 2012 US preventive services task force recommendations. European Urology Focus 2017.

21. Gaylis FD, Choi JE, Hamilton Z, Dato P, Cohen E, Calabrese R, et al., editors. Change in prostate cancer presentation coinciding with USPSTF screening recommendations at a community-based urology practice. Urologic Oncology: Seminars and Original Investigations; 2017: Elsevier.

22. Bhindi B, Mamdani M, Kulkarni GS, Finelli A, Hamilton RJ, Trachtenberg J, et al. Impact of the U.S. preventive services task force recommendations against prostate specific antigen screening on prostate biopsy and cancer detection rates. J Urol. 2015;193(5):1519–24.

23. Banerji JS, Wolff EM, Massman JD, Odem-Davis K, Porter CR, Corman JM. Prostate needle biopsy outcomes in the era of the US preventive services task force recommendation against prostate specific antigen based screening. J Urol. 2016;195(1):66–73.

24. Gershman B, Van Houten HK, Herrin J, Moreira DM, Kim SP, Shah ND, et al. Impact of prostate-specific antigen (PSA) screening trials and revised PSA screening guidelines on rates of prostate biopsy and postbiopsy complications. Eur Urol. 2017;71(1):55–65.

25. Halpern JA, Shoag JE, Artis AS, Ballman KV, Sedrakyan A, Hershman DL, et al. National Trends in prostate biopsy and radical prostatectomy volumes following the US preventive services task force guidelines against prostate-specific antigen screening. JAMA surgery. 2017;152(2):192–8.

26. Misra-Hebert AD, Hu B, Klein EA, Stephenson A, Taksler GB, Kattan MW, et al. Prostate cancer screening practices in a large, integrated health system: 2007–2014. BJU Int. 2017;

27. Hu JC, Nguyen P, Mao J, Halpern J, Shoag J, Wright JD, et al. Increase in prostate cancer distant metastases at diagnosis in the United States. JAMA oncology. 2017;3(5):705–7.

28. Barocas DA, Mallin K, Graves AJ, Penson DF, Palis B, Winchester DP, et al. Effect of the USPSTF grade D recommendation against screening for prostate cancer on incident prostate cancer diagnoses in the United States. J Urol. 2015;194(6):1587–93.

29. Jemal A, Ma J, Siegel R, Fedewa S, Brawley O, Ward EM. Prostate cancer incidence rates 2 years after the US preventive services task force recommendations against screening. JAMA oncology. 2016;2(12):1657–60.

30. Force USPST. Screening for prostate cancer: us preventive services task force recommendation statement. JAMA. 2018;319(18):1901–13.

30

Observation versus treatment among men with favorable risk prostate cancer in a community-based integrated health care system: a retrospective cohort study

Furaha Kariburyo[1]*, Yuexi Wang[1], I-Ning (Elaine) Cheng[2], Lisa Wang[3], David Morgenstern[4], Lin Xie[1], Eric Meadows[5,6], John Danella[6] and Michael L. Cher[7]

Abstract

Background: The objective of this study was to describe overall survival and the management of men with favorable risk prostate cancer (PCa) within a large community-based health care system in the United States.

Methods: A retrospective cohort study was conducted using linked electronic health records from men aged ≥40 years with favorable risk PCa (T1 or 2, PSA ≤15, Gleason ≤7 [3 + 4]) diagnosed between January 2005 and October 2013. Cohorts were defined as receiving any treatment (IMT) or no treatment (OBS) within 6 months after index PCa diagnosis. Cohorts' characteristics were compared between OBS and IMT; monitoring patterns were reported for OBS within the first 18 and 24 months. Cox Proportional Hazards models were used for multivariate analysis of overall survival.

Results: A total of 1425 men met the inclusion criteria (OBS 362; IMT 1063). The proportion of men managed with OBS increased from 20% (2005) to 35% (2013). The OBS group was older (65.6 vs 62.8 years, $p < 0.01$), had higher Charlson comorbidity index scores (CCI ≥2, 21.5% vs 12.2%, $p < 0.01$), and had a higher proportion of low-risk PCa (65.2% vs 55.0%, $p < 0.01$). For the OBS cohort, 181 of the men (50%) eventually received treatment. Among those remaining on OBS for ≥24 months ($N = 166$), 88.6% had ≥1 follow-up PSA test and 26.5% received ≥1 follow-up biopsy within the 24 months. The unadjusted mortality rate was higher for OBS compared with IMT (2.7 vs 1.3/100 person-years [py]; $p < 0.001$). After multivariate adjustment, there was no significant difference in all-cause mortality between OBS and IMT groups (HR 0.73, $p = 0.138$).

Conclusions: Use of OBS management increased over the 10-year study period. Men in the OBS cohort had a higher proportion of low-risk PCa. No differences were observed in overall survival between the two groups after adjustment of covariates. These data provide insights into how favorable risk PCa was managed in a community setting.

Keywords: Prostate cancer, Active surveillance, Overall survival, Monitoring patterns

* Correspondence: fkariburyo@statinmed.com
[1]STATinMED Research, 211 N. Fourth Avenue, Suite 2B, Ann Arbor, MI 48104, USA
Full list of author information is available at the end of the article

Background

The widespread adoption of prostate-specific antigen (PSA)-based screening has led to a substantial increase in the detection of favorable risk prostate cancer (PCa) [1]. PSA-based screening has been shown to reduce prostate-specific mortality by 21–30% [2, 3]. However, the use of PSA screening has resulted in considerable over-diagnosis and over-treatment, with 15–20% of men receiving a PCa diagnosis during their lifetime but only 3% dying from the disease [4].

Observation strategies (OBS) such as active surveillance (AS) and watchful waiting (WW) are alternatives to immediate treatment (IMT) for men diagnosed with favorable risk PCa. The primary motivation for these strategies is to avoid or delay treatment-related adverse events [5].

AS strategies also reduce immediate health care expenditures by avoiding aggressive treatment costs, including treatment complications, but they imply recurrent costs for biopsies and other tests that accumulate over the patient's lifetime [5]. The risk vs benefit consideration of AS also includes the possibility of disease progression to the point that a cure is less likely or not possible.

Recent studies indicate increased adoption of AS. However, most published reports are from academic centers [6] or prospective trials with defined AS protocols. Some studies have examined updated observational strategies, finding that those who chose to undergo OBS tended to be older with lower risk disease. The number of men diagnosed with low-risk PCa who chose AS in these studies was low, suggesting that AS may have been underused in the management of very low-risk PCa [7, 8]. The objectives of this study were to compare overall survival and the clinical characteristics and management trends (OBS vs IMT) among men with favorable risk PCa from a large community practice, as well as to identify factors associated with choosing OBS and to describe monitoring patterns used for OBS.

Methods

Data source

A retrospective study was conducted from January 2004 to April 2015 using linked electronic medical records (EMRs), oncology registry data, and enrollment information from the Geisinger Health System (GHS) – a community-based integrated health care organization serving residents in central, south, and northeast Pennsylvania. The EMR infrastructure contains longitudinal clinical patient data including patient demographics and encounter details from inpatient, outpatient, and office-based settings such as diagnoses, medications orders, procedures, and laboratory results.

Patient identification

Men aged ≥40 years and diagnosed with favorable risk PCa (International Classification of Diseases [ICD]-O3 site code C61.9 and morphology 81,403, T1 or 2, PSA ≤15 ng/mL, Gleason score ≤ 7 [3 + 4]) identified from January 2005–October 2013 and active in the GHS ≥12 months prior to and ≥ 18 months post-index date were selected. The first PCa diagnosis date was defined as the index date. Patient data were assessed until the earlier of death or April 2015.

Patients with evidence of a previous cancer diagnosis ≤5 years prior to the initial PCa diagnosis (except for non-melanoma skin cancer), any PCa treatment before the index PCa diagnosis, or other cancer diagnosis within 6 months after the initial PCa diagnosis (identified using ICD-O3-codes) were excluded.

PCa and other cancer diagnoses, Gleason score, and tumor stage were extracted from the oncology registry. Demographic, encounter, and PSA testing information were retrieved from EMR data. Cohorts were defined as receiving any PCa treatment (IMT) or no treatment within 6 months (OBS) after index PCa diagnosis date.

Prostate cancer risk categories were defined by D'Amico classification [9]: low (T1-T2A, PSA level ≤ 10 ng/mL, and Gleason score ≤ 6) [10] or intermediate (T1 or T2, PSA level > 10 and ≤ 20 ng/mL, and Gleason score = 7).

IRB approval

All patient information was de-identified at the source in accordance with 45 CFR 164.514(a) and (b) (Code of Federal Regulations Title 45, Public Welfare) and therefore independent review board approval was not required.

Study variables

Clinical characteristics Charlson Comorbidity Index (CCI) scores during the 12 months prior to index PCa diagnosis were measured. PCa-related characteristics were captured at the time of PCa diagnosis including tumor grade, Gleason score, and risk category based on the D'Amico risk classification. The index PSA was defined as the last PSA value before or on the index biopsy date.

Monitoring patterns Monitoring patterns included PSA test, biopsy, and urology visits.

Overall survival Overall survival was estimated per 100 person-years (PY).

Statistical methods

Clinical characteristics were examined descriptively and compared between the OBS and IMT cohorts. Chi-square and t-tests were used to calculate *p*-values, respectively, for categorical and continuous variables. Logistic regression was used to determine odds ratios and 95% confidence intervals (CIs) of factors associated with the selection of OBS versus IMT. Based on model fitting and clinical rationale, covariates adjusted in the model included age, race, marital status, insurance status, family history of PCa, prior diagnosis of chronic obstructive pulmonary disease, CCI score, and D'Amico risk categories. The use and frequency of monitoring patterns were assessed for patients utilizing OBS before switching to active treatment during the first, second, and third years following their index PCa diagnosis.

Unadjusted Kaplan-Meier (KM) and log rank tests were used to compare survival rates in OBS and IMT cohorts. Multivariate Cox proportional hazards models were used to examine Hazard Ratio (HR), and 95% CI of overall survival.

Statistical analyses were performed using SAS Version 9.3 (Cary, NC) with p-value < 0.05 considered significant. Standardized differences and clinical relevance were also considered.

Subgroup analyses
A subgroup analysis was conducted by reporting monitoring patterns among men whose treatment was managed with OBS: 1) for those who remained on OBS for at least 18 months and had ≥1 urologist visit (a proxy for active patient management), and 2) for those who remained on OBS for ≥24 months.

Chart review
Manual examination of de-identified EMR chart data was undertaken to explore why some OBS patients did not have follow-up visits. Charts were reviewed for all OBS patients without a follow-up visit in the urology department within the first year after PCa diagnosis ($N = 57$). The reasons were categorized as follow-up by another clinical department (eg, oncology), delayed treatment based on patients' preference, complicating comorbidities, and limited follow-up data.

Results
Patient characteristics
A total of 3342 men diagnosed with PCa and aged ≥40 years were identified from the oncology registry. After applying the exclusion criteria, the remaining 1425 men in this analysis included 362 patients (25.5%) in the OBS cohort vs 1063 patients (74.5%) in the IMT cohort (Fig. 1) with a median follow-up of 5 years.

There were no significant differences between the OBS and IMT groups in index PSA result, tumor stage, or body mass index (Tables 1 and 2). The OBS group was older (65.6 vs 62.8 years; $p < 0.01$), had higher CCI scores (CCI score ≥ 2: 21.5% vs 12.2%, $p < 0.01$), more patients whose marital status was "divorced" (9.1% vs 5.7%; $p = 0.03$), fewer patients whose marital status was "married" (72.9%

vs 80.9%; $p < 0.01$) and more Medicare beneficiaries (32.3% vs 24.2%; $p < 0.01$) (Table 1). The OBS cohort also had a lower proportion with Gleason score = 3 + 4 at diagnosis (22.9% vs 35.5%, $p < 0.01$), and a higher proportion of low-risk PCa (65.2% vs 55.0%, $p < 0.01$) (Table 2).

Factors associated with the selection of OBS vs IMT
Figure 2 shows the factors associated with OBS vs IMT using a logistic regression model. Older age (65–74 years; OR = 1.6 or 75+ years; OR = 4.3), marital status (single; OR = 1.6 or divorce/separated; OR = 1.9), high CCI score (≥2; OR = 1.6), and low-risk PCa (intermediate-risk vs low-risk, OR = 0.5) were significant predictors of choosing OBS over IMT, after adjusting for other covariates.

Prostate Cancer management trends
The proportion of men managed with OBS increased from 20% in 2005 to 35 and 52% in 2013 for patients with favorable risk PCa, or low-risk PCa, respectively (Fig. 3). A similar increase was observed in patients with intermediate-risk PCa up to 2012 (from 19% in 2005 to 30% in 2012) but the proportion decreased to 14% in 2013 (Fig. 3).

Time to active treatment
The median time to treatment of all OBS patients was ~ 4 years (Fig. 4). Of 181 OBS patients who switched to active treatment, the average time from initial PCa diagnosis to treatment was 459 days (1.3 years).

For the subgroup analysis according to D'Amico risk classification: 29% (236/821) of low-risk versus 20% (117/578) of intermediate-risk PCa patients received OBS. Among men managed by OBS, 50% of low-risk versus 53% of intermediate-risk PCa patients eventually received treatment during the follow-up period.

Monitoring patterns for men managed with OBS
Monitoring patterns were assessed among the patients remaining on OBS in year 1 ($n = 239$), year 2 ($n = 166$) and year 3 ($n = 116$) (Fig. 5). In the OBS cohort, the percentage of patients with at least one urology visit decreased during the first 3 years post-index PCa diagnosis from 86.6% in year 1 to 65.1% in year 2 and 54.3% in year 3. However, PSA testing rates remained similar in the first 3 years of diagnosis, with approximately 70% of men receiving ≥1 PSA test each year. Approximately 7.1, 18.7, and 10.3% of men in the OBS cohort received a prostate biopsy in the first, second, and third year, respectively (Fig. 5).

Among men remaining on OBS for ≥18 months and with ≥1 urology visit ($N = 212$), 85.8% received ≥1 PSA tests and 19.3% were administered one biopsy within the 18 months. Among those remaining on OBS for ≥24 months ($N = 166$), 88.6% received ≥1 PSA tests and 26.5% received one biopsy within the 24 months. A chart review of 57 patients in the

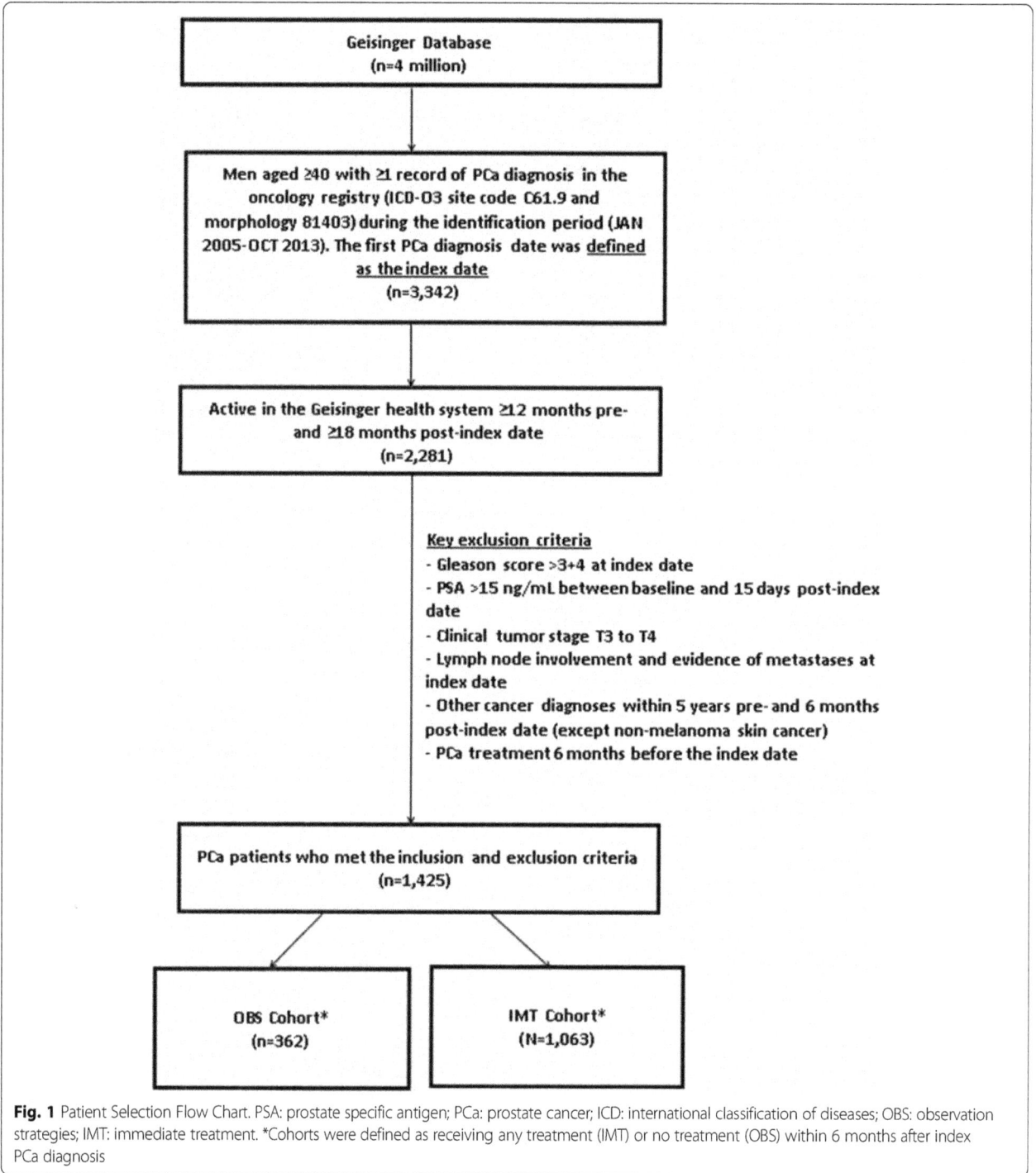

Fig. 1 Patient Selection Flow Chart. PSA: prostate specific antigen; PCa: prostate cancer; ICD: international classification of diseases; OBS: observation strategies; IMT: immediate treatment. *Cohorts were defined as receiving any treatment (IMT) or no treatment (OBS) within 6 months after index PCa diagnosis

OBS cohort without follow-up urology visits within the first 360 days post-diagnosis indicated that in 49 of 57 cases (86%) of PCa-related care by other GHS departments were identified with oncology as the most common specialty.

Overall survival

Median follow-up time from PCa diagnosis in the entire study cohort was approximately 5 years. The unadjusted all-cause mortality rate was higher for OBS compared with IMT (2.7 vs 1.3/100 PY; $p < 0.001$). The cumulative hazard plot for overall survival indicated that after the sixth year of PCa diagnosis, the risk of all-cause mortality was higher in the OBS cohort than in the IMT cohort (Fig. 6). However, after multivariate adjustment, there was no significant difference in all-cause mortality between the OBS and IMT cohorts (IMT vs OBS, HR = 0.73, $p = 0.138$;

Table 1 Socio-demographic characteristics of men with favorable risk PCa in OBS vs IMT cohorts

	OBS (n = 362)		IMT (n = 1063)			
	N/Mean	%/SD	N/Mean	%/SD	P-value	Standardized difference [a]
Age (Mean)	65.6	9	62.8	8	<.01	33.10
Age Group						
40–64	166	45.9%	601	56.5%	<.01	21.47
65–74	137	37.9%	390	36.7%	0.69	2.39
75+	59	16.3%	72	6.8%	<.01	21.47
Race						
White	347	95.9%	1044	98.2%	0.01	13.91
Black or African American	14	3.9%	11	1.0%	<.01	18.37
Native Hawaiian	1	0.3%	4	0.4%	0.78	1.75
Asian	0	0.0%	1	0.1%	0.56	4.34
Unknown	0	0.0%	3	0.3%	0.31	7.52
Marital Status						
Single	33	9.1%	68	6.4%	0.08	10.17
Married	264	72.9%	860	80.9%	<.01	18.99
Widow	30	8.3%	67	6.3%	0.20	7.63
Divorced	33	9.1%	61	5.7%	0.03	12.89
Separated	2	0.6%	7	0.7%	0.83	1.37
Insurance Status						
Medicare	117	32.3%	257	24.2%	<.01	18.15
Veterans Affairs	2	0.6%	2	0.2%	0.26	5.99
Medicaid	8	2.2%	19	1.8%	0.61	3.02
Commercial	227	62.7%	782	73.6%	<.01	23.44
Other	4	1.1%	3	0.3%	0.05	9.91
Unknown	4	1.1%	0	0.0%	<.01	14.93

OBS observation, IMT immediate treatment, SD standard deviation, CCI Charlson Comorbidity Index
[a]SD = standardized difference (SD is defined as the difference in sample means or proportions divided by standard error; reported as 100*|actual standardize difference|. Standardize differences >|10| are considered significant

Fig. 7). Multivariate analysis also indicated that older age, divorce or separated status; prior diagnosis of COPD, and congestive heart failure were risk factors for all-cause mortality.

Discussion

In this study, we described overall survival and the characteristics and management patterns in men with favorable risk PCa within a large community-based health care system in the United States. While no single source provides comprehensive data for most US patients, the major strength of this study is its large community-based setting. In addition to the real-world use of EMR, the claims oncology registry and unstructured information from charts maximized the available data for each patient, while also yielding a large sample size. Each of the data sources provided complementary information.

In the current analysis, we found that patients who were managed by OBS strategies were on average over age 65 years and had higher CCI scores when compared to patients who received definitive treatment after index PCa diagnosis. Factors associated with the selection of OBS were similar with Liu et al. [11]. Similarly, prior research has reported that OBS strategies focus on deferring PCa treatment in older, sicker patients diagnosed with a prostate tumor that is less aggressive than their underlying comorbidities [10, 12].

Because of these known demographic and clinical differences in patients who were managed by OBS compared to those who underwent IMT, the unadjusted all-cause mortality rate was higher in OBS patients compared to IMT. These findings are similar to a previously published study comparing radical prostatectomy with WW in early PCa patients [13]. After adjusting for these known differences in baseline demographic and clinical characteristics

Table 2 Clinical characteristics of men with favorable risk PCa in OBS vs IMT cohorts

	OBS (n = 362)		IMT (n = 1063)		p-value	Standardized difference [a]
	N	%	N	%		
Comorbid Indices (CCI)						
0	225	62.2%	750	70.6%	<.01	17.83
1	59	16.3%	183	17.2%	0.69	2.45
2+	78	21.6%	130	12.2%	<.01	25.04
Comorbid Conditions						
Hypertension	153	42.3%	405	38.1%	0.16	8.50
Diabetes	61	16.9%	134	12.6%	0.04	11.99
COPD	43	11.9%	82	7.7%	0.02	14.03
Congestive Heart Failure	13	3.6%	27	2.5%	0.30	6.09
Dementia	0	0.0%	3	0.3%	0.31	7.52
Benign Prostatic Hyperplasia	130	35.9%	388	36.5%	0.84	1.22
Body Mass Index						
Underweight (< 18.5)	1	0.3%	5	0.5%	0.62	3.18
Normal (18.5–24.9)	42	11.6%	102	9.6%	0.27	6.52
Overweight (25.0–29.9)	118	32.6%	342	32.2%	0.88	0.90
Obese (≥30)	112	30.9%	336	31.6%	0.81	1.44
Unknown	89	24.6%	278	26.2%	0.56	3.60
Family History of Prostate Cancer						
Yes	74	20.4%	262	24.7%	0.10	10.07
No	208	57.5%	598	56.3%	0.69	2.43
Unknown	80	22.1%	203	19.1%	0.22	7.42
Family History of Cancer	109	30.1%	339	31.9%	0.53	3.85
Prostate Cancer Characteristics						
Index PSA (Mean, SD)	5.8	2.5	5.7	2.5	0.31	6.31
< 4 ng/mL	69	19.1%	208	19.6%	0.83	1.28
4–10 ng/mL	256	70.7%	758	71.3%	0.83	1.30
> 10 ng/mL	30	8.3%	77	7.2%	0.52	3.90
Unknown	7	1.9%	20	1.9%	0.95	0.38
Index Clinical Stage [b]						
Stage 1	303	83.7%	855	80.4%	0.17	8.52
Stage 2	55	15.2%	184	17.3%	0.35	5.73
Unknown	4	1.1%	24	2.3%	0.17	8.97
Index Total Gleason Score = 3 + 4	83	22.9%	377	35.5%	<.01	27.82
Risk Category [c]						
Low-risk	236	65.2%	585	55.0%	<.01	20.84
Intermediate-risk	117	32.3%	461	43.4%	<.01	22.91
Unknown	9	2.5%	17	1.6%	0.28	6.27

OBS observation, IMT immediate treatment, SD standard deviation, COPD chronic obstructive pulmonary disease

[a]SD = standardized difference (SD is defined as the difference in sample means or proportions divided by standard error; reported as 100*|actual standardize difference|. Standardize differences >|10| are considered significant

[b]Clinical stage: anatomic Extent of the disease based on the clinical T, N and M element

[c]Risk Categories: Low risk (T1-T2A, PSA level ≤ 10 ng/mL, and Gleason score ≤ 6) and intermediate-risk (T1 or T2, PSA level > 10 and ≤ 20 ng/mL, and Gleason score = 7)

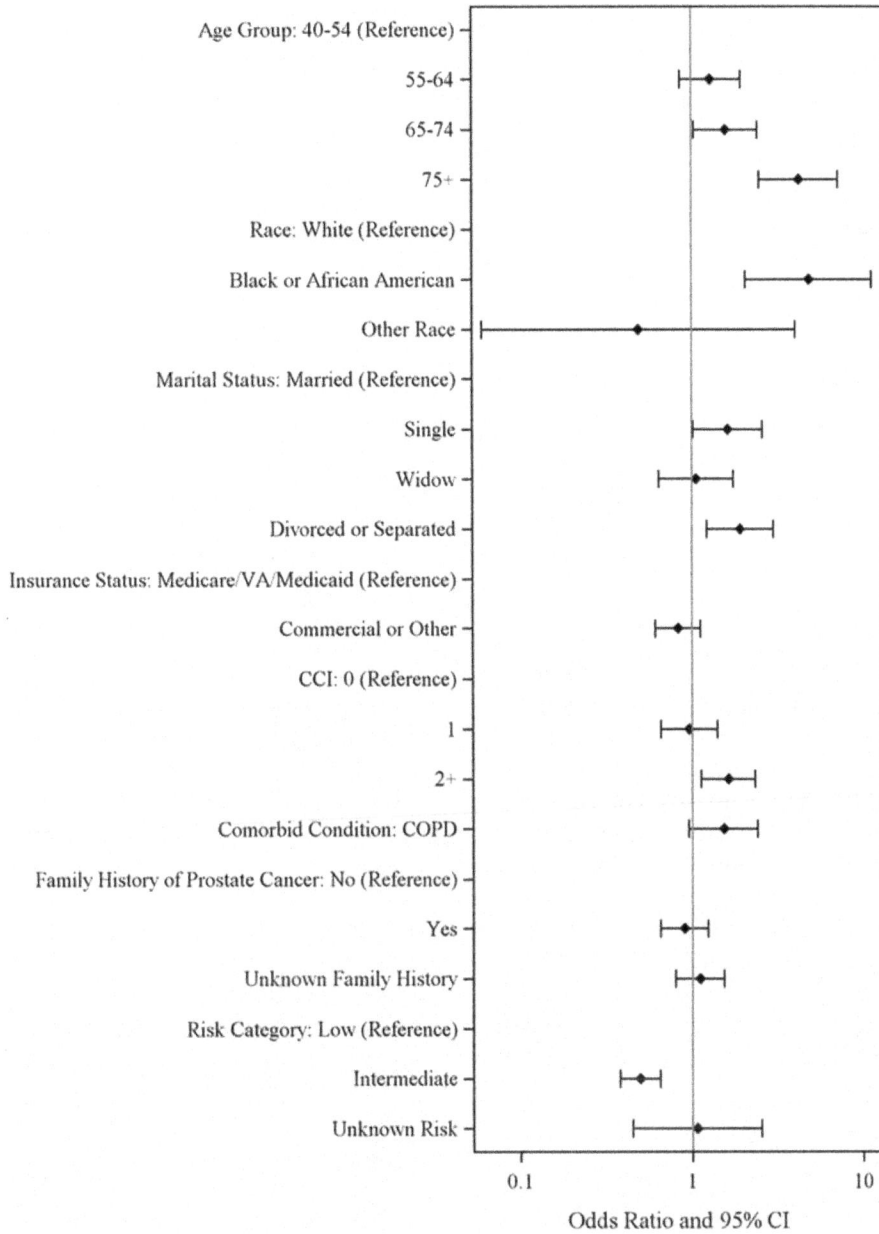

Fig. 2 Logistic Regression: Risk Factors Associated with OBS vs IMT. CCI: Charlson comorbidity index; CI: confidence interval; COPD: chronic obstructive pulmonary disease; VA: veterans affairs

between the OBS and IMT cohorts in a multivariate analysis, there was no longer a significant difference in all-cause mortality between the OBS and IMT cohorts. However, longer follow-up is needed to more convincingly assess all-cause mortality. We also evaluated deaths due to PCA or complication from PCA. However, the results were not conclusive because we could not identify the cause of death with certainty. There were a total of nine patients (2.5%) with deaths possibly or probably due to PCa in the OBS group vs 15 deaths (1.4%) possibly or probably due to PCa in the IMT group (results not shown). In addition,

PCa-specific mortality in favorable risk cancer is relatively low and we do not have sufficient numbers of patients followed for a long enough period to appreciate the differences between the OBS and IMT groups.

Other studies have shown that the presence of significant others in a patient's life often influences treatment decisions and our results suggest that even adjusting for other factors such as race and type of insurance, that men who were divorced or separated (or single) were more likely to be treated with OBS vs IMT. However, in this study, marital status was only captured as single, married,

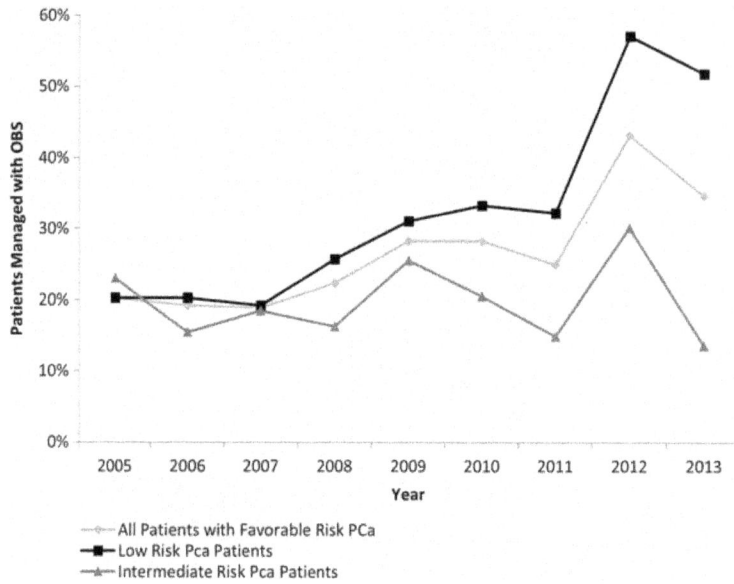

Fig. 3 Annual Prostate Cancer Management Trends for Favorable Risk and Low Risk PCa Patients. PCa: prostate cancer; OBS: observation strategies

widow, divorced, and separated, and data on whether men who were divorced, separated, or single were actually living alone or living with a significant other was not captured [14]. In addition, health insurance plans were identified from the data including Medicare, commercial, Medicaid, self/other, Veterans Affairs, and unknown. We observed from our study that the risk of choosing OBS was significantly lower among the patients enrolled in commercial/other types of health insurance plans (34.5%) compared to those enrolled in Medicare/VA/Medicaid health insurance plans.

Regarding the adoption of OBS, we found an increased use of OBS in the GHS over time. This trend was consistent with American Urological Association (AUA) guideline changes and was similar with the trend in the adoption of AS/WW from a large US national registry population with low-risk PCa [15]. Our study also indicated that patients who switched from OBS to IMT (64.6 years) were, on average, younger than patients who remained in the OBS (66.3 years) cohort with a median follow-up period of 5 years. Moreover, 50% of the men on OBS received active treatment eventually which is higher than in other studies [16–20]. This might be because the benefits of AS were not clearly discussed or due to lesser adoption of AS in community settings as opposed to academic institutions. This percentage is

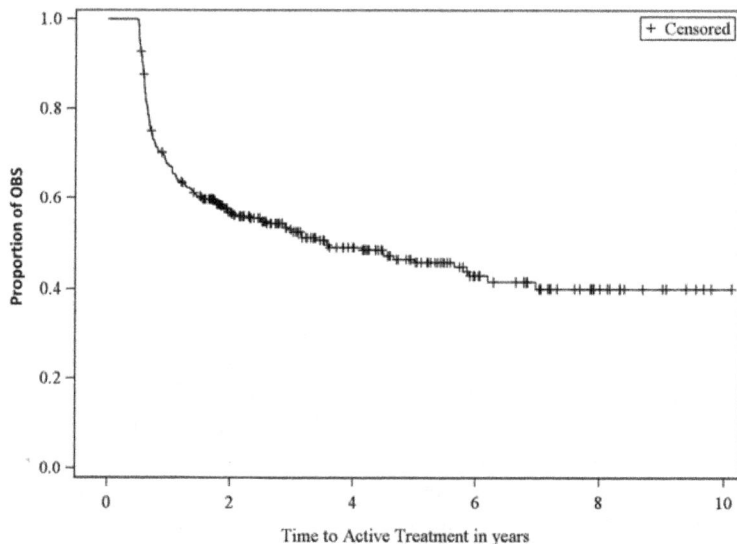

Fig. 4 Kaplan Meier for Time to Active Treatment in Men with Favorable Risk PCa Managed with OBS. OBS: observation strategies

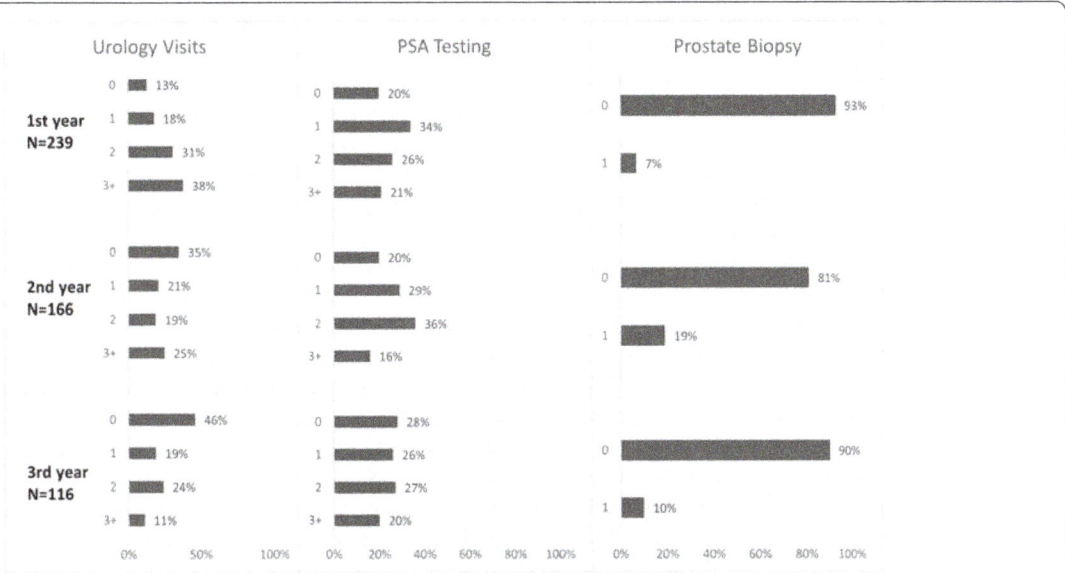

Fig. 5 Monitoring Patterns for PCa Patients Managed with OBS. PSA: prostate specific antigen

plausible given that during the timeframe of the study (January 2004 to April 2015), there were no existing AS guidelines to inform decisions on conversion of patients to active treatment.

The proportion of OBS patients converting to treatment within the first 12 months and the second 12 months after the index date is substantial. The most likely reason for the large drop during the first 12 months is patients simply deferred treatment. A chart review of 20 randomly-selected OBS patients showed that 10 of 20 (50%) patients were considered for IMT. One additional patient received brachytherapy 10 months after diagnosis, but there were limited encounters with urology; therefore, details of the complete treatment plan were not available. Eight of these 11 men (73%) had intentional delays in their

treatment date due to comorbid medical conditions to be addressed prior to surgery or to better align with personal commitments such as a seasonal work schedule.

Several AS schedules for the management of favorable risk PCa have been used in various studies including the 2017 National Comprehensive Cancer Network NCCN guideline [21] and Cancer Care Ontario's guideline on AS for the management of favorable risk PCa endorsed by the American Society of Clinical Oncology (ASCO) [22]. In comparison to these guidelines, we found that serial monitoring in GHS was relatively low.

Among the OBS patients who were active in the GHS for ≥2 years and who remained on OBS treatment in the first 2 years, only 61.5% had 3 or more PSA tests and only 26.5% had a prostate biopsy, which differs from

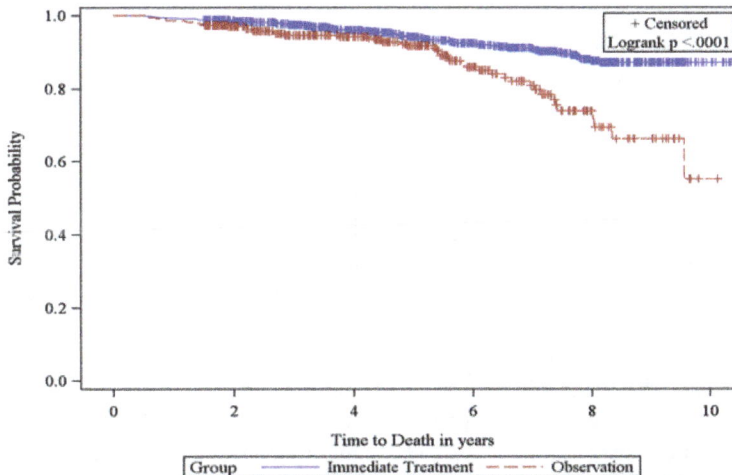

Fig. 6 Kaplan Meier Curve for Overall Survival Among Men With Favorable Risk PCa

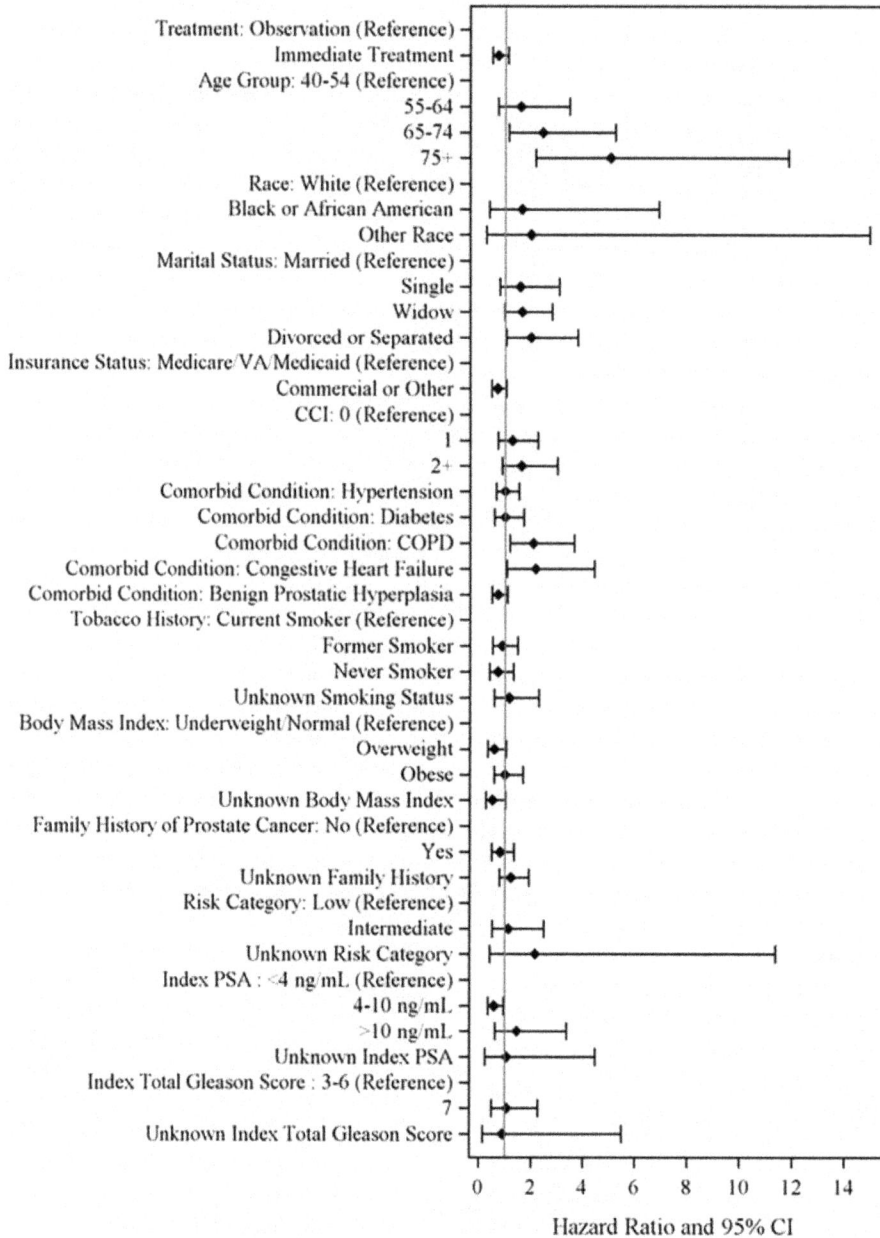

Fig. 7 Multivariate Cox Regression Model for All-cause Mortality Among. Men With Favorable Risk PCa. PCa: prostate cancer; VA: veterans affairs; CCI: Charlson comorbidity index; COPD: chronic obstructive pulmonary disorder; PSA: prostate specific antigen; CI: confidence interval

ASCO guidelines and most prospective AS protocols. Our data also showed a relatively stable PSA testing rate but a decrease in urology visits over time. In our study, 7.7, 20.5, and 10.8% of patients had one prostate biopsy in the first, second, and third year, respectively. Magnetic resonance imaging (MRI) use is an increasingly important tool in clinical practice for the diagnosis and monitoring of PCa patients, especially the multi-parametric (mp) MRI [23]. Using Current Procedural Terminology (CPT) codes to identify MRI use during the study period, we observed that only 8.56% of the patients who

were in the OBS group and 8.75% of the patients with IMT had prostate-related MRI during the follow-up period (results not shown). It is worth mentioning that MRI, including mpMRI, was not routinely used during the timeframe of this study (January 2004 to April 2015). Although MRI was not routinely carried out in the management of PCa in these patients, we do not believe that any of these patients had their cancer management affected by not using mpMRI.

The low monitoring rates observed in this study may reflect a greater proportion of WW versus AS, which we are unable to distinguish in our OBS population. In addition, a large proportion of patients included in this analysis were managed or treated prior to 2010 when AS was not yet widely adopted as a management strategy for patients with clinically-localized PCa and there were no consensus/guidelines for monitoring of AS or WW. Low monitoring rates for AS and WW in the community setting have been reported by Herden and Weissbach [24] and Auffenberg et al. [25] as well, suggesting a need for research into the factors associated with departure from guideline-recommended monitoring practices.

This study was a retrospective review of community practice intended to reflect the real-world implementation of routine management. The inclusion and exclusion criteria were primarily based on the patient having a lower-risk, early stage of cancer at diagnosis. To achieve the observational nature of the study, no requirements or exclusions were made based upon management protocol including the use of imaging data or biopsy results to address diagnosis or treatment among favorable risk PCa patients.

In sum, our data reveal significant opportunities for improvement in management strategies for favorable risk prostate cancer within our large community group setting. Educational activities should promote increased adoption of AS among favorable risk PCa patients as well as a clear distinction between AS and WW in individual patients. Community-based AS strategies should also focus on appropriate monitoring of patients placed on AS.

Limitations

All patients without definitive treatment in the first 6 months after PCa diagnosis were temporarily classified as receiving OBS. However, the OBS strategies, AS or WW, were not prospectively collected or always clearly noted by practitioners in the patient medical records. Therefore, we were not able to clearly distinguish between AS or WW from these real-world data. This limitation was also noted from other studies (Cooperberg et al., 2015) [15]. Furthermore, there also was some apparent misclassification in assigning patients to OBS strategies versus IMT by the 6-month threshold, as some patients planned for definitive treatment but waited longer than 6 months before receiving treatment. An additional limitation is that Geisinger serves patients in Central and Northeastern Pennsylvania; therefore, the study results may not be generalizable to the entire US PCa population. Finally, some patients may have received care outside of GHS.

Conclusion

The proportion of men managed by OBS increased over the 10-year study period although the rate of adoption might have been slightly slower in this large community setting compared with prospective AS protocols. Men in the OBS cohort had a higher proportion of low-risk PCa

but were older and had higher CCI scores. However, no differences were observed in overall survival between the two groups after covariates adjustment. These data provide insights into management patterns for favorable risk PCa within a community setting.

Analysis of monitoring patterns within the OBS cohort showed relatively low rates of repeat clinic visits and testing. Further research is necessary to focus on verifying the appropriate monitoring schedule to optimize patient outcomes and to encourage the adoption of AS in community settings.

Abbreviations

AS: Active surveillance; ASCO: American Society of Clinical Oncology; CCI: Charlson comorbidity index; CPT: Current procedural terminology; EMR: Electronic medical records; GHS: Geisinger Health System; IMT: Immediate treatment; mpMRI: Multi-Parametric magnetic resonance imaging; MRI: Magnetic resonance imaging; OBS: Observation strategies; PSA: Prostate specific antigen; PY: person years; WW: Watchful waiting

Acknowledgements
Editorial assistance was provided by Michael Moriarty of STATinMED research.

Funding
This study was funded by Roche Molecular Systems.

Authors' contributions
IC and DM conceptualized and designed the study. MFK and YW, LX, EM, JD, and MC verified and analyzed the data. MFK, YW, IC, LW, DM, LX, EM, MC and JD substantially contributed to the interpretation of the data, wrote the manuscript and/or substantially contributed to critical revisions of the intellectual content. All authors read and approved the final manuscript.

Competing interests
FK, YW, and LX are paid employees of STATinMED Research which is a paid consultant to Roche Molecular Systems. LW is a paid employee of Genentech which is a member of the Roche group. DM is a paid employee of Roche Diagnostics Operations. IC is a paid employee of Roche Molecular Systems. EM and JD are paid employees of Geisinger Health System which is a paid consultant to Roche Molecular Systems. MC has no conflicts to declare.

Author details
[1]STATinMED Research, 211 N. Fourth Avenue, Suite 2B, Ann Arbor, MI 48104, USA. [2]Diagnostics Information Solutions, F. Hoffmann-La Roche AG, Basel, Switzerland. [3]Genentech, Inc, South San Francisco, CA, USA. [4]Roche Diagnostics Operations, Indianapolis, IN, USA. [5]MedMining, Danville, PA, USA. [6]Geisinger Health System, Danville, PA, USA. [7]Wayne State University School of Medicine and the Barbara Ann Karmanos Cancer Institute, Detroit, MI, USA.

References

1. Polascik TJ, Passoni NM, Villers A, Choyke PL. Modernizing the diagnostic and decision-making pathway for prostate cancer. Clin Cancer Res. 2014;20(24):6254–7.
2. Schröder FH, Hugosson J, Roobol MJ, Tammela TL, Ciatto S, Nelen V, et al. Prostate-cancer mortality at 11 years of follow-up. N Engl J Med. 2012;366(11):981–90.
3. Roobol MJ, Kerkhof M, Schröder FH, Cuzick J, Sasieni P, Hakama M, et al. Prostate cancer mortality reduction by prostate-specific antigen-based screening adjusted for nonattendance and contamination in the European randomised study of screening for prostate Cancer (ERSPC). Eur Urol. 2009;56(4):584–91.
4. Mottet N, Bellmunt J, Bolla M, Joniau S, Mason M, Matveev V, et al. EAU guidelines on prostate cancer. Part II: treatment of advanced, relapsing, and castration-resistant prostate cancer. Actas Urol Esp. 2011;35(10):565–79.
5. Eldefrawy A, Katkoori D, Abramowitz M, Soloway MS, Manoharan M. Active surveillance vs. treatment for low-risk prostate cancer: a cost comparison. Urol Oncol. 2013;31(5):576–80.
6. Montironi R, Hammond EH, Lin DW, Gore JL, Srigley JR, Samaratunga H, et al. Consensus statement with recommendations on active surveillance inclusion criteria and definition of progression in men with localized prostate cancer: the critical role of the pathologist. Virchows Arch. 2014;465(6):623–8.
7. Ruseckaite R, Beckmann K, O'Callaghan M, Roder D, Moretti K, Millar J, et al. A retrospective analysis of Victorian and South Australian clinical registries for prostate cancer: trends in clinical presentation and management of the disease. BMC Cancer. 2016;16(1):607.
8. Barocas DA, Cowan JE, Smith JA Jr, Carroll PR, Investigators CPSURE. What percentage of patients with newly diagnosed carcinoma of the prostate are candidates for surveillance? An analysis of the CaPSURE™ database. J Urol. 2008;180(4):1330–5.
9. D'Amico AV, Whittington R, Malkowicz SB, Schultz D, Blank K, Broderick GA, et al. Biochemical outcome after radical prostatectomy, external beam radiation therapy, or interstitial radiation therapy for clinically localized prostate cancer. JAMA. 1998;280(11):969–74.
10. Filson CP, Marks LS, Litwin MS. Expectant management for men with early stage prostate cancer. CA Cancer J Clin. 2015;65(4):264–82.
11. Liu J, Womble PR, Merdan S, Miller DC, Montie JE, Denton BT, et al. Factors influencing selection of active surveillance for localized prostate Cancer. Urology. 2015;86(5):901–5.
12. Albertsen PC, Hanley JA, Gleason DF, Barry MJ. Competing risk analysis of men aged 55 to 74 years at diagnosis managed conservatively for clinically localized prostate cancer. JAMA. 1998;280(11):975–80.
13. Holmberg L, Bill-Axelson A, Helgesen F, Salo JO, Folmerz P, Haggman M, et al. A randomized trial comparing radical prostatectomy with watchful waiting in early prostate cancer. N Engl J Med. 2002;347:781–9.
14. Allen JD, Akinyemi IC, Reich A, Fleary S, Tendulkar S, Lamour N. African American women's involvement in promoting informed decision-making for prostate cancer screening among their partners/spouses. Am J Mens Health. 2018; https://doi.org/10.1177/1557988317742257.
15. Cooperberg MR, Carroll PR. Trends in management for patients with localized prostate cancer, 1990-2013. JAMA. 2015;314(1):80–2.
16. Newcomb LF, Thompson IM, Boyer HD, Brooks JD, Carroll PR, Cooperberg MR, et al. Outcomes of active surveillance for clinically localized prostate cancer in the prospective, multi-institutional Canary PASS cohort. J Urol. 2016;195(2):313–20.
17. Cooperberg MR, Cowan JE, Hilton JF, Reese AC, Zaid HB, Porten SP, et al. Outcomes of active surveillance for men with intermediate-risk prostate caner. J Clin Oncol. 2010;29(2):228–34.
18. Lang MF, Tyson MD, Alvarez JR, Koyama T, Hoffman KE, Resnick MJ. The influence of psychosocial constructs on the adherence to active surveillance for localized prostate cancer in a prospective, population-based cohort. Urology. 2017;103:173–8.
19. Loeb S, Folkvaljon Y, Makarov DV, Bratt O, Bill-Axelson A, Stattin P. Five-year nationwide follow-up study of active surveillance for prostate cancer. Eur Urol. 2015;67(2):233–8.
20. Aizer AA, Gu X, Choueiri TK, Martin NE, Efstathiou JA, Hyatt AS, et al. Cost implications and complications of overtreatment of low-risk prostate cancer in the United States. J Natl Compr Cancer Netw. 2015;13(1):61–8.
21. Mohler JL, Lee RJ, Antonarakis ES, Armstrong AJ, D-Amico AV, Davis BJ, et al. NCCN clinical practice guidelines in oncology (NCCN Guidelines): Prostate Cancer, Version 2.2018. National Comprehensive Cancer Network. 2018. https://www.nccn.org/professionals/physician_gls/pdf/prostate.pdf. Accessed 31 May 2018
22. Chen RC, Rumble RB, Loblaw DA, Finelli A, Ehdaie B, Cooperberg MR, et al. Active surveillance for the management of localized prostate cancer (Cancer Care Ontario guideline): American Society of Clinical Oncology clinical practice guideline endorsement. J Clin Oncol. 2016;34(18):2182–90.
23. Ahmed HU, El-Shater Bosaily A, Brown LC, Gabe R, Kaplan R, Parmar MK, et al. Diagnostic accuracy of multi-parametric MRI and TRUS biopsy in prostate cancer (PROMIS): a paired validating confirmatory study. Lancet. 2017;389(10071):815–22.
24. Herden J, Weissbach L. Utilization of active surveillance and watchful waiting for localized prostate cancer in the daily practice. World J Urol. 2018;36(3):383–91.
25. Auffenberg G, Luckenbaugh A, Hawken S, Dhir A, Linsell A, Kaul S, et al. MP25-12 Analysis fo active surveillance follow-up: how closely are patients monitored over time? J Urol. 2016;195(4):e283–4.

31

Hypocalcaemia in patients with prostate cancer treated with a bisphosphonate or denosumab: prevention supports treatment completion

Jean-Jacques Body[1]*, Roger von Moos[2], Daniela Niepel[3] and Bertrand Tombal[4]

Abstract

Background: Most patients with advanced prostate cancer develop bone metastases, which often result in painful and debilitating skeletal-related events. Inhibitors of bone resorption, such as bisphosphonates and denosumab, can each reduce the incidence of skeletal-related events and delay the progression of bone pain. However, these agents are associated with an increased risk of hypocalcaemia, which, although often mild and transient, can be serious and life-threatening. Here we provide practical advice on managing the risk of hypocalcaemia in patients with advanced prostate cancer who are receiving treatment with bone resorption inhibitors. Relevant references for this review were identified through searches of PubMed with the search terms 'prostate cancer', 'bone-targeted agents', 'anti-resorptive agents', 'bisphosphonates', 'zoledronic acid', 'denosumab', 'hypocalcaemia', and 'hypocalcemia'. Additional references were suggested by the authors.

Main text: Among patients with advanced cancer receiving a bisphosphonate or denosumab, hypocalcaemia occurs most frequently in those with prostate cancer, although it can occur in patients with any tumour type. Consistent with its greater ability to inhibit bone resorption, denosumab has shown superiority in the prevention of skeletal-related events in patients with bone metastases from solid tumours. Consequently, denosumab is more likely to induce hypocalcaemia than the bisphosphonates. Likewise, various bisphosphonates have differing potencies for the inhibition of bone resorption, and thus the risk of hypocalcaemia varies between different bisphosphonates. Other risk factors for the development of hypocalcaemia include the presence of osteoblastic metastases, vitamin D deficiency, and renal insufficiency. Hypocalcaemia can lead to treatment interruption, but it is both preventable and manageable. Serum calcium concentrations should be measured, and any pre-existing hypocalcaemia should be corrected, before starting treatment with inhibitors of bone resorption. Once treatment has started, concomitant administration of calcium and vitamin D supplements is essential. Calcium concentrations should be monitored during treatment with bisphosphonates or denosumab, particularly in patients at high risk of hypocalcaemia. If hypocalcaemia is diagnosed, patients should receive treatment with calcium and vitamin D.

Conclusion: With preventative strategies and treatment, patients with prostate cancer who are at risk of, or who develop, hypocalcaemia should be able to continue to benefit from treatment with bisphosphonates or denosumab.

Keywords: Bone-targeted agents, Bisphosphonate, Denosumab, Zoledronic acid, Prostate cancer, Hypocalcaemia

* Correspondence: jean-jacques.body@chu-brugmann.be
[1]Department of Medicine, CHU Brugmann, Université Libre de Bruxelles,
Place A.Van Gehuchten 4, 1020 Brussels, Belgium
Full list of author information is available at the end of the article

Background

Bone metastases are common in patients with prostate cancer and may develop in up to 90% of patients with advanced disease [1]. Skeletal-related events (SREs; including pathologic fracture, spinal cord compression, radiation to bone, and surgery to bone) are serious complications of bone metastases, are associated with increased pain, morbidity, and mortality, and therefore negatively affect patient quality of life [2]. Although bone metastases in patients with prostate cancer are frequently of the bone-forming osteoblastic type, biochemical and histological analyses suggest that there is also an excess of osteoclast activity in these lesions, leading to bone destruction and an increased risk of SREs [3]. Indeed, analysis of bone metastases type in 1487 patients with prostate cancer showed that 76.5%, 4.8%, and 18.7% of patients had osteoblastic, osteolytic, or mixed bone metastases, respectively (Amgen, data on file).

Inhibitors of bone resorption, such as the bisphosphonate zoledronic acid and the fully human monoclonal antibody against the receptor activator of nuclear factor kappa B ligand (RANKL) denosumab, reduce the incidence of SREs in patients with prostate cancer and bone metastases [3, 4]. Zoledronic acid and denosumab are indicated for the prevention of SREs in adults with advanced malignancies involving bone [5–7]. Therefore, the labels include prostate cancer patients with bone metastases irrespective of whether their disease is hormone-sensitive or castration-resistant. The development of bone metastases is a key event in the progression of castration-resistant prostate cancer and both agents can be used in men with this disease and bone metastases to prevent SREs [8]. The clinical effectiveness of these therapies in patients with castration-sensitive prostate cancer is yet to be demonstrated [9]. If not treated with an inhibitor of bone resorption, almost half of patients with prostate cancer and bone metastases could develop a SRE [4]. Denosumab is a more efficacious inhibitor of bone resorption than zoledronic acid and has shown superiority in the prevention of SREs [3, 10]. Both agents have been associated with an increased risk of hypocalcaemia, but the risk is greater with denosumab than with zoledronic acid, consistent with the greater efficacy of denosumab to inhibit bone resorption and reduce skeletal morbidity [3, 11]. Hypocalcaemia may lead to discontinuation of denosumab treatment; in a retrospective real-world study of 104 patients with bone metastases from solid tumours who were receiving denosumab, four patients discontinued treatment because of hypocalcaemia [12].

Patients with prostate cancer and osteoblastic metastases who are receiving treatment with inhibitors of bone resorption are at a particularly high risk of hypocalcaemia [11]. Although often mild and transient, hypocalcaemia

can also present as a serious and life-threatening condition, which can lead to treatment interruption or cessation. However, with proper patient monitoring, hypocalcaemia can be prevented and treated. In this review, we provide practical advice on managing the risk of hypocalcaemia in patients with advanced prostate cancer who are receiving treatment with bone resorption inhibitors. Relevant references for this review were identified through a literature search of PubMed (limited to English-language publications) with the search terms 'prostate cancer', 'bone-targeted agents', 'anti-resorptive agents', 'bisphosphonates', 'zoledronic acid', 'denosumab', 'hypocalcaemia', and 'hypocalcemia'. Additional references relevant to the topics of focus in the review were suggested by the authors based on their expert knowledge of the therapy area.

Main text
Diagnosing hypocalcaemia

Calcium homeostasis is mediated by the effect of active vitamin D (calcitriol) and parathyroid hormone (PTH) on the gastrointestinal (GI) absorption of calcium, renal excretion of calcium, and osteoclast/osteoblast activity in the skeleton (which is the main calcium sink in the body) [13]. Consequently, hypocalcaemia has many potential causes, such as vitamin D deficiency (which can lead to secondary hyperparathyroidism), abnormal magnesium or phosphate levels, and partial or complete hypoparathyroidism [14, 15]. Hypocalcaemia can range in severity from mild asymptomatic cases to acute life-threatening crises [16]; the Common Terminology Criteria for Adverse Events (CTCAE) define grades of hypocalcaemia from mild (grade 1) to severe (grade 5) (Table 1) [17].

Extracellular calcium is required for the normal functioning of muscles and nerves. Thus, signs and symptoms of hypocalcaemia include muscle twitching, spasms, tingling, and numbness, and patients with severe hypocalcaemia may develop tetany, seizures, and cardiac dysrhythmias [18]. The development of neuromuscular excitability depends on both the absolute concentration of calcium and how rapidly the concentration

Table 1 Common Terminology Criteria for Adverse Events grading of hypocalcaemia [17]

Grade	Total corrected calcium concentration, mmol/l (mg/dl)
1	2.0–2.1 (8.0–LLN)
2	1.75 to < 2.0 (7.0 to < 8.0)
3	1.5 to < 1.75 (6.0 to < 7.0)
4	< 1.5 (< 6.0)
5	If death occurs as a result of hypocalcaemia

LLN lower limit of normal

has fallen. Patients who experience a rapid fall in serum calcium concentration are often symptomatic, whereas those who develop hypocalcaemia gradually may be asymptomatic, with hypocalcaemia being diagnosed as an incidental biochemical finding [18]. However, if asymptomatic hypocalcaemia is not treated, long-term consequences can include neuropsychiatric symptoms, cataract formation, and raised intracranial pressure [18]. Such cases predominantly occur in patients with chronic hypoparathyroidism [19].

Measuring calcium concentrations

Approximately 50% of serum calcium exists in an unbound ionized form, and 50% is bound to protein (predominantly albumin) [18]. Only unbound ionized calcium is physiologically active; therefore, serum calcium concentration must be corrected for albumin concentration in order to confirm a diagnosis of hypocalcaemia [16]. This is particularly important in patients with advanced cancer in whom albumin levels are frequently low [20]. Hypocalcaemia is defined as a corrected serum total calcium concentration below 2.1 mmol/l (ionized calcium < 1.1 mmol/l) [21]. Corrected calcium can be calculated using the following formula: measured total calcium (mmol/l) + 0.02 × [40 − measured albumin level (g/l)] [22]. Analysis of unbound ionized calcium concentration provides the most accurate measurement of serum calcium and is recommended in patients who are seriously ill [16]: unfortunately, ionized calcium measurements are not often routinely available. Analysis of creatinine, phosphate, magnesium, vitamin D, and PTH levels is also recommended when diagnosing hypocalcaemia in order to identify other underlying causes of low serum calcium concentrations [16].

Identifying patients who are at high risk of hypocalcaemia

It is rare for patients with cancer to develop hypocalcaemia as a direct result of the primary tumour [23]. However, low calcium concentrations are quite frequently observed in individuals with osteoblastic bone metastases, in whom rapid mineralization of newly formed bone sequesters calcium from the bloodstream [24, 25]. In retrospective analyses, conducted before the introduction of bisphosphonate or denosumab treatment, hypocalcaemia was reported in 5–13% of patients with bone metastases, depending on the formula used to correct for albumin levels. Among these patients, 35% had hypocalcaemia of grade 1, 60% grade 2, and 5% grade 3 or higher [25]. Prevalence was highest among individuals with prostate cancer and bone metastases; 13–27% of these patients developed hypocalcaemia [25].

Hypocalcaemia has been reported as an adverse event associated with the use of bisphosphonates (such as zoledronic acid) and denosumab. Bisphosphonates are analogues of a natural regulator of bone metabolism, pyrophosphonate. They localise to the extracellular bone matrix from where they may prevent osteoclast differentiation, induce osteoblasts to produce osteoclast inhibitory factors, and cause apoptosis of osteoclasts [26]. Denosumab is a monoclonal antibody against RANKL that disrupts signalling through RANK, thus preventing tumour-mediated activation of osteoclasts [27]. Bisphosphonates and denosumab lead to reduced osteoclast activity, thus reducing bone resorption and the release of calcium from bone into the bloodstream [11]. Preclinical and clinical data indicate that denosumab is a more efficacious inhibitor of osteoclast activity than zoledronic acid [11] and has shown superiority in the prevention of SREs compared with zoledronic acid [3, 10]. Consistent with the potent action of denosumab, in a combined analysis of three clinical trials comparing denosumab and zoledronic acid in patients with bone metastases from solid tumours (including prostate cancer) or multiple myeloma, hypocalcaemia of any grade occurred more frequently with denosumab than with zoledronic acid (9.6% vs. 5%, respectively) (Fig. 1) [11].

Real-world data suggest that the incidence of hypocalcaemia associated with bisphosphonates or denosumab may be higher than has been reported in clinical trials. Retrospective studies of patients treated with denosumab have reported an incidence of 9–22% for hypocalcaemia of grade 2 or higher [21, 28–30]. A 12-month observational study of 125 patients with bone metastases (including 92 patients with prostate cancer) who were receiving zoledronic acid showed that hypocalcaemia of any grade occurred in 18.5% of the patients with prostate cancer. Of patients with any tumour type, hypocalcaemia of grade 3 or 4 occurred in 4% [31]. The higher incidence of hypocalcaemia encountered in real-world studies compared with clinical trials may reflect poor adherence to guidelines for calcium supplementation and monitoring of patients in clinical practice [12]. Although both clinical trial data and real-world evidence suggest that severe hypocalcaemia is a relatively rare occurrence, it can be a serious, life-threatening condition that requires hospitalization and administration of intravenous calcium [28]. However, hospital admissions due to hypocalcaemia associated with inhibitors of bone resorption remain low, suggesting that such cases are often mild [30].

Analysis of data from phase III clinical trials has identified several factors that increase the risk of hypocalcaemia [11]. Hypocalcaemia associated with inhibitors of bone resorption has been shown to occur in patients with bone metastases from a variety of primary tumour types, but is most frequently seen in those with prostate cancer or small-cell lung cancer [11]. Additionally, male sex and the presence of osteoblastic metastases have been shown to

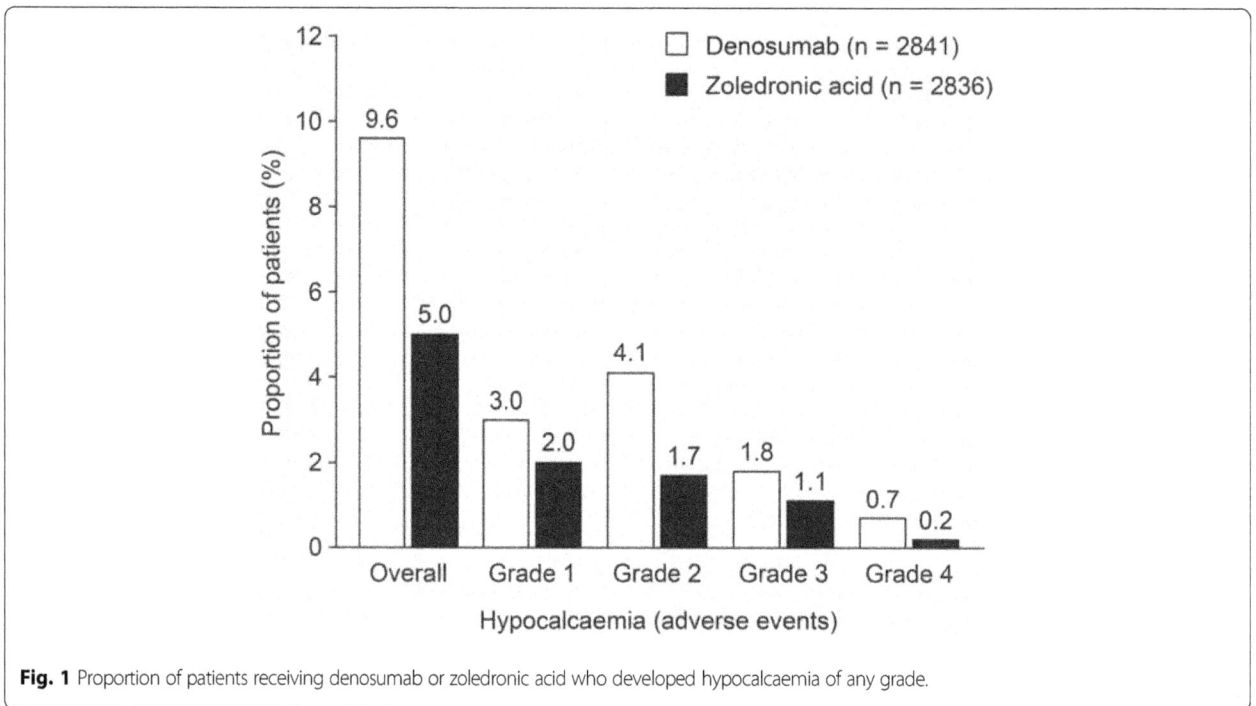

Fig. 1 Proportion of patients receiving denosumab or zoledronic acid who developed hypocalcaemia of any grade.

associate significantly with an increased risk of hypocalcaemia [11]. By inhibiting bone resorption and preventing the release of calcium from bone, bisphosphonates and denosumab further increase the bone mineralization and calcium sequestration associated with osteoblastic metastases [32].

Hypocalcaemia in patients with cancer frequently relates to a poor nutritional status, and these individuals often have low albumin and/or vitamin D concentrations [24]; therefore, as discussed above, it is important to correct serum calcium measurements for albumin levels. Moreover, vitamin D deficiency is associated with an increased risk of hypocalcaemia following treatment with inhibitors of bone resorption [33, 34] and is common in elderly people and those with cancer [35, 36]. Hence, vitamin D deficiency is a concern in men with prostate cancer, given that their median age at diagnosis is 66 years [37]. Indeed, more than 40% of men have been shown to be deficient in vitamin D (serum calcidiol < 20 ng/ml) at the time of diagnosis of prostate cancer [38].

Patients with severe renal insufficiency (glomerular filtration rate < 30 ml/min) or stage 4 or 5 chronic kidney disease (CKD) have an increased risk of hypocalcaemia associated with treatment involving inhibitors of bone resorption [21, 29]. This increased risk of hypocalcaemia likely results from CKD-induced secondary hyperparathyroidism [21]. Additionally, CKD causes a reduction in the activity of 1-α-hydroxylase and conversion of vitamin D to the active form (calcitriol), resulting in the reduced intestinal absorption of calcium [39]. Denosumab is a useful therapeutic option for patients with advanced

cancer and renal insufficiency or CKD because, in contrast to zoledronic acid, it is not excreted by the kidneys and requires no dose adjustment for renal insufficiency [6, 40]. However, owing to the high risk of hypocalcaemia in patients with severe renal insufficiency, we advise caution when considering such patients for treatment with denosumab, and if treatment is administered, such patients should be closely monitored [29].

Patients with high levels of bone turnover markers (i.e. urinary N-telopeptide of type I collagen and bone-specific alkaline phosphatase) at baseline are also at an increased risk of hypocalcaemia [11]. Additionally, patients with pre-existing hypocalcaemia, associated with impaired parathyroid function, have a high risk of developing hypocalcaemia following treatment with inhibitors of bone resorption [41].

Preventing hypocalcaemia

Hypocalcaemia associated with inhibitors of bone resorption is avoidable in most cases (Fig. 2). With proper management, patients should be able to continue to benefit from treatment with these agents, significantly reducing the risk of developing SREs, which may be painful or associated with increased mortality [2].

Although hypocalcaemia can occur at any time during therapy, it is most frequently reported within 6 months of treatment initiation (Fig. 3) and occurs earlier in patients receiving denosumab than in those receiving zoledronic acid; in phase III trials, the median time to hypocalcaemia of grade 2 or higher was 3.8 months with denosumab and 6.5 months with zoledronic acid [11].

Recommendations for the prevention of hypocalcaemia

- Measure serum vitamin D and albumin-corrected (or ionized) calcium concentrations before treatment initiation with a bisphosphonate or denosumab and correct any pre-existing hypocalcaemia

- For patients with ≥ 3 bone lesions, prescribe prophylactic calcium and vitamin D 1 week before starting treatment with inhibitors of bone resorption
    - Patient adherence to and tolerance of these supplements should be assessed during this week

- Measure serum calcium concentration within 2 weeks of the initial treatment dose in patients who are at a high risk of hypocalcaemia (e.g. patients who are critically ill or have renal insufficiency)

- Measure calcium levels in at-risk patients prior to administering the second dose of a bisphosphonate or denosumab

- Counsel patients on the signs and symptoms of hypocalcaemia and encourage them to report symptoms indicative of this condition

- Provide patients receiving denosumab with concomitant calcium (≤ 500 mg) and vitamin D (≤ 400 IU) daily

- Provide patients who experience unmanageable adverse events with calcium supplements with dietary advice on how to increase calcium intake

- Regularly measure vitamin D levels in patients who are at a high risk of hypocalcaemia and in those for whom poor adherence to supplementation is suspected

Recommendations for the treatment of hypocalcaemia

Mild hypocalcaemia (asymptomatic grade 1)
- Continue treatment with inhibitors of bone resorption
- Treat patients with oral calcium and vitamin D supplements: calcium (1 g) and vitamin D (cholecalciferol at least 800 IU) twice daily
    - Patients who are vitamin D deficient and who do not respond to this therapy can be given ≤ 25,000 IU orally once a week for 8 weeks or 7 mg intramuscularly every 3 months
- Check patients for hypomagnesaemia; if a patient is hypomagnesaemic:
    - Precipitating drugs should not be administered
    - Intravenous magnesium at a dose of 24 mmol should be administered over 24 hours to normalise magnesium concentration

Severe hypocalcaemia (grade ≥ 2)
- Delay treatment with inhibitors of bone resorption
    - Treatment can be continued once a patient has normal calcium levels for ≥ 4 weeks
    - Calcium levels should be measured 2 weeks after reinitiating treatment with an inhibitor of bone resorption, and monthly thereafter
- For symptomatic or at-risk patients, or those possibly/probably non-compliant with oral calcium supplement, administer intravenous calcium if corrected serum calcium concentration falls below 1.9 mmol/l (ionized calcium < 1.0 mmol/l; i.e., grade ≥ 2)
    - Calcium gluconate (10%) is preferred to calcium chloride
    - Phosphate and bicarbonate should not be infused with the calcium
    - Cardiac monitoring during intravenous calcium administration is recommended
- Provide oral calcium supplements and vitamin D (for example, 50,000 IU each week for 8 weeks or calcitriol 0.5–1 µg/day for patients with hypoparathyroidism) as needed
- Repeat calcium and vitamin D treatment until symptoms have subsided
- If a patient is hypomagnesaemic, magnesium replacement should also be given (as described above)
- Once a stable calcium concentration has been achieved, calcium concentrations should be monitored 1 week after hospital discharge
    - If satisfactory, further follow-up measurements should be taken monthly for 6 months

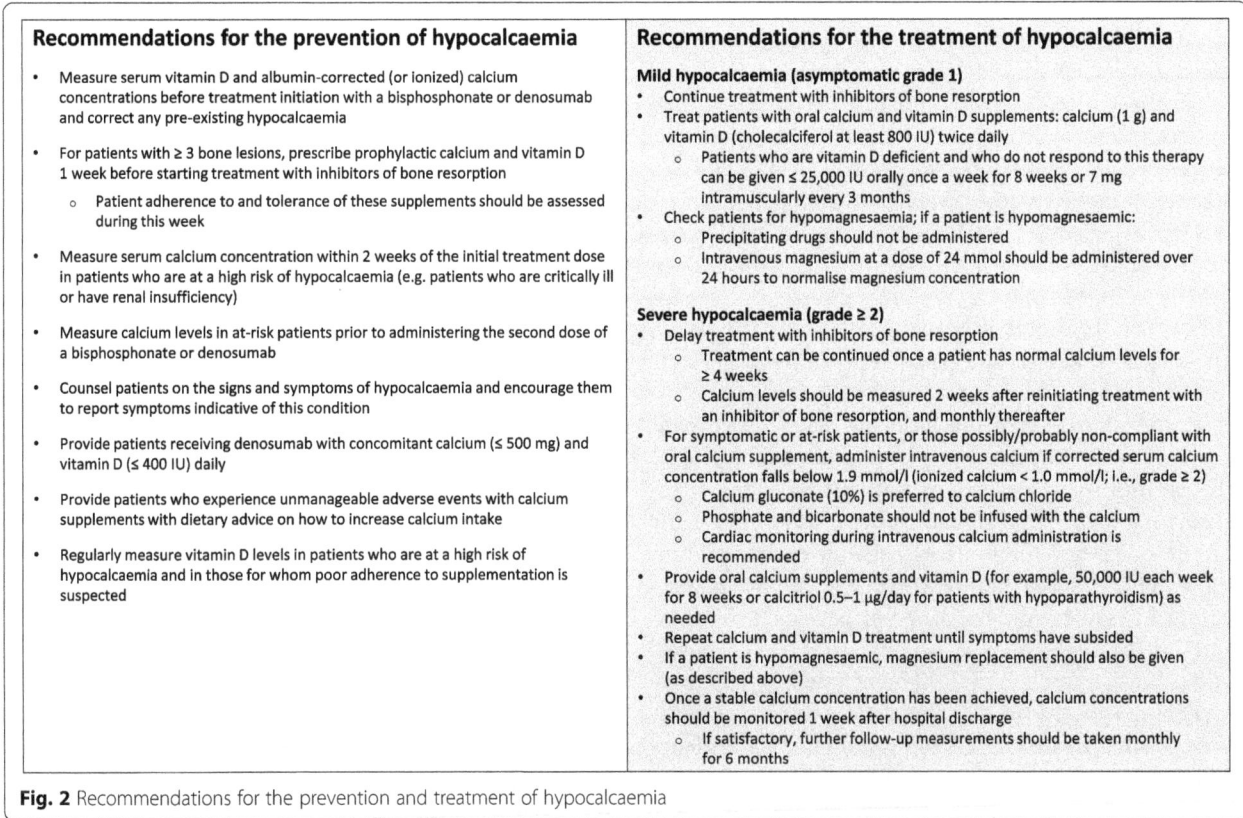

Fig. 2 Recommendations for the prevention and treatment of hypocalcaemia

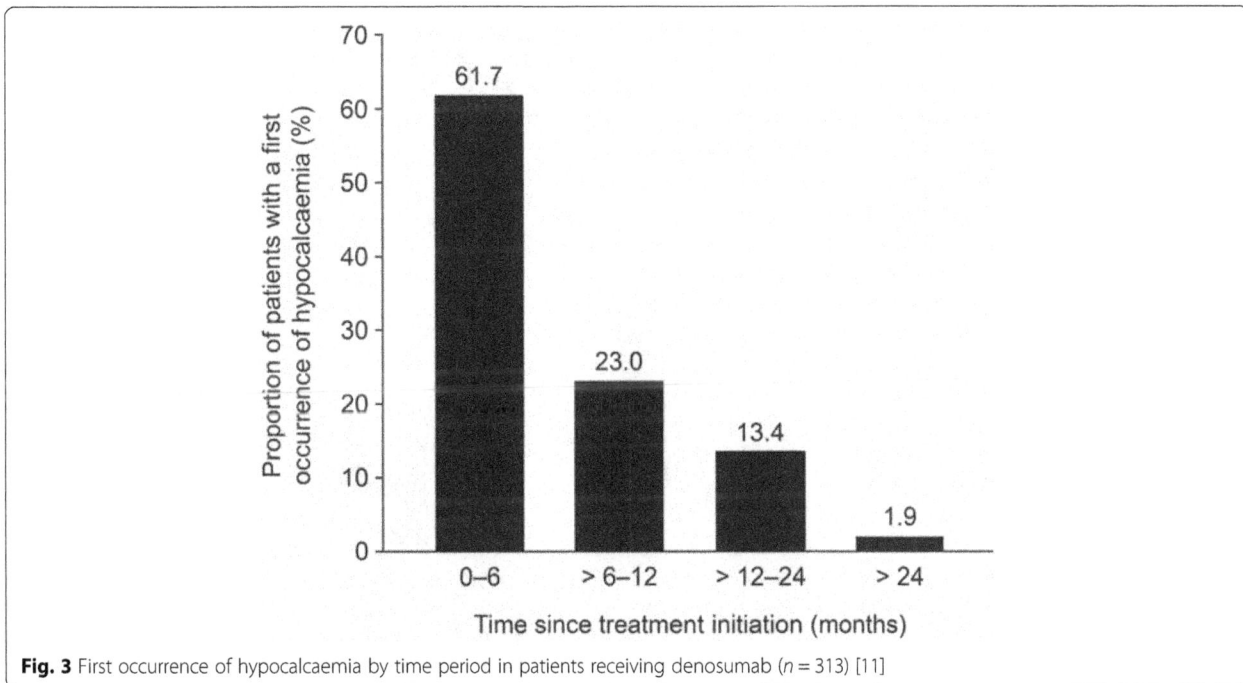

Fig. 3 First occurrence of hypocalcaemia by time period in patients receiving denosumab ($n = 313$) [11]

Similar findings have been reported in real-world studies; a retrospective chart review of 55 patients with advanced cancer who were receiving denosumab found that, in most patients, hypocalcaemia developed shortly after treatment administration (median 16 days) and after a median of one injection (range 1–14) [28]. Another retrospective study, conducted in 66 patients with cancer who received a median of 3–6 cycles of denosumab, found that the incidence of hypocalcaemia of any grade was higher during the first course of therapy (16.7%) than in second or later courses (6.1%) [29]. However, long-term clinical trial safety data on denosumab in patients with bone metastases from breast cancer or prostate cancer showed that the incidence of hypocalcaemia did not increase with longer exposure to denosumab [42].

To prevent hypocalcaemia in patients receiving a bisphosphonate or denosumab, serum vitamin D and albumin-corrected (or ionized) calcium concentrations should be measured before treatment initiation. Pre-existing hypocalcaemia must be corrected before treatment initiation [5, 6]. For patients with a substantial tumour burden in the bone (≥ 3 bone lesions), prophylactic calcium and vitamin D should be prescribed 1 week before starting treatment with a bisphosphonate or denosumab. During this week, patient adherence to and tolerance of these supplements should be assessed. The denosumab label recommends that serum calcium concentration should be measured within 2 weeks of the initial dose in all patients and that additional monitoring should be conducted in patients with suspected symptoms of hypocalcaemia and in those at high risk of hypocalcaemia [6]. However, in clinical practice, we recommend such monitoring following the initial dose of a bisphosphonate or denosumab only in patients who are at a high risk of hypocalcaemia, such as those who are critically ill or who have renal insufficiency. Nevertheless, we do recommend measuring calcium levels in at-risk patients [11] prior to administering the second dose of a bisphosphonate or denosumab. Additionally, patients should be counselled on the signs and symptoms of hypocalcaemia and encouraged to report symptoms indicative of this condition [6]. Monitoring allows early detection of hypocalcaemia and hence the correction of serum calcium concentration before administering further doses of a bisphosphonate or denosumab.

Calcium and vitamin D supplements

Preventative supplementation with calcium and/or vitamin D is associated with fewer hypocalcaemia adverse events for patients receiving zoledronic acid or denosumab. Use of these supplements [recommended doses: calcium ≥ 500 mg/day; vitamin D ≥ 400 International Units (IU) /day] has been shown to lower the risk of developing hypocalcaemia by 27% or 40% in patients receiving zoledronic acid or denosumab, respectively (Fig. 4) [11]. This reduction in risk is impressive given that, in this analysis, patients were considered to be receiving supplements if they had reported taking oral calcium and/or vitamin D at any time during the study (excluding those who reported supplement use only after their first hypocalcaemia event) [11].

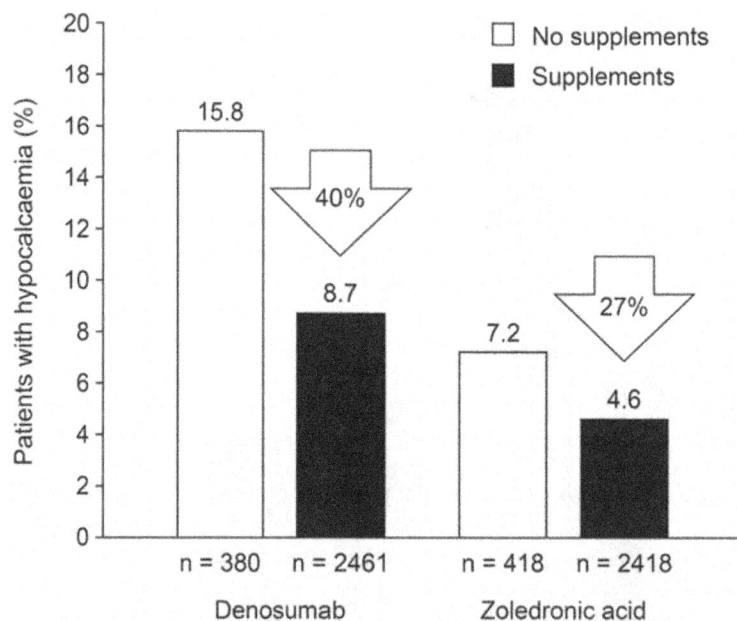

Fig. 4 Hypocalcaemia risk in patients receiving calcium and/or vitamin supplementation versus those who were not [11]

Adequate supplementation is necessary in all patients treated with a bisphosphonate or denosumab [5, 6]. For patients receiving denosumab, concomitant supplementation with a minimum of 500 mg calcium daily and 400 IU vitamin D daily is required [6]. When managing hypocalcaemia risk in patients with bone metastases from prostate cancer, it is important to note that those receiving androgen-deprivation therapy should also receive calcium and vitamin D supplements as part of the preventative treatment for cancer treatment-induced bone loss [43].

The recommended daily intake of calcium varies by guideline and by patient population. To avoid calcium deficiency, the British Dietetic Association recommends that adults consume 700 mg of calcium daily [44]. The National Institutes of Health recommends a daily intake of calcium of 1000 mg for adults aged up to 70 years (1200 mg for women aged 51–70 years) and 1200 mg for those aged over 70 years [45]. Elderly patients have an increased requirement for calcium due to age-associated reduction in intestinal calcium absorption [46]. For all patients, the percentage of calcium absorbed depends on the total amount of elemental calcium consumed at one time. The percentage absorption decreases as the amount of calcium increases: absorption is maximal when doses of 500 mg or less are consumed at one time [45].

The two main forms of calcium in supplements are carbonate and citrate [47, 48]. Calcium carbonate should be taken with food because absorption is dependent on stomach acid, whereas calcium citrate is absorbed equally well when taken with or without food and is the preferred form for patients receiving proton pump inhibitors [48]. Other calcium forms in supplements include calcium gluconate, calcium chloride, calcium lactate, calcium phosphate, and calcium citrate malate [45, 46].

The main circulating form of vitamin D is calcidiol [49]. Vitamin D also exists in two inactive forms, namely vitamin D_2 (ergocalciferol) and vitamin D_3 (cholecalciferol), which are hydroxylated in the liver to form calcidiol and then in the kidneys to form the biologically active form, calcitriol [49]. Vitamin D deficiency is defined as a serum calcidiol concentration below 20 ng/ml (50 nmol/l), and insufficiency is defined as a calcidiol level of 21–29 ng/ml (52–72 nmol/l) [49]. Patients with a calcidiol concentration below 10 ng/ml (25 nmol/l) can be considered to be severely deficient [50]. Vitamin D deficiency can be caused by reduced synthesis via the skin (owing to limited sun exposure, skin pigmentation or skin thinning as a result of ageing), decreased vitamin D absorption, and increased catabolism [16, 18, 49]. Calcitriol enhances intestinal absorption of calcium and promotes bone mineralization and remodelling [16]: there is a significant decrease in intestinal calcium absorption when serum vitamin D levels fall below 30 ng/ml [49].

Similar to calcium daily reference values, the recommended daily intake of vitamin D varies by guidelines and depends on the patient population being treated. The amount of vitamin D supplementation required to achieve adequate serum levels (> 30 ng/ml or > 75 nmol/l) depends on a variety of factors in addition to the baseline vitamin D levels including age, body mass index, sun-exposure history, and the use of medications that can affect vitamin D metabolism and intestinal absorption [51]. Among patients who are at risk of vitamin D deficiency, the Endocrine Society Clinical Practice Guidelines recommend that adults aged up to 70 years receive a preventative dose of vitamin D 600 IU daily, and those older than 70 years receive 800 IU daily [52]. The International Osteoporosis Foundation recommends that adults aged 60 years and over receive 800–1000 IU daily [53].

Many treatment regimens are available for patients with vitamin D deficiency. The Endocrine Society Clinical Practice Guidelines recommend that these patients should be treated with 50,000 IU of ergocalciferol or cholecalciferol weekly for 8 weeks or 6000 IU daily until a serum calcidiol level above 75 nmol/l is achieved. This should be followed with maintenance therapy of 1500–2000 IU daily [52]. NICE recommends that fixed loading doses of vitamin D (up to a total of 300,000 IU) be given as either weekly or daily split doses, followed by lifelong maintenance treatment of 800 IU daily [54]. Higher doses of up to 2000 IU daily, and occasionally much higher doses, may be used for certain groups of people (e.g., those with malabsorption disorders) [54]. Other treatment regimens include 50,000 IU once a week for 6 weeks (300,000 IU in total), 20,000 IU twice a week for 7 weeks (280,000 IU in total), or 4000 IU daily for 10 weeks (280,000 IU in total) [54]. For the treatment of vitamin D insufficiency, some guidelines recommend that maintenance doses should be started without the use of loading doses; however, we strongly recommend the use of vitamin D loading doses in patients who are deficient before starting therapy with an inhibitor of bone resorption [54].

Vitamin D can be given as ergocalciferol or cholecalciferol, or as the active metabolites alfacalcidol or calcitriol [55]. Ergocalciferol and cholecalciferol are both recommended for the treatment and prevention of vitamin D deficiency [52], although cholecalciferol is the more potent of the two agents [56] and is thus prescribed more commonly than ergocalciferol. The normal conversion of vitamin D to its active form is compromised in patients with severe renal insufficiency (glomerular filtration rate < 30 ml/min); therefore, calcitriol or alfacalcidol should be administered for the treatment of hypocalcaemia in these patients [57]. Treatment with calcitriol or alfacalcidol can lead to rapid changes in serum calcium levels, so patients should be monitored closely in order to avoid hypercalcaemia [58].

Adherence to supplements, particularly calcium supplements, is often low, which can have a negative impact on efficacy [47]. In patients receiving a bisphosphonate or denosumab, measures should be taken to maximise adherence to calcium and vitamin D supplements: the risk of hypocalcaemia and the importance of adherence to supplements should be discussed with patients, and serum calcium levels should be monitored to assess adherence. Regular patient follow-up to encourage treatment compliance may help to ensure that supplements are taken correctly.

Compliance may be enhanced by choosing a suitable dose and delivery method for calcium and vitamin D supplements. Calcium and vitamin D supplements are available as separate or combined formulations, as a variety of delivery compounds including oral tablets, capsules, soft-chews, powders, or as solution [46, 47]. Calcium carbonate, available as powder formulations, has been shown to have increased bioavailability compared with calcium citrate, most often given as tablet formulations [47]. However, patient preference studies of calcium and vitamin D supplements have shown that soft-chew tablets are preferred over powder formulations [59]. In addition, patients are more likely to be adherent with once-daily dietary supplements than with twice-daily supplements [60]. However, the advantages of once-daily supplementation depend on the dose required and should be considered in light of the reduced percentage absorption of calcium when it is given in doses above 500 mg [45]. As discussed above, vitamin D supplements can be given weekly or biweekly [54], which may improve adherence compared with daily supplements.

Calcium supplements are associated with a number of adverse events that may reduce patient compliance with treatment [61]. In particular, gastrointestinal (GI) adverse events are common in patients taking calcium supplements [61]. Compared with calcium citrate, calcium carbonate is more often associated with GI symptoms [48]. Although most GI adverse events are mild, a meta-analysis assessing the safety of calcium supplements in randomised trials found a significantly increased incidence of hospital admissions for GI adverse events in patients receiving calcium (6.8%) when compared with those receiving placebo (3.6%) [62]. For patients who experience unmanageable adverse events with calcium supplements, it is essential to provide dietary advice on how to increase calcium intake with calcium-rich foods (Table 2) [44, 63]. In contrast, vitamin D supplements are generally well tolerated [64], but we advise regular monitoring of vitamin D levels in patients who are at a high risk of hypocalcaemia and those for whom poor adherence to supplementation is suspected.

Table 2 Foods rich in calcium [44, 63]

Food type	Quantity	Calcium (mg)
Dairy sources of calcium		
Cow's milk (all types)	200 ml	240
Sheep's milk	200 ml	380
Hard cheese (e.g., cheddar, parmesan, emmental)	30 g	240
Fresh cheese (e.g., cottage cheese, ricotta, mascarpone)	200 g	138
Soft cheese (e.g., camembert, brie)	60 g	240
Feta	60 g	270
Mozzarella	60 g	242
Cream cheese	30 g	180
Yoghurt	120 g	200
Calcium-enriched fromage frais	50 g	125
Calcium-enriched low-fat spread	28 g	121
Malted milk drink	25 g serving in 200 ml milk	440–710
Hot chocolate (light)	25 g serving in 200 ml water	200
Rice pudding	200 g	176
Custard	120 ml	120
Non-dairy sources of calcium		
Sardines (with bones)	60 g	258
Pilchards (with bones)	60 g	150
Whitebait	50 g	130
White beans	80 g raw/200 g cooked	132
Wholemeal bread	100 g	100
Non-dairy calcium-fortified products		
Calcium-enriched milk alternatives (e.g., rice, soya, oat, nut, coconut)	200 ml	240
Soya bean curd/tofu[a]	60 g	200
Calcium-enriched orange juice	250 ml	195
Calcium-fortified cereals	30 g	137
Calcium-fortified bread	40 g	191

[a]Only if set with calcium chloride (E509) or calcium sulphate (E516)

Treating hypocalcaemia
Mild hypocalcaemia
Patients with mild hypocalcaemia (asymptomatic grade 1) should be treated with oral calcium and vitamin D supplements: calcium (1 g) and vitamin D (cholecalciferol at least 800 IU) should be given twice daily [65]. Patients who are vitamin D deficient and who do not respond to this therapy can be given higher doses of vitamin D: at least 25,000 IU orally once a week for 8 weeks or, where available and if needed, 7 mg intramuscularly every 3 months [65]. It is important to check whether a patient is hypomagnesaemic, which induces

functional hypoparathyroidism leading to low serum calcium levels [66]. If a patient is hypomagnesaemic, precipitating drugs should not be administered. To normalise magnesium concentration, intravenous magnesium at a dose of 24 mmol should be administered over 24 h [67]. We recommend that treatment with inhibitors of bone resorption be continued in patients who experience grade 1 hypocalcaemia.

Severe hypocalcaemia

For symptomatic or at-risk patients [11], or those possibly/probably non-compliant with oral calcium supplement, intravenous calcium should be administered if corrected serum calcium concentration falls below 1.9 mmol/l (ionized calcium < 1.0 mmol/l; i.e., grade $\geq$ 2) [16]. Asymptomatic patients with a corrected serum calcium below 1.9 mmol/l can rapidly become critically ill, and so it is important to treat and monitor these patients closely [18].

Intravenously administered calcium gluconate (10%) is preferred to calcium chloride, which is a strong irritant. It can be given as repeated 50–100 ml boluses in 5% dextrose or by continuous infusion [16, 67]. If calcium chloride is given, it should be administered via a central line to prevent irritation of veins [67]. In order to avoid precipitation of calcium salts, phosphate and bicarbonate should not be infused with the calcium [16]. Patients with severe hypocalcaemia should also receive oral calcium supplements (as described above) and vitamin D (e.g., 50,000 IU each week for 8 weeks or calcitriol 0.5– 1 µg/day for patients with hypoparathyroidism) as needed [18]. Treatment should be repeated until symptoms have subsided. It should be noted that hypocalcaemia can be prolonged, so continuous administration of a dilute solution of calcium for a few days may be required [18, 68]. Magnesium replacement should also be given (as described above) to those who are hypomagnesaemic [18, 67]. Cardiac monitoring during intravenous calcium administration is recommended because the rapid elevation of serum calcium concentration required to correct hypocalcaemia can result in cardiac arrhythmia [18].

Retrospective analysis of patients treated for denosumab-associated hypocalcaemia found that the median time from detection of hypocalcaemia to normocalcaemia was 33 days (range: 9–92 days) [28]. However, the time to normalization of serum calcium levels depends on the baseline calcium concentration, the treatment regimen, and how frequently calcium levels are measured. Once a stable calcium concentration has been achieved, calcium concentrations should be monitored 1 week after hospital discharge. If satisfactory, further follow-up measurements should be taken monthly for 6 months [18, 67]. We recommend that treatment with inhibitors of bone resorption be delayed in patients who experience grade 2 or higher hypocalcaemia; treatment can be continued once a patient has had a stable normal calcium level for a minimum of 4 weeks. In patients who have experienced severe hypocalcaemia, serum calcium levels should be measured 2 weeks after reinitiating treatment with an inhibitor of bone resorption, and monthly thereafter. Our recommendations for the treatment of hypocalcaemia are summarised in Fig. 2.

Conclusion

Hypocalcaemia associated with the use of bisphosphonates and denosumab can be serious; however, it is both preventable and treatable. Given the reduction in skeletal morbidity and the potential improvements to quality of life that inhibitors of bone resorption offer patients with cancer and bone metastases, potential barriers to their use should be properly understood and addressed. With appropriate patient monitoring and preventative measures, patients with advanced prostate cancer, including those with additional risk factors for hypocalcaemia, should be able to continue to benefit from treatment with these agents.

Abbreviations
CKD: Chronic kidney disease; CTCAE: Common Terminology Criteria for Adverse Events; GI: Gastrointestinal; PTH: Parathyroid hormone; RANKL: Receptor activator of nuclear factor kappa B ligand; SREs: Skeletal-related events

Acknowledgements
Medical writing support, funded by Amgen (Europe) GmbH, was provided by Kelly Soady PhD from Oxford PharmaGenesis, Oxford, UK. Editorial support was provided by Stéphane Gamboni of Amgen (Europe) GmbH.

Funding
Medical writing support for development of this manuscript was funded by Amgen (Europe) GmbH. An author (DN) employed by the funding body (Amgen [Europe] GmbH) was involved in the conception of the manuscript and in the identification, recommendation and interpretation of the published literature included in the review.

Authors' contributions
J-JB and DN made substantial contributions to conception of the objective of the manuscript. All authors made substantial contributions to literature identification and recommendation (acquisition of data), interpreted data from published sources, and were involved with drafting and critically revising the manuscript. All authors read and gave final approval of the version to be published, and agreed to be accountable for all aspects of the work.

Competing interests
J-JB has received speaker and consulting fees from Amgen. DN is an employee of Amgen and holds stocks. RvM has received research grants from Amgen and Bayer, has acted as a consultant for Amgen, Bayer, Bristol Myers Squibb, GlaxoSmithKline, Merck Sharp and Dohme, Novartis, and Roche, and has received honoraria from Amgen, Bayer, and GlaxoSmithKline. BT is an advisor and an investigator for Amgen, Astellas, Janssen, Medivation, and Sanofi.

Author details

[1]Department of Medicine, CHU Brugmann, Université Libre de Bruxelles, Place A.Van Gehuchten 4, 1020 Brussels, Belgium. [2]Kantonsspital Graubünden, Loëstrasse 170, CH-7000 Chur, Switzerland. [3]Global Medical Affairs, Amgen (Europe) GmbH, Zug, Switzerland. [4]Institute of Clinical Research, Université Catholique de Louvain, Avenue Mounier 50, 1200 Brussels, Belgium.

References

1. Parker C, Nilsson S, Heinrich D, Helle SI, O'Sullivan JM, Fossa SD, et al. Alpha emitter radium-223 and survival in metastatic prostate cancer. N Engl J Med. 2013;369(3):213–23.

2. Body JJ, Casimiro S, Costa L. Targeting bone metastases in prostate cancer: improving clinical outcome. Nat Rev Urol. 2015;12(6):340–56.

3. Fizazi K, Carducci M, Smith M, Damiao R, Brown J, Karsh L, et al. Denosumab versus zoledronic acid for treatment of bone metastases in men with castration-resistant prostate cancer: a randomised, double-blind study. Lancet. 2011;377(9768):813–22.

4. Saad F, Gleason DM, Murray R, Tchekmedyian S, Venner P, Lacombe L, et al. Long-term efficacy of zoledronic acid for the prevention of skeletal complications in patients with metastatic hormone-refractory prostate cancer. J Natl Cancer Inst. 2004;96(11):879–2.

5. European Medicines Agency. Zometa® (zoledronic acid) Summary of Product Characteristics. 2016; Available at: http://www.ema.europa.eu/docs/en_GB/document_library/EPAR_-_Product_Information/human/000336/WC500051730.pdf. Accessed 27 Apr 2018.

6. European Medicines Agency. XGEVA® (denosumab) Summary of Product Characteristics. 2018; Available at: http://www.ema.europa.eu/docs/en_GB/document_library/EPAR_-_Product_Information/human/002173/WC500110381.pdf. Accessed 6 Jun 2018.

7. European Medicines Agency. Xgeva (denosumab) summary of opinion (post authorisation). 2018; Available at: http://www.ema.europa.eu/docs/en_GB/document_library/Summary_of_opinion/human/002173/WC500244274.pdf. Accessed 6 Jun 2018.

8. Heidenreich A, Bastian PJ, Bellmunt J, Bolla M, Joniau S, van der Kwast T, et al. EAU guidelines on prostate cancer. Part II: treatment of advanced, relapsing, and castration-resistant prostate cancer. Eur Urol. 2014;65(2):467–79.

9. European Association of Urology. European Association of Urology guidelines – prostate cancer. 2018. Available at: http://uroweb.org/guideline/prostate-cancer/#6. Accessed 27 Apr 2018.

10. Lipton A, Fizazi K, Stopeck AT, Henry DH, Brown JE, Yardley DA, et al. Superiority of denosumab to zoledronic acid for prevention of skeletal-related events: a combined analysis of 3 pivotal, randomised, phase 3 trials. Eur J Cancer. 2012;48(16):3082–92.

11. Body JJ, Bone HG, de Boer RH, Stopeck A, Van Poznak C, Damiao R, et al. Hypocalcaemia in patients with metastatic bone disease treated with denosumab. Eur J Cancer. 2015;51(13):1812–21.

12. Manzaneque A, Chaguaceda C, Mensa M, Bastida C, Creus-Baro N. Use and safety of denosumab in cancer patients. Int J Clin Pharm. 2017;39(3):522–6.

13. Qi WX, Lin F, He AN, Tang LN, Shen Z, Yao Y. Incidence and risk of denosumab-related hypocalcemia in cancer patients: a systematic review and pooled analysis of randomized controlled studies. Curr Med Res Opin. 2013;29(9):1067–73.

14. Body JJ, Niepel D, Tonini G. Hypercalcaemia and hypocalcaemia: finding the balance. Support Care Cancer. 2017;25(5):1639–49.

15. Body JJ, Bouillon R. Emergencies of calcium homeostasis. Rev Endocr Metab Disord. 2003;4(2):167–75.

16. Fong J, Khan A. Hypocalcemia: updates in diagnosis and management for primary care. Can Fam Physician. 2012;58(2):158–62.

17. National Cancer Institute. Common Terminology Criteria for Adverse Events v4.0 2009; Available at: https://evs.nci.nih.gov/ftp1/CTCAE/CTCAE_4.03/CTCAE_4.03_2010-06-14_QuickReference_5x7.pdf. Accessed 27 Apr 2018.

18. Cooper MS, Gittoes NJL. Diagnosis and management of hypocalcaemia. BMJ. 2008;336(7656):1298–302.

19. Velasco PJ, Manshadi M, Breen K, Lippmann S. Psychiatric aspects of parathyroid disease. Psychosomatics. 1999;40(6):486–90.

20. Tanaka T, Taguri M, Fumita S, Okamoto K, Matsuo Y, Hayashi H. Retrospective study of unplanned hospital admission for metastatic cancer patients visiting the emergency department. Support Care Cancer. 2017;25(5):1409–15.

21. Huynh AL, Baker ST, Stewardson AJ, Johnson DF. Denosumab-associated hypocalcaemia: incidence, severity and patient characteristics in a tertiary hospital setting. Pharmacoepidemiol Drug Saf. 2016;25(11):1274–8.

22. Goltzman D. Approach to hypercalcaemia. 2016; Available at: https://www.ncbi.nlm.nih.gov/books/NBK279129/. Accessed 27 Apr 2018.

23. Blomqvist CP. A hospital survey of hypocalcemia in patients with malignant disease. Acta Med Scand. 1986;220(2):167–73.

24. Fallah-Rad N, Morton AR. Managing hypercalcaemia and hypocalcaemia in cancer patients. Curr Opin Support Palliat Care. 2013;7(3):265–71.

25. Riancho JA, Arjona R, Valle R, Sanz J, Gonzalez-Macias J. The clinical spectrum of hypocalcaemia associated with bone metastases. J Intern Med. 1989;226(6):449–52.

26. Rogers MJ, Gordon S, Benford HL, Coxon FP, Luckman SP, Monkkonen J, et al. Cellular and molecular mechanisms of action of bisphosphonates. Cancer. 2000;88(12 Suppl):2961–78.

27. Kostenuik PJ, Nguyen HQ, McCabe J, Warmington KS, Kurahara C, Sun N, et al. Denosumab, a fully human monoclonal antibody to RANKL, inhibits bone resorption and increases BMD in knock-in mice that express chimeric (murine/human) RANKL. J Bone Miner Res. 2009;24(2):182–95.

28. Lechner B, DeAngelis C, Jamal N, Emmenegger U, Pulenzas N, Giotis A, et al. The effects of denosumab on calcium profiles in advanced cancer patients with bone metastases. Support Care Cancer. 2014;22(7):1765–71.

29. Ikesue H, Tsuji T, Hata K, Watanabe H, Mishima K, Uchida M, et al. Time course of calcium concentrations and risk factors for hypocalcemia in patients receiving denosumab for the treatment of bone metastases from cancer. Ann Pharmacother. 2014;48(9):1159–65.

30. Yerram P, Kansagra S, Abdelghany O. Incidence of hypocalcemia in patients receiving denosumab for prevention of skeletal-related events in bone metastasis. J Oncol Pharm Pract. 2016;23(3):179–84.

31. Kmetec A, Hajdinjak T. Evaluation of safety and analgesic consumption in patients with advanced cancer treated with zoledronic acid. Radiol Oncol. 2013;47(3):289–95.

32. Ho JW. Bisphosphonate stimulation of osteoblasts and osteoblastic metastasis as a mechanism of hypocalcaemia. Med Hypotheses. 2012;78(3):377–9.

33. Breen TL, Shane E. Prolonged hypocalcemia after treatment with zoledronic acid in a patient with prostate cancer and vitamin D deficiency. J Clin Oncol. 2004;22(8):1531–2.

34. Muqeet Adnan M, Bhutta U, Iqbal T, AbdulMujeeb S, Haragsim L, Amer S. Severe hypocalcemia due to denosumab in metastatic prostate cancer. Case Rep Nephrol. 2014;2014:565393.

35. Segal E, Felder S, Haim N, Yoffe-Sheinman H, Peer A, Wollner M, et al. Vitamin D deficiency in oncology patients--an ignored condition: impact on hypocalcemia and quality of life. Isr Med Assoc J. 2012;14(10):607–12.

36. Gloth F, Gundberg CM, Hollis BW, Haddad JG, Tobin JD. Vitamin D deficiency in homebound elderly persons. JAMA. 1995;274(21):1683–6.

37. Droz JP, Albrand G, Gillessen S, Hughes S, Mottet N, Oudard S, et al. Management of prostate cancer in elderly patients: recommendations of a task force of the International Society of Geriatric Oncology. Eur Urol. 2017; 72(4):521–31.

38. Murphy AB, Nyame Y, Martin IK, Catalona WJ, Hollowell CMP, Nadler RB, et al. Vitamin D deficiency predicts prostate biopsy outcomes. Clin Cancer Res. 2014;20(9):2289–29.

39. Killen JP, Yong K, Luxton G, Endre Z. Life-threatening hypocalcaemia associated with denosumab in advanced chronic kidney disease. Intern Med J. 2016;46(6):746–7.

40. Baron R, Ferrari S, Russell RG. Denosumab and bisphosphonates: different mechanisms of action and effects. Bone. 2011;48(4):677–92.

41. Domschke C, Schuetz F. Side effects of bone-targeted therapies in advanced breast cancer. Breast Care. 2014;9(5):332–6.

42. Stopeck AT, Fizazi K, Body JJ, Brown JE, Carducci M, Diel I, et al. Safety of long-term denosumab therapy: results from the open label extension phase of two phase 3 studies in patients with metastatic breast and prostate cancer. Support Care Cancer. 2016;24(1):447–55.

43. Body JJ, Terpos E, Tombal B, Hadji P, Arif A, Young A, et al. Bone health in the elderly cancer patient: a SIOG position paper. Cancer Treat Rev. 2016; 51:46–53.

44. The British Dietetic Association. Food fact sheet: calcium. 2017; Available at: https://www.bda.uk.com/foodfacts/Calcium.pdf. Accessed 27 Apr 2018.

45. National Institutes of Health. Calcium. 2016; Available at: https://ods.od.nih.gov/factsheets/Calcium-HealthProfessional/#h5. Accessed 27 Apr 2018.

Hypocalcaemia in patients with prostate cancer treated with a bisphosphonate or denosumab: prevention...

269

46. British National Formulary. Calcium supplements. 2016. Available at: https://bnf.nice. org.uk/treatment-summary/minerals.html. Accessed 27 Apr 2018.

47. Wang H, Bua P, Capodice J. A comparative study of calcium absorption following a single serving administration of calcium carbonate powder versus calcium citrate tablets in healthy premenopausal women. Food Nutr Res. 2014;58:23229.

48. Institute of Medicine. Dietary reference intakes for calcium and vitamin D. Washington, DC: The National Academies Press; 2011. https://doi.org/10. 17226/13050

49. Holick MF. Vitamin D deficiency. N Engl J Med. 2007;357(3):266–81.

50. Kennel KA, Drake MT, Hurley DL. Vitamin D deficiency in adults: when to test and how to treat. Mayo Clinic Proc. 2010;85(8):752–8.

51. British Medical Journal. Best practice: vitamin D deficiency. 2017; Available at: http://bestpractice.bmj.com/best-practice/monograph/641/treatment/ step-by-step.html. Accessed 27 Apr 2018.

52. Holick MF, Binkley NC, Bischoff-Ferrari HA, Gordon CM, Hanley DA, Heaney RP, et al. Evaluation, treatment, and prevention of vitamin D deficiency: an Endocrine Society clinical practice guideline. J Clin Endocrinol Metab. 2011; 96(7):1911–30.

53. International Osteoporosis Foundation. Vitamin D. Available at: https://www. iofbonehealth.org/osteoporosis-musculoskeletal-disorders/osteoporosis/ prevention/vitamin-d. Accessed 27 Apr 2018.

54. National Institute for Health and Care Excellence. Vitamin D deficiency in adults - treatment and prevention. 2016; Available at: https://cks.nice.org.uk/ vitamin-d-deficiency-in-adults-treatment-and-prevention#!topicsummary. Accessed 27 Apr 2018.

55. British National Formulary. Vitamin D. 2016; Available at: https://bnf.nice.org. uk/treatment-summary/vitamins.html. Accessed 27 Apr 2018.

56. Glendenning P, Chew GT, Seymour HM, Gillett MJ, Goldswain PR, Inderjeeth CA, et al. Serum 25-hydroxyvitamin D levels in vitamin D-insufficient hip fracture patients after supplementation with ergocalciferol and cholecalciferol. Bone. 2009;45(5):870–5.

57. Buonerba C, Caraglia M, Malgieri S, Perri F, Bosso D, Federico P, et al. Calcitriol: a better option than vitamin D in denosumab-treated patients with kidney failure? Expert Opin Biol Ther. 2013;13(2):149–51.

58. International Society of Nephrology. KDIGO 2017 clinical practice guideline update for the diagnosis, evaluation, prevention, and treatment of chronic kidney disease–mineral and bone disorder (CKD-MBD). 2017. Available at: http://kdigo. org/wp-content/uploads/2017/02/2017-KDIGO-CKD-MBD-GL-Update.pdf. Accessed 26 Apr 2018.

59. den Uyl D, Geusens PP, van Berkum FN, Houben HH, Jebbink MC, Lems WF. Patient preference and acceptability of calcium plus vitamin D3 supplementation: a randomised, open, cross-over trial. Clin Rheumatol. 2010;29(5):465–72.

60. Saini SD, Schoenfeld P, Kaulback K, Dubinsky MC. Effect of medication dosing frequency on adherence in chronic diseases. Am J Manag Care. 2009;15(6):e22–33.

61. Reid IR, Bristow SM, Bolland MJ. Calcium supplements: benefits and risks. J Intern Med. 2015;278(4):354–68.

62. Lewis JR, Zhu K, Prince RL. Adverse events from calcium supplementation: relationship to errors in myocardial infarction self-reporting in randomized controlled trials of calcium supplementation. J Bone Miner Res. 2012;27(3): 719–22.

63. International Osteoporosis Foundation. Calcium content of common foods. 2017; Available at: https://www.iofbonehealth.org/osteoporosis- musculoskeletal-disorders/osteoporosis/prevention/calcium/calcium- content-common-foods. Accessed 27 Apr 2018.

64. Peppone LJ, Huston AJ, Reid ME, Rosier RN, Zakharia Y, Trump DL, et al. The effect of various vitamin D supplementation regimens in breast cancer patients. Breast Cancer Res Treat. 2011;127(1):171–7.

65. Malabanan A, Veronikis IE, Holick MF. Redefining vitamin D insufficiency. Lancet. 1998;351(9105):805–6.

66. Singh R, Bhat MH, Bhansali A. Hypomagnesaemia masquerading as hypoparathyroidism. J Assoc Physicians India. 2006;54:411–2.

67. Walsh J, Gittoes N, Selby P. Society for Endocrinology clinical C. SOCIETY FOR ENDOCRINOLOGY ENDOCRINE EMERGENCY GUIDANCE: Emergency management of acute hypercalcaemia in adult patients. Endocr Connect. 2016;5(5):G9–G11.

68. Milat F, Goh S, Gani LU, Suriadi C, Gillespie MT, Fuller PJ, et al. Prolonged hypocalcemia following denosumab therapy in metastatic hormone refractory prostate cancer. Bone. 2013;55(2):305–8.

Permissions

All chapters in this book were first published in UROLOGY, by BioMed Central; hereby published with permission under the Creative Commons Attribution License or equivalent. Every chapter published in this book has been scrutinized by our experts. Their significance has been extensively debated. The topics covered herein carry significant findings which will fuel the growth of the discipline. They may even be implemented as practical applications or may be referred to as a beginning point for another development.

The contributors of this book come from diverse backgrounds, making this book a truly international effort. This book will bring forth new frontiers with its revolutionizing research information and detailed analysis of the nascent developments around the world.

We would like to thank all the contributing authors for lending their expertise to make the book truly unique. They have played a crucial role in the development of this book. Without their invaluable contributions this book wouldn't have been possible. They have made vital efforts to compile up to date information on the varied aspects of this subject to make this book a valuable addition to the collection of many professionals and students.

This book was conceptualized with the vision of imparting up-to-date information and advanced data in this field. To ensure the same, a matchless editorial board was set up. Every individual on the board went through rigorous rounds of assessment to prove their worth. After which they invested a large part of their time researching and compiling the most relevant data for our readers.

The editorial board has been involved in producing this book since its inception. They have spent rigorous hours researching and exploring the diverse topics which have resulted in the successful publishing of this book. They have passed on their knowledge of decades through this book. To expedite this challenging task, the publisher supported the team at every step. A small team of assistant editors was also appointed to further simplify the editing procedure and attain best results for the readers.

Apart from the editorial board, the designing team has also invested a significant amount of their time in understanding the subject and creating the most relevant covers. They scrutinized every image to scout for the most suitable representation of the subject and create an appropriate cover for the book.

The publishing team has been an ardent support to the editorial, designing and production team. Their endless efforts to recruit the best for this project, has resulted in the accomplishment of this book. They are a veteran in the field of academics and their pool of knowledge is as vast as their experience in printing. Their expertise and guidance has proved useful at every step. Their uncompromising quality standards have made this book an exceptional effort. Their encouragement from time to time has been an inspiration for everyone.

The publisher and the editorial board hope that this book will prove to be a valuable piece of knowledge for researchers, students, practitioners and scholars across the globe.

Contributors

Lucio Gnessi, Stefania Mariani, Carla Lubrano, Sabrina Basciani and Mikiko Watanabe
Department of Experimental Medicine, Section of Medical Pathophysiology, Food Science and Endocrinology, Sapienza University of Rome, Policlinico Umberto I, 00161 Rome, Italy

Filomena Scarselli, Maria Giulia Minasi, Pier Francesco Greco and Ermanno Greco
Centre for Reproductive Medicine, European Hospital, Rome, Italy

Giorgio Franco
Department Gynaecological-Obstetrical and Urological Sciences, Sapienza University of Rome, Policlinico Umberto I, 00161 Rome, Italy

Alessio Farcomeni
Department of Public Health and Infectious Diseases, "Sapienza" University of Rome, Rome, Italy

Tsuzumi Konishi, Satoshi Washino, Yuhki Nakamura, Masashi Ohshima, Kimitoshi Saito and Tomoaki Miyagawa
Department of Urology, Jichi Medical University Saitama Medical Center, 1-847 Amanuma-cho, Omiya-ku, Saitama 330-8503, Japan

Yoshiaki Arai
Department of Urology, Nishi-Omiya Hospital, 1-1173 Mihashi, Omiya-ku, Saitama 330-0856, Japan

Lisa M. DeMaria, Diana Tamondong-Lachica, Jhiedon Florentino, M. Czarina Acelajado, Othman Ouenes and Trever Burgon
QURE Healthcare, 450 Pacific Ave, Suite 200, San Francisco, CA, USA

John W. Peabody
QURE Healthcare, 450 Pacific Ave, Suite 200, San Francisco, CA, USA
University of California, San Francisco, 500 Beale Street, San Francisco, CA, USA

Jerome P. Richie
Metamark Genetics, 245 First Street, 10th Floor, Cambridge, MA, USA

Weiguo Hu, Boxing Su, Bo Xiao, Xin Zhang, Song Chen, Yuzhe Tang, Yubao Liu, Meng Fu and Jianxing Li
Department of Urology, Beijing Tsinghua Changgung Hospital, Tsinghua University, No. 168 Litang Road, Changping District, Beijing 102218, China

Andrea Gallioli, Elisa De Lorenzis, Luca Boeri, Stefano Paolo Zanetti, Fabrizio Longo and Emanuele Montanari
Fondazione IRCCS Ca' Granda Ospedale Maggiore Policlinico, Department of Urology, University of Milan, Via della Commenda 15, 20122 Milan, Italy

Maurizio Delor
Istituto Europeo di Oncologia, Department of Urology, University of Milan, Via Giuseppe Ripamonti 435, 20141 Milan, Italy

Alberto Trinchieri
Department of Urology, Ospedale Alessandro Manzoni Lecco, Via dell'Eremo 9/11, 23900 Lecco, Italy

Jeffrey A. Albaugh and Jacqueline Petkewicz
John and Carol Walter Center for Urological Health, NorthShore University HealthSystem, 2180 Pfingsten Road, Suite 3000, Glenview, Illinois 60026, USA

Nat Sufrin
The Doctoral Program in Clinical Psychology, The City College of the City University of New York, New York, NY, USA

Brittany R. Lapin
Cleveland Clinic, Cleveland, OH, USA

Sandi Tenfelde
The Marcella Niehoff School of Nursing, Loyola University of Chicago, Maywood, IL, USA

Yuji Hakozaki, Hisashi Matsushima, Taro Murata, Tomoko Masuda and Yoko Hirai
Department of Urology, Tokyo Metropolitan Police Hospital, #4-22-1 Nakano, Nakano-ku, Tokyo 164-0001, Japan

Mai Oda and Nobuo Kawauchi
Department of Radiology, Tokyo Metropolitan Police Hospital, Tokyo, Japan

Munehiro Yokoyama
Department of Pathology, Tokyo Metropolitan Police Hospital, Tokyo, Japan

Jimpei Kumagai and Yukio Homma
Department of Urology, The University of Tokyo Graduate School of Medicine, Tokyo, Japan

Shimpei Yamashita, Yasuo Kohjimoto, Takashi Iguchi, Akinori Iba, Takahito Wakamiya, Satoshi Nishizawa and Isao Hara
Department of Urology, Wakayama Medical University, 811-1 Kimiidera, Wakayama City, Wakayaka 641-0012, Japan

Yasuo Hirabayashi
Department of Urology, Hashimoto Municipal Hospital, 2-8-1 Ominedai, Hashimoto City, Wakayama 648-0005, Japan

Masatoshi Higuchi
Department of Urology, Kinan Hospital, 46-70 Shinjyo, Tanabe City, Wakayama 646-8588, Japan

Hiroyuki Koike
Department of Urology, Rinku General Medical Center, 2-23 Rinkuouraikita, Izumisano City, Osaka 598-8577, Japan

Sung Dae Kim
Department of Urology, Graduate School of Medicine, Jeju National University, Jeju, South Korea

Kang Jun Cho and Joon Chul Kim
Department of Urology, Bucheon St. Mary's hospital, College of Medicine, The Catholic University of Korea, Sosa-Ro 327, Wonmi-gu, Bucheon-si, Gyeonggi-do, Seoul 14647, South Korea

Chanjuan Zhang, Zhiying Xiao, Xiulin Zhang, Liqiang Guo, Wendong Sun, Zhaoqun Jiang and Yuqiang Liu
Department of Urology, The Second Hospital of Shandong University, 247 Beiyuan Street, Jinan 250033, China

Changfeng Tai
Department of Urology, University of Pittsburgh, Pittsburgh, PA, USA
Department of Pharmacology and Chemical Biology, University of Pittsburgh, Pittsburgh, PA 15213, USA

Andy W. Yang, Aydin Pooli, Subodh M. Lele, Ina W. Kim, Judson D. Davies and Chad A. LaGrange
Division of Urologic Surgery, University of Nebraska Medical Center, Omaha, NE, USA

Ferdinando Fusco, Massimiliano Creta, Nicola Longo, Francesco Persico, Marco Franco and Vincenzo Mirone
Department of Neurosciences, Human Reproduction and Odontostomatology, University of Naples, Federico II - Via Pansini 5, 80131 Naples, Italy

Makito Miyake, Nobumichi Tanaka, Shunta Hori, Yosuke Morizawa, Yasushi Nakai, Takeshi Inoue, Satoshi Anai, Kazumasa Torimoto, Katsuya Aoki and Kiyohide Fujimoto
Department of Urology, Nara Medical University, 840 Shijo-cho, Nara 634-8522, Japan

Yoshihiro Tatsumi
Department of Urology, Nara Medical University, 840 Shijo-cho, Nara 634-8522, Japan
Department of Pathology, Nara Medical University, Nara, Japan

Isao Asakawa and Masatoshi Hasegawa
Department of Radiation Oncology, Nara Medical University, Nara, Japan

Tomomi Fujii and Noboru Konishi
Department of Pathology, Nara Medical University, Nara, Japan

Joo Yong Lee, Won Sik Ham and Young Deuk Choi
Department of Urology, Severance Hospital, Urological Science Institute, Yonsei University College of Medicine, Seoul, South Korea

Seong Uk Jeh
Department of Urology, Gyeongsang National University Hospital, Gyeongsang National University School of Medicine, Jinju, South Korea

Man Deuk Kim
Department of Radiology, Severance Hospital, Research Institute of Radiological Science, Yonsei
University College of Medicine, Seoul, South Korea

Dong Hyuk Kang
Department of Urology, Inha University School of Medicine, Incheon, South Korea

Jong Kyou Kwon
Department of Urology, Severance Check-Up, Yonsei University Health System, Seoul, South Korea

Kang Su Cho
Department of Urology, Gangnam Severance Hospital, Urological Science Institute, Yonsei University College of Medicine, 211 Eonju-ro, Gangnam-gu, Seoul 06273, South Korea

Satoshi Kurokawa
Department of Urology, Nagoya Tokushukai General Hospital, 2-52, Kouzouji-cho-kita, Kasugai 487-0016, Japan
Department of Nephro-urology, Nagoya City University Graduate School of Medical Sciences, 1, Kawasumi, Mizuho-cho, Mizuho-ku, Nagoya 467-8601, Japan

Yukihiro Umemoto, Kentaro Mizuno, Atsushi Okada, Akihiro Nakane, Hidenori Nishio, Shuzo Hamamoto, Ryosuke Ando, Noriyasu Kawai, Keiichi Tozawa, Yutaro Hayashi and Takahiro Yasui
Department of Nephro-urology, Nagoya City University Graduate School of Medical Sciences, 1, Kawasumi, Mizuho-cho, Mizuho-ku, Nagoya 467-8601, Japan

Huibo Lian, Junlong Zhuang, Wei Wang and Hongqian Guo
Department of Urology, Drum Tower Hospital, Medical School of Nanjing University, 321 Zhongshan Road, Nanjing 210008, Jiangsu, People's Republic of China
Institute of Urology, Nanjing University, Nanjing 210008, Jiangsu, People's Republic of China

Bing Zhang and Danyan Li
Department of Radiology, Drum Tower Hospital, Medical School of Nanjing University, 321 Zhongshan Road, Nanjing 210008, Jiangsu, People's Republic of China

Jiong Shi and Yao Fu
Department of Pathology, Drum Tower Hospital, Medical School of Nanjing University, 321 Zhongshan Road, Nanjing 210008, Jiangsu, People's Republic of China

Xuping Jiang and Weimin Zhou
Department of Urology, the Affiliated Yixing people's Hospital of Jiangsu University, Yixing, Jiangsu 212000, China

Dong Fang, Shiming He, Gengyan Xiong, Zhenpeng Cao, Lei Zhang, Xuesong Li and Liqun Zhou
Department of Urology, Peking University First Hospital, Institute of Urology, Peking University, National Urological Cancer Centre, No. 8 Xishiku St, Xicheng District, Beijing 100034, China

Nirmish Singla
Department of Urology, University of Texas Southwestern Medical Center, Dallas, TX, USA

Kian Asanad
David Geffen School of Medicine at the University of California Los Angeles, 300 Stein Plaza, Suite 348, Los Angeles, California 90095, USA.

Andrew T. Lenis, Nicholas M. Donin and Karim Chamie
David Geffen School of Medicine at the University of California Los Angeles, 300 Stein Plaza, Suite 348, Los Angeles, California 90095, USA
Department of Urology, Health Services Research Group, David Geffen School of Medicine at UCLA, Los Angeles, California, USA
Jonsson Comprehensive Cancer Center, David Geffen School of Medicine at UCLA, Los Angeles, California, USA

Maher Blaibel
Riverside School of Medicine, University of California, Riverside, California, USA

Sezim Agizamhan, Feng Qu, Ning Liu, Hongqian Guo and Weidong Gan
Department of Urology, Nanjing Drum Tower Hospital, The Affiliated Hospital of Nanjing University Medical School, No. 321 Zhongshan Road, Nanjing 210008, Jiangsu Province, China

Jing Sun
Department of Oncology, Jiangsu Province Hospital, The First Affiliated Hospital of Nanjing Medical University, Nanjing, Jiangsu, China

Wei Xu
Department of Pathology, Jiangsu Cancer Hospital, The Affiliated Cancer Hospital of Nanjing Medical University, Nanjing, Jiangsu, China

Lihua Zhang
Department of Pathology, Zhongda Hospital Southeast University, Nanjing, Jiangsu, China

Neil M. Schultz, Bruce A. Brown and Scott C. Flanders
Astellas Pharma, Inc., 1 Astellas Way, Northbrook, IL 60062, USA

Neal D. Shore
Carolina Urologic Research Center, Myrtle Beach, SC, USA

Simon Chowdhury
Guy's, King's, and St. Thomas' Hospitals, London, UK

Laurence H. Klotz
Sunnybrook Health Sciences Centre, University of Toronto, Toronto, ON, Canada

Raoul S. Concepcion
Urology Associates, P.C, Nashville, TN, USA

David F. Penson
Vanderbilt University Medical Center, Nashville, TN, USA

Lawrence I. Karsh
The Urology Center of Colorado, Denver, CO, USA

Hongbo Yang
Analysis Group, Inc., Boston, MA, USA

Arie Barlev
Medivation, Inc., San Francisco, CA, USA
Pfizer, Inc., New York, NY, USA

Véronique Ouellet
Institut du cancer de Montréal and Centre de recherche du Centre hospitalier de l'Université de Montréal, 900, St-Denis St, room R10-464, Montréal, Québec H2X 0A9, Canada

Jean-Baptiste Lattouf and Fred Saad
Institut du cancer de Montréal and Centre de recherche du Centre hospitalier de l'Université de Montréal, 900, St-Denis St, room R10-464, Montréal, Québec H2X 0A9, Canada
Department of Surgery, Université de Montréal, Montréal, Québec, Canada

Mathieu Latour and Dominique Trudel
Institut du cancer de Montréal and Centre de recherche du Centre hospitalier de l'Université de Montréal, 900, St-Denis St, room R10-464, Montréal, Québec H2X 0A9, Canada
Department of Pathology and Cellular Biology, Université de Montréal, Montréal, Québec, Canada

Anne-Marie Mes-Masson
Institut du cancer de Montréal and Centre de recherche du Centre hospitalier de l'Université de Montréal, 900, St-Denis St, room R10-464, Montréal, Québec H2X 0A9, Canada

Department of Medicine, Université de Montréal, Montréal, Québec, Canada

Armen Aprikian and Simone Chevalier
Research Institute of McGill University Health Center and Department of Surgery (Urology), McGill University, Montréal, Québec, Canada

Alain Bergeron and Louis Lacombe
CHU de Québec-Université Laval and Department of Surgery, Université Laval, Québec City, Québec, Canada

Fadi Brimo
Department of Pathology, McGill University Health Centre, Montréal, Québec, Canada

Robert G. Bristow
Department of Medical Biophysics and Department of Radiation Oncology, University of Toronto, Toronto, ON, Canada
University Health Network, Toronto, ON, Canada

Theodorus van der Kwast
University Health Network, Toronto, ON, Canada

Neil E. Fleshner
University Health Network, Toronto, ON, Canada
Division of Urology, Department of Surgery of University Health Network, University of Toronto, Toronto, ON, Canada

Darrel Drachenberg
University of Manitoba and Manitoba Prostate Centre, Winnipeg, MB, Canada

Ladan Fazli
Vancouver Prostate Centre, Vancouver, BC, Canada

Martin Gleave
Vancouver Prostate Centre, Vancouver, BC, Canada
Department of Urologic Sciences, Vancouver, BC, Canada

Pierre Karakiewicz
Cancer Prognostics and Health Outcomes Unit, Centre hospitalier de l'Université de Montréal, Montréal, Québec, Canada
Department of Surgery, Université de Montréal, Montréal, Québec, Canada

Laurence Klotz
Sunnybrook Health Sciences Centre, Toronto, ON, Canada

Jeremy A. Squire
Department of Pathology and Molecular Medicine, Queen's University, Kingston, ON, Canada
Department of Genetics and Pathology, Ribeirão Preto Medical School, University of São Paulo, Ribeirão Preto, Brazil

Shuichi Morizane, Masashi Honda, Takehiro Sejima and Atsushi Takenaka
Department of Urology, Tottori University Faculty of Medicine, Yonago, Japan

Kuniyasu Muraoka
Department of Urology, Tottori University Faculty of Medicine, Yonago, Japan
Division of Urology, Department of Surgery, Tottori University Faculty of Medicine, 36-1 Nishi-cho, Yonago 683-8504, Japan

Keisuke Hieda
Department of Urology, Hiroshima University Faculty of Medicine, Hiroshima, Japan

Gen Murakami
Division of Internal Medicine, Iwamizawa Kojin-kai Hospital, Iwamizawa, Japan

Shin-ichi Abe
Department of Anatomy, Tokyo Dental College, Tokyo, Japan

P. Anheuser and M. Kulejewski
Albertinen-Krankenhaus Hamburg, Klinik für Urologie, Hamburg, Germany

K.-P. Dieckmann
Albertinen-Krankenhaus Hamburg, Klinik für Urologie, Hamburg, Germany
Asklepios Klinik Altona, Urologische Abteilung, Hodentumorzentrum Hamburg, Hamburg, Germany
Asklepios Klinik Altona, Hodentumorzentrum Hamburg, Paul Ehrlich Strasse 1, 22763 Hamburg, Germany

R. Gehrckens
Albertinen-Krankenhaus Hamburg, Klinik für Diagnostische Radiologie, Hamburg, Germany

B. Feyerabend
MVZ Hanse Histologikum, Hamburg, Germany

Minyao Jiang, Bowei Li, Guo Chen, Yanru Zeng and Yuxiang Liang
Department of Urology, Guangdong Key Laboratory of Clinical Molecular Medicine and Diagnostics, Guangzhou First People's Hospital, Guangzhou Medical University, Guangzhou 510180, China

Jianheng Ye
Department of Urology, Guangdong Key Laboratory of Clinical Molecular Medicine and Diagnostics, Guangzhou First People's Hospital, Guangzhou Medical University, Guangzhou 510180, China

Departments of Urology and Pathology, Massachusetts General Hospital and Harvard Medical School, Boston, MA 02114, USA

Weide Zhong
Department of Urology, Guangdong Key Laboratory of Clinical Molecular Medicine and Diagnostics, Guangzhou First People's Hospital, Guangzhou Medical University, Guangzhou 510180, China
Department of Urology, Guangzhou First People's Hospital, Guangzhou Medical University, Guangzhou 510180, China

Huichan He
Department of Urology, Guangdong Key Laboratory of Clinical Molecular Medicine and Diagnostics, Guangzhou First People's Hospital, Guangzhou Medical University, Guangzhou 510180, China
Urology Key Laboratory of Guangdong Province, The First Affiliated Hospital of Guangzhou Medical University, Guangzhou Medical University, Guangzhou 510230, China

Shulin Wu, Zongwei Wang and Chin-Lee Wu
Departments of Urology and Pathology, Massachusetts General Hospital and Harvard Medical School, Boston, MA 02114, USA

Yanqiong Zhang
Departments of Urology and Pathology, Massachusetts General Hospital and Harvard Medical School, Boston, MA 02114, USA
Institute of Chinese Materia Medica, China Academy of Chinese Medical Sciences, Beijing 100700, China

Zhiduan Cai
Southern Medical University, Guangzhou 510515, China

Mona Abdelrahim, Mahmoud Laymon, Mamdouh Elsherbeeny, Mohammed Sultan, Ahmed Shokeir, Ahmed Mosbah, Hassan Abol-Enein and Amira Awadalla
Urology and Nephrology Center, Mansoura University, Mansoura, Egypt

Ahmed M. Mansour
Urology and Nephrology Center, Mansoura University, Mansoura, Egypt
University of Texas Health Science Center, San Antonio, USA

Eunho Cho and Vikram Sairam
University of California Los Angeles, Los Angeles, CA, USA

Jayoung Kim
University of California Los Angeles, Los Angeles, CA, USA
Departments of Surgery and Biomedical Sciences, Samuel Oschin Comprehensive Cancer Institute, Cedars Sinai Medical Center, 8700 Beverly Blvd, Los Angeles, CA 90048, USA

Taeeun D. Park
University of California, Berkerly, CA, USA

Muhammad Shahid
Departments of Surgery and Biomedical Sciences, Samuel Oschin Comprehensive Cancer Institute, Cedars Sinai Medical Center, 8700 Beverly Blvd, Los Angeles, CA 90048, USA

Cosimo De Nunzio, Fabrizio Presicce, Riccardo Lombardo, Alberto Trucchi, Mariangela Bellangino and Andrea Tubaro
Department of Urology, Ospedale Sant'Andrea, "Sapienza" University of Rome, Rome, Italy

Egidio Moja
Unit of Clinical Psychology, Department of Health Sciences, University of Milan, San Paolo Hospital, Milan, Italy
CURA Centre, University of Milan, Milan, Italy

Kevin Rhee and Paul Lee
Section of Urologic Oncology, Rutgers Cancer Institute of New Jersey, 195 Little Albany Street, New Brunswick, NJ 08903, USA

Young Suk Kwon and Isaac Yi Kim
Section of Urologic Oncology, Rutgers Cancer Institute of New Jersey, 195 Little Albany Street, New Brunswick, NJ 08903, USA
Division of Urology, Rutgers Robert Wood Johnson Medical School, New Brunswick, NJ, USA

Nicholas Farber, Christopher Han and Nikhil Gupta
Division of Urology, Rutgers Robert Wood Johnson Medical School, New Brunswick, NJ, USA

Ji Woong Yu
Samsung Medical Center, Sungkyunkwan University School of Medicine, Seoul, Korea

Patrick Ney
Department of Biostatistics, Rutgers School of Public Health, Piscataway, NJ, USA

Jeong Hee Hong
Department of Urology, Dankook University College of Medicine, Chungnam, Korea

Wun-Jae Kim
Department of Urology, Chungbuk National University College of Medicine, Cheongju, Korea

Huan Yang and Shaogang Wang
Dartment of Urology, Tongji Hospital,Tongji Medical School, Huazhong University of Science and Technology, Wuhan 430030, China

Jianxing Li
Department of Urology, Beijing Tsinghua changgung Hospital, Beijing, China

Gang Long
YouCare Technology Co., Ltd, Wuhan, China

Ahmed S. Zakaria, Alice Dragomir, Wassim Kassouf, Simon Tanguay and Armen Aprikian
Department of Surgery, Division of Urology, McGill University, McGill University Health Centre, 1001 Boulevard Decarie, Montreal, Quebec H4A 3J1, Canada

Fadi Brimo
Department of Pathology, McGill University, Montreal, Quebec, Canada

Furaha Kariburyo, Yuexi Wang and Lin Xie
STATinMED Research, 211 N. Fourth Avenue, Suite 2B, Ann Arbor, MI 48104, USA

I-Ning (Elaine) Cheng
Diagnostics Information Solutions, F. Hoffmann-La Roche AG, Basel, Switzerland

Lisa Wang
Genentech, Inc, South San Francisco, CA, USA

David Morgenstern
Roche Diagnostics Operations, Indianapolis, IN, USA

Eric Meadows
MedMining, Danville, PA, USA
Geisinger Health System, Danville, PA, USA

John Danella
Geisinger Health System, Danville, PA, USA

Michael L. Cher
Wayne State University School of Medicine and the Barbara Ann Karmanos Cancer Institute, Detroit, MI, USA

Jean-Jacques Body
Department of Medicine, CHU Brugmann, Université Libre de Bruxelles, Place A.Van Gehuchten 4, 1020 Brussels, Belgium

Roger von Moos
Kantonsspital Graubünden, Loëstrasse 170, CH-7000 Chur, Switzerland

Daniela Niepel
Global Medical Affairs, Amgen (Europe) GmbH, Zug, Switzerland

Bertrand Tombal
Institute of Clinical Research, Université Catholique de Louvain, Avenue Mounier 50, 1200 Brussels, Belgium

Index

www.ingramcontent.com/pod-product-compliance
Lightning Source LLC
Chambersburg PA
CBHW061315190326
41458CB00011B/3812